PHYSICON
The Reliable Icon in
PHYSIOLOGY

PHYSICON
The Reliable Icon in PHYSIOLOGY

(Exam Preparatory Manual for Undergraduates)

Second Edition

Sanoop KS MBBS MD (Internal Medicine)
Registrar
Internal Medicine
Kerala Institute of Medical Sciences
Thiruvananthapuram, Kerala, India

Mridul GS MBBS MS (General Surgery)
Assistant Divisional Medical Officer
Southern Railways

Nishanth PS MBBS MD (Pulmonary Medicine)
Senior Resident
Department of Pulmonary Medicine
BLK Super Speciality Hospital
New Delhi, India

Foreword
N Geetha

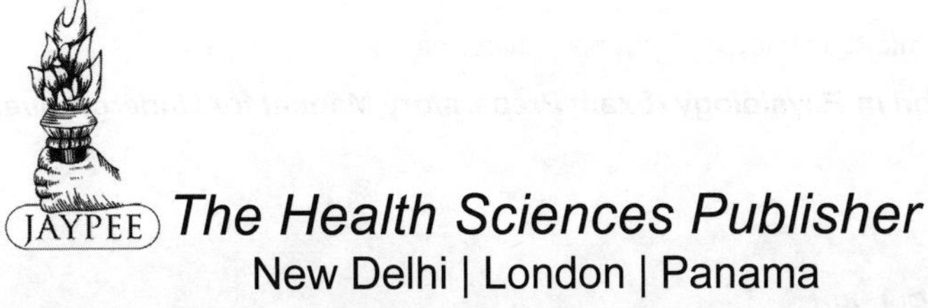
The Health Sciences Publisher
New Delhi | London | Panama

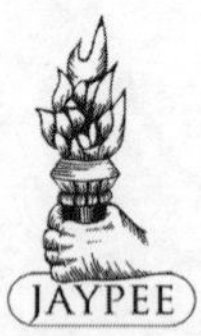

Jaypee Brothers Medical Publishers (P) Ltd

Headquarters

Jaypee Brothers Medical Publishers (P) Ltd
4838/24, Ansari Road, Daryaganj
New Delhi 110 002, India
Phone: +91-11-43574357
Fax: +91-11-43574314
Email: jaypee@jaypeebrothers.com

Overseas Offices

J.P. Medical Ltd
83 Victoria Street, London
SW1H 0HW (UK)
Phone: +44 20 3170 8910
Fax: +44 (0)20 3008 6180
Email: info@jpmedpub.com

Jaypee-Highlights Medical Publishers Inc
City of Knowledge, Bld. 235, 2nd Floor, Clayton
Panama City, Panama
Phone: +1 507-301-0496
Fax: +1 507-301-0499
Email: cservice@jphmedical.com

Jaypee Brothers Medical Publishers (P) Ltd
17/1-B Babar Road, Block-B, Shaymali
Mohammadpur, Dhaka-1207
Bangladesh
Mobile: +08801912003485
Email: jaypeedhaka@gmail.com

Jaypee Brothers Medical Publishers (P) Ltd
Bhotahity, Kathmandu
Nepal
Phone: +977-9741283608
Email: kathmandu@jaypeebrothers.com

Website: www.jaypeebrothers.com
Website: www.jaypeedigital.com

Inquiries for bulk sales may be solicited at: jaypee@jaypeebrothers.com

PHYSICON—The Reliable Icon in Physiology (Exam Preparatory Manual for Undergraduates)

First Edition: 2012
Second Edition: **2019**
ISBN: 978-93-5270-283-1

Printed at: Sterling Graphics Pvt. Ltd.

Dedicated to

Our Parents

Whose blessings and love have always been our precious resource

Our beloved teacher, Dr Swarnalatha PK

Who laid the foundation for our interest in the subject and kept the flame glowing against all winds

Almighty

Whose mighty grace strengthens all our weaknesses from day one to this day and for the days to come ...

Contributors

Shameez Muhammed Salim MBBS MS
MVJ Medical College and Research Hospital
Karnataka, India

Rashma S MBBS DCH
Government Medical College
Goa, India

Ninumol PK MBBS
Al Ahalia Hospital
Abu Dhabi, UAE

What readers have to say about the book

We have found this book very useful for undergraduate students of MBBS and other paramedical courses. Considering the reduced duration of MBBS course and the time available for first year MBBS course, it has become difficult for students to go through physiology books especially by Western authors. Still students want to get better marks in the subject. With this scenario, *Physicon* appears to be a best resource to revise physiology, just prior to the examination within shortest possible time.

The book includes theory, practical, MCQs, and question bank also. Therefore, in a single sitting entire physiology can be revised by the students.

Dr AR Joshi, Professor and Head
Dr AV Phadke, Assistant Professor
Department of Physiology
Bharati Vidyapeeth Medical College
Pune, Maharashtra, India

Physicon covers all topics, easy to read and reproduce in exam, very important for revision as it covers everything from theory to practical. Reference from standard books and includes latest concepts. One of a kind book, MCQs + theory + practical. I will recommend the book to my students.

Dr Devendra Patil, Associate Professor
KJ Somaiya Medical College
Sion, Mumbai, Maharashtra, India

Coverage of contents is adequate with good illustrations. Language is lucid and clarity of subject is very nice. Good for quick revision and last-minute reading.

Dr Lakshmi S Patel, Additional Professor
Department of Physiology
Lokamanya Tilak Muncipal Medical College
Sion, Mumbai, Maharashtra, India

Nice book. I want to know about the authors. What pushed them to write a book to simplify the problems that we all face in our first year MBBS, but they decided to solve them for others.

Dr Saurabh Swaroop Verma
MBBS Student, AIIMS
Raipur, Chhattisgarh, India

Nice during exam time because of less amount of time and vast number of portions. Covers Ganong and Guyton. Little errors are there, mainly typing mistakes. It will be good if we read standard textbook once and then go through. Great Effort!

Dr Sarath RS
MBBS Student, AIIMS
Bhopal, Madhya Pradesh, India

Foreword

There are two kinds of people in the world—one who complains about what is lacking and the other who does something to make things better. So when a group of students got together to bring out a book which aimed to aid the students of first year medicine with a short and exam-oriented book, they were choosing to side with the latter kind, by doing something to make things better. The result was *PHYSICON—The Reliable Icon in Physiology*, a book which was purely exam-oriented, which aimed at helping the students pass the first year MBBS exams with a good score. The authors of the book were very clear in their objectives from day one. The book never professed to be an encyclopedia of knowledge. It was a simple yet elegant, exam-oriented literature. In a world of Guyton's and Ganong's, they carved out their own little niche and the book is brilliant simply because it delivers on what it promises.

At the outset itself, a word of caution. It is very important to go deep into the subject if you aim to be a good doctor. No one text can give you all the information that you need on a subject in medicine. By reading detailed references, you not only pick up on the topic you are deliberating but also on multiple other topics you read through in the process of research. As a doctor, it is your moral obligation to be informed and knowledgeable. Ours is a profession that does not give second chances. The first year of MBBS lays the foundation of your career. The importance of building a strong foundation cannot be overstated.

But when it comes to the exam, we all could use a little help. You might have read vastly on a topic but would not mind refreshing the same with a concise material. You might have failed to prepare on another area and would be desperately searching for a capsule to help you gain at least a peripheral idea on the same. That is where this book delivers. This could be your go to guide for brushing up topics right before the exams. It definitely serves the purpose of those lazier doctors in the making who are looking for instant and short-lived enlightenment. As you can clearly see, the book you hold in your hand is a tool, which can be used by the most studious and most lazy first year students. The former uses it to fine tune and revise while the latter sees it as their 'Messiah' to scrape through.

Let me record my sincere appreciation for Sanoop KS, Mridul GS and Nishanth PS for taking up this tremendous challenge and coming out with such a beautiful work which manages to do justice to the topics explored while still being a capsule for students in their exam time. It is a proud moment for me as a teacher when students excel in any sphere. I sincerely hope and pray that the book will be received with the same enthusiasm by the first year students as it was in its previous *avatars*. I also hope that the book will be utilized by them to fine tune and perfect their knowledge rather than as a last-minute mugging up for clearing the exam.

N Geetha MD
Professor and HOD
Department of Physiology
Government Medical College
Thiruvananthapuram, Kerala, India

Preface to the Second Edition

First of all, thanks to our readers for their overwhelming response and acceptance to the previous edition of this book which is really a great appreciation for us. We are happy to note that this book has become essential and readyreckoner for students in their preparation for MBBS examination. Exam preparatory manuals are often revised every 3 to 4 years as new information becomes available. Occasionally, revision involves a cursory review of the original material with relatively minor changes to the content. In our naiveté, we imagined revising the first edition would be matter of a few weeks of intense work. Instead, over the course of 10–12 months, we found ourselves overhauling the entire book, rewriting chapters, adding new diagrams and clinical boxes.

As the duration of first MBBS course is reduced from its original one-and-half years to one year, medical students are confronted with the daunting task of assimilating a vast quantity of information for their exams. It has become impossible for the MBBS students to read the bulky textbooks in each subject for want of time especially during exam days. This exam preparatory manual comes handy, prepared just as per the ABC (Accurate, Brief and Clear) of good teaching. Only less than 80% of topics from a standard textbook are needed for any examination. These 80% topics are covered in such a readable student-friendly synopsis form in this book that it can be read in 20% of the time involved. This book aims to facilitate the learning process by providing a concise yet comprehensive account of important topics. Certain restrictions become necessary in a compact book with some topics being deliberately omitted.

As per the readers feedback, we have improved upon an already successful formula. As with the first edition, our strategy was to teach the subject in an integrated fashion with respect to the basic sciences as well as in a clinical context wherever possible. We believe this new edition represents significant improvement from the first edition for a variety of reasons.

- **Text:** In the second edition, the content has been entirely reorganized and updated. Each chapter has been extensively revised and made clear and concise with emphasis on imparting a conceptual understanding.
- **Tables and illustrations:** A picture speaks 1000 times more than words. New diagrams, flowcharts and tables are added to make learning still easier. Not only it helps to memorize and recap the topics, but also, presenting the text along with flowcharts and diagrams in exams helps the examiner easily assess the knowledge of the students. Usually, presentation with flowcharts and diagrams are more marks-fetching.
- **Two-color design:** The layout has been largely re-worked to make it easier for the eye. Colored text and headings make studying more efficient and pleasing.
- **Clinical boxes:** Dispersed throughout the book. Stress the clinical significance of the underlying physiology which facilitates comprehension and makes the material more enjoyable.
- **Clinical questions:** The inclusion of clinical questions at the end of chapters will not only allow the students to test their knowledge of the subject, but also to focus their attention on areas most commonly addressed in the examinations.
- **Calculations:** A new chapter on calculations has been added in this edition. It includes essential calculations in physiology with sample questions.

We have tried our level best to make *PHYSICON*—a very student-friendly and updated compendium because we strongly believe in order to have the best; you have to read the best. We have kept an eagle eye for any inaccuracies, but if you find any, you can mail at physiconphysiology@gmail.com. Finally, we wish that 'This book would be the first book that any first year MBBS students must read for their exam preparation and this would be the last choice to revise before they appear for exam'. Your success is the ultimate reward that we get for our work and we wish you all the best in your success. Happy reading...

Sanoop KS
Mridul GS
Nishanth PS

Preface to the First Edition

PHYSICON—The Reliable Icon in Physiology (Preparatory Manual for Undergraduates), designed to provide a concise knowledge of the subject, is finally at your reach. The purpose of this book is to serve as a companion during the first MBBS Physiology examination preparation. A student must have good command over the subject, as Physiology forms the basis of General Medicine, so the subject has to be learnt as it is from its roots. Many standard books for Physiology are available; both by Indian as well as Foreign authors. In these books, certain chapters are dealt clearly with appropriate illustrations while leaving the rest. So, students need to refer more than one textbook to master the subject, this is difficult particularly during the examination periods. This inspired us to bring forth a single comprehensive and examination-oriented companion in Physiology, which could provide all the information, an undergraduate need to know, so as to appear for an examination with confidence.

A concerted effort has been made to provide concise and comprehensive coverage of the subject with simple language, self-explanatory diagrams, flowcharts and illustrations. Practicals are also covered in a systematic manner with complete viva questions. We have also included wide collections of MCQs and reasoning type questions. A question bank containing the previous university examination questions has been included taking advantage of the fact that most questions are generally repeated.

We are very much indebted to our beloved teacher, Dr Swarnalatha PK (Associate Professor, Department of Physiology, Kannur Medical College, Kannur, Kerala, India), whose guidance and inspiration helped us throughout the tedious task of making this project a reality. She has been with us in all stages from day one.

We hope our efforts would meet the expectations of the students. We are sure that the students will find the book in this present form more useful. The book is primarily intended for undergraduate MBBS students, though we believe it should prove useful to other health professionals like BDS, Ayurveda, Homeopathy, Nursing, BPT, etc. because of its simplicity. This material is in no way a substitute for any standard textbook. As this is an examination-oriented book, you should read your textbooks first, before reading this book.

Sincere attempts have been made to maintain the accuracy and correctness of the subject. But we request all the readers to send their valuable suggestions and feedback to kmcphysicon@gmail.com or log on to www.facebook.com/Physicon and it will be acknowledged. As we conclude, we would like to bow in front of Almighty's grace with which we are blessed abundantly so as to make the dream called *Physicon* into a reality.

Wishing you all the best

Sanoop KS
Mridul GS
Nishanth PS

Acknowledgments

The gratitude we feel for all those mentioned below is too great and is quite impossible to express our feelings in words. We urge the readers to take a few minutes to read this section before moving on to the rest of the book. There are numerous people we want to thank them.

We thank Dr PP Venugopalan (Former Medical Director and Dean), Dr Shivasubrahmanyam (Former Associate Professor, Department of Biochemistry), Kannur Medical College, Kannur, Kerala, India, and our families for their constructive criticism, advice and their moral support.

We are extremely grateful to Dr AR Joshi (Professor and Head, Department of Physiology), Dr (Mrs) AV Phadke (Assistant Professor, Department of Physiology), Bharati Vidyapeeth Medical College, Pune, for their constructive criticism and valuable suggestions. They contributed clinical questions for some topics. We would like to thank Dr Neeraja Sanoop for her support and assistance in the preparation of this edition. She lent her support in updating the topics and sketching of new diagrams and flowcharts for *PHYSICON.*

We are also grateful to the MBBS 2007 batch of Kannur Medical College for their indispensable help, encouragement and support without which '*PHYSICON*' would have never reached its present state. We owe our special thanks to our Juniors—2008, 2009 and 2010 MBBS of Kannur Medical College for their continuous support and valuable suggestions.

We express our sincere gratitude to Shri Jitendar P Vij (Group Chairman) and Mr Ankit Vij (Managing Director) of M/s Jaypee Brothers Medical Publishers (P) Ltd, New Delhi, for publishing the book and materialize our dreams. Special mention to Mr Sujeesh VS (Branch Manager-Kochi branch), Mr Arun Kumar C (SSPO Incharge-Thiruvananthapuram Branch) and Ms Payal Bharti (Senior Manager) for their support in bringing up this edition; this would have been a rather difficult task to accomplish.

Last but not least, we thank Dr Amit Darwin, Dr Rejith Sreenivasan (2006 MBBS, Kannur Medical College), Dr Shijin PK, Dr Arun Ramesh (2007 MBBS, Kannur Medical College), Dr Muneer A (2008 MBBS, Kannur Medical College), Dr Saneesh PS, Sanu S, Deepthi S Johnson (2009 MBBS, Kannur Medical College), Sibi, Sumit and Jithu (Midas offset, Kannur).

How to Use this Book

How to Prepare for University Examination?

Going through the e-mails, we get to know some common queries like—How to prepare for exams? Is there any need to read other books for physiology, if we read *PHYSICON*? Can we get through by reading only *PHYSICON*?

Each and every student has his own style of preparation but here are some useful tips, which we would like to recommend. You need proper planning and a good schedule to study and should relax at appropriate times. We are giving a schema to tackle this subject.

The best way to start the subject is to start as early as possible. Whenever you read any subject in MBBS, you need to decide two books for that subject—one with the details and one to get you through the examination. The book with details should be good enough to give you the basics and a grasp of subject with in-depth discussion of all the topics important for learning the subject. On the other hand, you also need a book to help in rapid revision and quick accumulation of various exam-oriented topics in the subject according to the university examination scheme to get you through the examination.

Ganong and Guyton are considered standard descriptive books on physiology and are excellent to gain in-depth knowledge, but difficult to digest and revise at examination time. The list also extends to include GK Pal, AK Jain, N Geetha and many more. During examination, when you have to revise these books, it is a tough task to complete, also with the thought in mind that you have other subjects to look after.

Begin early, read a descriptive book that suits you from the above options as a reference and a book like '*PHYSICON*' since you start reading and not just as a last resort book. This pattern of study will give you the necessary confidence that, you know the basics and orient yourselves to all the important topics of the subject. While reading, preferably use highlighters. Highlighting the facts and important points will help you to concentrate on salient points on the day before exams. Apply this pattern to all the subjects to gain maximum benefit.

How this Book will Help you in your Preparation of Physiology?

This is the most simplified book to understand the concepts and to revise even at the eleventh hour. *Physicon* provides everything for examination—theory, practicals, MCQs, reasoning type questions, question bank and clinical questions; one of its kind, not seen in any other books. Searching different books during exam days creates unnecessary waste of time and stress. It will help you in gaining the requisite knowledge of all important topics of physiology as per the last 20 years of university papers and to clear the examinations without much stress.

All topics including the difficult to understand are discussed in such an easy-to-follow method that they are no longer unlearnable for the average students. Thus, complex topics have become easier to grasp and quicker to recollect. So, no matter how much an odd-man out feel an average student has among the high-end students, it is possible to equal them in performance if the student meticulously follows this book. So, it is guaranteed that the student choosing this book is likely to enjoy learning physiology.

In the end, we would just like to mention that there are no shortcuts to success. So, keep working hard and keep revising as frequently as you can. Trusting yourselves is as important as preparing hard for the examinations.

Contents

Section 1: Theory

Section 2: Practicals

Section 3: Extra Mile

Section 1

THEORY

CHAPTER 1

General Physiology

INTRODUCTION

Human physiology is concerned with the way various systems function and the way each contributes to the functions of the body as a whole. General physiology forms the foundation in the learning of physiology principles. It consists of molecular mechanisms that underlie the functioning of our organ systems. Learning of such mechanisms is a critical aspect in our understanding of disease processes. For instance, it includes the transport processes through our cell membranes. One such transport mechanism is sodium-potassium pump, an active transport through all our cell membranes. Many of the disease processes are linked, at the cellular level, to the sodium-potassium pump functioning or loss of its function.

TRANSPORT ACROSS CELL MEMBRANE

Transport across the cell membrane can be classified into active and passive transport, based on whether it is along the concentration gradient or against the concentration gradient (Tables 1.1 and 1.2).

Passive Process (Flowchart 1.1)

Passive transport across the cell membrane is a physical process and depends entirely on physical factors such as concentration gradient, electrical gradient and pressure gradient depending upon the type of passive transport. It is not a biological process (activity of enzyme), therefore does not require energy expenditure. It is in the direction of concentration gradient, i.e. downhill movement (from high concentration to low concentration). Examples are: 1. Without carriers—simple diffusion, osmosis and 2. Through carrier—facilitated diffusion.

Table 1.2: Transport mechanism

Transport mechanism	Examples
Simple diffusion	Movement of fats, oxygen, CO_2 through lipid portion of membrane
Facilitated diffusion	Movement of glucose and some amino-acids
Osmosis	Movement of water into and out of the cell
Primary active transport	Ions K^+, Ca^{2+}, H^+
Secondary active transport	Glucose or amino-acid into the cell along Na^+ (symport or cotransport) Ca^{2+}, H^+ out of the cell against Na^+ (antiport or countertransport)

Flowchart 1.1: Passive process

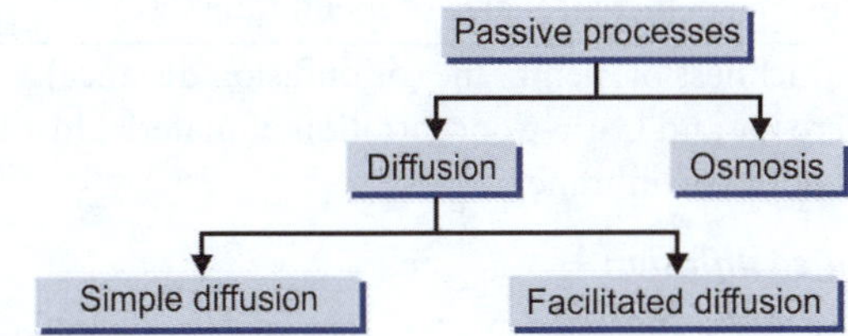

Table 1.1: Types of transport across cell membrane

	Carrier protein involved	Energy required	Concentration gradient
Simple diffusion	No	No	Along (downhill)
Osmosis (diffusion of H_2O)	No	No	Along (downhill)
Facilitated diffusion	Yes	No	Along (downhill)
Active transport	Yes	Yes	Against (uphill)
Exocytosis	No	Yes	N/A (not applicable)
Endocytosis			
• Pinocytosis and phagocytosis	No	Yes	N/A
• Receptor mediated endocytosis	Yes	Yes	N/A

Diffusion

It is a passive process by which molecules move from areas of high concentration to areas of low concentration. This can be of two types—simple diffusion and facilitated diffusion.

Simple diffusion

Simple diffusion refers to diffusion of molecules across the membrane following a concentration gradient or chemical gradient, but without the help of any carrier protein.

It occurs because the heat content of the solution keeps the solvent and the solute particles of the solution in constant motion. The examples of substances that pass through cell membranes by simple diffusions are transport of O_2, CO_2, urea, ammonia and ions.

Factors affecting diffusion

- *Distance:* The greater the distance, the longer the time required.
- *Size of gradient:* The larger the concentration gradient, faster the diffusion.
- *Temperature:* The higher the temperature, faster the diffusion rate.
- *Molecular size:* The permeability of cell membrane to a substance falls rapidly with increase in molecular weight in the range between 10,000 and 60,000. This is why glucose diffuses faster than large proteins.
- *Lipid solubility:* Lipid soluble molecule diffuses rapidly.
- *Surface area:* The larger the surface area, faster the diffusion.

  The rate at which a material diffuses through the membrane is given by Fick's law of diffusion.

  Net rate of diffusion =

$$\frac{\text{Diffusion coefficient} \times \text{area of membrane} \times (C_{in} - C_{out})}{\text{Thickness of membrane (or diffusion distance)}}$$

Where C_{in} and C_{out} = Concentration of material inside and outside of the membrane.

Facilitated diffusion

It is a carrier - mediated process that enables molecules that are too large to flow through membrane channels by simple diffusion. The carrier molecule undergoes repetitive spontaneous configurational changes during which, the binding site for the substance is alternately exposed to the ICF and ECF (Fig. 1.1). For example:

- Glucose transport by the glucose transporter (GLUT) across intestinal epithelium.
- Transport of glucose into RBC, muscle and adipose tissue in presence of insulin.

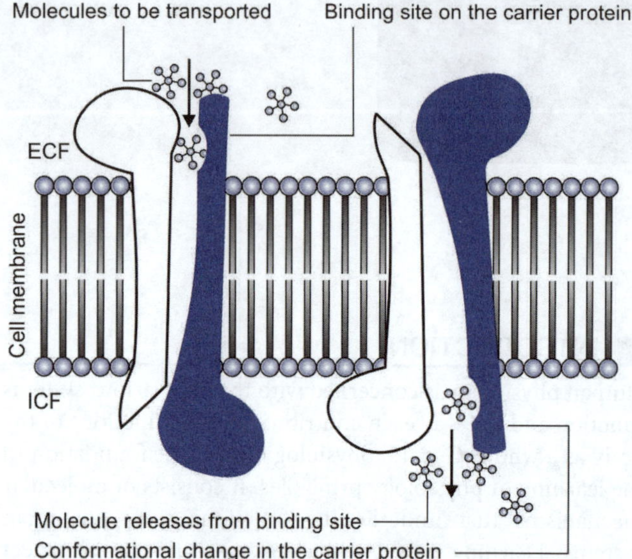

Fig. 1.1: Facilitated diffusion

Osmosis

Osmosis is the major passive transport mechanism after diffusion. In comparison to diffusion where the passive transport of solute occurs, osmosis is the passive transfer of solvent, especially water across the semipermeable membrane.

Water moves from area of its high concentration (low solute content) to area of its low concentration (high solute content). The mole is the standard unit for expressing the amount of substances in the SI unit system. One osmole (Osm) corresponds to the number of osmotically active substance. For example, NaCl would dissociate into Na^+ and Cl^- ions, so that each mole in solution would supply 2 Osm. Osmolarity is the number of osmoles per liter of solution (e.g. plasma). Osmolality is the number of osmoles per kilogram of solvent. Solutions that have the same osmolality as plasma are said to be isotonic; those with greater osmolality are hypertonic; and those with lesser osmolality are hypotonic. Normal serum osmolality is about 290 mOsm/L.

Active Transport Process (Flowchart 1.2)

Substances are transported against their chemical and electrical gradient (uphill movement). This form of transport require energy. It includes:

Flowchart 1.2: Active transport

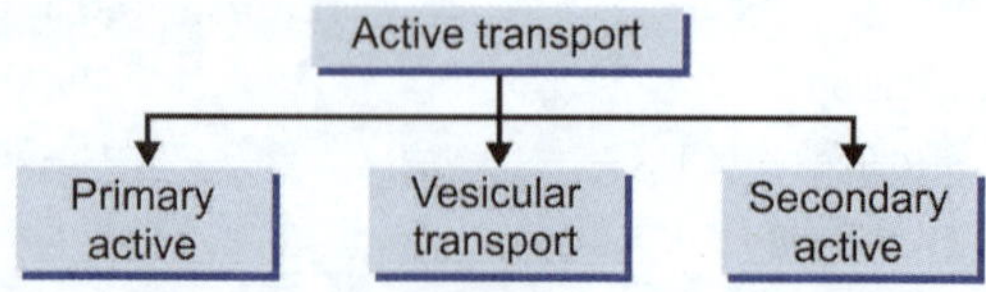

Primary Active Transport

In primary active transport, the energy is derived directly from hydrolysis (breakdown) of ATP (or related molecule). The most important example is $Na^+ - K^+$ pump ($Na^+ - K^+$ ATPase). It consists of:

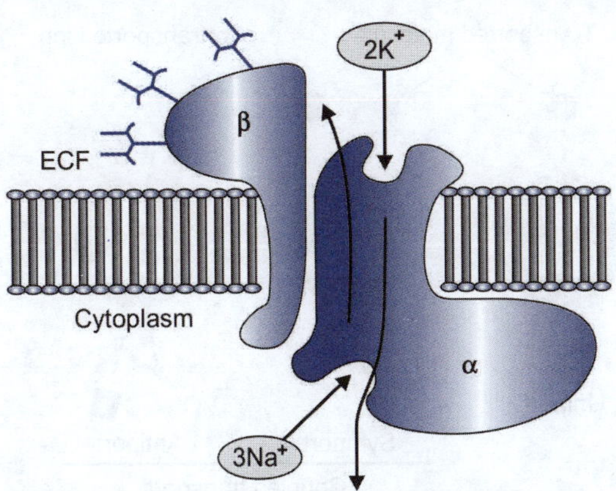

Fig. 1.2: Mechanism of operation of Na^+ – K^+ pump

Na^+- K^+ pump

It is an electrogenic pump. Here $3Na^+$ ions moves out and two K^+ ions moves in. It uses ATPase as the carrier molecule. ATPase is composed of 6 subunits, 3 α- and 3 β-subunits. Sodium and potassium transport occurs through α subunits. α subunit has ATPase enzymatic activity. Binding sites are present on its intracellular and extracellular faces.

Mechanism of action (Fig. 1.2): Binding of $3Na^+$ ions and ATP to a carrier protein inside the cell transfers high energy phosphate group from ATP to aspartic acid residue of α-subunit of ATPase (phosphorylation). This causes change in configuration of protein resulting in $3Na^+$ ions to move out of the cell.

When $2K^+$ ions bind to carrier protein on the outside of the cell, the aspartic acid - phosphate bond is hydrolyzed (dephosphorylation).This causes second change in configuration of protein resulting in $2K^+$ ions to move into the cell.

Clinical significance: Digitalis, a drug used for the treatment of heart failure, increases myocardial contractility by binding to α-subunit and interfering with the dephosphorylation step of transport process. This action is prominent in failing heart.

Ca^{2+} pump

It is present in sarcoplasmic reticulum of muscle to maintain intracellular Ca^{2+} concentration. It is also present in cell membrane and cell organelle membrane. In the cell membrane, the direction of Ca^{2+} is from cytoplasm to ECF. In the cell organelle membranes, it is from cytoplasm to the organelle lumen.

Potassium-hydrogen pump

It is present in cells of gastric mucosa and renal tubules where it causes secretion of H^+.

Some Channel Blockers

Na channels—TTX (tetrodotoxin), STX (saxitoxin)
K channels—TEA(tetraethylammonium)
Ca channels—verapamil, nifedipine
Na^+ – K^+ ATPase—ouabain, digitoxin.

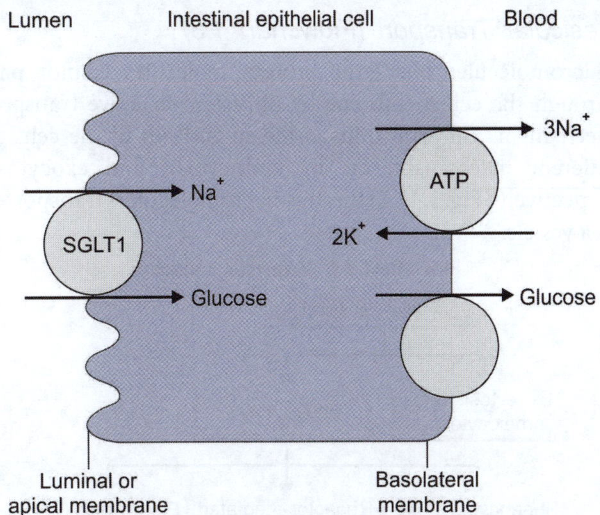

Fig. 1.3: Secondary active transport of glucose

Secondary Active Transport

In secondary active transport, the energy is derived from the store which has been created originally by primary active transport. Secondary active transport represents a combination of primary active transport and facilitated diffusion. It is a carrier-mediated active transport in which, the energy stored in the Na^+ concentration gradient is utilized for the transport of other molecules or ions. Hence, it uses energy indirectly. Energy/ATP is required to establish the Na^+ concentration gradient so that Na^+ concentration is higher in the ECF as compared to Na^+ in the ICF. Potential energy in this concentration gradient is then utilized for the movement of other substances. Thus, it is 'secondary' because ATP was utilized elsewhere (in the primary active transport). It is exemplified by glucose transport across intestinal mucosal epithelial cells and kidney tubules (Fig. 1.3).

The Na^+ – K^+ pump operates at the basolateral border of the cell and maintains intracellular concentration of Na^+ very low. The low intracellular Na^+ concentration provides the accessory concentration gradient for Na+ to diffuse in passively at the luminal border through facilitated cotransport with glucose. Thus, the Na^+ – K^+ pump (Na^+ – K^+ ATPase) indirectly powers the movement of glucose into the cell, and glucose can move in against a concentration gradient so long as Na^+ diffuses in along a concentration gradient. It is important to know that at luminal border, Na^+ is transported by facilitated diffusion (as it diffuses along a concentration gradient) while the glucose is transported actively (against a concentration gradient) and the energy is provided by Na^+ – K^+ ATPase at basolateral border. So, secondary active transport is a combination of active transport (glucose transport against concentration gradient) and facilitated diffusion (Na^+ transport along concentration gradient by carrier protein).

Vesicular Transport (Flowchart 1.3)

Macromolecules like large protein molecules cannot pass through the cell membrane by diffusion or active transport mechanism. They are transported in and out of the cells by different mechanism, i.e. by endocytosis and exocytosis respectively (Fig. 1.4). In this the macromolecule is transported as a vesicle.

Flowchart 1.3: Vesicular transport

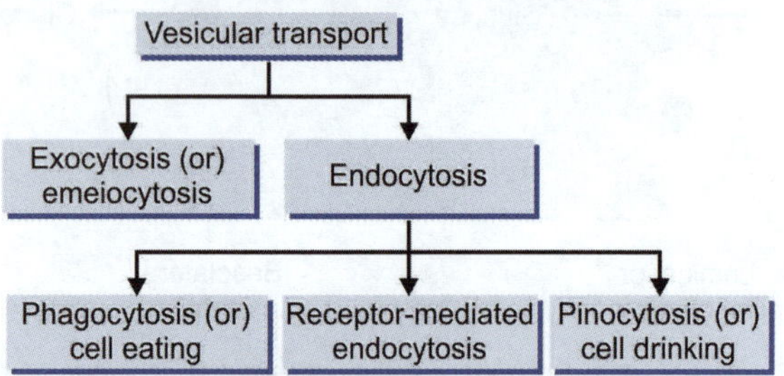

- *Endocytosis:* In endocytosis, the cell takes something in, into its cytoplasm from ECF. When a large molecule comes in contact with cell membrane, the membrane invaginates to include the macromolecule as a vesicle. The vesicle next gets pinched off to the interior of cell and the cell membrane is restored. Endocytosis may be:
  - *Phagocytosis:* Process by which extracellular substances (bacteria, dead tissue, foreign particles) are engulfed by the cells. The substance makes contact with the cell membrane, which then invaginates. The endocytic vesicle pinches off from the cell membrane and fuses with another intracellular vesicle. For example, a bacterium or a dead tissue. It occurs in a few cells like WBC and tissue macrophages.
  - *Pinocytosis:* When endocytosis of liquid occurs. It occurs in most of the cells.
  - *Receptor-mediated endocytosis:* It is an efficient process of endocytosis in which the extracellular molecule binds with the specific receptor on the cell membrane.

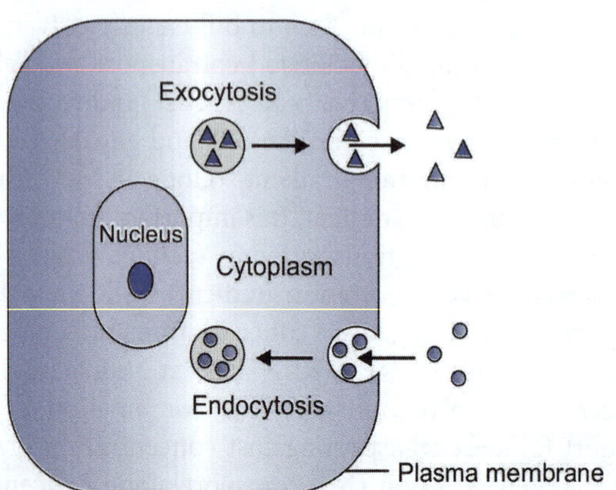

Fig. 1.4: Vesicular transport process

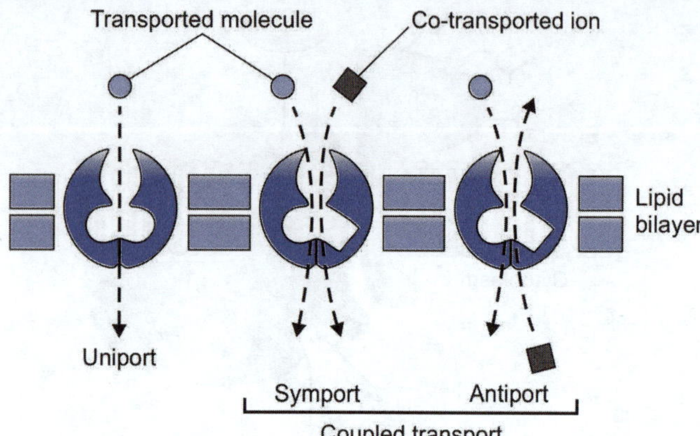

Fig. 1.5: Carrier type processes

Receptors are concentrated at a depression on membrane called coated-pits. Below these pits, on the inside of the cell membrane there is a fibrillar protein called clathrin. Once the particle combines with the receptors, the clathrin causes the pit to invaginate inward. It becomes deeper and deeper. The edges of the membrane come closer. The part of the membrane now pinches off into the cell in the form of an endocytic vesicle causing rapid internalization of the molecule. Hormones, growth factors, transport-proteins like transferring toxins, viruses, etc. enter cells by receptor mediated endocytosis.

- *Exocytosis:* Substance secreted by the cell are trapped within the vesicles or granules which fuse with the membrane and release their content into ECF. It is the reverse of endocytosis.

Types of Carrier Proteins

Carrier is a transport protein that binds ions and other molecules and then change their configuration, thus moving the bound molecule from one side of cell membrane to other (Fig. 1.5).

Types

1. *Uniporters*: Transport a single particle in one direction. For example, facilitated diffusion of glucose.
2. *Symporters*: Transport two particles together in same direction. For example, transport of glucose and amino acids into the epithelial cells of GI tract and the kidney tubules. Glucose cotransport with sodium is carried out by carrier proteins called 'SGLTs' (sodium - glucose transporters).
3. *Antiporters:* Transport molecules in opposite directions in which one substance is transported to the inside of the cell and other substance from inside the cell to the outside. For example, Na^+- K^+ pump, Na^+- Ca^{2+} exchangers, Na^+- H^+ exchangers.

Nonionic Diffusion

Some weak acids and bases are quite soluble in cell membranes in the undissociated form, whereas they cannot cross membranes in the charged (i.e. dissociated) form. Molecules of the undissociated substance diffuse from one side of the membrane to the other and then dissociate is called nonionic diffusion. The main process by which NH^3 is secreted into the urine and then changed to NH^{4+}, is an example of nonionic diffusion.

BODY FLUID COMPARTMENTS

Water constitutes approximately 60% of total body weight. Of this 60%, 40% is present in the cell, i.e. intracellular fluid (ICF) and 20% is present outside the cells constituting extracellular fluid (ECF). 20% of body weight of water in ECF is divided into interstitial fluid (15% of body weight) and plasma (5% of body weight). An adult weighing 70 kg contains 42 liters of water. Of these 42 liters, 28 liters are present inside the cell as ICF and remaining 14 liters are present outside the cell as ECF. The ECF is present as interstitial fluid (10.5 L) and blood plasma (3.5 L) (Fig. 1.6). Composition of fluid in ECF and ICF is significantly different. In ECF, most abundant cation is Na^+ and most abundant, anion is Cl^-. On the other hand, in ICF most abundant cation is K^+ and most abundant anion is PO_4^{-2} followed by protein.

Extracellular Fluid

This is the fluid contained in the spaces outside the cell. Extracellular fluid (ECF) compartment includes plasma, interstitial fluid and transcellular fluid.

Plasma

It is the fluid portion of the blood. It represents 25% of the ECF. Its volume can be calculated from blood volume and PCV.

Plasma volume = blood volume × (100 – hematocrit/100)
where, blood volume = 80 ml/kg of body weight.

Interstitial Fluid

It is that part of ECF that is outside the vascular system. It surrounds all cells except blood cells and includes lymph.

Transcellular Fluid

It represents fluid in the lumen of structures lined by epithelium. It includes digestive secretions, sweat, CSF, pleural, peritoneal, synovial, intraocular, pericardial fluids, bile and luminal fluids of the gut, thyroid, cochlea.

Intracellular Fluid

This is the fluid containing within the body cells. Its volume varies.

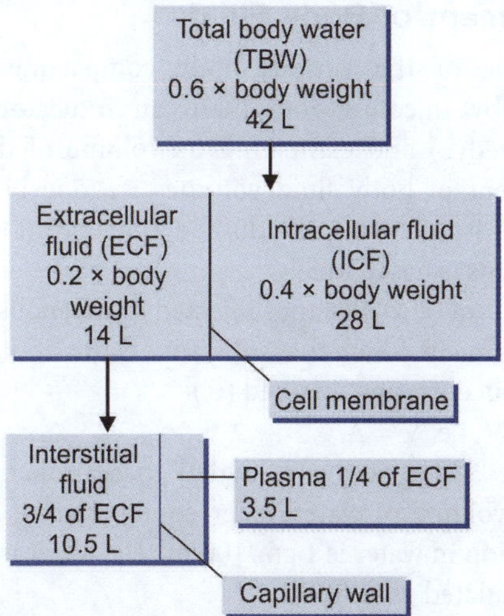

Fig. 1.6: Distribution of total body water (normal 70 kg man)

> **Clinical Note**
>
> Dehydration is common and rapid in children. Ratio of ECF volume to ICF volume is larger in infants and children than in adults. However, the total volume of ECF is much smaller in children than in adults. In addition, the regulatory mechanisms for maintaining ECF volume are not well developed in infants and children. Therefore, dehydration is more common and occurs rapidly in these age groups.

Major Cations and Anions of ECF and ICF (Fig. 1.7)

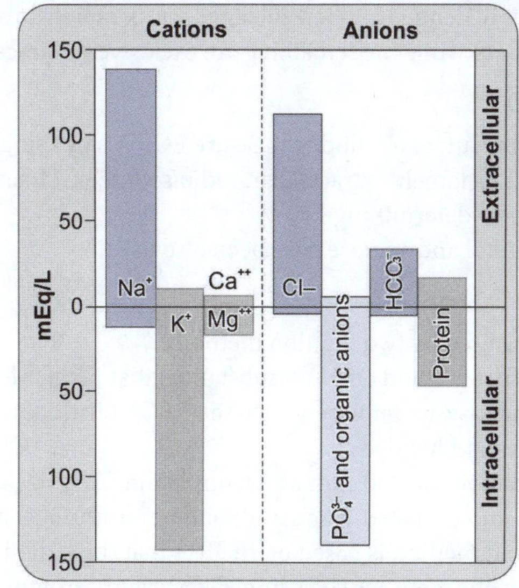

Compartment	Major cation	Major anion
ECF	Sodium (Na^+)	Chloride (Cl)
ICF	Potassium (K^+)	Phosphates (PO_4^{3-})

Fig. 1.7: Major cations and anions of ECF and ICF

Measurement of Body Fluids

The volume of the various body compartments can be measured by injecting into them an indicator substance (marker or dye) and estimating its volume of distribution. Measurement of body fluid volumes is done by 'dilutional method', i.e by knowing the diluted concentration of dye in the fluid. This is based on:

- The amount of a substance injected intravenously (A)
- The volume in which that substance is distributed (V)
- Final concentration attained (C)
  C = A/V, i.e. V = A/C.

Suppose 5 gm of dye is added to a beaker containing unknown volume of water. After equilibrium, if the marker concentration in water is 1 gm/100 ml, the water in the beaker can be calculated as follows:

Volume of water = Total amount of marker/Concentration of marker in water = 5 gm/1 gm per 100 ml = 500 ml.

Characteristics of Indicator

- Should be easy to measure
- Nontoxic
- Must mix evenly
- Must remain in compartment being measured
- Must not alter water distribution
- Must be unchanged by the body.

Extracellular Fluid Measurement

The ECF volume is difficult to measure as the limits of this space are ill defined and few substances mix rapidly in all parts of the space while the remaining are exclusively extracellular.

Methods

- Most accurate method to measure ECFV is by using inulin.
- As Cl^- is largely extracellular, radioisotope of Cl have been used for determining ECFV.
- Mannitol and sucrose have been also used.

Plasma volume

It is measured by two dilution methods.

1. The first method employs substances that neither leave the vascular system nor penetrate the RBC. It includes:
   - Evan's blue dye
   - Radioiodinated human serum albumin
   - Radioiodinated gamma-globulin and fibrinogen.
2. Second method is based on the fact that the radio isotopes of the phosphorous (P^{32}), iron ($Fe^{56, 57}$) and chromium(Cr^{51}) penetrate and bind to RBC. Therefore the red cell volume, i.e. volume occupied by all the circulating RBC in the body can be measured by injecting tagged RBCs intravenously and after mixing has occurred, measuring the fraction of the RBCs that is tagged. Commonly used tag is Cr^{51} that is attached to the cells by incubating them in a suitable 'Cr' solution. Then,

$$\text{Plasme volume} = \text{Blood volume} \times \frac{100 - \text{PCV}}{100}$$

(practically PCV = volume)

Interstitial fluid volume

It cannot be measured directly because as it is difficult to sample and no substance is distributed exclusively in this compartment. Interstitial fluid volume is determined as the difference between ECFV and plasma volume.

Intracellular Fluid Volume Measurement

Intracellular fluid volume (ICFV) cannot be measured directly by dilution, because no substance is confined exclusively to this compartment after intravenous administration. It is determined indirectly as:

$$\text{ICFV} = \text{TBW} - \text{ECFV}$$

Total body water can be measured by *indicator dilution principle.* Deuterium oxide (heavy water) has properties that are slightly different from water, but in equilibration experiments for measuring TBW, it gives accurate results. Tritium oxide and aminopyrine have also been used to measure TBW.

INTERCELLULAR CONNECTIONS

Two types of junctions form between the cells that makes up tissues (Flowchart 1.4 and Fig. 1.8).

Flowchart 1.4: Intercellular connections

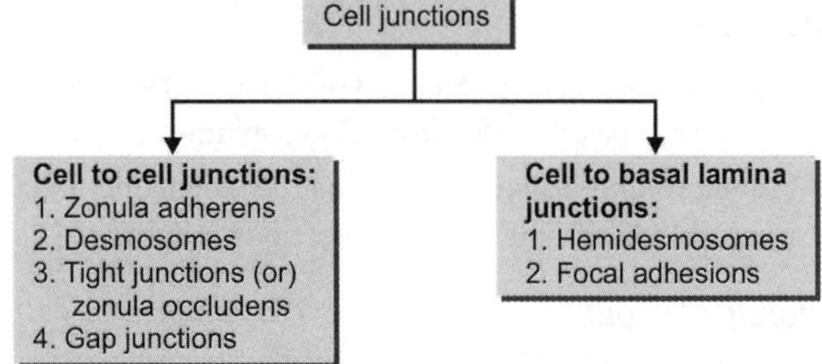

Tight Junction (Zonula Occludens)

It is the region where the cell membranes of the adjacent cells fuse together firmly. It is present in the apical margins of epithelial and endothelial cells in the intestinal mucosa, wall of renal tubule, capillary wall and choroid plexuses. It is made up of two ridges one half of ridge is from one cell and the other half from the other cell. It provide strength and stability to the tissues, prevents lateral movements of proteins and lipids in the cell membrane, in brain capillaries it forms blood brain barrier.

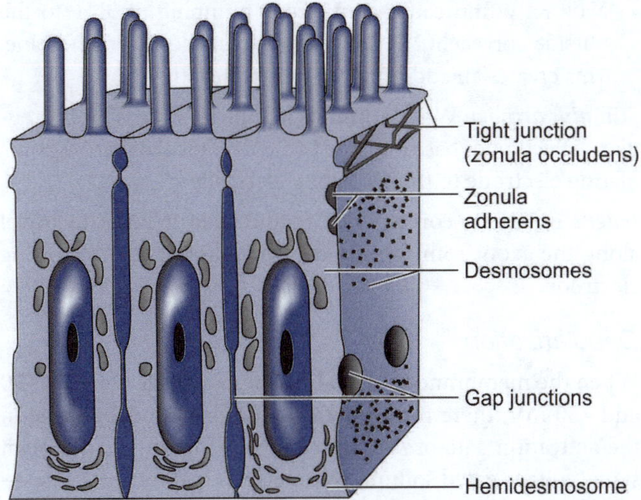

Fig. 1.8: Intercellular connections

Zona Adherens

It is a continuous structure on the basal side of zona occlundens, and it is a major site for the attachment of intracellular microfilaments.

Desmosomes

They are patches characterized by apposed thickenings of the membranes of two adjacent cells. This holds adjacent cells firmly together in areas that are subjected to stretching, such as skin.

Hemidesmosomes

It looks like half-desmosomes that attach cells to the underlying basal lamina and are connected intracellularly to intermediate filaments.

Gap Junctions

It is present in heart, basal part of epithelial cells of intestinal mucosa. Here, the cytoplasm of the two cells is connected by the channels formed by the membranes of both cells. Each channel consist of two halves. Each half belongs to one of the adjacent cells. It helps in the exchange of chemical messengers between the cells and in rapid propagation of AP (action potential) from one cell to another.

ACTION POTENTIAL

Action potential can be defined as sequence of changes in the membrane potential of an excitable cell due to opening and closure of different ion channels after the application of a threshold stimulus. Each action potential begins with a sudden change from the negative resting membrane potential (–70 mV) to a positive potential (+35 mV) and then ends with an almost equally rapid change back to the negative potential. To conduct a nerve signal, the action potential moves along the nerve fiber until it comes to the fiber's end (Figs 1.9 and 1.10).

Resting Membrane Potential (RMP)

When two electrodes are connected through a suitable amplifier and placed on the surface of a single axon, no potential difference is observed. However, if one electrode is inserted into the interior of the cell a constant potential difference is observed. The inner surface of cell membrane is usually charged negative with respect to its outer surface. The potential of the inner surface of the membrane with respect to its outer surface is called membrane potential. The membrane potential is produced by the passive diffusion of ions. When cell is not stimulated the potential is called resting membrane potential.

Genesis of RMP

The cell membrane is selectively permeable. Due to presence of potassium leak channels, K^+ ions are freely permeable, but

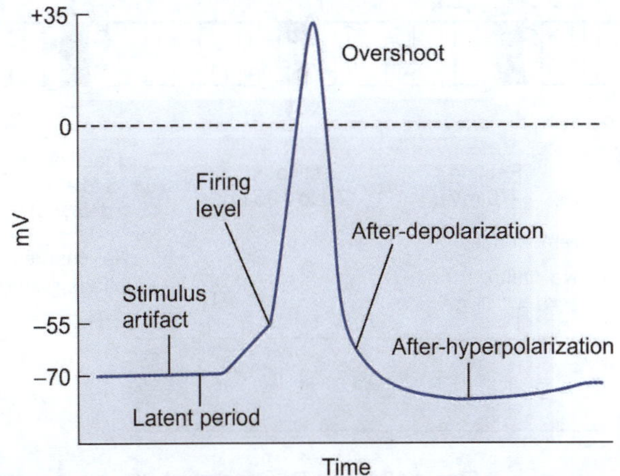

Fig. 1.9: Action potential in a neuron

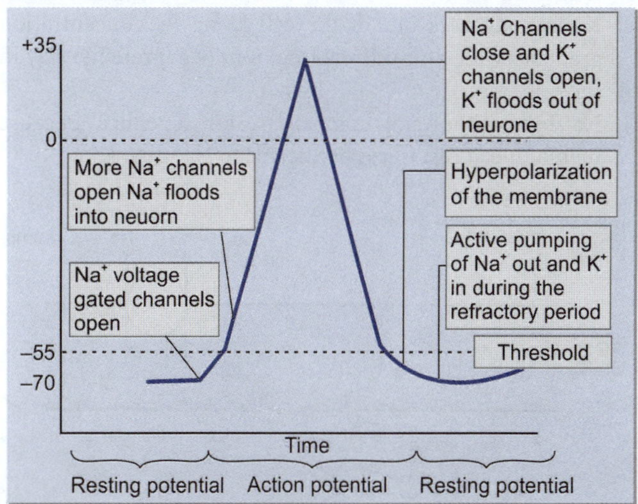

Fig. 1.10: Stages of action potential

PHYSICON—The Reliable Icon in Physiology

permeability of Na^+ is much less. In the generation of RMP, following sequence of events occur:

- K^+ diffuses out of cell along its concentration gradient (K^+ concentration is very high inside the cells and very low in ECF).
- The diffusion of K^+ produces an intracellular negativity (due to nondiffusible protein anion in the cells) which is not nullified by the diffusion of Na^+ in the opposite direction (membrane is impermeable to Na^+) or diffusion of Cl^- in same direction (Cl^- concentration is already very high in ECF in comparison to ICF).
- So, intracellular negativity is produced which opposes outward diffusion of K^+ and when the equilibrium is reached, the inward force on K^+ due to electrical gradient balances and outward force on K^+ due to concentration gradient.
- Finally, at equilibrium inner side of cell is negatively charged with respect to outer side, and resting membrane potential is produced. So, the RMP is principally due to concentration difference (chemical difference) of K^+ in ECF and ICF. In neurons, the resting membrane potential is usually about –70 mV, which is close to the equilibrium potential for K^+. Here, it is worth noting that RMP is close to the equilibrium potential of K^+, but the value of RMP is exactly same as equilibrium potential of Cl^-. It is because other ions also diffuse through membrane, though their effect is very little.

Phases

Resting Membrane Potential Stage

Here inside of nerve is negative and the outside of nerve is positive (Fig. 1.11). RMP = –70 mV. Membrane is maintained in polarized state by:

- Due to distribution of ions across the cell membrane. Some K^+ ions diffuses out of the cell along its concentration gradient while non-diffusable an ions (e.g. proteins) stay in the cell.
- Na^+ influx does not compensate for K^+ efflux, because membrane at rest is less permeable to Na^+ than K^+.

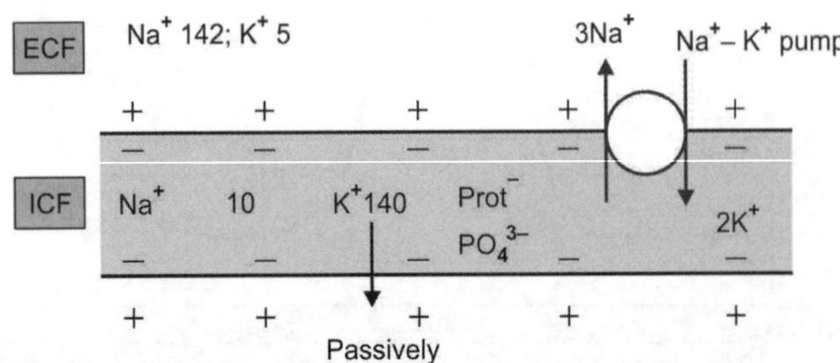

Fig. 1.11: Resting membrane potential

- Na^+- K^+ pump cause continuous pumping of $3Na^+$ to the outside for each $2K^+$ ion pumped inside the membrane. This creates an additional degree of negativity.

Stimulus artifact: When stimulus is applied there is brief irregular deflection of base line due to a current leakage from stimulating electrode to the recording electrode.

Latent period: It corresponds to the time it takes to travel along the axon from the site of stimulation to the recording electrode.

Depolarization

When the membrane potential reaches a voltage between –70 and –50 mV, there occurs sudden conformational change in the activation gate of sodium channels, flipping it into open state (voltage gated sodium channels has two separate gates—activation and inactivation gate) called as activated state and sodium ions moves in Figures 1.12A and B. The tracing rises rapidly till +35m V. Now inside of the nerve becomes positive and the outside of nerve is negative.

Repolarization

After sodium channel has remained open for 10,000 of a second, it suddenly closes. At this point the membrane potential begins to recover back to RMP. Repolarization starts with K^+ efflux due to opening up of voltage gated K^+ channels (Fig. 1.13). A very important characteristic of sodium channel inactivation process is that the inactivated gate will not reopen until the membrane potential returns to RMP.

After Depolarization

The phase of rapid rise (in depolarization) and of rapid fall (in repolarization) is called the spike potential. At the termination of spike potential K^+ conduction is slowed down and thus a few

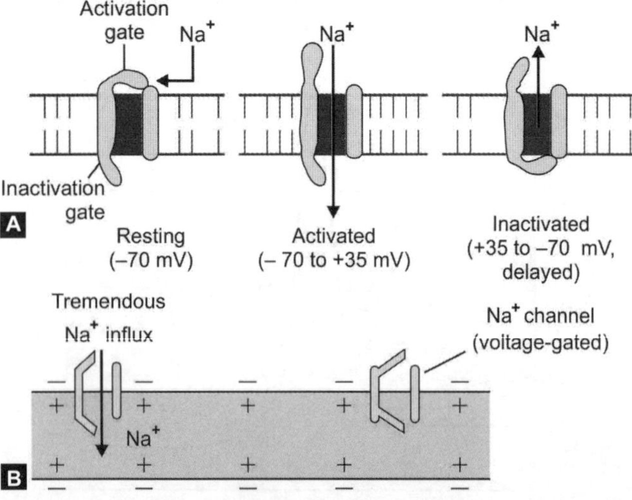

Figs 1.12A and B: Depolarization

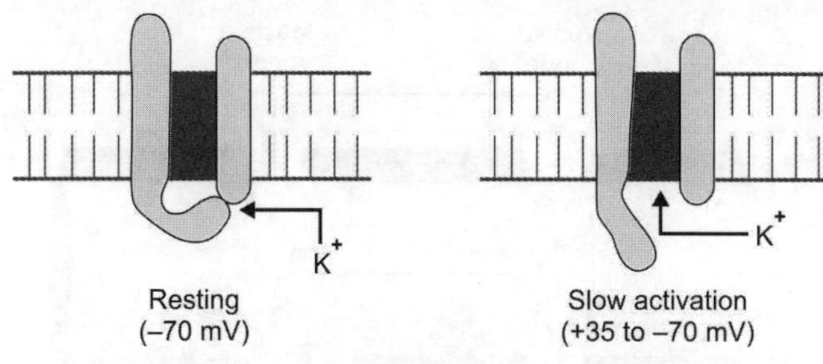

Fig. 1.13: Repolarization

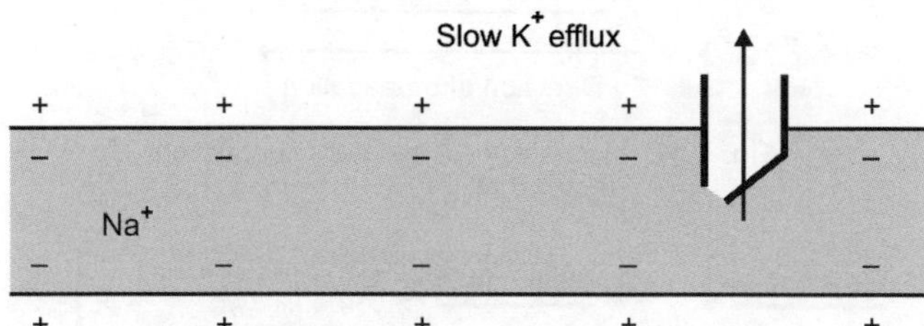

Fig. 1.14: After depolarization

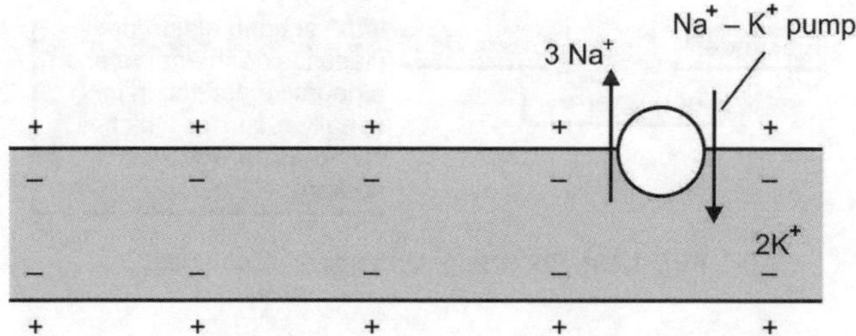

Fig. 1.15: After hyperpolarization

milliseconds are delayed in restoring the membrane potential. This last phase of slow K^+ efflux is called after depolarization (Fig. 1.14).

After Hyperpolarization

Resting membrane potentials is achieved by the active Na^+ – K^+ pump mechanism which transport $3Na^+$ out and $2K^+$ in (Fig. 1.15). During repolarization phase K^+ channels open and there is K^+ efflux. The membrane voltage falls back (repolarizes) to resting potential, i.e. –70 mV. At this voltage, K^+ channels close, but quite slowly. Therefore, more K^+ ions leak out, causing a brief period in which the voltage falls below 70 mV, i.e. hyperpolarization. Then Na^+ – K^+ pump works to reestablish resting potential by pumping Na^+ ions back out and K^+ ions back into the cells.

Properties of Action Potential

Threshold Stimulus

It is the minimum intensity of stimulating current that after acting for a given duration will just produce an action potential.

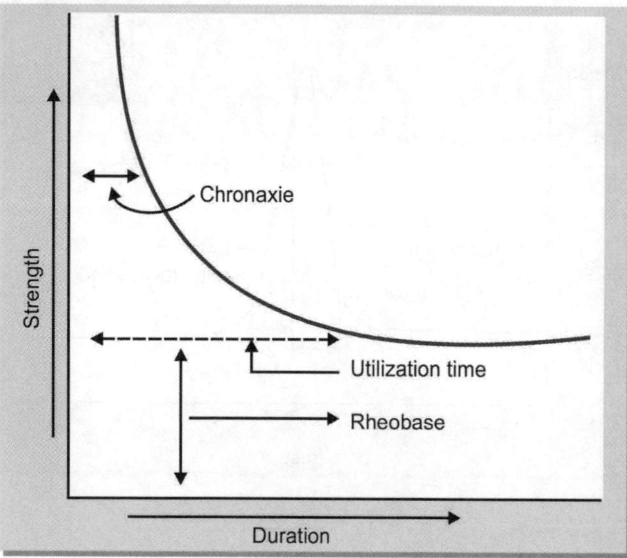

Fig. 1.16: Strength-duration curve

Note: The relationship between the strength and duration of a stimulus has been studied by varying the duration of stimulus and finding out threshold strength for each duration. Following information can be gathered from strength-duration curve.

Rheobase and Chronaxie (Fig. 1.16)

In general, the stronger the stimulus, less the duration required it to excite an action potential. The weakest current strength which can excite a tissue, if allowed to flow through it for an adequate time is called rheobase. The time for which it is applied is called utilization time. The minimum duration for which a stimulus double the rheobase has to be applied for it to excite an action potential is called chronaxie.

All or None Response

The action potential is an all or none response to stimuli, i.e. if the stimulus is subthreshold (not adequate), no action potential is produced. Once threshold is reached, a full-fledged action potential is produced. Further increase in the intensity of a stimulus produces no increment in the height of the action potential provided the other experimental condition remains the same.

Accommodation

If an excitable cell is applied with a constant strength of current, the site of membrane under stimulation fails to produce AP, i.e. the membrane adapts to the applied stimulus. This is due to slower opening and delayed closing of the voltage gated K^+ channels.

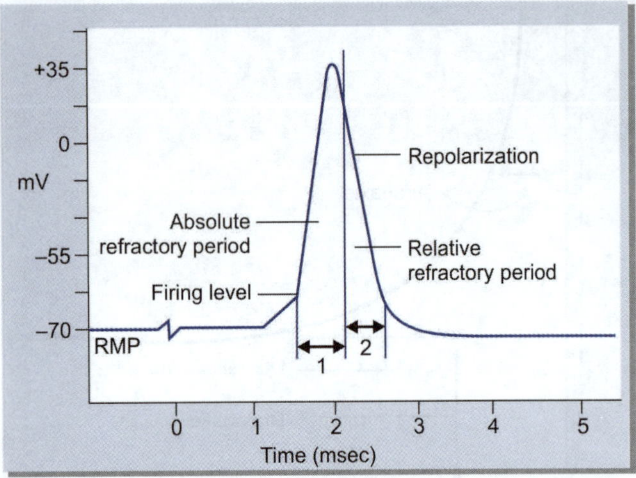

Fig. 1.17: Refractory periods

Conductivity

The action potential developed at one location on the excitable cell acts as a stimulus for the production of an AP in the adjacent region of the membrane. The excitation impulse is conducted along the cell membrane as a wave of depolarization.

Refractory Period

If two successive stimuli of more than threshold intensity are applied to an excitable cell, it is found that for sometime after the first stimulus, the cell becomes refractory. There are two types of refractory period (Fig. 1.17).

1. *Absolute refractory period:* Begins from the time the firing level is reached till the repolarizatoin is approx 1/3rd complete. During this period no strong stimulus can initiate the fresh impulse.
2. *Relative refractory period:* Begins at the end of ARP to the start of the after depolarization. During this stimuli stronger than normal stimulus can cause excitation.

Saltatory Conduction

Depolarization in myelinated axons jumps from one node of Ranvier to the next. This jumping of depolarization from node to node is called saltatory conduction. It is a rapid process, and myelinated axons conduct up to 50 times faster than the fastest unmyelinated fibers (Fig. 1.18).

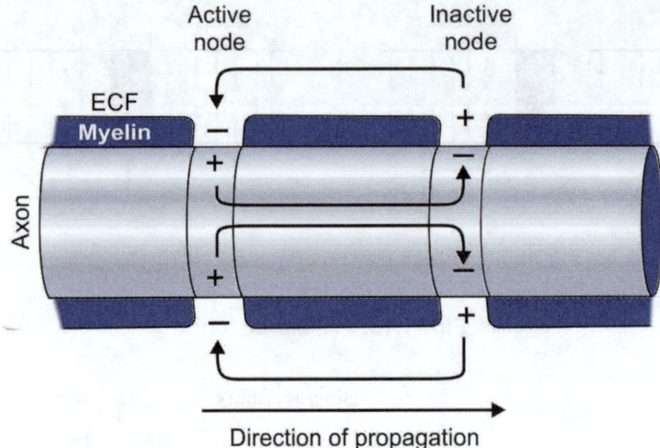

Fig. 1.18: Mechanism of saltatory conduction

RECORDING OF MEMBRANE POTENTIAL

The description of the resting membrane potential and action potential outline above is based on recording with two electrodes, one in the extracellular space (on surface of neuron) and one in the intracellular space (in the interior of neuron) (Fig. 1.19).

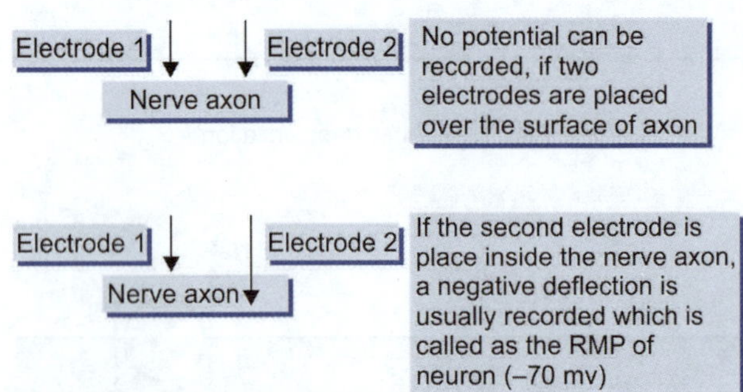

Fig. 1.19: Recording of membrane potential

Monophasic Action Potential

In this one microelectrode is placed inside the nerve fiber and the other electrode on the outer surface. These electrodes are then connected to the cathode ray oscilloscope (CRO). Monophasic record has following components:

- Depolarization
- Repolarization

Biphasic Action Potential

Here both the electrode are placed on the outer surface of nerve fibers, and they are connected to a CRO. When nerve is stimulated a record of alternate deflection one positive above the baseline and one negative below the baseline is depicted. As the wave of depolarization reaches the first electrode, this electrode becomes negative and an upward deflection is recorded. When the impulse passes to the portion of nerve between the two electrodes, the potential returns to zero and no deflection is recorded finally it passes the second electrodes and the first electrode becomes positive. Thus a downward deflection is recorded. This sequence is called biphasic action potential.

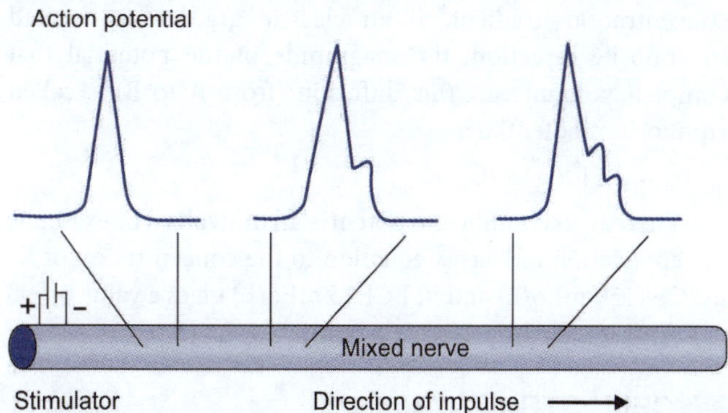

Fig. 1.20: Compound action potential: Record obtained with recording electrodes at various distances from the stimulating electrodes along a mixed nerve

Compound Action Potential

Compound action potential is the monophasic recording of action potential from a mixed nerve which contains different types of nerve fibers with varying diameter. Therefore, the compound action potential represents an algebraic summation of the all or none action potential of many axons (Fig. 1.20).

Causes of Compound Action Potential

A mixed nerve is made up of families of fibers with varying speed of conduction. Therefore

1. When all the fibers are stimulated, the activity in fast conducting fibers arrives at the recording electrodes sooner than the activity in slower fibers.
2. The farther away from the stimulating electrodes the action potential is recorded, the greater is the separation between the fast and slow fiber peaks (Fig. 1.21).

In general, group 'A' fibers make maximum contribution to compound action potential and group 'C' to the least.

GIBBS-DONNAN EFFECT

If two compartments are separated by a semipermeable membrane and one of the compartments contains diffusible ions, the ions will soon distribute themselves equally across the two compartments. If, however, one of the compartments contains nondiffusible (impermeable) anions (like protein) along with diffusible ions, the typical equilibrium (with equal number of ion on both side of the membrane) does not occur. Instead, a different type of equilibrium called the Gibbs-Donnan equilibrium will occur in which two conditions must be satisfied.

1. Both the compartment must be electroneutral.
2. The product of diffusible ions (anions and cations) must be equal in both compartments.

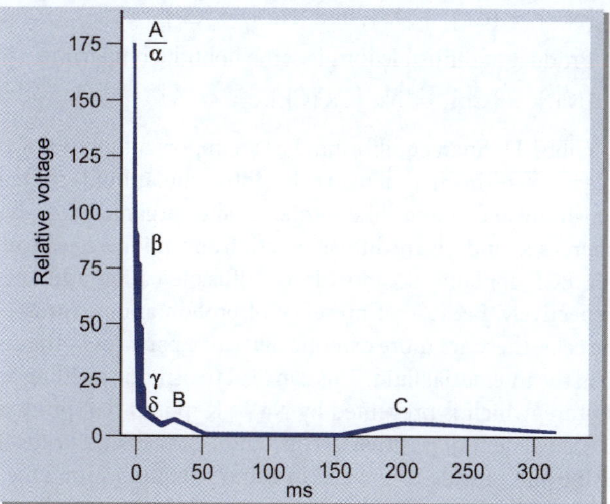

Fig. 1.21: Reconstruction of a compound action potential to show relative sizes and time relationships of the components

For example, there are 2 compartments, 'A' and 'B' which are separated from semipermeable membrane. 'A' contans 10 moles of NaCl and 5 moles of NaX (where X is non-diffusible anion).

Compartment A	Compartment B
10 NaCl	
5 NaX	

In compartment A, Na^+, Cl^- are diffusible while X is nondiffusible. Compartment A has 15 moles of Na^+ (10 from NaCl and 5 from NaX), 10 moles of Cl^- and 5 moles of X^-. Na^+ and Cl^- are diffusible, whereas X^- is non-diffusible. Now the question arises, how much ions will diffuse into compartment B and the answer is Donan-Gibbs equilibrium:

Compartment A	Compartment B
9 Na^+	6 Na^+
4 Cl^-	6 Cl^-
5 X^-	

	Compartment A	Compartment B
Total (+ve) charge	9 (due to 9 Na^+)	6 (due to 6 Na^+)
Total (-ve) charge	9 (4 Cl^- + 5 X^-)	6 (6 Cl^-)
Product of diffusible ions $[Na^+] \times [Cl^-]$	36 (9 Na^+ × 4 Cl^-)	36 (6 Na^+ × 6 Cl^-)
Total number of ions	18 (9 + 4 + 5)	12 (6 + 6)

This results in asymmetrical distribution of ions across the cell membrane. So, at Donnan-Gibbs equilibrium the total number of ions are different, but:

- Both compartments are electroneutral, i.e. negative and positive charge is same, e.g. compartment 'A' is electroneutral because it has 9 positive and 9 negative charges.

$[Na^+]_A = [Cl^-]_A + [X^-]_A$ and $[Na^+]_B = [Cl^-]_B$

- Product of diffusible ions is same in both compartments.

  $[Na^+]_A \times [Cl^-]_A = [Na^+]_B \times [Cl^-]_B$

Gibbs-Donnan equilibrium has an important physiological role in cells. The mammalian cells (intracellular fluid) contains non-diffusible anion like proteins and organic phosphate whereas K^+ and Cl^- are diffusible cation and anion, respectively. The ECF contains K^+ and Cl^- as diffusible cation and anion respectively. Because of presence of protein anions (prot-) in the cells, there are more osmotically active particles in the cells than the interstitial fluid. This can lead to osmotic swelling and rupture, which is prevented by $Na^+ - K^-$ pump that produces net movement of positive charge out of the cell and keeps the inside and outside of the cell in osmotic equilibrium. Due to Gibbs-Donnan equilibrium:

- Concentration of K^+ is greater in ICF than ECF (concentration of diffusible cation is greater in compartment with non-diffusible anion).
- Concentration of Cl^- is greater in ECF than ICF.
- Total number of ions is greater in ICF than ECF.

All these effects help to maintain the shape and volume of cells by distributing diffusible ions across the membrane according to physiological demand. The Gibbs-Donnan effect also makes a small contribution to the value of the resting membrane potential.

Nernst Equation

When two ionic solution (ions) A and B of different concentration (C_A and C_B) of an ion separated by a permeable membrane, the ions tend to diffuse along their concentration gradient. Since ions are charged particles, their diffusion can be stopped by an appropriate electrical potential (E) applied across the membrane. The magnitude and polarity of the potential (equilibrium potential) that must be applied to side A of the membrane for stopping the diffusion of ions (E_A) is given by Nernst equation, i.e. the equilibrium potential (E_m) for an ion is calculated by Nernst equation.

As described above, in accordance with Gibbs-Donnan equilibrium, asymmetrical distribution of diffusible ions occurs across the cell membrane with more cation (K^+) present inside. Therefore, K^+ will try to diffuse into the ECF from ICF, which is opposed by the electrical gradient, created by presence of non-diffusible anions inside the cell. Thus, finally equilibrium is reached between the concentration gradient and the electrical gradient resulting in diffusion potential (equilibrium potential) across the cell membrane. The degree of this equilibrium potential is determined by Nernst equation.

For example, if solution A contains an ion with negative charge in more concentration than the concentration of same ion in solution B, the ion will diffuse from A to B along concentration gradient. If an electric gradient is created in opposite direction, the magnitude of the potential that completely counteract this diffusion (from A to B) is called equilibrium potential.

$$E_M = \pm 61 \log C_A/C_B$$

Where E_M is equilibrium potential in milivolts. For example, the application of Nernst equation to the concentration of K^+ in ICF (150 mEq/L) and in ECF (5 mEq/L) gives a value of -90 mV. This is called the Nernst potential for K^+ (E_K).

CELL STRUCTURE

The cells are functional unit of living organisms. There are approximately 100 trillion cells in a human. For descriptive purpose, structure of a cell is divided into (Fig. 1.22):

- Cell membrane
- Cytoplasm and its organelles
- Nucleus

Cell Membrane (Plasma Membrane)

The membrane that surrounds the cell is called cell membrane. It is approximately 7.5–20 nanometer thick. It is composed almost entirely of proteins and lipids. Carbohydrates are minimal and occurs almost invariably in combination with proteins or lipids in the form of glycoproteins or glycolipids. Fluid Mosaic model proposed by Singer and Nicholson explains the components of cell membrane and their functions. According to this model, the fluid component of membrane is the lipids and the mosaic component is the membrane proteins. Proteins are the major constituents of cell membrane. Inner mitochondrial membrane has maximum protein concentration. The only exception where lipids outnumber proteins is myelin sheath of nerve cell membrane.

Membrane Lipids

Three types of lipids are seen in cell membrane:

1. Lipids with phosphate group attached—Phospholipids.
2. Lipids with carbohydrate group attached—Glycolipids.
3. Sterols—Cholesterol.

Phospholipids are the most abundant lipids in cell membrane. Most lipids are distributed unequally (membrane asymmetry). Some lipids are present on the outer surface of membrane (glycolipids). Some lipids are present on the inner surface of membrane (phosphatidylinositol and phosphatidylserine).

Membrane Proteins

Membrane proteins are the maximum constituents in all cell membranes. They are the mosaic components of fluid mosaic model (Fig. 1.23). They can be of the following three types:

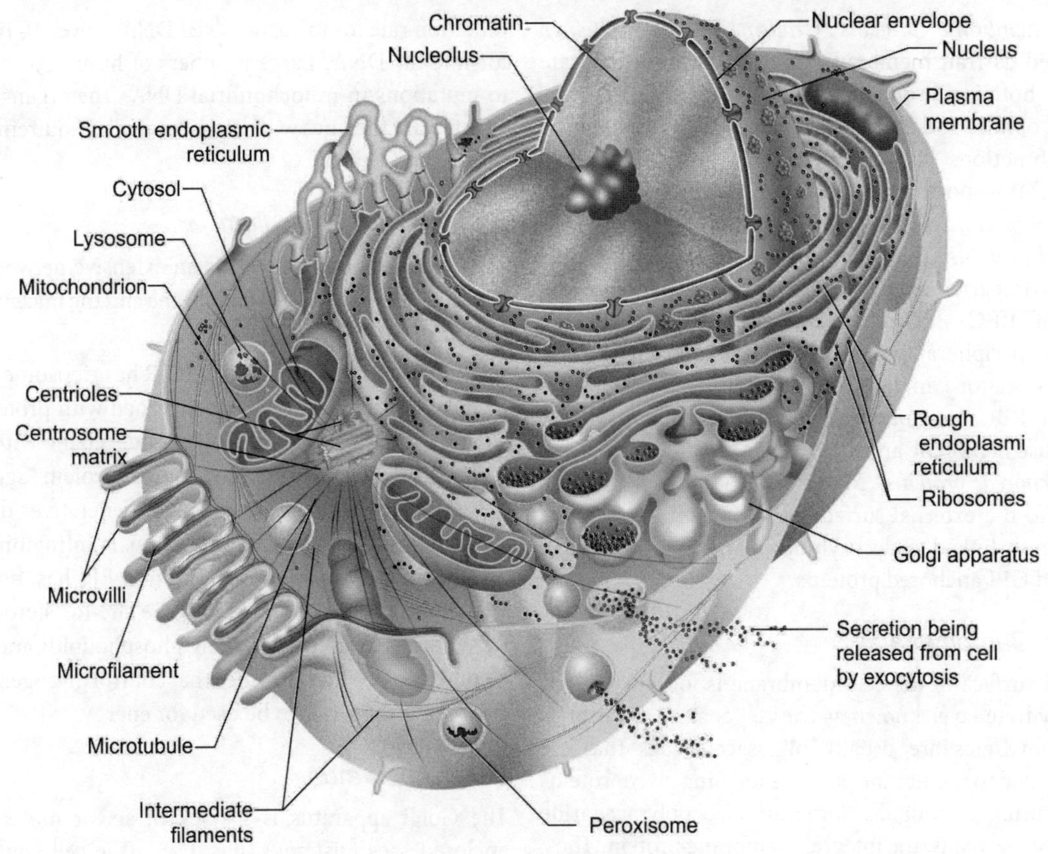

Fig. 1.22: Parts of a cell

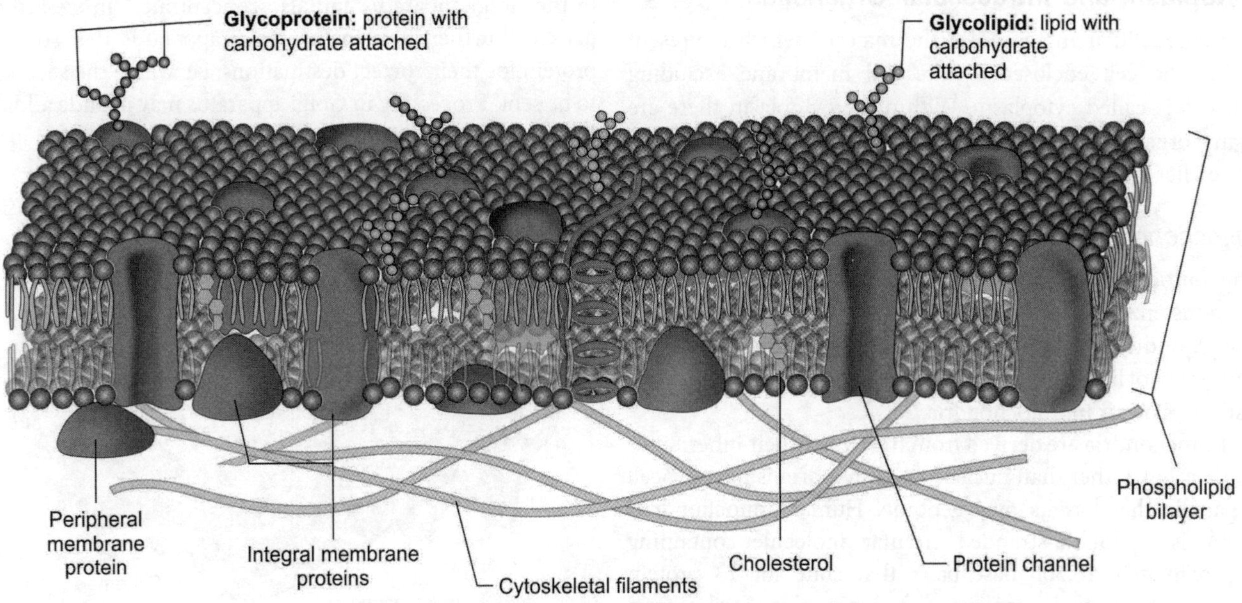

Fig. 1.23: Fluid mosaic model

1. *Integral membrane proteins (transmembrane proteins):* Also called as transmembrane proteins because they are present in both inside and outside of membrane. They have both hydrophilic and hydrophobic regions (amphipathic). Mainly functions as receptors (G protein coupled receptors), transporters - as carriers (or) channel proteins [sodium potassium ATPase ($Na^+ - K^+$ Pump].
2. *Peripheral proteins:* They are mainly supportive and gives structural integrity. Seen on one side of the membrane. Shapes of RBCs are biconcave disks because of the important peripheral proteins spectrin, ankyrin, band-3 protein. Mutations in these proteins leads to change in shapes of RBCs to spherical (hereditary spherocytosis) which cause hemolytic anemia.
3. *Lipid anchored proteins*: Many lipid-anchored proteins attached to the external surface of the plasma membrane are covalently linked to glycosylphosphatidylinositol (GPI); also called GPI anchored proteins.

Membrane Carbohydrates

The external surface of the cell membrane is loosely covered by a carbohydrate layer known as the cell coat or glycocalyx. These carbohydrates are usually oligosaccharides that are covalently linked to membrane proteins forming glycoproteins or lipids forming glycolipids. Some are also polysaccharide chains of proteoglycans, the integral membrane protein. Thus, the outer surface of the lipid bilayer is covered by a layer of glycoproteins and glycolipids.

Cytoplasm and Intracellular Organelles

The intracellular material, i.e. the material which is present inside the cell enclosed by the cell membrane excluding nucleus is called cytoplasm. Within the cytoplasm there are many organelles. The fluid that is present in between the organelles is called cytosol.

Mitochondria

The mitochondria are the 'powerhouses of cell' because it contains enzymes for energy metabolism and ATP synthesis. Mitochondria are spherical or cylindrical bodies which are composed of lipid bilayer protein membranes. Many metabolic pathways occur in mitochondria.

Mitochondria are derived from the ovum, their inheritance is maternal. Other than nucleus, mitochondria is the only cell organelle that has its own genome. Human mitochondrial DNA is a double-stranded circular molecule containing approximately 16,500 base pairs that code for 13 protein subunits to form 4 enzyme complexes plus 2 ribosomal and 22 transfer RNAs involved in mitochondrial functions. Mitochondria have an ineffective DNA repair system, and the mutation rate for mitochondrial DNA is over 10 times the rate for nuclear DNA. Large numbers of human diseases are due to mutations in mitochondrial DNA. The organs particularly affected are the ones with high metabolic requirements namely muscle and heart.

Endoplasmic Reticulum

The endoplasmic reticulum is an extensive network of tubules running between the cell membrane and the nucleus (Fig. 1.24). Two varieties of ER are known:

1. *Rough or granular ER:* Rough ER has ribosomes attached to its cytoplasmic side. It is concerned with protein synthesis and initial folding of polypeptide chain with formation of disulyphide bond. Misfolded protein aggregates are responsible for many neurodegenerative diseases like Alzheimer's disease, Prion disease, Huntington's disease.
2. *Smooth (agranular) ER:* Smooth ER has no ribosomes attached to it. Smooth ER is the site for steroid synthesis, synthesis of lipids especially phospholipids and cholesterol and also provide enzymes that control glycogen breakdown when glycogen is to be used for energy.

Golgi Apparatus

The Golgi apparatus is a stack of six or more membrane-enclosed sacs (cistems) (Fig. 1.25). The cell contains one or more Golgi apparatus, usually near the nucleus. Proteins and polypeptides synthesized in the rough ER are passed on to the Golgi apparatus. These secretions (polypeptide) are stored in the Golgi apparatus and also concentrated, processed and packed. Further, it is in the Golgi apparatus that sorts out protein for their correct destinations, i.e. where the secretions to be sent. Processing in Golgi apparatus may include addition of the carbohydrate moiety to proteins (glycosylation) to

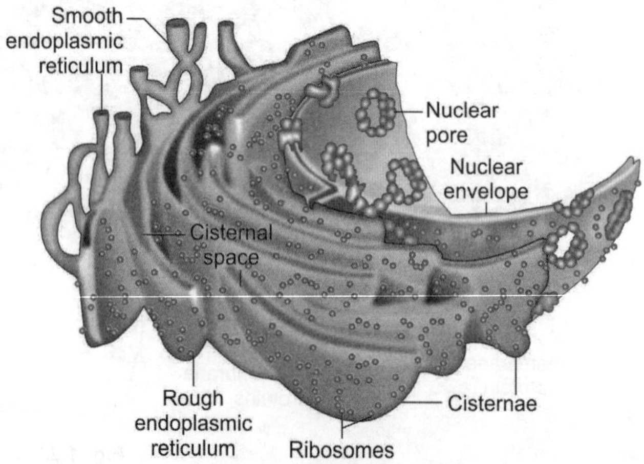

Fig. 1.24: Endoplasmic reticulum

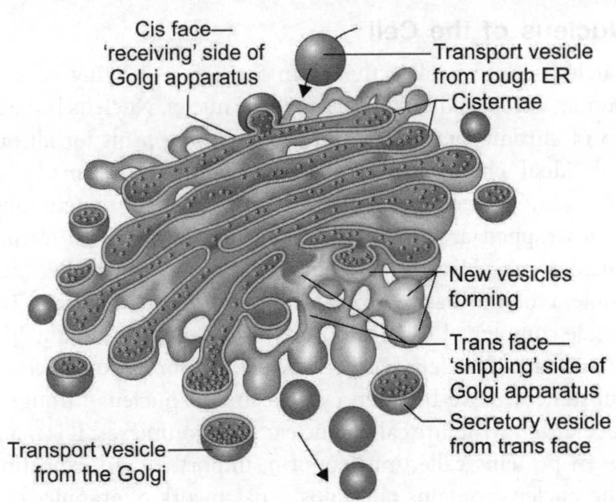

Fig. 1.25: Golgi apparatus

form glycoproteins; sulphation of mucopolysaccharides to form hyaluronic acid and chondroitin sulfate; cleavage of the polypeptide chain to form the active product, for example, proinsulin is cleaved by the Golgi apparatus to form insulin. Each Golgi apparatus is a polarized structure with a cis and a trans side. Cis end is the receiving end. Membrane vesicles containing newly synthesized protein bud off from the rough ER and fuse with cis side of GoIgi apparatus. Once processed, the vesicles are released in the form of exocytosis from trans end. So trans end is the secretory end.

Ribosomes

Ribosomes are the actual sites of protein synthesis. The ribosomes are small granules of RNAs. Ribosomes are usually occur in clusters called polyribosomes attached to one mRNA molecule, an arrangement that increases the rate of polypeptide synthesis. There are two types of polyribosomes:

1. *Free (cytosolic):* Present free in cytosol.
2. *Bound polyribosome:* Present on rough ER.

Both types can synthesize proteins.

Peroxisomes

Peroxisomes are cellular storehouses of metabolic enzymes. Peroxisomes matrix contains nearly 50 enzymes that catalyze a variety of metabolic reactions including detoxification of alcohol and other harmful compounds in liver. Peroxisomal membrane also has an elaborate mechanism for importing several enzymes into its matrix. A defect in peroxisomal membrane transport is the cause of Zellweger syndrome. Another similar genetic disorder is Refsum disease. Peroxisomes (or) microbodies are concerned with three vital functions in a cell namely.

1. *Generation and degradation of hydrogen peroxide (H_2O_2):* These organelles were named 'peroxisomes' because they are the site of synthesis and degradation of hydrogen peroxide, a highly reactive and toxic oxidizing agent. The defining characteristic of a peroxisome is the presence of catalase, an enzyme essential for the degradation of hydrogen peroxide. Hydrogen peroxide is a potentially toxic compound that is formed by a variety of oxidative reactions catalyzed by oxidases. Both catalase and the oxidases are confined to peroxisomes. Marker enzyme of peroxisomes is catalase.
2. *Fatty acid metabolism:* Oxidation of very long chain fatty acids (e.g. C20, C22) happens in peroxisomes. Peroxisomes shorten the side chain of cholesterol in bile acid formation. Peroxisomes are the sites for synthesis of plasmalogens and platelet activating factor. Plasmalogens are very abundant in the myelin sheaths that insulate axons in the brain. Abnormalities in the synthesis of plasmalogens can lead to severe neurological dysfunction. Platelet-activating factor aggregates platelets.
3. *Detoxification of harmful chemicals:* Peroxisomal enzymes such as superoxide dismutase, catalase and peroxidases detoxify reactive oxygen species, ethanol, formic acid, formaldehyde, nitrites and phenols. Peroxisomes rich in liver and kidney perform this function.

Lysosomes

Lysosomes are membranous bags containing hydrolytic enzymes for digesting large molecules of proteins, polysaccharides, fats and nucleic acids. Lysosomes bud off from trans face of the Golgi apparatus. Lysosomal enzymes are synthesized in rough ER and then processed by Golgi apparatus. The marker enzyme offer lysosome is acid phosphatase. Other enzymes found in lysosome (but are not markers) are ribonuclease, deoxyribonuclease, glucosidase, arylsulfatase, collagenase. Lysosomes are called 'suicidal bags of the cell', because the interior of lysosomes are always acidic. The lysosomes that pinched off from Golgi complex are called primary lysosomes. After a primary lysosome has fused with the vacuole or vesicle containing the material to be digested, it forms the secondary lysosome. After the process of digestion has been completed, a secondary lysosome forms the residual body. The residual body generally discharges its contents by exocytosis. Sometimes, however, residual bodies containing some indigestible substances may be retained in the cell. Such collections of residual bodies gradually increase with age, and are believed to contribute to impairment of physiological function associated with the process of aging.

Cytoskeletal Filaments—'Bones of the Cell'

Cytoskeletal filaments are involved in providing strength, support, shape of the cell. It also allows appropriate change in

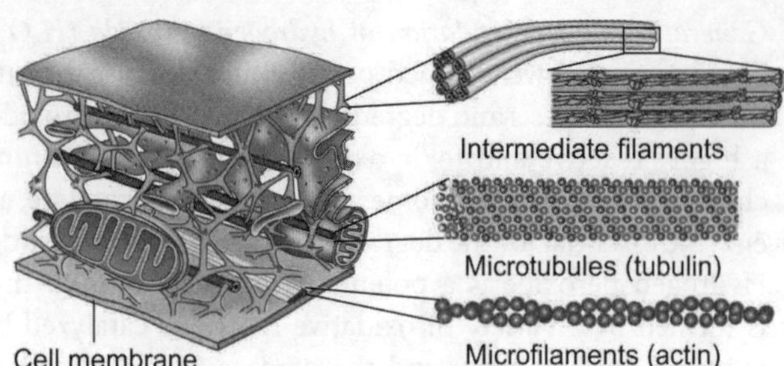

Fig. 1.26: Cytoskeleton

cell shape for cell mobility and participation of cell in various physiological activities. They are of the following three types: a. Microtubules, b. Intermediate filaments and c. Microfilaments (Fig. 1.26).

Microtubules (Diameter: 25 nm)

Microtubules are hollow fine tubules made up of a protein called tubulin. They are made up of two globular subunits α and β tubulin. A third subunit, γ tubulin, plays on an important role in assembly and is specifically localized to centrosome. Microtubules are necessary for the formation and function of mitotic spindle. Microtubules form the major structural components of cilia and flagella. Microtubules are a major component of axons and dendrites, where they maintain structure and participate in the axoplasmic flow of material along this neural process.

Microfilaments (Actin, Diameter: 7–9–5 nm)

All eukaryotic cells contain microfilaments that contribute to the maintenance of and change in cell shape and regulation of cell functions. Microfilaments are filamentous structures, made of two F-actin (filamentous actin) strands that are coiled helically. Actin is the most abundant protein in mammalian cells. Actin is most often associated with muscle contraction. Bundles of microfilaments are also present in the core of microvilli of epithelial cells of intestinal mucosa.

Intermediate Filaments (Diameter: 10–12 nm)

These are filamentous structures made up of various subunits. The average diameter of these filaments varies from 8 to 14 nm. Atleast 4 classes of intermediate filaments are found—lamins, keratins, vimentin, neurofilaments. They connect the nuclear membrane to the cell membrane and also membranes of cell organelles. Therefore, the major function of these filaments is to integrate the organelles within the cytoplasm. They form supple skeletal network for the cell and resist rupture of cell from external pressure. In the absence of microfilaments, cells easily rupture. Blister formation in skin is common in humans when these filaments are absent or abnormal.

Nucleus of the Cell

Nucleus controls all activities in the cell. All living cells in human except red blood cells contain nuclei. Nucleus is made up of chromosomes which carries the blue print for all our individual characteristics. Each chromosome is made up of a giant molecule of DNA, which is about 2 meters long. It is wrapped around a core of histone proteins to form a nucleosome. Histone protein possess an unusually high content of the basic amino acids arginine and lysine. The whole complex of DNA and proteins is called chromatin. The membrane of nucleus is called nuclear membrane, or envelope. Substances move between cytoplasm and nucleus through a specialized structure called nuclear pore complexes. It is made up of proteins called nucleoporin, importins and exportins. The nucleus contains nucleolus, a patchwork of granules rich in RNA. There may be multiple nucleoli in a nucleus. They synthesize ribosomes (Table 1.3).

Table 1.3: Parts of cell and their functions

Parts of a cell	Functions
Cell membrane (or) plasma membrane	Selectively permeable barrier
Nucleus	Controls all activities in the cell
Mitochondria	Synthesis of ATP
Rough endoplasmic reticulum	Synthesis of proteins
Golgi apparatus	Processing and sorting of proteins
Smooth endoplasmic reticulum	Synthesis of steroids, detoxification
Lysosomes	Digestion of substances in cell
Peroxisomes	Detoxification, liquid metabolism, generation and degradation of free radicals
Cytoplasm	Intracellular fluid compartment of cell
Cytoskeletal filaments	Support to the cell

HOMEOSTASIS

Imagine what happens to our blood glucose levels after food intake? It rises but not indefinitely. It is immediately sensed by beta cells of pancreas and insulin is released which brings back blood glucose to near normal levels. The concept here is constancy. All our body parameters have to be maintained at near normal levels. This concept of constancy is called *homeostasis*, the term coined long ago by Walter Cannon. Homeostasis is defined as the maintenance of constancy of internal environment of the body. Now what maintains it? Well yes, we have control systems.

Control Systems

Homeostatic regulation is mainly achieved through the feedback mechanisms. There are three types of feedback regulations—negative feedback, positive feedback, feed-forward control (Flowchart 1.5).

Flowchart 1.5: Homeostasis

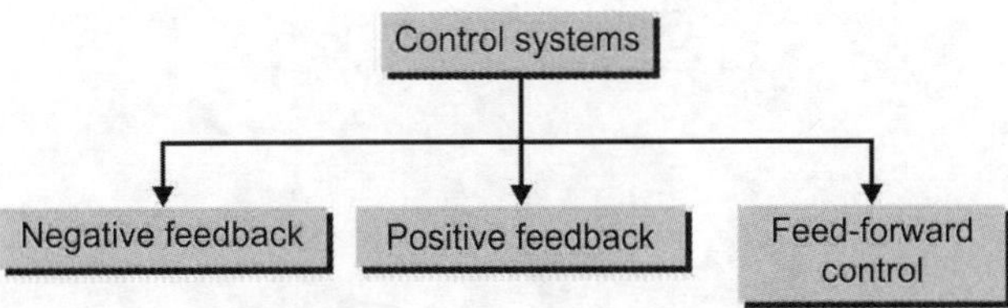

Negative Feedback

In this type of control system, an increased level of that particular parameter is immediately followed by a decrease. The classical example is blood pressure (BP) regulation by baroreflex. Baroreceptors sense the increase in BP because they are stretch receptors. Once they sense the increase in BP, they send the impulse to medulla, which immediately decreases the BP as a part of reflex called baroreflex. Another good example for negative feedback control system is endocrine hormone regulation.

Positive Feedback

Most control systems operate by negative feedback and not positive feedback because of a simple reason. Imagine a person experiencing hemorrhagic shock. The amount of blood in the body is decreased to such a low level that not enough blood is available for the heart to pump effectively. This scenario results in weakening of the heart, further diminished pumping, and a further decrease in coronary blood flow, and still more weakness of the heart; the cycle repeats itself again and again, until death occurs. Positive feedback, once started, it enhances or amplifies the effect on its own. That is why positive feedback is also called vicious cycle. Shock is one example of positive feedback.

We discussed before that all endocrine hormone regulations falls under negative feedback. Only time where the endocrine hormone regulation comes under a positive feedback is LH surge and the hormone responsible is estrogen. Exactly around 24-36 hours before ovulation, estrogen increases the levels of LH and that's why it's positive feedback. LH surge is raising levels of LH. At one-time point, LH reaches its peak value which is called LH peak and it happens 8-12 hours before ovulation. Entry of calcium into sarcoplasmic reticulum of muscle is another example for positive feedback is seen in muscle. Sarcoplasmic reticulum (SR) is the store house of calcium. This SR has a channel protein which takes up calcium and is called Sarcoplasmic Reticulum Calcium ATPase (SERCA Pump). Once small amount of calcium enters SR using SERCA, it increases more and more calcium influx and that's why its positive feedback. This phenomenon is entirely responsible for muscle relaxation.

In parturition, once labor is initiated, the uterine contractions dilate the cervix, and this dilation in turn sets up signals in afferent nerves that increase oxytocin secretion. The plasma oxytocin level rises and causes further uterine contraction ultimately leading to the delivery of fetus. The name of this positive feedback reflex seen during parturition is called Ferguson reflex.

Opening of sodium channels during depolarization phase of action potential increases sodium influx leading to a sharp overshoot. The name of this positive feedback cycle is called Hodgkin cycle. Blood coagulation process is called coagulation cascade. The word cascade simply means amplification of subsequent steps. When a blood vessel is ruptured dotting factors are activated. Once activated, these factors activate remaining clotting factors ultimately leading to blood coagulation.

Feed-Forward Control

In positive and negative feedback, we need a stimulus to get a response. But there is a control system in our body when no stimulus is required but still the system anticipates and makes corrective changes. Such a system is called feed-forward or anticipatory or adaptive control.

Examples includes cephalic phase of gastric secretion—just thinking about food increases gastric acid production, thinking about exercise itself increases heart rate (anticipatory tachycardia) and respiratory rate, role of cerebellum in motor coordination.

CHAPTER

2

Circulating Body Fluids

BLOOD

The circulating system is the transport system that supplies O_2 and substances absorbed from the tissues, returns CO_2 to the lungs and products of metabolism to the kidney, functions in the regulation of body temperature, distributes hormones and other agents that regulate cell function. The blood is the carrier of these substances.

The cellular elements of the blood represents 45% of the total blood volume. It includes white blood cells, red blood cells, platelets and are suspended in the plasma. Plasma is a clear, straw colored fluid portion of the blood and represents 55% of the total blood volume. It contains 91–92% water, 8–9% solids. The solids comprise both organic [8%; plasma proteins, carbohydrates, enzymes, fats, hormones, nonprotein nitrogenous (NPN) substances] and inorganic (1%; sodium, calcium, potassium, magnesium, bicarbonate, chloride, phosphate, copper, iron). The thin middle layer that separates the upper plasma and lower red cell mass after centrifugation of blood is the buffy coat (Fig. 2.1).

The normal total circulating volume is 5600 ml in a 70 kg man (about 8% of body weight). The pH is 7.35–7.45 (average 7.4) and the specific gravity is 1055–1062. Blood is five times more viscous than water. Salinity of blood is 0.9 N.

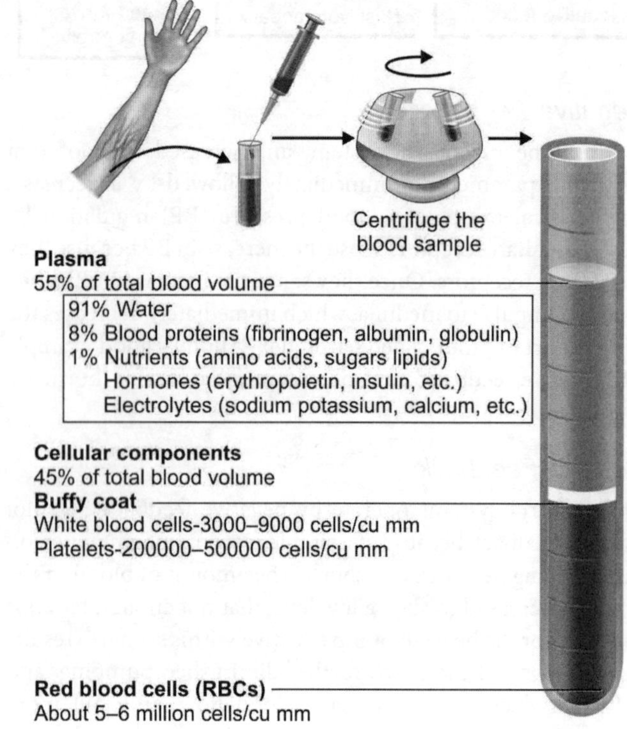

Fig. 2.1: Appearance of centrifuged blood and its constituents

Functions of Blood

- *Respiratory:* Helps in the transport of O_2 and CO_2
- *Nutritive:* Distribute various nutrients to all parts of the body
- *Excretory:* Transports waste materials to the organs of excretion
- *Defense mechanism:* Due to the presence of antibody.
- *Storage function:* Acts as storehouse for different materials like nutrients, water, electrolytes, etc.
- Regulation of body temperature (due to high specific heat of blood).
- *Regulation of acid-base balance:* Plasma proteins and Hb acts as buffers.
- Plays a major role in homeostasis.

PLASMA PROTEINS

The plasma proteins include albumin, globulin, fibrinogen, prothrombin. The total amount of plasma proteins in the blood is 6.4–8.3 gm %. The further details about each of them are given in Table 2.1. Normal A/G (albumin–globulin) ratio is 1.7:1. It is reversed in liver disorders. Plasmapheresis/Whipple's experiment is an experimental procedure done in animals to demonstrate the importance of plasma proteins.

Functions of Plasma Proteins

- *Coagulation of blood:* Due to the presence of fibrinogen, prothrombin and clotting factors.
- *Defense mechanism of body:* Gamma-globulins produce antibodies.
- *Maintain colloidal osmotic pressure (COP):* Eighty-percent of COP is due to albumin (COP is inversely proportional

Table 2.1: Types of plasma proteins and functions

Type	Molecular weight	Normal plasma level	Site of production	Function
Albumin	69000	3.5–5 gm%	Liver	Binding and carrier protein, osmotic regulation
Globulin	90000–156000	2–3 gm%	Recticuloendothelial cells, plasma cells	Mediates immunity, transport proteins like transferin, ceruloplasmin, hemopexin are different forms of globulin
Fibrinogen	350000	0.2–0.4 gm%	Liver	Important for clotting of blood, responsible for major part of viscosity
Prothrombin	68000	0.1 gm%	Liver	Important for clotting of blood

to molecular size and directly related to concentration of molecule).

- *Transport:* Albumin and globulin transports various hormones, enzymes, bilirubin and metals like Cu, Fe, etc.
- *Acid-base regulation:* Due to buffering action.
- *Provides stability to blood:* This is due to the presence of globulin and fibrinogen. If blood loose viscosity RBC will pile upon each other and leads to *Rouleaux formation.*
- *Maintains systemic arterial BP constant:* Viscosity of the blood is mostly due to fibrinogen. Arterial BP depends on viscosity of the blood.
- Acts as protein store.

Hyperproteinemia

Increase in level of plasma proteins and is seen in conditions which causes hemoconcentration (diabetes insipidus).

Hypoproteinemia

Decrease in level of plasma proteins. It is seen in malnutrition, burns, malabsorbtion, hemorrhages. This causes decrease in COP; therefore increase in filtration occurs at arterial end and decrease in absorption at venous end, resulting in edema.

In Liver Disorders, A/G Ratio Reverses

When body tissues are damaged, though plasma albumin falls, plasma immunoglobulin increases as a result of plasma cell hyperplasia causing A/G ratio reversal.

Multiple Myeloma

Increase in the level of globulin due to malignant growth of plasma cells.

Clinical Box

Plasma is separated by centrifuging anticoagulated blood. The serum separated from blood by allowing the blood to coagulate. (serum = blood-fibrinogen and other clotting factors)

HEMOGLOBIN

Hemoglobin (Hb) is the most important red cell constituent. Major function of hemoglobin is uptake of oxygen in lung and delivery of it to tissues. Hemoglobin starts appearing in developing RBC at intermediate normoblastic stage. The hemoglobin molecule is an assembly of four subunits.

Structure of Hb (Fig. 2.2)

Each subunit is composed of a protein (polypeptide) part, i.e. globin and a nonprotein part, i.e. heme. Heme is an iron containing porphyrin derivative. Each hemoglobin molecule contains four heme units and two pairs of similar polypeptides (globin). The heme part of globular protein is same in all types of hemoglobin. The protein part vary in different hemoglobin. For example, Hb A consists of two identical α chains and two identical β chains, Hb F consists of two identical α chains and two identical γ chains. The iron atom in each subunit of heme is in ferrous form (Fe^{2+}) and has a bond available for loose union with oxygen molecule. So, one Hb molecule can combine with four molecules of O_2 (Fig. 2.2A).

Normal Values

Males: 14 –18 gm% (avg -15.5 gm%)
Females: 12–15.5 gm% (avg -14 gm%)

Types of Hb

Normal Varieties

- Adult Hb are of two types:
  1. Hemoglobin A ($\alpha_2\beta_2$)
  2. Hemoglobin A2 ($\alpha_2\delta_2$)
- Fetal Hb ($\alpha_2\gamma_2$)

Abnormal Varieties

- *Hemoglobinopathies;* here abnormal polypeptides are produced.
  - HbS: In the β chain, glutamine at the 6th position is replaced by valine. When HbS is reduced, it precipitates into crystals within RBCs leading to sickling of RBCs. Sickle shaped RBCs are more fragile resulting in sickle cell anemia (Fig. 2.2B).
  - HbC
  - HbE
  - HbI, etc.

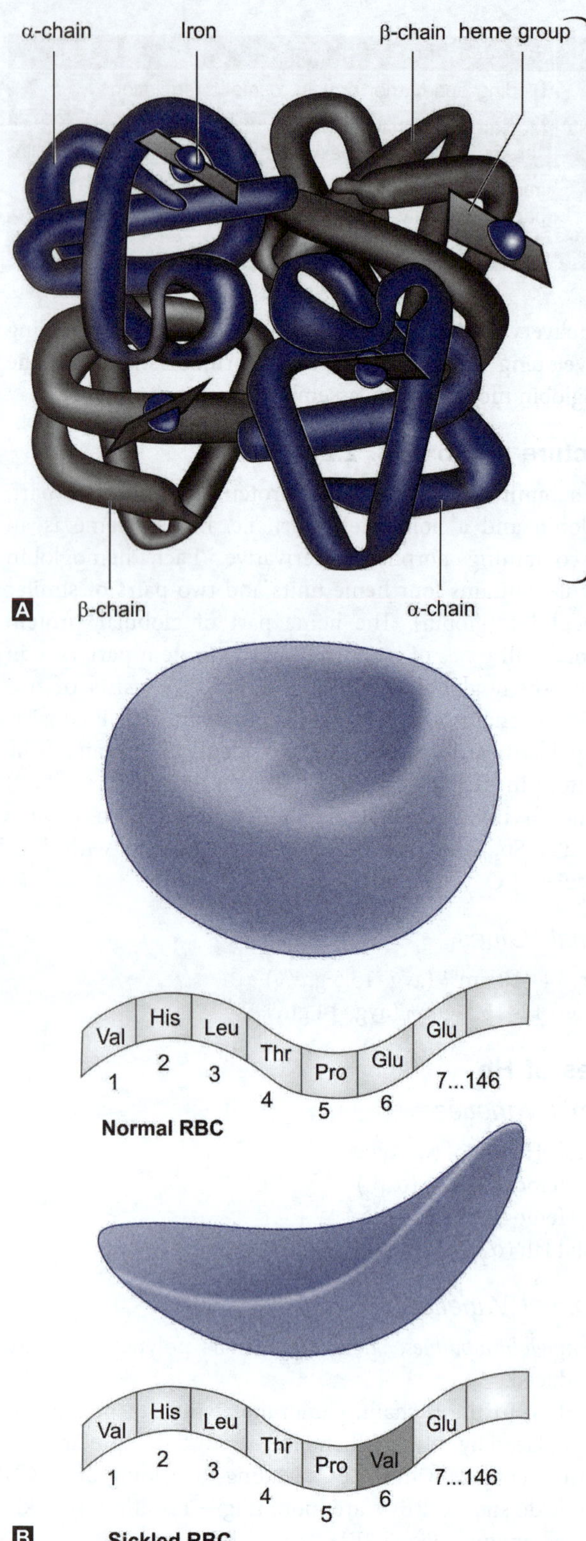

Figs 2.2A and B: A. Structure of hemoglobin; **B.** Comparison of normal erythrocyte to a sickled erythrocyte. Part of its hemoglobin sequence is shown

- *Thalassemias (Flowchart 2.1):* Both α and β chains are present and are normal in structure, but produced in decreased amounts or absent.

Flowchart 2.1: Types of thalassemia

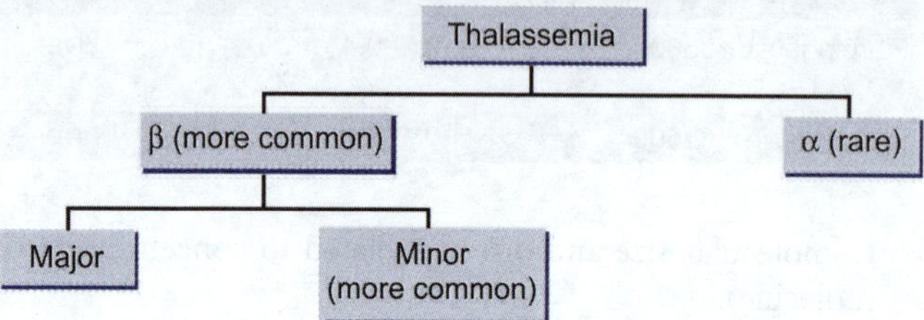

Major β thalassemia (Cooley's anemia or Mediterranean anemia):

- Less common
- Total absence of chain synthesis
- Homozygous transmission
- Victim usually dies.

Minor β thalassemia

- More common
- Partial synthesis of β chain
- Heterozygous transmission.

Heme-Heme Interaction

In the initial phase of oxygenation the combination of heme and O_2 is a bit slow. But once a little of O_2 has combined with heme further interactions are facilitated. This is called heme-heme interaction and this explains the sigmoid shape of O_2 dissociation curve *(See Chapter 3)*.

Catabolism of Hb (Flowchart 2.2)

When the RBCs become old their walls become weak and their shape changes and finally the RBC are broken down. RBCs are destroyed mainly in the spleen by the reticuloendothelial cells. Hb is then released from RBC, which splits into heme and globin.

The end products of heme catabolism are bile pigments. Bilirubin has no function in the body so excreted through bile. Globin is broken into amino acids within the RE (reticuloendothelial) cells, which will be later utilized for synthesis of body proteins. Iron is then released into plasma and is transported by transferrin to the storage sites. The porphyrin ring is broken down in RE cells of liver, spleen and bone marrow where it gets converted into biliverdin (green pigment).

Bilirubin metabolism can be discussed under the following headings (Fig. 2.3).

- Normal sources of bilirubin
- Transport of bilirubin

Flowchart 2.2: Catabolism of hemoglobin

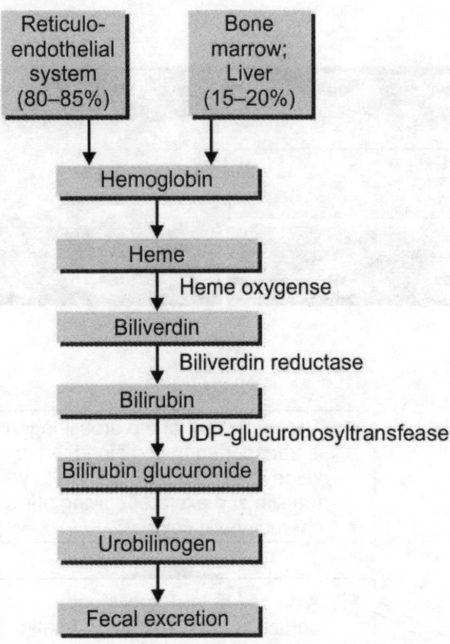

- Hepatic metabolism
- Intestinal phase of bilirubin metabolism
- Renal excretion of bilirubin

Normal Sources of Bilirubin

- 80–85% of bilirubin is derived from catabolism of hemoglobin of senescent red blood cells.
- 15–20% is derived from bone marrow due to destruction of maturing cells and from liver due to turnover of heme and heme containing precursors (cytochromes, myoglobin, etc.).
- In plasma, Hb binds with haptoglobin. The Hb-haptoglobin complex is transported to liver, where heme of Hb is oxidized to biliverdin by enzyme heme oxygenase to iron and biliverdin. Heme liberated from other sources are also oxidized to biliverdin by enzyme heme oxygenase.
- Biliverdin is then reduced to bilirubin by the enzyme biliverdin reductase.

Transport of Bilirubin

Unconjugated bilirubin is liberated into plasma. This unconjugated bilirubin is tightly bound to albumin in a fully reversible manner. Thus, unconjugated bilirubin is transported in the plasma and bound to albumin. Unbound unconjugated bilirubin can cross blood brain barrier and cause kernicterus in neonates with hyperbilirubinemia. Conjugated bilirubin is also bound to albumin, but both in reversible and irreversible manner.

Hepatic Metabolism

It has three distinct phases: Hepatic uptake, conjugation, excretion into bile.

Hepatic Uptake

Unconjugated bilirubin—albumin complex is subjected to the liver cell, i.e. hepatocyte. Albumin dissociates and the unconjugated bilirubin enters the cell. In the cell, unconjugated bilirubin gets bound to several of the glutathione-S-transferases. This binding prevents the efflux of unconjugated bilirubin back into plasma.

Conjugation

In the hepatocyte, the unconjugated bilirubin is conjugated by the enzyme bilirubin UDP-glucuronosyl-transferase. The cosubstrate for bilirubin conjugation is UDP-glucuronic acid, ubiquitous intracellular substance derived from glucose. Conjugation is a two-step reaction resulting first in the formation of bilirubin monoglucuronide and then bilirubin diglucuronide. *Why conjugate?* Unconjugated bilirubin is water insoluble and so not excreted into bile. So, it must be converted to a water soluble derivative (i.e. conjugated bilirubin or bilirubin glucuronide) in order to be excreted by liver cell into bile.

Excretion or Secretion into Bile

This is the rate limiting step of bilirubin metabolism. This step is the one that is most susceptible to impairment when liver cell is damaged. The secretion across the plasma membrane is by ATP dependent transport process mediated by a membrane protein. So conjugated bilirubin is secreted into bile. Normal bile contains 90% of bilirubin diglucuronide and 7% of bilirubin monoglucuronide with remaining 2–3% as unconjugated bilirubin. When this step is comprised two consequences occur: 1) Decreased excretion of bilirubin into bile, and 2) Regurgitation or reentry of conjugated into the blood-stream (conjugated hyperbilirubinemia).

Intestinal Phase of Bilirubin Metabolism

Conjugated bilirubin (bilirubin diglucuronide and bilirubin monoglucuronide) reaches the intestinal lumen through bile. Conjugated bilirubin as such is not reabsorbed by intestinal mucosa. This conjugated bilirubin has got two fates:

1. Part of this conjugated bilirubin is excreted in the stool as such, i.e. bilirubin diglucuronide and bilirubin monoglucuronide.
2. Rest of the conjugated bilirubin is metabolized in the lumen to urobilinogen by the action of intestinal bacteria. This urobilinogen has three fates:
   a. Part of this urobilinogen is reabsorbed from small intestine into portal circulation, thus reaching liver (enterohepatic circulation). The liver reexcretes this urobilinogen into bile.

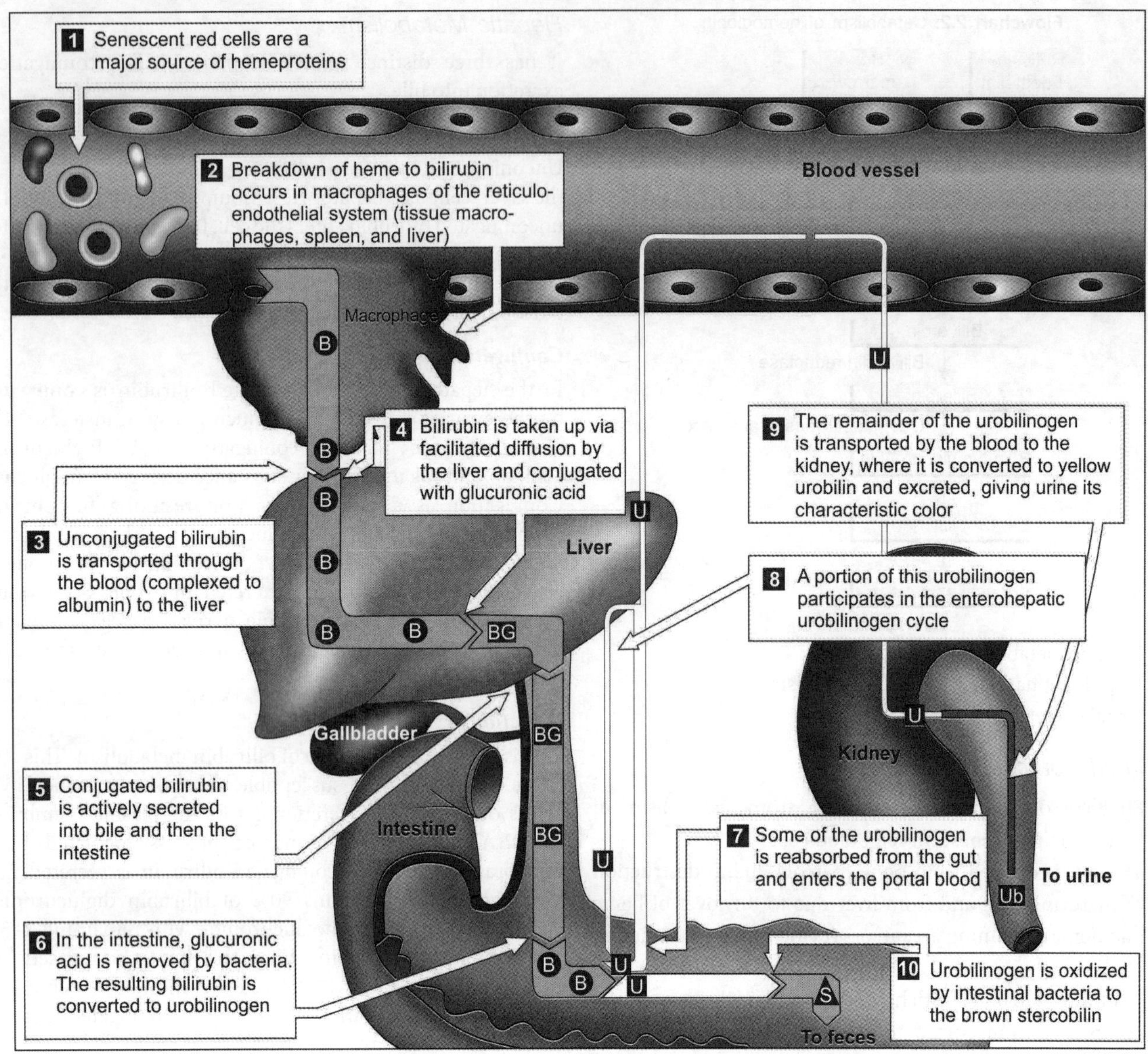

Fig. 2.3: Summary of catabolism of heme. B = bilirubin, BG = bilirubin diglucoronide, U = urobilinogen, Ub = urobilin, S = stercobilin

b. Part of the urobilinogen is transported by blood to kidneys, where it is reabsorbed and oxidized to yellow urobilin and excreted in the urine giving the urine its color.
c. Part of the urobilinogen in the intestine is oxidized by intestinal bacteria to excrete in the stool as stercobilinogen. Stercobilinogen gives the stool its normal color. In obstructive jaundice stercobilinogen is absent in the stool, and hence stools are pale or clay colored.

Renal Excretion of Bilirubin

In normal individuals, there is no bilirubin in urine since unconjugated bilirubin is tightly bound to albumin and hence not filtered by glomeruli. But with regard to conjugated bilirubin, a small fraction (5%) is less tightly bound to albumin and another small fraction is unbound. This unbound fraction is filtered and appears in the urine as bilirubin. So in contrast to unconjugated hyperbilirubinemia, bilirubin appears in the urine in conjugated hyperbilirubinemia.

Clinical Box

Plasma haptoglobin indicates hemolysis. In intravascular hemolysis, Hb-haptoglobin complex clears haptoglobin from plasma. Therefore, haptoglobin content of the plasma is decreased in hemolysis and the degree of decrease is apparently proportionate to the rate of hemolysis. Therefore, estimation of plasma haptoglobin level is an index of hemolysis.

ERYTHROCYTES (RBC)

Normal count	: *Males*—5–6 million cells/mm^3 (average 5.4 million cells/mm^3) *Females*—4.5–5.5 million cells/mm^3 (average 4.8 million cells/mm^3)
Diameter	: 7.2 µm (avg)
Thickness	: 2 µm (avg)
Volume	: 78 – 94 µm^3
Hematocrit (PCV)	: Males 47% and Females 42%
Lifespan	: 120 days
Site of production	: Bone marrow
Site of destruction	: Tissue macrophage system.

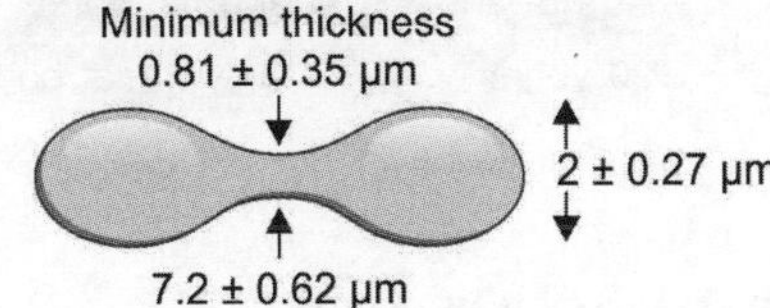

Fig. 2.4: RBC

Advantages of Biconcave Shape

- Can squeeze through capillaries very easily
- Can withstand endosmosis
- Large surface area is provided which help in quick exchange of gases.

Functions

- Gas transport
- Acid-base balance
- Formation of bilirubin
- Responsible for major portion of viscosity of whole blood
- Helps in identifying blood groups as it contains antigen on its surface.

Red Cell Fragility

Red blood cells shrink in solutions with an osmotic pressure > normal plasma (0.9N). In solutions with a lower osmotic pressure they swell, becoming spherical and lose their Hb (hemolysis). The tendency to hemolyze is called fragility. In hereditary spherocytosis (congenital hemolytic icterus) cells hemolyze more readily than normal cells in hypotonic NaCl solutions. Fragility is high in G6PD deficiency. Red cells can also be lysed by drugs and infections.

Hereditary Spherocytosis

Common cause of hereditary hemolytic anemia. The membrane of RBC is made of spectrin and is anchored to transmembrane protein band 3 by the protein ankyrin. Hereditary spherocytosis is caused by defects in band 3, spectrin and ankyrin.

RBC Indices

The number, shape, volume and color of RBCs indicate the quality of blood. Blood indices have got a diagnostic value in determining the type of anemia. These are:

Mean Corpuscular Volume (MCV)

It is the volume of a single RBC in cubic microns.

$$\text{MCV} = \frac{\text{PCV per 100 ml blood} \times 10\ \mu\text{m}^3}{\text{RBC count in million/cu mm}}$$

Normal value: 87 µm^3

Mean Corpuscular Hemoglobin (MCH)

It is the average amount of Hb in a single RBC in pictogram.

$$\text{MCH} = \frac{\text{Hb in gm\%} \times 10\ \text{pg}}{\text{RBC count in million/cu mm}}$$

Normal value: 29 pg

Mean Corpuscular Hemoglobin Concentration (MCHC)

It is the Hb concentration in a single RBC or it is the amount of Hb expressed as % of the volume of a RBC.

$$\text{MCHC} = \frac{\text{Hb in gm\%} \times 100}{\text{PCV per 100 ml blood}}$$

Normal value: 34%

Color Index

It denotes the ratio of Hb to RBC.

$$\text{Color index} = \frac{\text{Hb\%}}{\text{RBC\%}}$$

Normal value: 1

Packed cell volume (hematocrit), erythrocyte sedimentation rate (ESR) are discussed in practical section.

HEMOPOIESIS

Formation of blood cells is termed as hemopoiesis or hematopoiesis. In children, blood formation occurs in the marrow cavities of most of the bones. The well marked cellularity gives the red color to the marrow when seen with a naked eye. Red bone marrow contains various developing stages of red cells, white cells and platelets as well as some adipose tissue and connective tissue cells. By 21 years of age, the red bone marrow is limited to the axial skeleton (skull, vertebrae, ribs, sternum and pelvis) and the proximal ends of the femur and the humerus. In the remaining parts of long bones, the marrow consists of adipose tissue and some blood capillaries. Such marrow is known as yellow bone marrow. When the rate

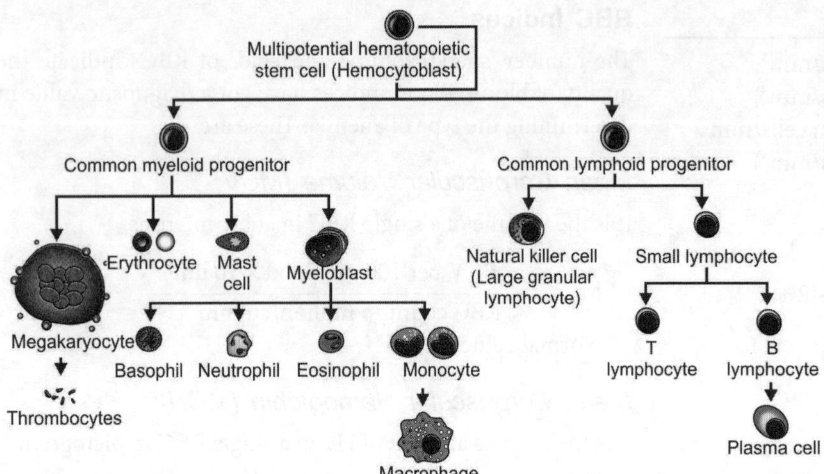

Age	Site of hematopoiesis
3 weeks–3 months	Yolk sac
3–5 months	Liver, spleen
5–9 months	Red bone marrow in long and flat bones
After birth till 20 years of age	Red bone marrow in long and flat bones
>20 years	Only in flat bones like ilia

Fig. 2.5: Hemopoiesis

of formation of red cells (erythropoiesis) is to be markedly accelerated (e.g. after severe hemorrhage or in hemolytic anemia), the yellow marrow is converted to red marrow. Thus yellow marrow acts as a reserve for increased blood formation in case of situations requiring rapid erythropoiesis.

The red marrow contains pluripotent/multipotent stem cells (hemocytoblast) which give rise to all types of blood cells (Fig. 2.5). Certain humoral substances like erythropoietin, colony stimulating factors, thrombopoietin push the stem cells into respective line of development. Pluripotent stem cells give rise to two specialized stem cells. The myeloid cell gives rise to still other cells, which become red blood cells, platelets, and all the whole blood cells except lymphocytes. The lymphatic stem cells gives rise to lymphoblasts, which become lymphocytes. The process of differentiation from stem cell to mature erythrocyte is called **erythropoiesis**, to mature leukocyte is called **leukopoiesis** and development of platelets is called **thrombopoiesis**. The rates at which the blood cells produced are regulated in healthy individuals to match the rates at which they leave the circulation. The balance between production and elimination is disturbed in pathological condition.

Erythropoiesis

Formation of red blood cells is called erythropoiesis. In normal adult human, the site of production is bone marrow (red bone marrow). In the first-three months of intrauterine life, blood cells develop from mesoderm of yolk sac or area vasculosa (mesoblastic stage). After 3 months, up to 5 months of fetal life red blood cells are developed from liver and spleen (hepatic stage). From 5th month onwards up to birth and up to adulthood from red bone marrow (myeloid stage).

In children erythropoiesis occurs in:
- All bones with red marrow (mainly)
- Liver and spleen

In adults erythropoieses occurs in red bone marrow which includes:
- Ends of long bones (shaft is converted to yellow marrow)
- Flat bones (skull, vertebrae, ribs, sternum, pelvis).

Stages of Erythropoiesis (Fig. 2.6)

Hemocytoblast
- It is considered as a pleuripotent stem cell (noncommitted)
- Diameter: 18–20 µm
- Nucleated with thin rim of basophilic cytoplasm
- Nucleus may contain two or more nucleoli with open chromatin.
- They proliferate extensively and give rise to committed stem cell.

Committed Stem Cells
- Develop from pleuripotent stem cells.
- Two types—myeloid and lymphoid.
- They have become committed to give rise to a particular line of cells (either erythrocytes, platelets, monocytes, etc.).
- Committed stem cells of myeloid series gives rise to all types of blood cells except lymphocytes.

Progenitor Cells
- Develop from committed stem cells
- Progenitor cells are of two types:
  - BFU-E (burst forming unit of erythrocyte series)
  - CFU-E (colony forming unit of erythrocyte series)
- BFU-E give rise to CFU-E cells.

Proerythroblast
- The first blast cell (immature cells) belonging to red blood series

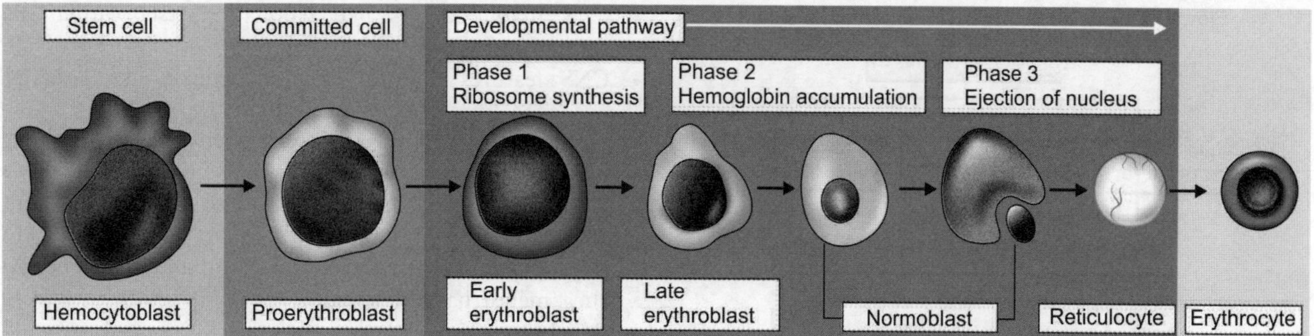

Fig. 2.6: Phases of erthrocyte differentiation

- They are formed from CFU-E stem cells
- Large nucleus, distinct nucleoli, open chromatin
- Basophilic cytoplasm
- Shows active mitosis.

Early Normoblast

- Size further decreases
- No nucleoli, condensed chromatin threads
- Cytoplasm is basophilic
- Shows active mitosis.

Intermediate Normoblast

- Cell size reduces
- Chromatin thread further condenses
- Hb starts appearing
- Cytoplasm becomes polychromatic
- In the later part mitosis stops.

Late Normoblast

- Further reduction in cell size
- Nucleus moves to periphery
- Further condensation of chromatin threads
- In the later part nucleus becomes pyknotic
- Further increase in concentration of Hb
- Cytoplasm is mostly eosinophilic (acidic).

Reticulocyte

- Cell size reduces and almost same size of matured RBC (7–9 µm)
- No nucleus
- When stained with dyes like brilliant cresyl blue, cytoplasm shows a small reticulum (due to the presence of RNA) and hence the name
- Cytoplasm is eosinophilic.

Erythrocyte

- Fully eosinophilic
- Non-nucleated, biconcave
- *Diameter*: 7.2 µm.

Factors Affecting Erythropoiesis

General Factors

Erythropoietins

- Glycoprotein in nature, also called hemopoietin or erythrocyte stimulating factor.
- It is secreted by interstitial cells in peritubular capillaries of kidney and by hepatocytes in the liver. In adults 85% of secretion comes from kidney, 15% from liver.
- It acts from the stage committed stem cell. It causes early differentiation of erythropoietin sensitive stem cells to proerythroblast and subsequently to mature RBCs. It prevents apoptosis of red cells. It increases synthesis of RNA, DNA, globin, ferritin which increases heme synthesis. It increases the release of reticulocytes from bone marrow.
- Stimulants for secretion includes hypoxia (most important), androgens, cobalt salts, catecholamines, alkalosis.
- Estrogen decreases the production of erythropoietin. This is the reason for decreased red cell count in females.

Lack of O_2

The role of hypoxia on erythropoietin is in Flowchart 2.3.

Hormones

Testosterone, thyroxine, corticosteroids, growth hormone favors and estrogen inhibits erythropoiesis.

Hemopoietic Growth Factors

These are interleukins and stem cell factor. Generally these factors induce the proliferation of pleuripotent stem cells.

Maturation Factors

- *Vitamin B_{12} and folic acid:* They are called extrinsic factors and are necessary for DNA synthesis. Erythroblast need them before every mitosis and deficiency leads to failure in maturation and reduction in cell divisions.
- *Iron:* It is necessary for Hb synthesis.

Flowchart 2.3: Role of hypoxia on erythropoiesis

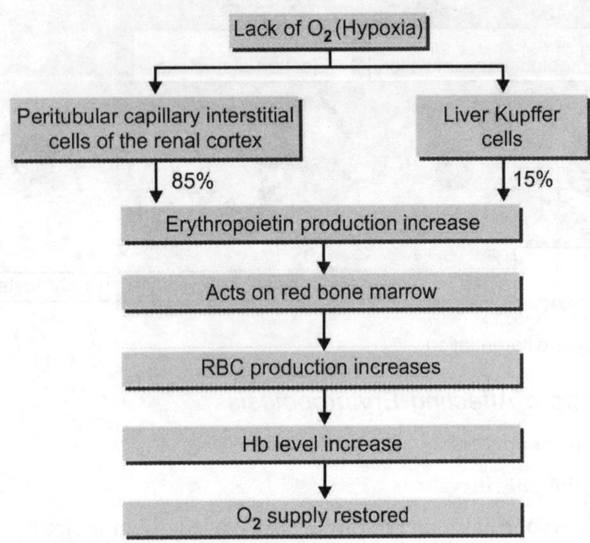

- *Castle's intrinsic factor:* It is produced by parietal cells of the stomach. It is essential for the absorption of vitamin B_{12}.
- *Dietary factors:* Proteins help in globin formation. Fe, Mn, Cu, Co helps in heme formation. Vitamin C and Ca increases iron absorption from gut.

Note: Androgens has stimulating effect on erythropoietin. Estrogen decreases hepatic synthesis of globulin. They also depress the erythropoietic response to hypoxia. That is why in females, RBC count is less as compared to males.

Clinical Box

Reticulocyte indicate bone marrow activity. Reticulocytes are the immediate precursors of red cells. Therefore, when the demand for red cells in the body is increased, the reticulocyte formation and release are also increased.

Anemia

Anemia is a clinical condition characterized by decrease in O_2 carrying capacity of blood due to either decrease in the number of RBCs or their content of Hb or both.

Grading

Mild anemia: Hb 8–12 gm%
Moderate anemia: Hb 5–8 gm%
Severe anemia: Hb < 5 gm%

General Clinical Features of Anemia

- Generalized weakness, tenderness and fatigability.
- Pallor of skin and mucous membrane.
- Respiratory symptoms like breathlessness.
- CVS manifestations like palpitation, tachycardia and cardiac murmurs.
- CNS features due to cerebral hypoxia like lethargy, headache, tinnitus and confusion.
- Ocular manifestations like visual disturbances, retinal hemorrhage.
- Gastrointestinal symptoms like anorexia, nausea, constipation.
- Reproductive system: Menstrual disturbances like amenorrhea, menorrhagia in females.
- Renal system involvement.
- BMR increases in severe anemia.

Classification

Morphological/Wintrobe's classification

Based on the size and color of RBC (i.e. based on MCV and MCHC):

- Normocytic normochromic
- Normocytic hypochromic
- Macrocytic normochromic
- Macrocytic hypochromic
- Microcytic normochromic
- Microcytic hypochromic.

Etiological/Whitby's classification (Table 2.2)

Based on the cause of anemia:

- Hemorrhagic: Due to blood loss
- Hemolytic: Due to destruction
- Nutritional deficiency
- Aplastic due to decreased formation.

Pernicious Anemia/Addison's Anemia

(Pernicious Means Destructive or Injurious)

Causes

This is due to lack of intrinsic factor. Consequently there will be failure in the absorption of vitamin B_{12}. Production of intrinsic factor is affected due to atrophy of gastric mucosa.

RBCs are macrocytic normochromic. Excessive destruction of RBCs produces mild hemolytic jaundice. Bone marrow becomes hyperplasic due to increased hypoxic stimulation for erythropoiesis. Neurological disorders are seen in extreme conditions.

Reticulocyte Response

Increase in number of reticulocytes after vitamin B_{12} therapy. This is due to proliferation of bone marrow and numerous young RBC pass into circulation.

Folic Acid Deficiency Anemia

Anemia is megaloblastic as seen with vitamin B_{12} deficiency. But neurological disorders may not develop.

Table 2.2: Etiological/Whitby's classification of anemia

Types of anemia	Causes	Morphology of RBC
Hemorrhagic	• Acute loss of blood • Chronic loss of blood	• Normocytic normochromic • Normocytic hypochromic
Hemolytic	• Hypersplenism • Infections (malaria) • Drugs (quinine, aspirin) • Poisons (snake venom) • Congenital/Acquired default in shape of RBC	• Normocytic normochromic • Sickle cell anemia: Sickle shaped • Thalassemia: Microcytic hypochromic
Nutrition deficiency	• Iron • Protein • Vitamin B_{12} • Folic acid	• Microcytic hypochromic • Macrocytic hypochromic • Macrocytic normochromic • Macrocytic normochromic
Aplastic	• X-ray irradiation • Bone marrow disorder	• Normocytic normochromic

Causes of Folic Acid Deficiency

- Less dietary intake.
- Poor absorption, e.g. in steatorrhea and sprue (absorption defect is due to lack of digestive enzymes and in part due to folic acid deficiency).
- Increased demand as in pregnancy.
- Antifolate drugs, e.g. anticancer drugs (methotrexate).

Iron Deficiency Anemia

It is the most common nutritional deficiency disorder present throughout the world. Iron deficiency anemia is the most common anemia in India. Iron deficiency anemia can be defined as any anemia which responds to adequate dosages of iron. With long standing severe anemia, thinning, flattening and eventually 'spooning' (koilonychia) of finger nails sometimes appears (Fig. 2.7).

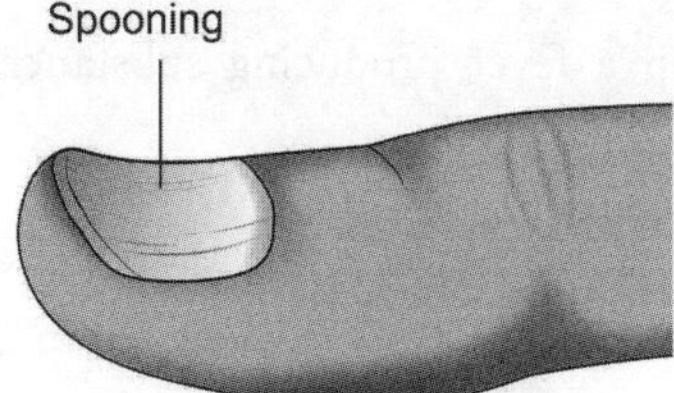

Fig. 2.7: Koilonychia

Causes

- Decreased intake, cow milk fed infants.
- Increased loss in acute or chronic hemorrhage (e.g. worm infestation, peptic ulcer, piles, increased menstrual blood loss).
- *Increased demand:* Infancy, childhood, pregnancy and menstruation.
- Defective utilization due to decreased absorption in diseases of stomach and duodenum.

Clinical Box

Renal disease causes anemia. As the kidney is the major source of erythropoieten, chronic renal diseases that reduce renal mass significantly produce anemia.

Blood Indices in Anemia's (Table 2.3)

Effects of Anemia on Circulatory System

The viscosity of the blood depends on the blood concentration of red blood cells. In severe anemia, the blood viscosity may fall to as low as 1.5 times that of water. This decreases the resistance to blood flow in the peripheral blood vessels, so that far greater than normal quantities of blood flows through the tissues and return to the heart. This greatly increases the cardiac output. Hypoxia resulting from diminished transport of oxygen by the blood causes the peripheral tissue blood vessels to dilate, allowing further increase in the return of blood to the heart and increasing the cardiac output to a still higher level. Thus, one of the major effects of anemia is greatly

Table 2.3: Blood indices in anemia

Index	Hypochromic microcytic iron deficiency anemia	Normochromic macrocytic megaloblastic anemia	Normochromic normocytic anemia
MCV	↓	↑	—
MCH	↓	↓	—
MCHC	↓	—	—
Hb	↓	↓	↓
RBC	↓	↓	↓
Mean diameter	↓	↑	—
PCV	↓	↓	↓
↓ Decrease ↑ Increase — Normal			

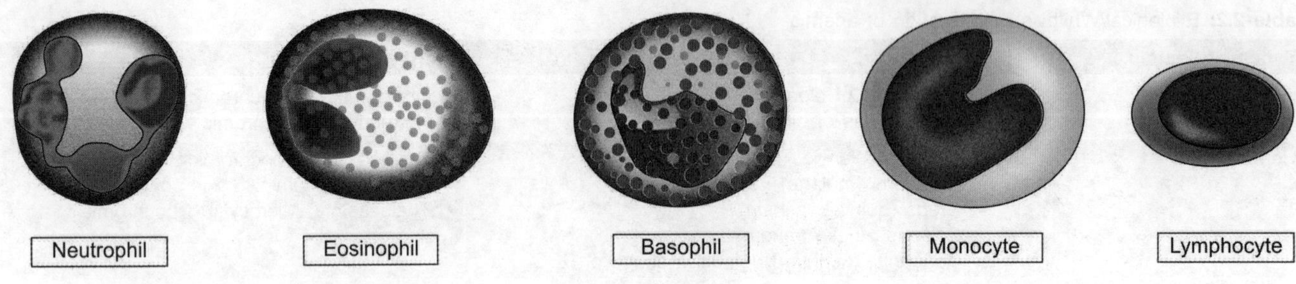

Fig. 2.8: Leukocytes

increased cardiac output and increased pumping workload on the heart.

Clinical Box

Anemia occurs after gastrectomy because gastric secretions play an important role in dissolving the iron, thereby permitting it to form soluble complexes with ascorbic acid and other substances that aids its reduction to Fe^{2+} form. This is very important for absorption of iron in the duodenum even though only traces of iron absorption occur in stomach.

Polycythemia

Abnormal increase in RBC count. Classified into two:

1. *Primary type (Polycythemia Vera/Erythremia):* Increase in RBC count more than 7–8 million cells/mm^3. It may be due to neoplastic growth of stem cell.
2. *Secondary type:* Rise in RBC count (6–7 millon/mm^3) occurs due to some disease or altered physiologic state (high altitude), which cause rise of erythropoietin concentration (due to hypoxia).

Effects on Circulatory System

- Cardiac output is not far from normal due to the balance between the increased viscosity of blood and greatly increased blood volume.
- Arterial pressure is also normal in most people with polycythemia.
- In polycythemia vera, the skin is cyanotic.

LEUKOCYTES

The leukocytes are also called white blood corpuscles or simply the white cells of the blood (Fig. 2.8). They are colorless and they defend the body against diseases by fighting against infections, malignancies, etc. The normal total white cell count is 4000–11000 cells/ mm^3 blood (average 9000). Leukocytes are classified as in Flowchart 2.4.

Flowchart 2.4: Classification of leukocytes

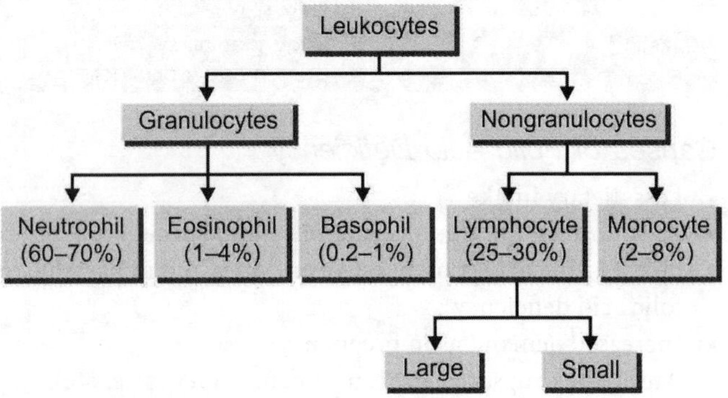

Classification

Neutrophil

Normal count: 5400 cells/cu mm blood (3000–6000)
Size: 10–14 μm diameter.
They are called first-line of defense.
Nucleus is multilobed
Cytoplasm contains fine pink granules.

Functions

- Phagocytosis
- They contain a fever producing substance, endogenous pyrogen.

Neutrophilia

Increase in neutrophils.

Causes

- Acute infections
- Following tissue destruction
- Pregnancy, menstruation, lactation.

Neutropenia

Decrease in neutrophils.

Causes

- Viral infection
- Typhoid fever
- Bone marrow depression.

Eosinophil

Normal count: 275 cells/cu mm (150–300).
Size: 10–14 μm diameter.
Nucleus is bilobed.
Cytoplasm contains coarse brick red granules.

Functions

- During allergic conditions, eosinophils are collected at the sites and limits the intensity by degrading the effects of mediators.
- Mild phagocytosis.

Eosinophilia

Increase in eosinophil.

Causes

- Allergic conditions (bronchial asthma).
- Parasitic infestation (hook worm).

Eosinopenia

Decrease in eosinophils.

Causes

- After injection of corticosteroids.
- Acute pyogenic infections.

Basophil

Normal count: 35 cells/cu mm of blood (0–100).
Size: 10–14 μm diameter.
S shaped nucleus.
Cytoplasm contains coarse bluish black granules which may mask the nucleus.

Functions

- Mild phagocytosis.
- They are responsible for inflammatory changes.
- They liberates histamine and heparin.

Basophilia

Increase in basophils.

Causes

- Chickenpox
- Tuberculosis
- Influenza

Basopenia

Decrease in basophils.

Causes

- After administration of glucocorticoids.
- Drug induced reactions.

Monocytes

Normal count: 540 cells/cu mm of blood (300–600).
Size: 10–18 μm diameter.
They are called second-line of defense.
Kidney-shaped nucleus and placed eccentrically.

Functions

- Active phagocytosis.
- All tissue macrophages come from monocytes.
- They synthesize prostaglandin E and clot promoting factors.
- They kill tumor cells.

Monocytosis

Increase in monocytes.

Causes

- Tuberculosis
- Syphilis

Monocytopenia

Decrease in monocytes.

Causes

Hypoplastic bone marrow.

Lymphocytes

Normal count: 2750 cells/cu mm of blood (1500–4000)
Size: Large lymphocytes: 10–14 μm diameter
Small lymphocytes: 7–10 μm diameter
Nucleus is round, oval and central in position.

Functions

Produce antibodies.

Lymphocytosis

Increase in lymphocytes.

Causes

- Lymphatic leukemia
- Viral infections.
- Tuberculosis.

Lymphopenia

Decrease in lymphocytes.

Causes

- Hypoplastic bone marrow
- AIDS.

Steps of Phagocytosis

Margination

In the area of infection neutrophils get attached to the capillary endothelium.

Diapedesis

Neutrophils and monocytes can squeeze through pore of blood vessels, a process called diapedesis.

Chemotaxis

Bacterial products interact with plasma proteins. They produce chemotactic agents which attract neutrophil to site of infection. This is called chemotaxis. Chemotactic agents are components of complement system, leukotrienes, polypeptides from lymphocytes, basophil, mast cells.

Opsonization

Opsonins are antibodies against bacteria. These antibodies cover bacteria along with component of complementary system, a process called opsonization.

Phagocytosis

This coated bacteria attaches to receptors on neutrophil and they are engulfed by neutrophil by endocytosis (Fig. 2.9).

Degranulation

Inside neutrophil, it becomes phagosome/phagocytic vacuole. Granules of neutrophil move towards phagocytic vacuole and discharge its contents into it and kills the bacteria. During this NADPH oxidase system is activated and there is sharp increase in O_2 uptake and metabolism, (respiratory burst) with generation of superoxide radical and H_2O_2. Free radical superoxide and H_2O_2 are both oxidants and react to form hydroxyl radical, a potent bactericidal agent.

Notes

- *Agranulocytosis:* Decrease in granulocytes
- *Myeloid leukemia:* Presence of immature WBCs in circulation.

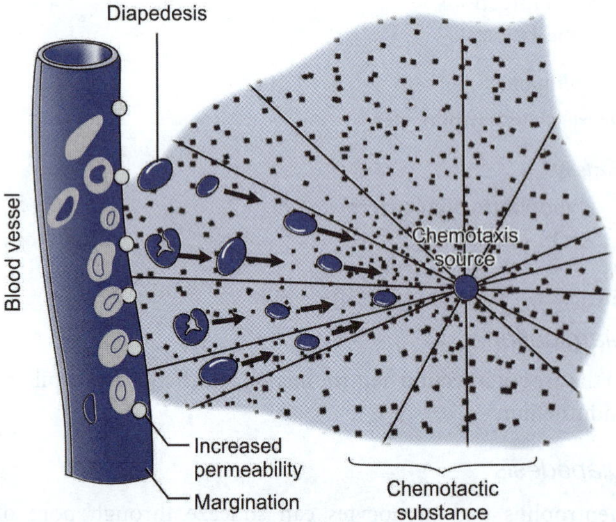

Fig. 2.9: Steps of phagocytosis

- *Lymphocytosis:* Increase in lymphocytes. Seen in chronic infections, viral infections, lymphoma, etc.
- *Leukocytopenia:* Decrease in WBC count.
- *Leukemias:* Uncontrolled production of WBC caused by cancerous mutation of myelogenous or lymphogenous cell.

Arneth Count

It is the count of the neutrophils according to the number of lobes present in there nuclei (Table 2.4). Normal values are as follows.

Number of lobes in the nuclei of a neutrophil inreases with the age. In circulation if there are more neutrophils with less lobes, it means more young cells are there (and vice versa). When there are more young cells, it indicates increased rate of production and more old cells means decreased rate of production. These may be due to different diseases and can be diagnosed by Arneth count.

Table 2.4: Arneth count

Groups	I	II	III	IV	V
No. of lobes in nuclei	1 lobe	2 lobes	3 lobes	4 lobes	5 lobes
Percentage (%)	5–10	25–30	45–47	16–18	≥2

PLATELETS

Platelets or thrombocytes are the formed elements of blood. Platelets are small colorless, non-nucleated and moderately refractive bodies. These formed elements of blood are considered to be the fragments of cytoplasm.

Normal count: 300000 cells/cu mm (200000–500000)
Lifespan: 8–12 days
Site of formation: Bone marrow
Site of destruction: Spleen and other reticuloendothelial cells.

Stages of Formation

The stages of formation are given in Flowchart 2.5.

Flowchart 2.5: Stages of formation

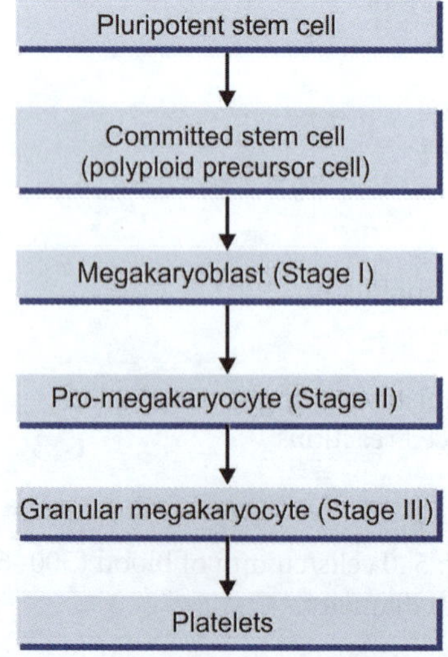

PHYSICON—The Reliable Icon in Physiology

Functions of Platelets

- Hemostasis
- Role in blood clotting.
- Role in clot retraction
- Phagocytic action
- Storage and transport function.

Hemostasis

Spontaneous arrest or stoppage of bleeding by forming clots in the walls of damaged blood vessels while maintaining blood in a fluid state within the vascular system is called hemostasis. It occurs in three stages (Flowchart 2.6 and Fig. 2.10):

- Vasoconstriction
- Platelet plug formation
- Coagulation of blood (conversion of platelet plug into definitive hemostatic clot).

Flowchart 2.6: Stages of hemostasis

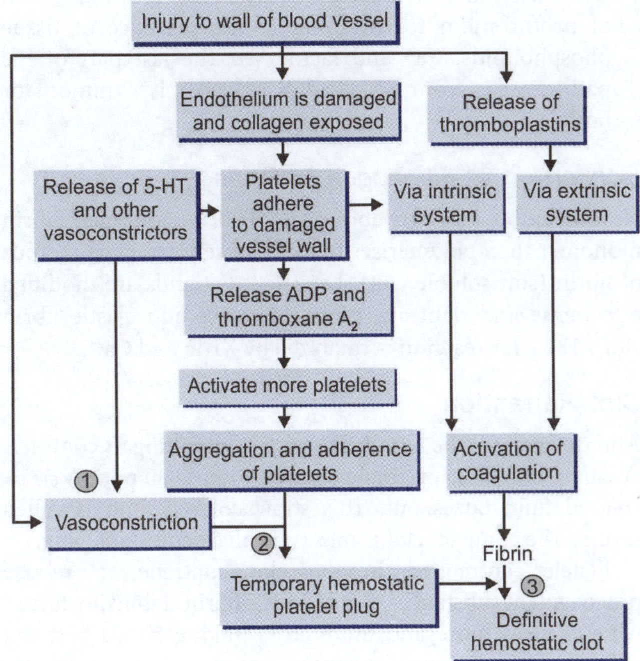

Mechanism of Hemostasis

Vasoconstriction

Following an injury, the first event that takes place in hemostatic mechanism is vasoconstriction.

Vasoconstriction is due to:

- Local myogenic spasm.
- Vasoconstrictor agents released by traumatized tissues and platelets.
- Nervous reflexes.

Platelet Plug Formation

When blood vessel is injured, platelets adhere to the exposed collagen and von Willebrand factor. Binding produces platelet activation which releases the contents of their granules. The released ADP acts on the ADP receptors in the platelet membranes to produce further accumulation of more platelets (platelet aggregation). Aggregation is also facilitated by platelet activating factor (secreted by neutrophils, monocytes and platelets).

Platelet aggregation causes the production of arachidonic acid derivatives like thromboxane A_2 and prostacyclin. Thromboxane A_2 further increases platelet aggregation and helps in the formation of *temporary hemostatic plug.* Thromboxane A_2 causes the release of norepinephrine and 5-HT (vasoconstrictor agents). Prostacyclin inhibits thromboxane A_2 and prevents further platelet aggregation (keeping platelet plug localized).

Clinical Box

Administration of aspirin in low dosage shifts the balance towards prostacyclin (by inhibiting thromboxane A_2) and inhibits platelet aggregation. Aspirin in low doses prevents MI and stroke.

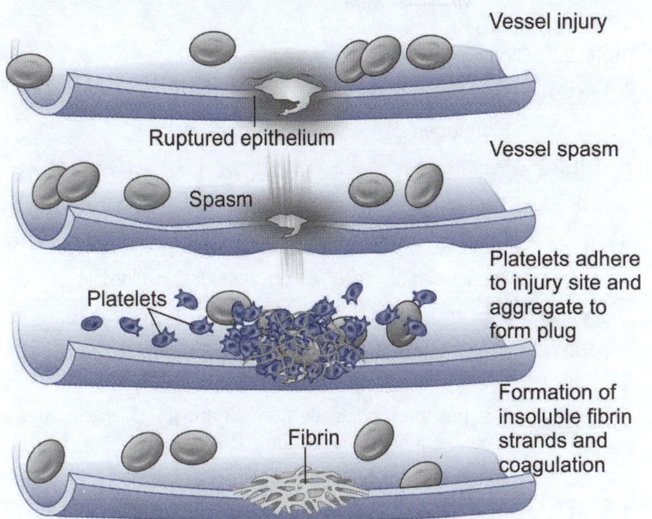

Fig. 2.10: Role of platelets in hemostasis

Coagulation of Blood (Flowchart 2.7)

It is a physiochemical change by which the liquid blood is converted into a jelly like mass called clot. Substances necessary for clotting are called clotting factors (Table 2.5).

Process of Coagulation

Clotting of blood occurs in three stages:

- Formation of prothrombin activator
- Conversion of prothrombin into thrombin
- Conversion of fibrinogen into fibrin.

Flowchart 2.7: Clotting mechanism: Intrinsic and extrinsic

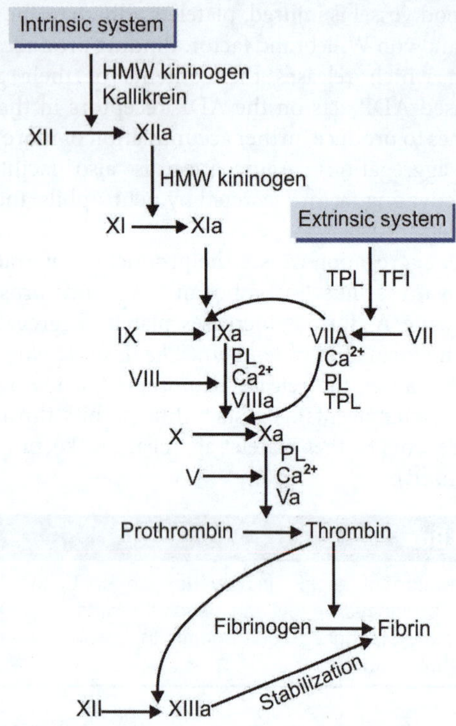

Table 2.5: Clotting factors

Factor	Names
I	Fibrinogen
II	Prothrombin
III	Thromboplastin
IV	Calcium
V	Proaccelerin, labile factor, accelerator globulin
VII	Proconvertin, SPCA, stable factor
VIII	Antihemophilic factor (AHF), antihemophilic factor A, antihemophilic globulin (AHG)
IX	Plasma thromboplastic component (PTC), Christmas factor, antihemophilic factor B
X	Stuart-Prower factor
XI	Plasma thromboplastin antecedent (PTA), antihemophilic factor C
XII	Hageman factor, Glass factor
XIII	Fibrin-stabilizing factor, Laki-Lorand factor

Formation of Prothrombin Activator

Prothrombin activator is formed by two ways:

1. *Intrinsic pathway:* Intrinsic system is triggered when blood is exposed (trauma to blood vessel) to the subendothelial collagen tissue resulting in formation of 'intrinsic prothrombin activator'. It occurs *in vivo* (inside body) and *in vitro* (in test tube).

   . The factor XII comes in contact with subendothelial collagenous tissue and is converted to factor XII a (active form of factor XII) and this reaction is catalyzed by high molecular weight kininogen and kallikrein. Active factor XII then activates factor XI and active factor XI activates factor IX. Factor VIII is activated when it is separated from von Willebrand factor. Now activated factors IX and VIII along with phospholipids, Ca^{2+} activates factor X. In the presence of tissue phospholipids Ca^{2+} and factor V, activated factor X catalyzes the conversion of prothrombin to thrombin.

   Note: Xa plus Va plus platelet phospholipid together form prothrombin activator.

2. *Extrinsic pathway:* Injury of the extravascular tissue and blood vessel causes release of substance called tissue thromboplastin (which is a complex of phospholipid and protein) from the injured tissue which activates factor VII to factor VIIa. It occurs *in vivo* only (inside body). Tissue thromboplastin and factor VII activate factors IX and X. Ultimately activated factor X catalyzes the conversion of prothrombin to thrombin in the presence of tissue phospholipids, Ca^{2+} and factor Va. The last part of the pathway, i.e. from activated X onwards is common for both.

Conversion of Fibrinogen to Fibrin

Now thrombin converts fibrinogen to fibrin monomer. Fibrin monomer then polymerises to form loosely arranged strands of fibrin (soft soluble clot). Later loose strands are modified into dense and tight aggregate (insoluble and elastic fibrin clot). The later reaction is catalyzed by XIIIa and Ca^{2+}.

Clot Retraction

After formation, the blood clot starts contracting. It contracts down to 40% of its original volume within 5–30 min. A straw colored fluid oozes out. This straw colored fluid is called serum. The compact clot is more effective hemostatic plug.

Platelet entrapped in the clot continue to release procoagulant substances. For example, fibrin stabilizing factor, which causes more and more cross linking bonds between adjacent fibrin fibers. Platelet themselves contribute directly to clot retraction by activating platelet thrombosthenin, actin and myosin.

Actions of Thrombin

Thrombin is the principal enzyme of hemostasis. It catalyzes the conversion of fibrinogen to fibrin and activates procoagulant factors V, VIII, XI, and XIII. Additionally, when bound to thrombomodulin, it activates protein C, an anticoagulant. Thrombin also activates platelets, regulates endothelial cell function. Thrombin contains binding site which binds fibrinogen and thrombomodulin.

Actions of Calcium

- It accelerates the conversion of X to Xa and VII to VIIa.
- The conversion of prothrombin to thrombin requires Ca^{2+}.
- The conversion of soft soluble fibrin clot to firm insoluble clot is catalyzed by Ca^{2+}. But Ca^{2+} deficiencies do not produce coagulation disorders because only traces of Ca^{2+} are required for coagulation.

Limiting Reactions

These reactions are:

- Prevent intravascular thrombosis
- Maintains blood in fluid state.

These reactions include:

- Antithrombin III is a circulating protease inhibitor. It inhibits active forms of factors IX, X, XI, XII.
- The platelet aggregating effect of thromboxane A_2 is balanced by antiaggregating effect of prostacyclin, which causes clots to form at the site when a blood vessel is injured but keeps the vessel lumen free of clot.
- Heparin (a naturally occurring anticoagulant) facilitates the action of antithrombin III.
- Removal of activated clotting factors by the liver.
- Smoothness of endothelium prevents platelet adhesion and extension of clot into blood vessel.
- Negatively charged particles present over endothelial lining, repel the clotting factors.
- Continuous movement of blood does not allow clot formation.
- Simultaneous activation of fibrinolytic system along with clotting mechanism.

Fibrinolytic System

This system keeps lumen of blood vessels patent by dissolving clot. Plasmin (fibrinolysin) is the active component of fibrinolytic system. The endothelium of blood vessels (except those in cerebral microcirculation) produce thrombomodulin (a thrombin - binding protein). Thrombin binds to thrombomodulin and forms a complex. Thrombomodulin - Thrombin complex activates protein C.

Activated protein C along with its cofactor protein S, in activates factors V, VIII and inactivates an inhibitor of tissue plasminogen activator. Plasmin is formed from plasminogen by the action of thrombin and tissue plasminogen activator (Flowchart 2.8). Thus formation of plasmin is enhanced. Plasmin lyses fibrin and fibrinogen, with the production of fibrinogen degradation products that inhibit thrombin.

Anticoagulants

Heparin

It is a mucopolysaccharide, natural anticoagulant, secreted by granules of mast cells and basophils. It facilitates the action of antithrombin III and thereby inhibits active forms of factors IX, X, XI, XII.

Flowchart 2.8: Steps involved in the formation of plasmin (fibrinolysin)

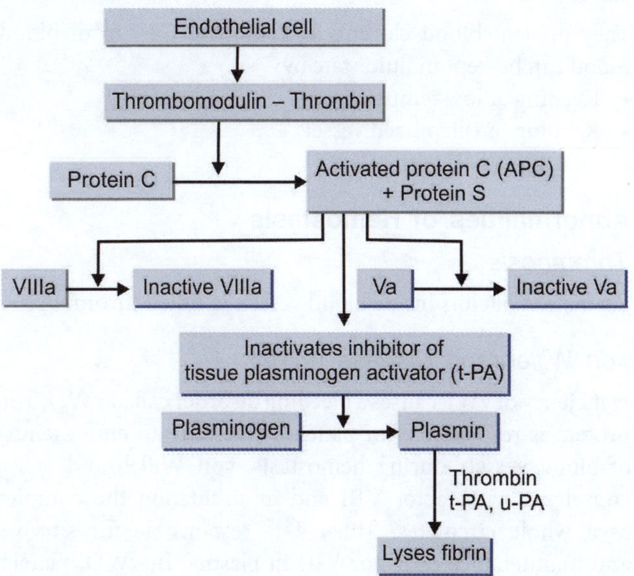

Vitamin K Antagonists

- Dicumarol
- Warfarin
- Phenindione.

Vitamin K is essential for liver formation of clotting factors like II, VII, IX, X. All these factors are synthesized by the liver as inactive zymogens.

> **Clinical Box**
>
> Bleeding tendency occurs in obstructive jaundice. In obstructive jaundice, there is no release of bile from liver into the intestine, so no absorption of fat soluble vitamin, i.e. vitamin K, thereby vitamin K deficiency.

Oxalate Compounds

They prevent coagulation by forming calcium oxalate. Thus Ca^{2+} is removed from blood. A mixture of ammonium oxalate and potassium oxalate in the ratio of 3:2 is used. Potassium oxalate alone causes shrinkage of RBCs. Ammonium oxalate alone causes swelling of RBCs. But together these substances do not alter cellular activity.

Citrates

Citrates combine with Ca^{2+} in blood to form calcium citrate. Reduction in Ca^{2+} level prevents coagulation.

Na, K and NH_3 citrates are used.

EDTA

They prevent blood clotting by removing Ca^{2+} from blood. Blood can be kept in fluid state by:
- Keeping at low temperature
- Keeping in siliconized vessels
- Diluting blood with saline.

Abnormalities of Hemostasis

Thrombosis

Formation of clots inside blood vessels is called thrombosis.

von Willebrand Disease (vWD)

Deficiency of vWF causes a bleeding disorder called vWD. This protein is responsible for platelet adherence to endothelium of blood vessels during hemostasis. von Willebrand factor complexes with factor VIII and in circulation the complex as a whole circulates. Thus, it is responsible for survival and maintenance of factor VIII in plasma. In vWD, platelet adhesion is reduced and thus hemostasis is affected.

Hemophilia

Hemophilia is a group of sex-linked inherited blood disorders, characterized by prolonged clotting time. However, the bleeding time is normal. Usually, it affects the males, with the females being the carriers. Here clotting time is prolonged (normal: 3–8 min) but bleeding time is normal (normal: 2–5 min). Because of prolonged clotting time, even a mild trauma causes excess bleeding which can lead to death. Damage of skin while falling or extraction of a tooth may cause excess bleeding for few weeks. Easy bruising and hemorrhage in muscles and joints are also common in this disease. Hemophilia occurs due to lack of formation of prothrombin activator. That is why the coagulation time is prolonged. The formation of prothrombin activator is affected due to the deficiency of factor VIII, IX (Figs 2.11 and 2.12).

Treatment

- Fresh blood transfusion (factor VIII is lost on storage).
- Injecting factor VIII and IX.
- Injecting thrombin or thromboplastin. It is of two types:
  a. Hemophilia A (classical hemophilia)
     Factor VIII is absent. It is relatively common.
  b. Hemophilia B (Christmas disease)
     Factor IX is deficient.

Purpura

It is a condition characterized by spontaneous hemorrhages beneath the skin, mucous membrane and in the internal organs. Bleeding time is prolonged (normal: 2–5 min). Clotting time is normal (normal: 3–8 min).

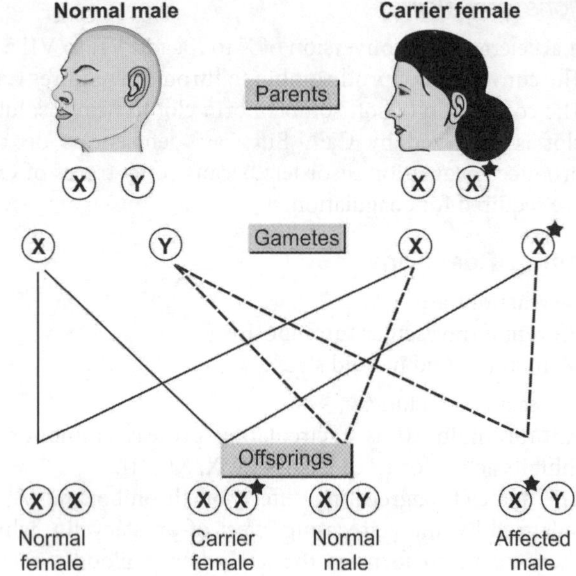

Fig. 2.11: Transmission of hemophilia

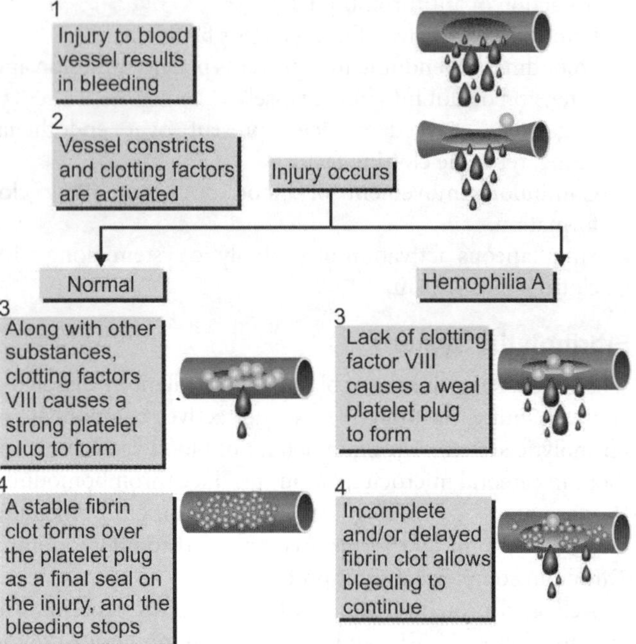

Fig. 2.12: Hemophilia

It may be due to:
- Decreased platelet count (thrombocytopenic purpura)
- Drug induced (quinine, ergot, iodine, etc.).
- Defective capillary contractility.

Forms

- Thrombocytopenic purpura (decreased platelet count)
- Athrombocytopenic purpura (normal platelet count)
- Thromboasthenic purpura (abnormal circulating platelet but platelet count is normal).

Treatment

- Injecting corticosteroids or ACTH
- Splenectomy.

BLOOD GROUPS

ABO Blood Groups Systems

The ABO blood groups systems are given in Table 2.6.

Table 2.6: ABO blood groups

Blood group	Erythrocyte contains (agglutinogen)	Plasma contains (agglutinin)
A	A	anti-B (β)
B	B	anti-A (α)
AB	A and B	Nil (o)
O	Nil	anti-A and anti-B (α and β)

Landsteiner's Law

- If a particular agglutinogen (antigen) is present in the RBCs, the corresponding agglutinin (antibody) must be absent in the plasma (Fig. 213).
- If a particular agglutinogen is absent in the RBCs, the corresponding agglutinin must be present in the plasma.
- The second part of the law is not applicable to Rh, M and N blood groups.

Compatibility between Different Groups

The compatibility between different groups are given in Table 2.7.

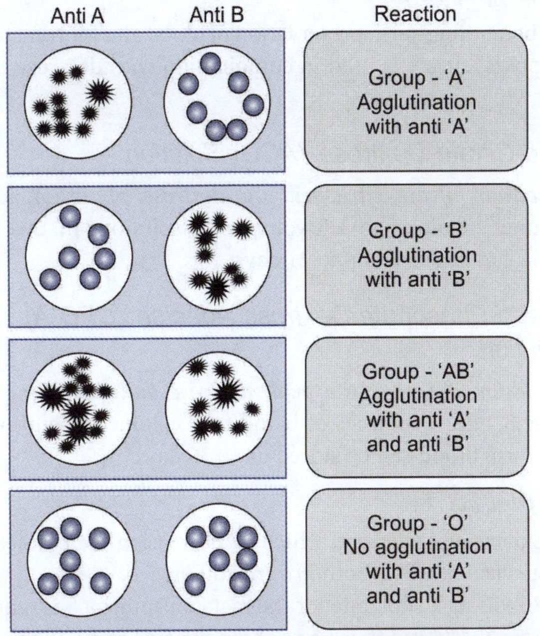

Fig. 2.13: Determination of blood groups

Table 2.7: Blood groups compatibility

Donor's group	Recipient's group			
	A (Aβ)	B (Bα)	AB (AB nil)	O (nil αβ)
O	✓	✓	✓	✓
A	✓	×	✓	×
B	×	✓	✓	×
AB	×	×	✓	×

✓ = no mismatching; × = mismatching

Cross Matching

In clinics, cross matching is always done before blood transfusion. There are two types of cross matching—major (direct) and minor (indirect).

1. *Direct cross matching:* Here donors RBCs are mixed with recipients plasma and checked for agglutination. The donor's plasma get diluted with recipients plasma so that agglutination of recipients RBCs occur rarely.
2. *Indirect cross matching:* Here the donor's plasma is reacted with recipients RBC and checked for agglutination. If agglutination occurs during either of the both tests, the blood from that person is not used for transfusion.

Note

- H antigen is normally present in all individuals of all blood types.
  Bombay blood group: Individuals with Bombay phenotype (hh) do not express H. Since there is no H antigen, there is no antigen A or antigen B on red cells. However, the plasma contains anti-A, anti-B and anti-H antibodies. As a result such a person can receive blood only from a person having Bombay blood type.
- ABO incompatibility does not cause hemolytic diseases of newborns: The antibodies of ABO blood group are of the IgM variety. They cannot cross the placenta. So there are no complications due to ABO incompatibility.

The Rh System

Rh factor is an antigen present in RBC. This system primarily comprises of C, D and E antigens. D is the most antigenic compound and the term Rh+ve generally means that the individual has agglutinogen D. The antibody in this system is called anti-D and it is produced only when a Rh -ve individual receives the D antigen. The antibodies are of IgG variety. Rh factor is an inherited dominant factor.

Hemolytic Disease of Newborn (HDN)

When an Rh-ve mother carries an Rh+ve fetus, small amount of blood leak into the maternal circulation at the time of delivery. During postpartum period, the mother develops Rh antibody in her blood. When the mother conceives for the second time and if the fetus happens to be Rh+ve again, the Rh antibody from mother's blood crosses the placental barrier and enters fetal blood (only Rh antigen cannot cross the placental barrier whereas the Rh antibody can cross it). The Rh antibodies which enter the fetus cause agglutination of fetal RBCs resulting in hemolysis. The changes in the fetus are termed as hemolytic diseases. The various forms of hemolytic disease of newborn (HDN) are:

- *Erythroblastosis fetalis:* The disease is also called icterus gravis neonatorum. The infant is jaundiced due to excessive destruction of RBC. Due to severe hemolysis, anemia develops and fetal body tries to compensate and as a result large number of premature red cells (erythroblasts) appear in peripheral circulation of fetus.
- *Hydrops fetalis:* If hemolysis is more severe, death of the fetus occurs in the uterus or may develop severe jaundice, anemia and edema.
- *Kernicterus:* It is a condition which develops when bilirubin deposition occurs in basal ganglia of brain (as BBB is not developed in fetus and newborn infants) producing abnormalities in the functions of basal ganglia.

Treatment of HDN

- *Phototherapy:* Neonatal jaundice can be treated by phototherapy (bilirubin is photoisomerized to lumirubin which can be excreted in bile).
- Drugs like phenobarbitone.
- Exchange blood transfusion soon after birth, i.e. to replace the neonates blood with Rh –ve blood.

Prevention of HDN

Administration of anti-Rh antibodies (anti-D antibody) soon after child birth, if Rh –ve mother gives birth to Rh +ve child. It is also administered to expectant mother starting at 28–30 week of gestation.

Blood Transfusion

Indications

Blood loss, blood disorders, blood diseases, poisoning, acute infections, shock, etc.

Complications of Blood Transfusion

Due to Mismatched Transfusion

The antibodies in the recipient's serum attach to the antigens of donor's RBC. This antigen-antibody reaction leads to agglutination (forming clumps). The RBCs are first agglutinated and then undergo hemolysis. The clumps of cells may block smaller blood vessels in the coronary/pulmonary/renal circulation. This may result in shock. The hemolyzed RBCs causes increased release of Hb which gets metabolized to bilirubin and may lead to jaundice. If the amount of Hb in the renal tubules is sufficiently high, kidney failure can develop.

Flowchart 2.9: Hazards of blood transfusion

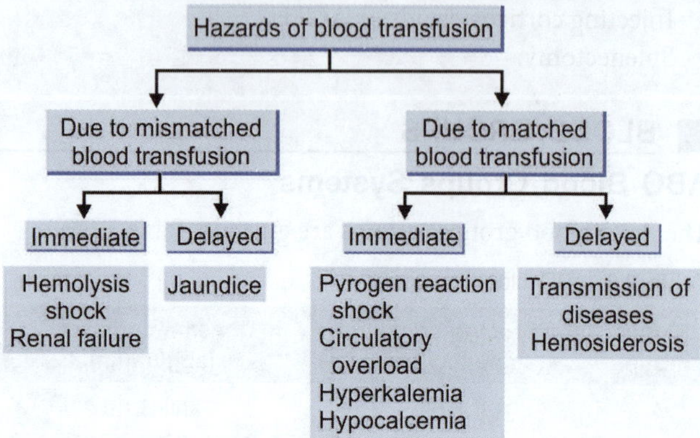

Which are not due to mismatched transfusion (Flowchart 2.9)

- Excess volume of transfusion can cause hypervolemia. As stored blood cells lose K^+ to the external plasma, hyperkalemia results.
- Blood is stored using citrates and transfused blood contains enough citrates. With massive transfusion of citrated blood, citrate removes the Ca^{2+} ions of recipient's blood. This results in hypocalcemia.
- Hemosiderosis (due to excess Fe).
- Pyrogenic reactions like fever.
- Allergic reactions and shock.
- Transmission of diseases like AIDS, malaria, syphilis, etc.

Blood Storage

For better long-term preservation of blood and for transfusion purposes, citrate is used in combination with dextrose in the following forms.

Acid-Citrate-Dextrose (ACD) Solution

Trisodium citrate, citric acid and dextrose: pH is 5.4, add 10 volumes of blood to 1.5 volumes of solution. In this form blood can be stored up to 21 days.

Citrate-Phosphate-Dextrose-Adenine (CPD-A) Solution

Trisodium citrate, citric acid, dextrose and adenine: pH is 5.6–5.8, add 7 volumes of blood to 1 volume of solution. In this form blood can be stored up to 35 days.

Dextrose acts by

- Liberating lactic acid which by decreasing the pH helps in survival of RBCs both *in vitro* and *in vivo*.
- Providing a substrate for the metabolism which is required even at 4°C and thus helps in the survival of cell (Table 2.8).

Table 2.8: Lifespan of constituents of blood

Cell	Lifespan
Neutrophils	2–5 days
Eosinophils	7–12 days
Basophils	12–15 days
Lymphocytes	1 days
Monocytes	2–5 days
Macrophages	Months (longest)
Platelets	10 days

Changes in the Stored Blood (Preservation Injuries)

Blood stored in the blood bank suffers some changes.

- Decrease in 2, 3 DPG, so increased affinity of Hb to O_2.
- Increase in K^+ concentration in plasma so chance of hyperkalemia.
- Increase in concentration of Na^+ in RBC.
- Decreased viability of RBCs, so they cannot work for longer time due to decreased ATP in them.
- Decrease in platelet count.
- Increased fragility.

IMMUNITY

Resistance of body against pathogenic agents is known as immunity. Immunity is of two types:

1. *Innate immunity (Nonspecific):* It is the inborn capacity of the body to resist the entry of microorganisms into the body. It represents the first-line of defense against any pathogen. For example:
   - Phagocytosis of bacteria and other invaders by WBC and tissue macrophage system
   - Destruction of swallowed organisms by acids secreted from stomach and digestive enzymes
   - Destruction of foreign cells and tumor cells by natural killer cells.
2. *Acquired immunity (Specific):* It is the resistance developed in the body against any specific foreign body like bacteria, viruses, toxins, vaccines, etc. The key to acquired immunity is the ability of lymphocytes to produce antibodies that are specific to foreign bodies (antigen).Acquired immunity is of two types—active and passive.
   a. *Active immunity:* Acquired immunity developed by the individual as a result of antigenic stimulation like previous infections, vaccines, etc. This involves the active functioning of the person's immune system leading to the synthesis of antibodies or production of immunologically active cells.
   Active immunity can be induced naturally or artificially.
   – Natural active immunity—results from either subclinical or clinical infection
   – Artificial active immunity—by giving vaccines.
   b. *Passive immunity:* Acquired immunity developed by an individual through the transfer of blood, serum, antibody from an immune individual; in ready made form. Here, the recipients immune system plays no role. It gives immediate response and is transient. It can be natural or artificial.
   – *Natural passive immunity:* Antibody transmitted from mother to fetus either through placenta or through breast milk.
   – *Artificial passive immunity:* Resistance passively transmitted to recipient by administration of Ab. It is given in the form of serum; e.g. anti-tetanus serum (ATS).

Acquired immunity has two components: Humoral and cell mediated.

Lymphocytes

They are responsible for specific immune response. In fetus, lymphocytes develop from bone marrow.

The lymphocyte designed to develop the cellular immunity migrates into thymus gland and are transformed into T lymphocytes. The lymphocyte designed to develop the humoral immunity are processed in liver (during fetal life) and bone marrow (after birth) and are transformed into B lymphocytes (Fig. 214). There is a third variety of lymphocytes called natural killer cells (NK Cells).

Types of T Lymphocytes

- Helper T cells or inducer T cells (T4 cells/CD4)
- Cytotoxic T cells or killer cells (T8 cells/CD8)
- Suppressor T cells (T8 cells/CD8)
- Memory T cells.

Types of B Lymphocytes

- Plasma cells
- Memory cells.

Humoral Immunity

It is mediated by circulating Ig antibodies in the γ-globulin fraction of the plasma proteins. Ig antibodies are produced by B lymphocytes. B lymphocytes are stimulated directly by foreign organisms or through an antigen presenting cell. Some of B lymphocytes are converted to plasma cells, producing immunoglobulin. Each plasma cell continues to produce specific Ab for several days or weeks, till it dies. Some of the B lymphocytes are converted to blast-like cells and they remain as memory B cells. On exposure to same antigen

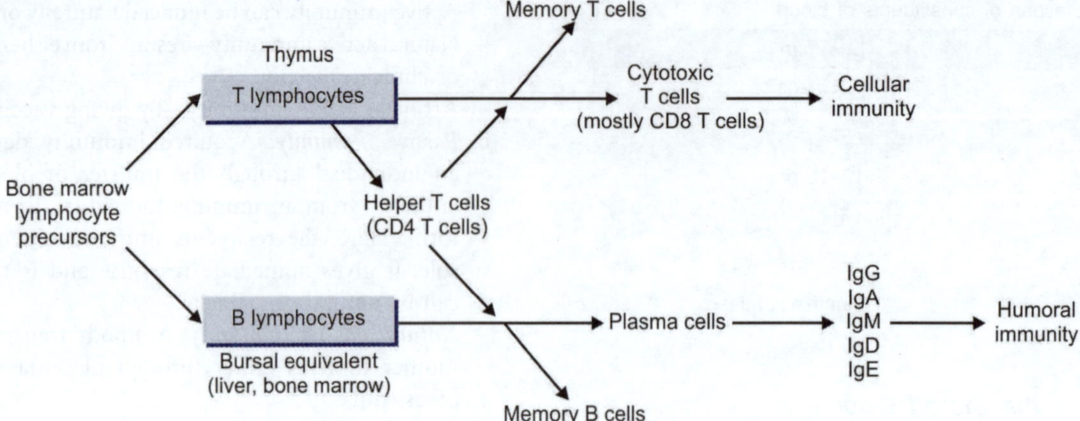

Fig. 2.14: Development of immune system from the common bone marrow stem cell

subsequently, initiate a rapid response due to the presence of memory B cells. Humoral immunity is major defense against bacterial infections.

Immunoglobulin

Immunoglobulin are produced by the plasma cells. It is composed of four polypeptide chains, linked by disulfide bonds. There are two heavy chains (H) and two light chains (L). Each light chain lies parallel to the terminal portion of heavy chain. There are two areas; Fab for antigen binding and Fc for complement binding (Fig. 2.15). Terminal portions of both heavy and light chains are called variable segment. Specificity of each Ab is due to specific amino acid pattern of variable segment. Thetr are of five basic types or classes:

1. *IgG:* It is the most abundant antibody present in our body. It can pass through the placental barrier and it provides natural passive immunity. They serve as opsonins and promotes phagocytosis of the bacteria. It is the antibody seen in secondary immune response.
2. *IgA:* It is formed by mucosal and submucosal aggregates of lymphoid tissue. From here it is transported to epithelial cells. This provides effective defense mechanism in mucosa of alimentary canal and lungs and genitourinary tracts.
3. *IgM:* Earliest Ig to be synthesized. It activates complement system. They are predominantly produced in primary immune response. Antibodies of ABO blood group system belongs to this class.
4. *IgE:* They mediate allergy, hypersensitivity and anaphylaxis. Chiefly produced in the lining cells of respiratory and intestinal tract. They releases histamine from basophils and mast cells.
5. *IgD:* Present on the surface of B lymphocytes and therefore involved in antigen recognition.

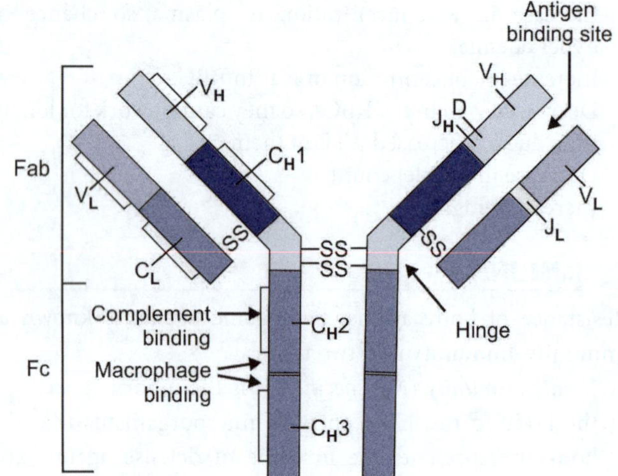

Fig. 2.15: Structure of an immunoglobin molecule

Mechanism of Antibody Action

An antibody exerts its action by two mechanisms:

1. Direct action
2. Indirect action (through activation of complement system).

Direct Action

There are multiple antigen sites on invading organisms. So antibodies can inactivate the invading agent in one of the following mechanisms:

- *Agglutination:* Antibodies bind with antigen and forms a clump.
- *Precipitation:* Molecular complex of antigens and antibodies becomes so large that is rendered insoluble and it precipitates.
- *Neutralization:* Antibodies cover toxic sites of antigenic agents and make it nontoxic.

- *Lysis:* Antibodies attack cell membrane of foreign organisms and cause destruction of organism or lysis.
- Ab enhances opsonization and phagocytosis.

Indirect Action

It is through activation of complement system. It is a system of about 20 proteins. Normally these are present in blood and tissue spaces and are inactive. They are activated by antigen-antibody reaction. When an antibody binds with an antigen, binding site on antibody for complement becomes activated and that will bind with complements. That will activate the complement system and activated complements produce certain effects. The effects are:

Opsonization and phagocytosis: Activated complement C3b strongly activate phagocytosis by neutrophils and macrophages. These neutrophils and macrophages phagocy-tose foreign antigen or foreign bacteria.

Lysis: One of the most important products of complement cascade is the lytic complex, which is a combination of multiple complement factors C5, C6, C7, C8, C9. Its directly cause lysis of foreign organism.

Agglutination: The complement products changes the surface of invading organism and causes them to adhere one another or agglutination.

Neutralization: The activated complements attack the structure of some viruses and make them nonvirulent or nontoxic. It leads to inflammatory changes, i.e. increased local blood flow, capillary leakage of proteins to interstitial space, coagulation of this proteins. These inflammatory changes immobilize the organism and prevent movement of organism from area of invasion to other part of the body.

Cellular Immunity

It is produced by T lymphocytes that can directly attack intracellular pathogenic microorganisms like virus, fungus, bacteria, etc. They can activate macrophages which phagocytose pathogenic microorganisms. T lymphocytes require an antigen presenting cell for its action. The antigen presenting cells are, macrophages, B lymphocytes, dendrite cells in spleen and Langerhans cell of skin. MHC2 is present on membranes of antigen presenting cell (Major Histocompatibility Complex: Gene that produces proteins MHC1 and MHC2. MHC1 is present on membranes of all nucleated cells and platelets).

T lymphocytes are activated through antigen presenting cell. Antigen presenting cell (APC) phagocytoses the foreign organism, digests it and separates portion responsible for antigenicity. This gets attached to the MHC2 proteins which protrude from the surface of APC. This MHC2 antigen complex is recognized by an appropriate T lymphocyte and T lymphocyte gets attached to this complex. This will activate the T lymphocyte (CD4 or helper T cells). The activated T cells proliferate and a clone of activated T cells is produced, some remain as memory T cells. The following effects are produced by activated T cells.

- Interleukins are produced and these activate further proliferation of T cells.
- Interleukins produced by activated T cells activate B lymphocyte.
- Activated T lymphocytes activate CD8 or cytotoxic T cells. Cytotoxic T cells cause cell lysis directly.
- Activated T cells lead to inflammation and delayed allergic reactions.

During the second exposure, the memory cells are stimulated and produce more quantity of antibodies at a faster rate, than the first exposure.

Summary

a. When an antigen enters the body, it is ingested by macrophages and is partially digested. Antigen peptide fragments then combine with MHC-2 and move to cell surface.
b. This processed antigen with macrophage then binds with CD4 cell. CD4 cell is activated and it secretes interleukin 2 (IL-2).
c. IL-2 cause the cell to multiply, forming a clone.
d. The CD4 cells then activate B lymphocytes causing them to proliferate and transform into memory B cells and plasma cells or it may activate cytotoxic CD8 cell. The plasma cells secrete large quantities of antibodies (immunoglobulins) into general circulation (Fig. 2.16).

The CD8 cell can also be activated by forming a synapse with an MHC 1 antigen presenting cell.

Reticuloendothelial System

They are special groups of cells scattered in different parts of the body which play an important role in the defense mechanism. The combination of monocytes, mobile macrophages, fixed macrophages and a few specialized endothelial cells in the bone marrow, spleen and lymph nodes is called reticuloendothelial system. It is also known as monocyte macrophage system (almost all these cells originate from monocytic stem cells). The macrophages can phagocytose abnormal body tissue, microbes and foreign particle. Tissue macrophages are of two types—fixed and wandering.

Site of Occurrence

Spleen and Bone Marrow

In both these tissues, macrophages have become entrapped by the reticular meshwork of the two organs. When foreign

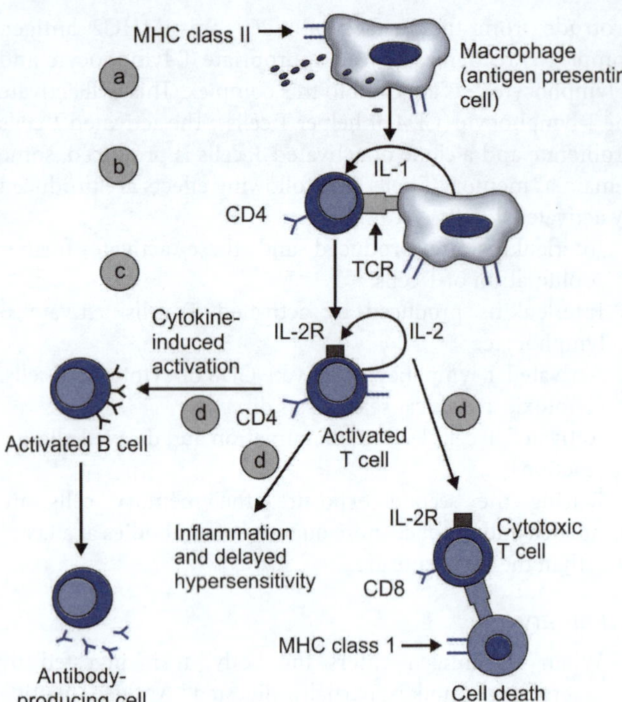

Fig. 2.16: Acquired immunity

particles come in contact with these macrophages, they are phagocytosed. They are present in both red and white pulp of spleen. Macrophages of the spleen and bone marrow are called reticulum cells. Reticulum cells of spleen can phagocytose RBC, platelets, parasite and bacteria. From the Hb of the RBC, these macrophages produce bilirubin.

Lungs

Macrophages found in the alveoli phagocytose the dust/ carbon particles.

Liver

Sinusoids of the liver are lined by macrophages called Kupffer cells. It removes bacteria of portal venous blood. Portal vein contains bacteria coming from the intestine. The presence of Kupffer cells ensure effective filtration so that hepatic venous blood is free from bacteria.

Lymph Nodes

If particles are not destroyed locally in the tissues they enter the lymph and flow to the lymph nodes. The foreign particles are entrapped in these nodes in a meshwork of sinuses lined by tissue macrophages. These macrophages phagocytose the particles entering the sinuses.

Warm and Cold Antibodies

Agglutinogens of ABO system and RH system can react with their corresponding antibodies at normal or near body temperature that is in warm environment. Therefore, this agglutinins are called warm antibodies.

But antibodies of some other blood group systems can react with their corresponding agglutinogens only at a temperature between 5 to 20°C. They are called cold antibodies.

LYMPHATIC SYSTEM

- Lymphatic system exists in all the organs with the exception of CNS and cornea.
- Lymph is a tissue fluid that enters the lymphatic vessels and then drains into the venous blood via the thoracic and right lymphatic duct.
- Lymph contains clotting factors and it clots on standing *in vitro*.
- It is transparent, yellowish in color, faintly alkaline and its colloidal osmotic pressure is less than that of plasma.
- *Rate:* Total estimated lymph flow is about 120 ml/hr or 2–3 L/day.

Formation

Formation is based on transcapillary exchange (Fig. 2.17). Lymph is derived from interstitial fluid that flows into the lymphatics. It enters terminal lymphatics (same composition as interstitial fluid). The protein concentration of the lymph is near 2 gm/dl which is the average protein concentration of interstitial fluid. Even large particles such as bacteria can push their way between the endothelial cells of lymphatic capillaries (thereby enter lymph).

Function

- Returns proteins, water and electrolytes from tissue spaces to the blood and thus controls concentration of proteins in the interstitial fluid, volume of interstitial fluid and interstitial fluid pressure.
- Absorption of nutrients especially fats from the GIT.
- Acts as transport mechanism to remove red blood cells that have lost into the tissues as a result of hemorrhage.
- Lymph nodes act as efficient filters. They have sinuses lined with phagocytic cells that engulf bacteria, red blood cells and other particulate matter (bacteria or toxins are carried to them through lymph).
- *Nutritive:* It supplies nutrition and O_2 to those parts where blood cannot reach.

Dynamics of Fluid Exchange at capillary Levels

At the arterial end of capillaries different forces cause movement of fluid out through capillary membrane. The low pressure at the venous end of capillaries leads to movement of fluid into the capillaries. Basically, there are two forces or pressures that are responsible for fluid movement: (1) Hydrostatic pressure and (2) Colloid osmotic pressure.

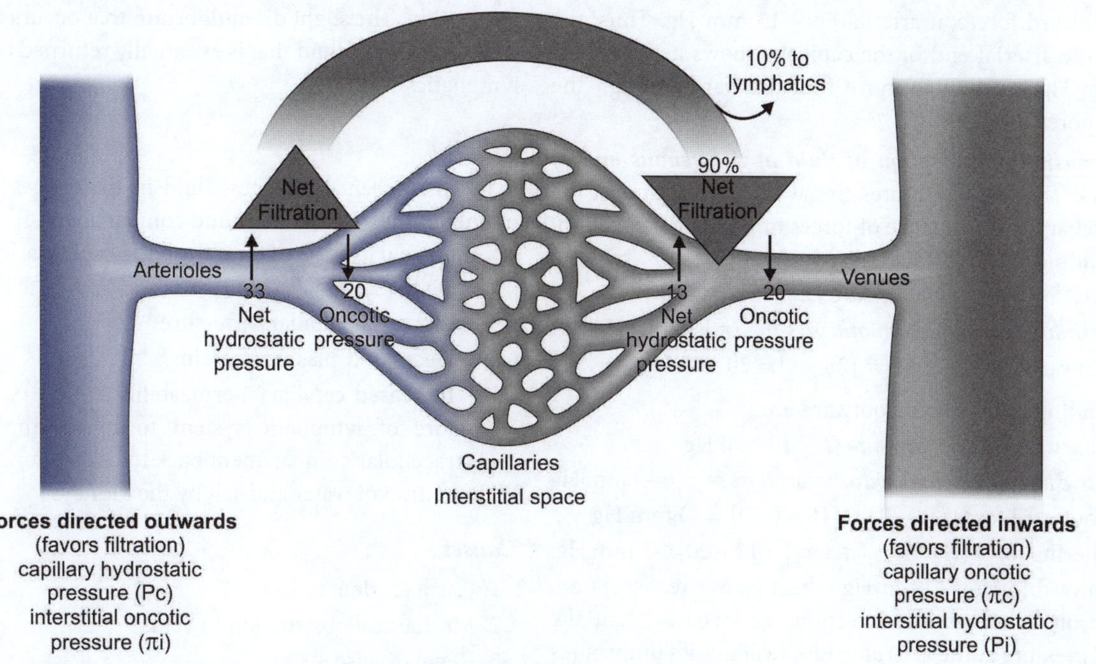

Fig. 2.17: Starling forces at capillary

1. ***Hydrostatic pressure:*** It is a force that pushes fluid or water away from it into the neighboring compartment. It is exerted by the accumulated fluid or water (*'hydro', 'static'*). It is proportional to the amount of the accumulated fluid; greater the accumulated fluid, greater will the hydrostatic pressure.
   a. *Capillary hydrostatic pressure (P_c):* It is exerted by the blood (plasma) within a capillary. It forces the plasma fluid out of the capillary.
   b. *Interstitial fluid hydrostatic pressure (P_i):* It is exerted by the interstitial fluid present within a tissue. It tends to push the fluid into the capillary. In loose subcutaneous tissue, interstitial fluid pressure measured is usually a few millimeters of mercury less than atmospheric pressure; that is, the values are called negative interstitial fluid pressure. In other tissues that are surrounded by capsules, such as kidneys, the interstitial pressure is generally positive (greater than atmospheric pressure).
2. ***Colloid osmotic pressure***: It is a force exerted by the proteins in a compartment. It tends to pull fluid or water into the compartment by osmosis.
   a. *Plasma colloid osmotic pressure (π_c):* It is exerted by the plasma proteins in the vascular compartment. It pulls water into the capillary by osmosis.
   b. *Interstitial fluid colloid osmotic pressure (π_i):* It is exerted by the proteins in the interstitial fluid. It tends to pull water out of the capillary into the interstitium.

Starling Forces

Pressures in the capillaries are the major forces that govern fluid movement in them. Such forces are commonly called Starling forces. Capillaries are called exchange vessels because exchange of fluid, nutrients, and gases happen between capillaries and the interstitial space. The rate of filtration and absorption at any point along a capillary wall depends on a balance of forces (Starling forces), which depends on:

- *Hydrostatic pressure gradient (P_c–P_i):* Hydrostatic pressure in the capillary minus the hydrostatic pressure in the interstitial space.
- *Oncotic pressure gradient (π_c–π_i):* Colloid osmotic pressure of the plasma minus the colloid osmotic pressure in the interstitial fluid.
- *Capillary permeability:* Capillary filtration coefficient (k) is proportional to the permeability of the capillary and surface area available for filtration.
  Fluid movement = $k [(P_c - P_i) - (\pi_c - \pi_i)]$

Factors causing filtration of fluid at the arterial end of capillaries: The forces that tend to cause movement of fluid out of the capillary are:

a. *Capillary hydrostatic pressure (P_c):* 30 mm Hg
b. *Negative interstitial fluid hydrostatic pressure (P_i):* –3 mm Hg
   Total outward force $(P_c - P_i) = [30 - (-3)] = 33$ mm Hg

Forces tending to move fluid inward are:

a. *Plasma colloid osmotic pressure (π_c):* 28 mm Hg
b. *Interstitial fluid colloid osmotic pressure (π_i):* 8 mm Hg
   Total inward force $(\pi_c - \pi_i) = [28 - 8] = 20$ mm Hg

So, net filtering force $[(P_c - P_i) - (\pi_c - \pi_i)] = 33 - 20 = 13$ mm Hg

PHYSICON—The Reliable Icon in Physiology

Net outward force (at arterial end) 13 mm Hg. Thus, the forces at the arterial end of the capillary shows net filtration of 13 mm Hg, tending to move fluid outward through the capillary pores.

Factors causing reabsorption of fluid at the venous end of capillaries: The low blood pressure at the venous end of the capillary changes the balance of forces in favor of absorption.

Forces tending to move fluid inward:

a. *Plasma colloid osmotic pressure* (π_c): 28 mm Hg
b. *Interstitial fluid colloid osmotic pressure* (π_i): 8 mm Hg
Total inward force (π_c - π_i) = [28 – 8] = 20 mm Hg

Forces tending to move fluid outward are:

a. *Capillary hydrostatic pressure* (P_c): 10 mm Hg
b. *Negative interstitial fluid hydrostatic pressure* (π_i): –3 mm Hg
Total outward force (P_c – P_i) = [10 – (–3)] = 13 mm Hg

So, net filtering force [(P_c - P_i) - (π_c - π_i)] = 13 – 20 = -7 mm Hg.

Net inward force is 7 mm Hg which causes reabsorption. The reabsorption pressure at venous end is less than the filtration pressure at the arterial ends of capillaries but venous capillaries are more numerous and more permeable than the arterial capillaries, so less pressure is required to cause inward movement. About nine-tenths of filtered fluid is absorbed at the venous end.

Starling's Equilibrium

EH starling pointed out that under normal condition a state of near equilibrium exists at capillary membrane. The amount of fluid filtering out from capillaries equals almost exactly the quantity of fluid that is returned to the circulation by absorption. The slight disequilibrium that occurs accounts for small amount of fluid that is eventually returned by way of the lymphatics.

Edema

It means presence of excess fluid in the tissues of the body mainly in the extracellular fluid compartment. It is due to:

- Abnormal leakage of fluid from the capillaries. This in turn is due to:
  - Increased capillary pressure
  - Decreased plasma proteins
  - Increased capillary permeability.
- Failure of lymphatic system to return the fluid from extracellular compartment back to circulation.
- Retention of water and salt by the kidneys.

Causes

1. Cardiac edema
2. Mechanical obstruction to veins
3. Renal disease
4. Inflammatory area (increased capillary permeability)
5. Malnutrition (lack of proteins)
6. Toxic substances (increased capillary permeability).

Clinical Box

Hypoproteinemia causes decrease in COP, therefore increased filtration occurs at arterial end and decrease in absorption of fluid at venous end, resulting in abnormal collection of fluid in interstitial spaces called edema.

CLINICAL QUESTIONS

1. **A RBC was placed in a saline (NaCl) solution and the cell volume increased to 1.5 times its original volume.**
   a. What is the nature of the saline solution? (isotonic/hypotonic/hypertonic)
   b. Define the transport mechanism responsible for the above effect.
   c. Name other mechanisms for transport across the cell membrane.
2. **A patient after receiving blood transfusion developed deep jaundice and hemoglobinuria within 48 hours.**
   a. Identify the condition.
   b. What is the cause of jaundice and hemoglobinuria?
   c. What is the preventive line of treatment?
3. **A patient came with the complaint of brownish spots under skin. On examination spleen was found to be enlarged. Investigations showed:**
   - **Bleeding time—10 min**
   - **Clotting time—6 min**
   - **Platelet count—30,000/mm^3**

   a. Identify the condition and give probable cause.
   b. Explain the features.
   c. Outline the physiological basis of treatment?
4. **A 16-year-old boy from Himachal Pradesh is found to have hemoglobin of 22 gm%. His physical examination and other routine investigations are within normal limits.**
   a. Identify the condition.
   b. What is the cause?
   c. Does he need treatment for this?

5. **A woman aged 30 years came with the complaints of weakness and breathlessness. On examination, pallor was present and nails were spoon shaped. Hemoglobin was 8 gm% and peripheral blood smear examination showed microcytic and hypochromic RBCs.**
   a. Identify the condition.
   b. Explain the features.
   c. What is the physiological basis of treatment?
6. **A healthy woman gave birth to a deeply jaundiced, edematous and anemic child. First baby was born normal.**
   a. Identify the condition.
   b. Why was the first baby healthy?
   c. What is the preventive and curative treatment?
7. **A 5 year old child from a poor slum dweller family is brought to the doctor with complaint of pica. On examination patient is having pallor, hemoglobin concentration is 8 gm%.**
   a. What is the likely cause of anemia?
   b. Enumerate other causes of anemia.
   c. What is the physiological basis of treatment? (Pica; persistant eating of non-edible substances like earth, paint charcoal; can lead to worm infestation and thus iron deficiency anemia)
8. **A male patient comes with persistent bleeding after tooth extraction. Investigations show:**
   - **Bleeding time—4 min**
   - **Clotting time—20 min**
   - **Platelet count—2 Lacs/mm³**

   a. What is the likely diagnosis?
   b. What is the physiological basis of treatment?
   c. Enumerate the mechanisms of hemostasis.
9. **A medical student went to a blood bank for voluntary blood donation.**
   a. What are the criteria for selection of the donor?
   b. At what frequency can a person donate blood?
   c. What precautions are necessary before blood transfusion?
10. **A patient came to the clinic with complaints of chronic weight loss with fever and diarrhea not responding to treatment. Investigations revealed that the CD4 count was decreased.**
    a. What is the probable diagnosis?
    b. What is the cause of this condition?
    c. Explain the patho-physiology of the symptoms.
11. **A patient after receiving blood transfusion developed deep jaundice and hemoglobinuria within 48 hours.**
    a. Identify the condition.
    b. What is the cause of jaundice and hemoglobinuria?
    c. What is the preventive line of treatment?
12. **A 35 year old female patient was taking radiotherapy for breast cancer. During routine checkup her blood examination showed the Hb concentration 7 gm%. WBC count—2,000/cumm. Platelet count—30,000/mm³.**
    a. Comment on these findings.
    b. Name other conditions leading to similar findings.

Answers for Clinical Questions are given in the Appendix

CHAPTER

3

Respiratory System

In most of the chemical reactions involved in the production of energy, oxygen is consumed and carbondioxide is produced. An adult consumes about 250 ml of oxygen and produces about 200 ml of carbon dioxide per minute.

The main function of respiratory system is to extract O_2 from the atmosphere, to deliver it to the tissues and to take CO_2 from the tissues and discharge it to the atmosphere. The entire respiration can be divided into two main divisions.

- *External respiration:* It deals with the absorption of O_2 and removal of CO_2 from the body as a whole.
- *Internal respiration:* It is the utilization of the O_2 and production of CO_2 by cells and the gaseous exchange between the cells in their fluid medium.

GENERAL PRINCIPLES

The respiratory tract is functionally divided into:

- ***Upper respiratory tract*:** Nasal and oral cavities, pharynx, larynx.
- ***Lower respiratory tract*:** From trachea to alveoli, i.e. tracheobronchial tree and the lung parenchyma.

In order to reach the lungs, air has to pass through a series of air passages (airways), such as the nose (or mouth), pharynx, larynx, trachea, bronchi, and bronchioles.

Weibel's Lung Model (Tracheobronchial Tree)

This was introduced by ER Weibel (1963). Between the trachea and alveolar sac, the air passage divides 23 times.

Trachea is designated as generation zero. First-two major divisions of trachea constitute the 'first' generation and so on. Atria or the alveolar sac is the 23rd generation (last generation). From the functional point of view tracheobronchial tree can be divided into two major zones (Fig. 3.1).

1. *Conducting zone*: The first 16 generation bronchioles form the conducting zone of air (no alveoli present). So no exchange of gases takes place here. This area forms the anatomical dead space. The 16th generation bronchioles are called terminal bronchioles.
2. *Respiratory zone:* On and from the 17th generation, few alveoli are seen. Here exchange of gases takes place, so called respiratory bronchioles.

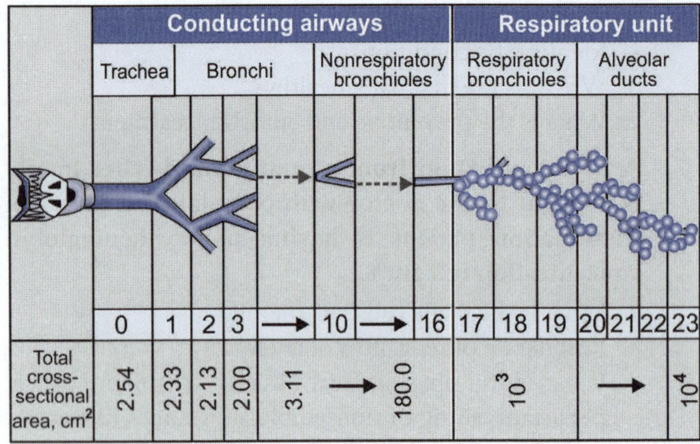

Fig. 3.1: Weibel's lung model

Advantages

These multiple divisions increase the total cross-sectional area of airways (from 2.5 to 11800 cm^2) in the alveoli. As a result the velocity of airflow in small airways is greatly reduced allowing better gaseous exchange. The alveoli are surrounded by pulmonary capillaries.

Respiratory Membrane

The air in the alveoli is separated from the blood in the pulmonary capillaries by a wall called 'respiratory membrane' (Fig. 3.2). Basically, it consists of alveolar wall and the capillary wall.

The following are the six layers of the respiratory membrane:

1. A layer of surfactant lining the alveolus.
2. The alveolar epithelium.
3. Basal lamina of alveolar epithelial cells.
4. A thin interstitial space between the alveolar epithelium and the capillary membrane.
5. Basal membrane of endothelial cells.
6. A capillary endothelial membrane.

Despite these large number of layers, the overall thickness of the membrane in some areas is as little as 0.2 micrometer (average about 0.6 micrometer), except where there are cell nuclei. The total surface area of the respiratory membrane is about 70 m^2 in the normal adult human male, which facilitates

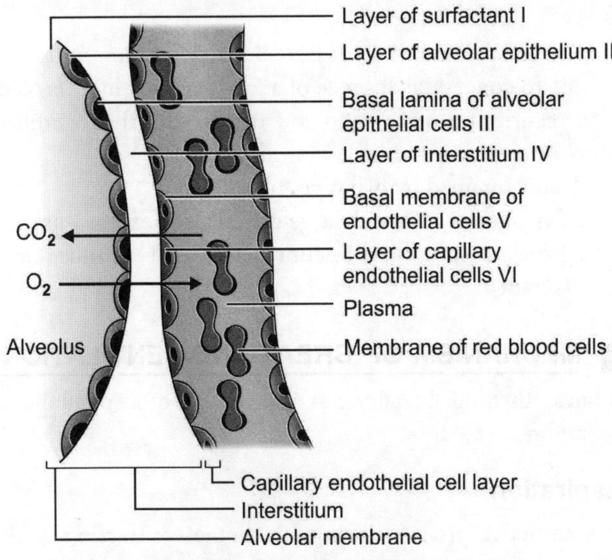

Fig. 3.2: Respiratory membrane

the rapidity of respiratory exchange of O_2 and CO_2. There are about 300 million alveoli in the two lungs.

Factors Affecting the Rate of Gas Diffusion

$$V_{gas} = A/T \times D \times (P_1 - P_2)$$

1. *The thickness (T) of the membrane:* Thickness increases in pulmonary edema and fibrosis of lung.
2. *The surface area (A) of the membrane:* Surface area decreases in pneumonectomy and emphysema.
3. *The diffusion coefficient (D) of the gas in the substance of the membrane:* Diffusion coefficient is directly proportional to the solubility of the gas and inversely proportional to the square root of molecular weight of gas.
4. The partial pressure difference of the gas between the two sides of the membrane (P_1–P_2).

Airway Resistance

When air flows through the airways, there is resistance to the air flow, which is referred to as airway resistance. Normal value is 1.5–2 cm H_2O/L/sec.

$$\text{Airway resistance} = \frac{\text{Pressure difference between atmosphere and alveolar pressure (cm } H_2O)}{\text{Airflow (L/sec)}}$$

Factors Affecting Airway Resistance

1. *Total cross-sectional area:* Resistance to the airflow is inversely related to the total cross-sectional area of the respiratory passage. Therefore, the resistance to the airflow is high in the 'conducting zone' whereas it is low in the 'respiratory zone'.
2. *According to Poiseuille: Hagen* formula, the relation between the flow in a long narrow tube, the viscosity of fluid and the radius of the tube is :
$$F = (P_A - P_B) \times (\pi/8) \times (1/\eta) \times (r^4/L)$$
where,
F = flow, $P_A - P_B$ = pressure difference between two ends of the tube, η = viscosity, L= length of the tube, r = radius of the tube.
Since flow = $\frac{P_A - P_B}{R}$ where, R = resistance
So, Resistance (R) $= \frac{8\,\eta\,L}{\pi\,r^4}$
i.e $R \propto 1/r^4$
Therefore, if the radius decreases by 'half' keeping the other factors constant, the resistance increases by '16' times; but this does not occur in our body because as diameter of the airways is large, there is no difficulty in breathing.
3. *Type of flow:* Airway resistance is more in 'turbulent' flow (i.e during rapid respiration) than in 'laminar' flow or streamline flow (i.e. in quiet breathing).

Nonrespiratory Functions of Lungs

The main function of the respiratory system in general and lungs is gas exchange. Nonrespiratory functions of the respiratory system includes:

1. Lung defense mechanisms

a. The respiratory passages not only serve as gas conduits, but also humidify and cool or warm the inspired air to make it attain the body temperature by the time it reaches the alveoli.
b. Bronchial secretions contain secretory immunoglobulin (IgA) and other substances that help to resist infections and maintain mucosal integrity.
c. Pulmonary epithelium contains an interesting group of protease activated receptors (PARs), which when activated triggers the release of PGE_2, which in turn protect the epithelial cells.
d. Pulmonary alveolar macrophages (PAMs): These cells come originally from bone marrow. They are important component of pulmonary defense mechanisms. They are actively phagocytic and ingest inhaled bacteria and small particles. They help in processing the inhaled antigens for immunological attack. They secrete substances that attract granulocyte to the lung as well as substances that stimulate granulocyte and monocyte formation in bone marrow.
e. Prevents foreign body from reaching alveoli.
   i. *Particles ≥ 10 μm in diameter*: The hair in the nostrils strain out many particles and they settle down on mucous membrane in the nose and pharynx.

ii. *Particles 2–10 μm diameter:* These particles when fall on the walls of the bronchi as airflow slows in smaller passages, initiates reflex bronchoconstriction and coughing, thereby the particles are moved away from lungs by ciliary escalator action.

iii. *Particles ≤ 2 μm in diameter:* Generally reach the alveoli, where they are ingested by the macrophages.

2. ***Functions of pulmonary circulation***
   a. *Reservoir for left ventricle:* If the LV output becomes transiently greater than systemic venous return, LV output can be maintained by drawing out blood stored in the pulmonary circulation (for few strokes only).
   b. *Role as a filter*: Pulmonary circulation act as a filter for many substances like fibrin clots, fat cells, detached cancer cells, agglutinated RBCs.
   c. *Fluid exchange and drug absorption:* Low pulmonary hydrostatic pressure tends to pull fluid from alveoli into pulmonary capillaries, thereby keeping the alveolar surface free from liquids. This facilitates the rapid entry of drugs into systemic circulation which rapidly pass through the alveolar-capillary barrier by diffusion. For example: (i) anesthetic gases (ii) aerosols.
3. ***Metabolic and endocrine functions of the lungs***
   a. Manufactures surfactant for local use, which prevents the development of surface tension between the fluid lining the alveoli and the alveolar air.
   b. Substances synthesized or stored and released into the blood. For example, prostaglandins (esp. PGE_2 and $PGF_{2\alpha}$)
   c. Contain a fibrinolytic system that lyses clots in the pulmonary vessels.
   d. The lungs also activate one hormone in the pulmonary circulation.

$$\text{Angiotensin I} \xrightarrow{ACE} \text{Angiotensin II}$$

   (This reaction occurs in other tissues also, but prominent in lungs)
   - Angiotensin I—Inactive decapeptide
   - Angiotensin II—A pressor, aldosterone stimulating octapeptide.

   Large amounts of ACE is located on endothelial cells of the pulmonary capillaries. Angiotensin converting enzyme (ACE) inactivates bradykinin.
   e. It helps in the removal of serotonin and norepinephrine, thereby reducing the amounts of vasoactive substances reaching the systemic circulation. However, many other vasoactive substances like epinephrine, dopamine, oxytocin pass through the lungs without being metabolized.

Note

1. *Kartagener's syndrome:* It is associated with immotile cilia (due to congenital absence of axonemal dynein). This leds to recurrent lung infections. Patients with this condition are infertile due to lack of sperm motility.
2. Alveoli are lined by two types of cells:
   a. Type I (Flat cells with large cytoplasmic extensions)
   b. Type II (granular pneumocytes, that produce surfactant).

MECHANISM OF BREATHING/VENTILATION

Eupnea: Rhythmic breathing at rest, consists of inspiration and expiration.

Inspiration

It is an active process during which the contraction of the inspiratory muscles increases the intrathoracic volume. The intrapleural pressure at the base of the lungs is normally about –2.5 mm Hg (relative to atmospheric pressure) at the start of inspiration and it decreases to about –6 mm Hg. Thus lungs are pulled into a more expanded position making the pressure in the airways slightly negative and air flows into the lung.

The movement of the *diaphragm* accounts for 75% of the change in the intrathoracic volume during quiet inspiration. The other inspiratory muscles are the external intercostal muscles, which run obliquely downward and forward from rib to rib. The ribs pivot as if hinged at the back, so that when the external intercostals contract they elevate the lower ribs which pushes sternum outward causing in increased anteroposterior (AP) diameter of the chest.

Inspiratory Mechanism

During inspiration the thorax is enlarged by:
- Rib movements (movement of ribs outwards and upwards)
- Diaphragmatic movements (descent of diaphragm).

Rib Movements

Pump handle movements: The 2nd to the 6th ribs slope obliquely downwards and forwards from their joints with the spinal column, on inspiration the ribs move upwards pushing the sternum more anteriorly (pump handle movements; Fig. 3.3) to assume a more horizontal position by contraction of external intercostals resulting in increase in AP diameter of the chest.

Bucket handle movement: The lower ribs (7th to 10th) also swing outwards and upwards in inspiration causing increase in the transverse diameter of the thorax (Fig. 3.4).

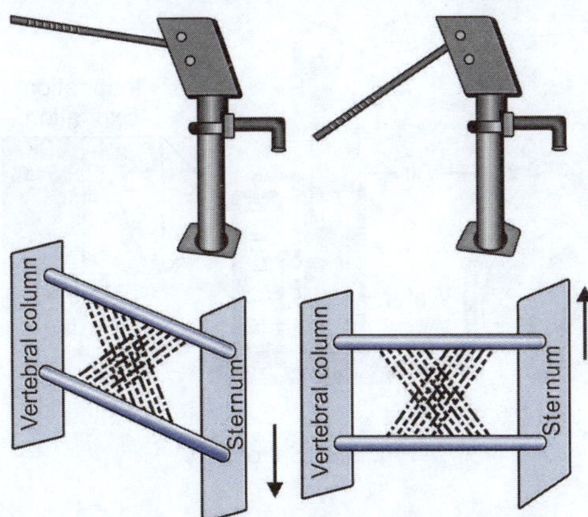

Fig. 3.3: Pump handle movement increases the anteroposterior diameter

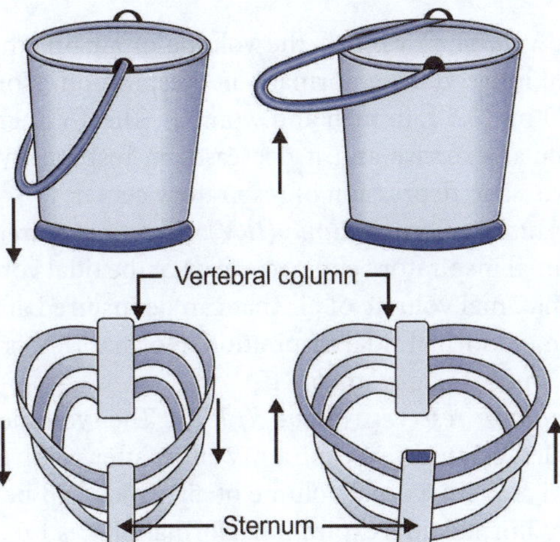

Fig. 3.4: Bucket handle movement increases the transverse diameter

Accessory muscles of inspiration

Scalene, Sternocleidomastoid

Active during voluntary static inspiratory efforts that help to elevate the thoracic cage during deep inspiration.

Intrinsic Muscles of Larynx

Abductor muscles of vocal cords (posterior cricoarytenoid) that contract early on inspiratory phase pulling the vocal cords apart, opening the glottis.

Expiratory Mechanism

Quiet breathing is a passive process. But during forced expiration, e.g. exercise, bronchial asthma, the muscles of expiration contract.

Expiratory muscles

- Anterior abdominal muscles (abdominal recti, transversus abdominus, internal and external oblique muscles
- Internal intercostal muscle
- Accessory muscles of expiration (adductor muscles of vocal cord).

Pressure Changes During Ventilation (Fig. 3.5)

Intrapulmonary Pressure/Intra-alveolar Pressure

Intrapulmonary pressure is defined as the pressure in the lung parenchyma. It reduces with the expansion of the lungs and facilitates the pull of air into the lungs via the tracheobronchial tree.

In normal quiet breathing, at end-expiration and end-inspiration, as no air is going in and coming out of the lungs, the intrapleural pressure = atmospheric pressure, i.e. 760 mm Hg.

With the beginning of inspiration, as volume increases pressure decreases and intrapulmonary pressure decreases to approx 3 mm Hg below the atmospheric pressure (i.e. 757 mm Hg), but regains the pressure value at end-inspiration. As expiration follows passively, the elastic recoil of the lungs causes the intrapulmonary pressure to swing to the positive side (i.e. 763 mm Hg).

Factors affecting intrapulmonary pressure

a. *Valsalva maneuver*: Forced expiration against a closed glottis, may produce a positive intrapulmonary pressure of 100 mm Hg above atmospheric pressure.
b. *Müller's maneuver*: Forced inspiration against a closed glottis, can reduce the intrapulmonary to 80 mm Hg below the atmospheric pressure.

Intrapleural (Intrathoracic) Pressure

The pressure in the 'space' between the lungs and the chest wall (intrapleural space) is called intrapleural pressure. This pressure is subatmospheric and is not uniform throughout the thoracic cavity due to the effect of gravity. It is –2 mm Hg at the base and –7 mm Hg at the apex.

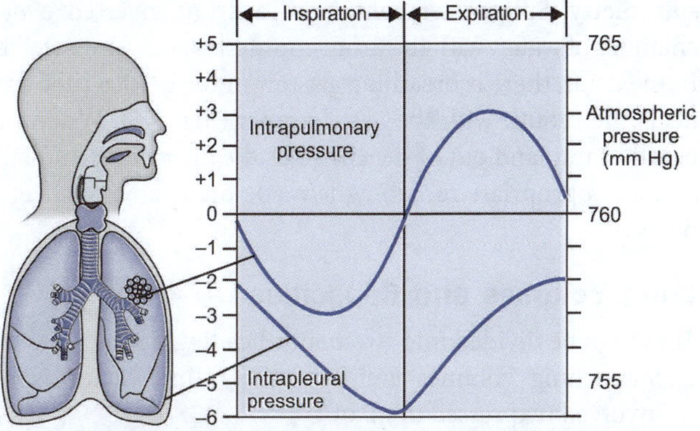

Fig. 3.5: Changes in the intrapulmonary and intrapleural pressure during the respiratory cycle

PHYSICON—The Reliable Icon in Physiology

The negative intrapleural pressure is directly proportional to amount of thoracic expansion. Therefore during quiet inspiration, the lungs are pulled into a more expanded position causing the intrapleural pressure to decrease to about -6 mm Hg. At the end of inspiration, the muscles of inspiration relax and the intrapleural pressure becomes less negative and the lungs recoil thereby intrapulmonary pressure increases.

Factors affecting intrapleural pressure

a. Deep inspiration decreases it as much as 30 mm Hg, subatmospheric (730 mm Hg).
b. *Effect of gravity:* The intrapleural pressure in standing position is more negative (–7 mm Hg) at the apices of the lungs compared to the bases (–2 mm Hg).

Transpulmonary Pressure

It is the difference between the alveolar pressure and the pleural pressure. It is the pressure difference between the pressure in the alveoli and that on the outer surfaces of the lungs. It is a measure of the elastic forces in the lungs that tend to collapse the lungs at each instant of respiration called the recoil pressure.

Clinical Significance

1. Since the transmural pressure, i.e. pressure gradient between intrapulmonary and intrapleural pressure is less at the bases, therefore, the lungs are less expanded at the bases.
2. Emphysema, i.e. loss or decrease in lung elasticity which increases intrapleural pressure thereby chest expands becomes barrel-shaped.
3. Injury to thorax causes entry of air between two layers of pleura, therefore intrapleural pressure equal to atmospheric pressure. Thereby lungs collapses (pneumothorax).

Spirometry

Pulmonary ventilation is studied by recording the volume movement of air into and out of the lungs—a process called spirometry. Spirometer consists of a drum inverted over a chamber of water, with the drum counterbalanced by a weight. In the drum there is breathing gas (air or oxygen); a tube connects the mouth with the gas chamber (Fig. 3.6). When one breathes into and out of the chamber the drum rises and falls, and an appropriate recording is made on a moving sheet of paper.

Lung Volumes and Capacities

These can be divided into two major headings:

1. Static lung volumes and capacities—time factor is not involved (expressed in ml or L).
2. Dynamic lung volumes and capacities—time dependent, (expressed in ml/min or L/min).

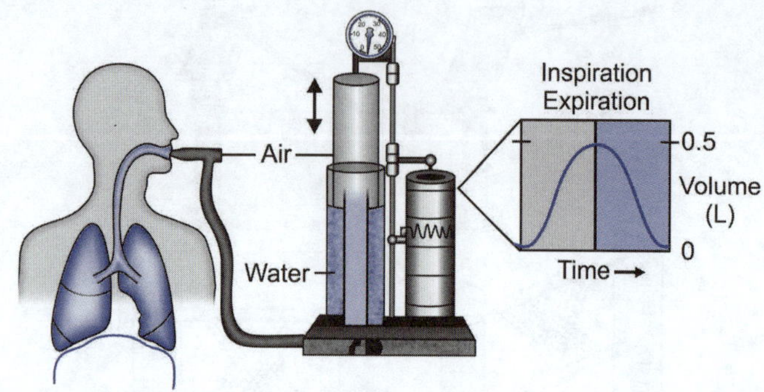

Fig. 3.6: Spirometry

Static Lung Volume and Capacities (Fig. 3.7, Table 3.1)

Volumes

1. *Tidal volume (TV):* It is the volume of air breathed in or out of lungs, during normal quiet respiration. Normal TV is 500 ml (0.5 L in men and women). The TV increases in muscular exercise and it decreases in respiratory muscle weakness or depression of respiratory center.
2. *Inspiratory reserve volume (IRV):* The air inspired with a maximal inspiratory effort in excess of the tidal volume, i.e. the maximal volume of air that can be inspired after completing a normal tidal inspiration. Normal IRV is 3.3 L in men and 1.9 L in women.
3. *Expiratory reserve volume (ERV):* The volume of air expelled by an active expiratory effort after passive expiration, i.e. the maximal volume of air which can be expired after a normal tidal expiration. Normal ERV is 1.0 L in men and 0.7 L in women.
4. *Residual volume (RV):* The air left in the lungs after a maximal expiratory effort. Normal RV is 1.2 L in men and 1.1 L in women.

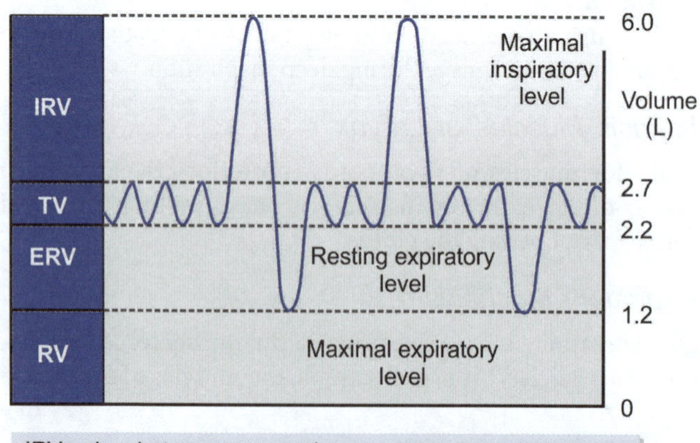

Fig. 3.7: Lung volumes and capacities

Table 3.1: Respiratory volumes and capacities for an average young adult male

Measurement	Typical value	Definition
		Respiratory volumes
Tidal volume (TV)	500 ml	Amount of air inhaled or exhaled in one breath during relaxed, quiet breathing
Inspiratory reserve volume (IRV)	3000 ml	Amount of air in excess of tidal inspiration that can be inhaled with maximum effort
Expiratory reserve volume (ERV)	1200 ml	Amount of air in excess of tidal expiration that can be exhaled with maximum effort
Residual volume (RV)	1200 ml	Amount of air remaining in the lungs after maximum expiration, keeps alveoli inflated between breaths and mixes with fresh air on next inspiration
		Respiratory capacities
Vital capacity (VC)	4700 ml	Amount of air that can be exhaled with maximum effort after maximum inspiration (ERV + TV + IRV), used to assess strength of thoracic muscles as well as pulmonary function
Inspiratory capacity (IC)	3500 ml	Maximum amount of air that can be inhaled after a normal tidal expiration (TV + IRV)
Functional residual capacity (FRC)	2400 ml	Amount of air remaining in the lungs after a normal tidal expiration (RV + ERV)
Total lung capacity (TLC)	5900 ml	Maximum amount of air the lungs can contain (RV + VC)

5. *Closing volume:* It is the lung volume above residual volume at which airways in the lower, dependent parts of the lung begin to close off because of the lesser transmural pressure in these areas.
6. *Pulmonary ventilation/Respiratory minute volume (RMV):* It is the amount of air inspired per minute. Normal RMV is 6.0 L (500 ml/breath × 12 breaths/min).

Capacities

1. *Inspiratory capacity (IC):* It is the maximal volume of air which can be inspired after completing tidal expiration, i.e. from the end-expiratory position. IC = TV + IRV. Normal IC is 3.8 L in men and 2.4 L in women. *Range:* 2.5 L–3.7 L.
2. *Expiratory capacity (EC):* It is the maximal volume of air which can be expired after completing tidal inspiration, i.e. from the end-inspiratory position. EC = TV + ERV. Normal EC is 1.5 L in men and 1.2 in women. *Range:* 1.25 L–1.5 L.
3. *Vital capacity (VC):* The largest amount of air that can be forcefully expired after a maximal inspiratory effort, which is frequently measured clinically as an index of pulmonary function.

Advantages of vital capacity

- It gives useful information about the strength of the respiratory muscles; therefore maximal inspiratory and expiratory efforts can be assessed.
- It gives useful information about other aspects of function through FEV1
  VC = TV + IRV + ERV. Normal VC is 4.8 L in men, 3.1 L in women.

Factors affecting vital capacity

Physiological

- Physical dimension, i.e. size and development of the subject. The VC more in males (2.6 L /m^2 BSA) than in females (2.1 L/m^2 BSA) because of large chest size, more muscle power, more body surface area (BSA).
- As age increases VC decreases due to loss of elasticity of lungs.
- Strength of respiratory muscles—VC increases in swimmers and divers.
- Pregnancy—VC decreases.
- Posture—in standing position VC is more than sitting or lying posture.

Pathological

- The VC decreases in diseases of the respiratory apparatus. For example, poliomyelitis, pulmonary fibrosis, pulmonary edema, pneumothorax, etc.
- Ascites, the accumulation of fluid in the abdominal cavity causes VC to decrease.
- *Functional residual capacity (FRC):* It is the volume of air which is contained in the lungs at end-expiratory position, i.e. after completion of tidal expiration. FRC = RV + ERV. Normal FRC is 2.2 L in men and 1.8 L in women.
- *Total lung capacity (TLC):* It is the volume of air contained in the lungs after a maximal inspiration. TLC = VC+ RV or TLC = TV + IRV + ERV + RV. Normal: TLC is 6.0 L in males and 4.2 L in women.
- *Maximal voluntary ventilation/Maximal breathing capacity (MVV):* It is the largest volume of air that can be moved into and out of the lungs in 1 min by voluntary effort. Normal MVV 125–170 L /min.

- *Breathing reserve (BR) or Pulmonary reserve (PR):* It is the maximum amount of air above the pulmonary ventilation, which can be breathed in or out of lungs in one minute. The BR = MVV–RMV.

Dynamic Lung Volumes and Capacities

Timed vital capacity (TVC) or forced vital capacity (FVC)

Forced vital capacity is the maximal volume of air that can be breathed out as 'forcefully' and 'rapidly' as possible following a maximum inspiration. The TVC similar to VC except that there is a special stress on rapid, forcible and complete exhalation.

Components of TVC (FVC)

a. *FEV_1 (Forced expiratory volume in 1 sec):* The fraction of the vital capacity expired during the 1st second of a forced expiration or it is the volume of FVC expired in 1st sec of exhalation. Normal: 80% of FVC (Fig. 3.8).
b. *FEV_2 (Forced expiratory volume in 2 sec):* The volume of FVC expired in first-two seconds of exhalation. Normal: 95% of FVC.
c. *FEV_3 (Forced expiratory volume in 3 sec):* The volume of FVC expired in first three seconds of exhalation. Normal: 98–100% of FVC.

Clinical significance of FVC

To distinguish between restrictive and obstructive lung disorders.

Lung volumes alter in many lung diseases as follows:

- *Obstructive lung diseases:* In obstructive lung diseases like COPD, bronchial asthma, obstruction of airways occurs mainly in expiration. So, air tends to enter the lung easily (as inspiration is less affected) but then becomes trapped in the lung over a period of months or year, this increases total lung capacity, residual volume (RV) and functional residual capacity (FRC). Due to obstruction, FEV1 is decreased and vital capacity is also decreased later. The characteristic feature of COPD is early decrease of FEV1 and out of proportion to vital capacity/ forced vital capacity. Therefore, FEV1/FVC is decreased. The most important COPD is emphysema.
- *Restrictive lung diseases:* These diseases are characterized by decreased lung compliance and constricted lungs. Therefore, all volumes and capacity are decreased. TLC, FEV1, VC/FVC, RV, FRC all are reduced. FEV1 is decreased in proportion or slightly less than FRV; therefore, FEV1/FVC is either normal or slightly increased. Interstitial lung diseases (like pneumoconiosis, interstitial pneumonitis, sarcoidosis) and pulmonary fibrosis, kyphoscoliosis, ankylosing spondylitis (affects vertebral column) are restrictive lung diseases (Fig. 3.9).

Note: The FEV_1 is much more sensitive index (i.e. most reproducible) of the severity of obstructive lung disorders, but it does not allow for the differentiation of the various causes for the obstruction.

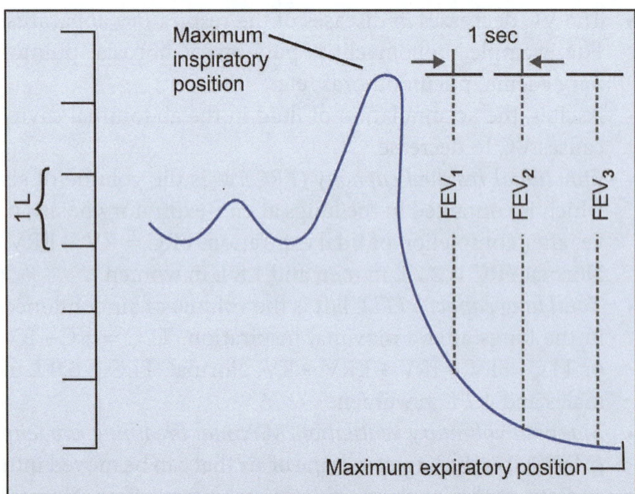

Fig. 3.8: Timed vital capacity

Surfactants

It is a lipid surface tension lowering agent lining the alveoli.

Composition

It is a mixture of protein-lipid complexes made up of mainly dipalmitoylphosphatidylcholine (DPPC) lipid along with other lipids (phosphatidyl glycine, phospholipids, neutral lipids) and proteins (Table 3.2).

Synthesis of Surfactant

Surfactant is produced by type II alveolar epithelial cells. Laminar bodies containing phospholipids are formed in these cell are secreted into the alveolar lumen by exocytosis in the form of tubes of lipids called tubular myelin. The lipid are later

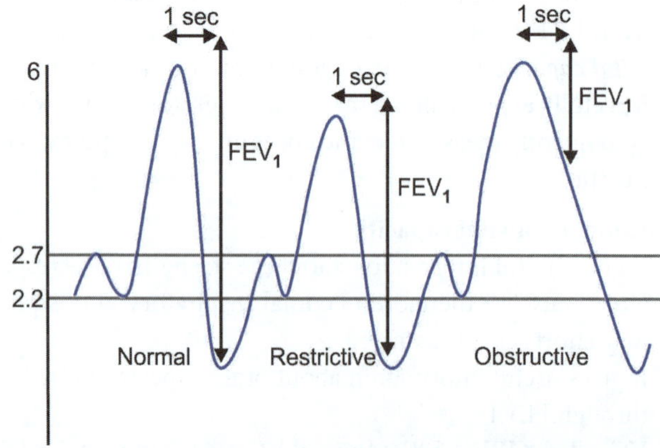

Fig. 3.9: FEV_1 in normal, restrictive and obstructive patients

Table 3.2: Composition of surfactant

Component	% Composition
Dipalmitoylphosphatidylcholine	62
Phosphatidylglycerol	5
Other phospholipids	10
Neutral lipids	13
Proteins	8
Carbohydrate	2

converted into phospholipids, which is the major constituent of surfactant. The surfactants are then taken by the alveolar macrophages. Some of the protein-lipid complexes are taken up by the type II alveolar cells and cycled (Fig. 3.10). Formation of the phospholipid film is greatly enhanced by the proteins in the surfactant. This material contains four unique proteins: SP-A, SP-B, SP-C and SP-D.

Factors Affecting Surfactant Synthesis

1. Thyroid hormone increases the production of surfactant.
2. Glucocorticoid influence production and maturation of surfactant.
3. Insulin inhibit synthesis of surfactant.
4. Smoking reduces surfactant.

Functions of Surfactant

1. *Reduction of surface tension:* According to the Law of Laplace in a spherical structure like alveoli, distenting pressure (P) equals to two times the tension, T (surface tension on walls) divide by the radius (R).

$$P = \frac{2T}{R}$$

Surface tension is due to the intermolecular attraction between the surface molecules and thus it tries to reduce surface area and collapses the lungs. Hence this surface tension must be reduced especially during expiration. Otherwise, the lungs will collapse.

Surface tension (T) is the inward force. Therefore, with 'P' constant if the 'T' is not reduced as 'R' is reduced during expiration, surface tension may overcome the distending pressure and then lungs will collapse. But in lungs, with reduction of radius, there is reduction of surface tension by a surface tension lowering agent called surfactant.

Surface tension is inversely related to the concentration of surfactant per unit area. Surfactant molecules are spread apart as alveolar size increases during inspiration but come closer during expiration thereby adjusting surface tension during breathing. Its action is more effective during expiration than during inspiration. Surface tension between the fluid and the air is 7–14 times more than between the surfactant and the air.

2. *It maintains stability of the alveoli:* Surfactant reduces surface tension so that alveoli do not collapse. In absence of surfactant air will tend to move from smaller alveoli (where pressure is more) to large aleveoli (where pressure is low) leading to collapse of small alveoli and overdistention of large alveoli (Fig. 3.11).
3. Surfactant also helps to prevent pulmonary edema by reducing surface tension.
4. Surfactant keeps the alveoli dry and thus helps in the exchange of gases.

Clinical Significance

1. *Infant respiratory distress syndrome (IRDS) or Hyaline membrane disease:* Infants especially premature and infants born to diabetic mother have deficiency of surfactant in their alveoli and there is increased surface tension. Surfactant normally appears at the 28th week of gestation and mature just before 36th week. After birth, the infant makes several strong inspiratory movements and the lung expand. Surfactant keeps them from collapsing again. So

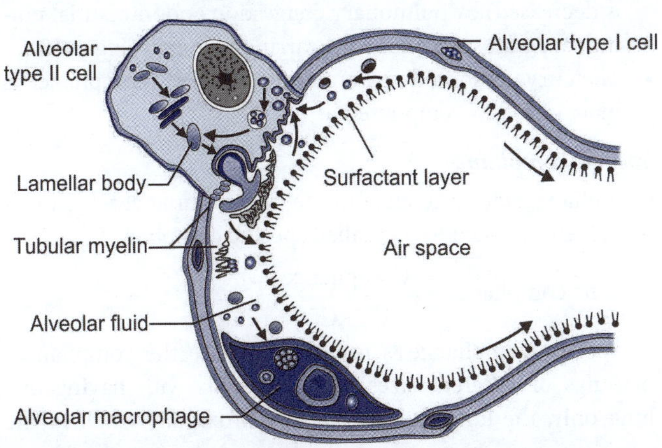

Fig. 3.10: Synthesis of surfactant

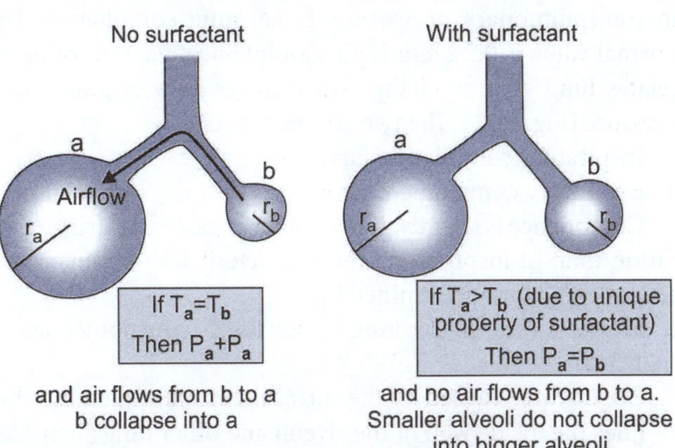

Fig. 3.11: Action of surfactant

deficiency of surfactant causes both collapsing of alveoli in many areas (atelectasis) and pulmonary edema. Other factors that cause IRDS are:

i. Low level of thyroid and glucocorticoids.
ii. During fetal life, Cl^- is secreted with fluid by the pulmonary epithelial cells. At birth, there is a shift to Na^+ absorption by these cells via epithelial Na^+ channels (ENaCs), and fluid is absorbed with the Na^+. Prolonged immaturity of the ENaCs contributes to the pulmonary abnormalities in IRDS.

2. *Patchy atelectasis:* Seen in patients who have undergone cardiac surgery, during which a pump oxygenator is used and the pulmonary circulation is interrupted.

Compliance

The lung and the thoracic cage are both elastic structures. Hence, they display a constant relationship between distending pressure and change in volume.

The change in lung volume per unit change in airway pressure ($\Delta V/\Delta P$) is the 'stretchability' (compliance) of the lungs and the chest wall.

Where, V= volume of the lung, P = airway pressure, Δ= the difference. It is expressed as liter/cm H_2O.

Factors Influencing Compliance

- Elasticity of lung
- Changes in lumen size
- Surfactants and surface tension
- Blood supply
- Interdependence
- Chest wall size, shape, deformity, infections and nerve damage

Compliance is studied under two headings:

1. Compliance of the lungs only
2. Compliance of the lungs and thoracic wall.

Compliance of Lung

The extent to which the lung will expand for each unit increase in transpulmonary pressure is called lung compliance. The normal value is 0.2 L/cm H_2O. Compliance diagram of lungs relates lung volume changes to changes in transpulmonary pressure (Fig. 3.12). The two curves are called

1. Inspiratory compliance curve
2. Expiratory compliance curve.

Compliance is slightly greater when measured during expiration than in inspiration. The characteristics of the compliance diagram are determined by:

a. Elastic forces of the lung tissue itself (contributes about 1/3rd).
b. Elastic force caused by the surface tension of the fluid that lines the inside wall of the alveoli and other lung air spaces (contributes about 2/3rd). Therefore, lowering of surface tension by the surfactant improves the distensibility of the lungs, i.e. surfactant increases the compliance of lungs.

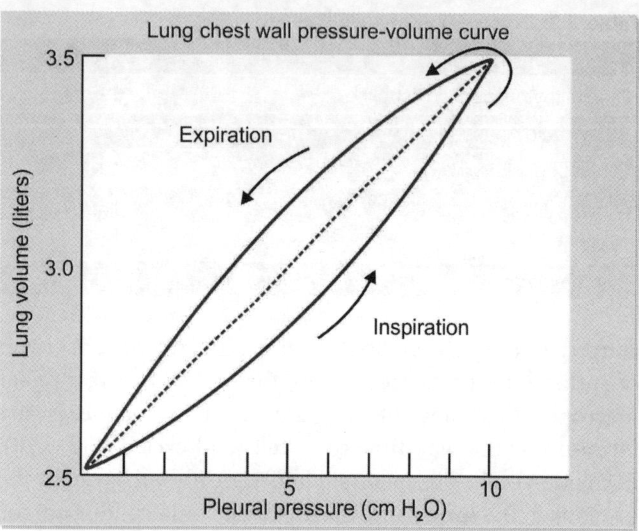

Fig. 3.12: Compliance of lung (Pressure/volume relationship)

Elastic force of the lung is determined mainly by elastin and collagen in the lung parenchyma.

Compliance of Lung and Thoracic Wall

It is the compliance of the entire pulmonary system. It is measured while expanding the lungs of a totally relaxed or paralyzed person. To inflate this total pulmonary system, almost twice as much pressure is needed as to inflate the same lungs after removal from chest cage. Normal value—0.11 liter/cm H_2O, it signifies that when there is an increase of airway pressure by 1 cm H_2O, then the volume of the lungs inside the thoracic wall increases by 0.13 liter.

Note

- The curve is shifted downward and to the right (compliance is decreased) by pulmonary congestion and interstitial pulmonary fibrosis (stiffening, scarring of lungs) (Fig. 3.13).
- The curve is shifted upward and to the left (compliance is increased) as in emphysema.

Specific compliance

Compliance with reference to the lung volume at which it is measured (i.e. the FRC) is called specific compliance.

$$\text{Specific compliance} = \frac{\text{Compliance}}{\text{FRC}}$$

Specific compliance is used to compare the compliances of lungs of different sizes. In individuals with having one lung only, the lung compliance is approximately half of the

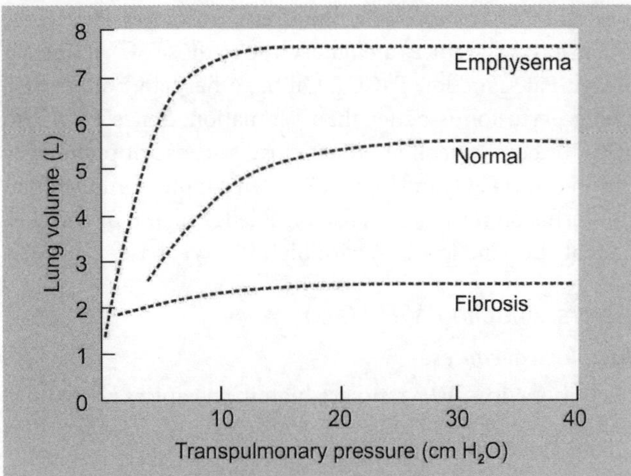

Fig. 3.13: Compliance in emphysema and fibrosis compared to normal

normal compliance. Similarly in children because of smaller lung volume, compliance will be below normal inspite of normal distensibility. This confusion is removed with specific compliance since 'FRC' is proportionately reduced and specific compliance remains essentially constant.

Dead Space and its Significance

It is the amount of air in the 'respiratory passage' which does not take part in exchange of gases.
It is of two types:

1. Anatomical Dead Space (150 ml)

It is the volume of air present in the 'conducting zone' of the respiratory passage which is from nose and mouth up to terminal bronchioles. It is the respiratory system volume exclusive of alveoli. Here there is no exchange of gases.

Normal value

Anatomical dead space value is approximately the body weight in pounds. For example, in a man who weighs 150 lb (68 Kg), only the first 350 ml of the 500 ml inspired with each breath at rest mixes with the air in the alveoli, i.e. the 150 ml of the expired gas is from the dead space.

2. Physiological Dead Space/Total Dead Space

It includes anatomical dead space plus volume of air in the alveoli which does not take part in exchange of gases (i.e wasted alveolar ventilation). It is the volume of gas not equilibrating with blood.

Note: Clinically anatomical and physiological dead spaces are same in healthy subjects. If ventilation and perfusion are not in equilibrium, then only they differ in volume.

Variations

Physiological

a. *Sex:* Dead space is more in males.
b. *Age:* Dead space increases as age increases (inflated lungs pull the airways, increasing the airway diameter).
c. *Body height:* Dead space is directly proportional body height.

Pathological

a. *Emphysema*—loss of elasticity of lungs decreases elastic recoil. Produces hyperinflation of lungs which causes increase in dead space.
b. *Bronchiectasis*—it is associated with dilated bronchi leading to increase in dead space.

Alveolar Ventilation

It is the amount of air ventilating the alveoli per minute. But dead space reduces the volume of air reaching the alveoli and participating gas exchange. So,

Alveolar ventilation =
(Tidal volume – Dead space) × Respiratory rate

i.e. normal alveolar ventilation = (500 – 150) × 12 = 4.2 L /min.

Alveolar ventilation represents the amount of air reaching the alveoli. This is the air that takes part in gas exchange. Even in the absence of lung diseases, if anatomic dead space volume is increased due to any cause, alveolar ventilation decreases. For example, a patient on mechanical ventilator, alveolar ventilation decreases due to increased dead space volume (by tubing, etc.). In such patients, if minute ventilation remains constant, alveolar gas exchange suffers.

Physiological Significance of Alveolar Ventilation

In rapid and shallow breathing, though minute ventilation does not change much, alveolar ventilation is grossly impaired because most of the air inhaled is utilized to occupy the anatomic dead space (the air available to enter into alveoli is less).

- Therefore, patients with rapid and shallow breathing develop hypoxia and hypercapnea.
- In contrast, a subject with deep and slow breathing will have adequate alveolar ventilation though the minute ventilation does not change much. Such subjects have alveolar ventilation even greater than subjects with normal breathing. Thus, to improve alveolar ventilation, it is important to increase the depth of breathing than to increase the frequency. In fact, during moderate to severe exercise, a trained athlete achieves the target alveolar ventilation by mainly increasing the depth rather than the frequency of breathing.

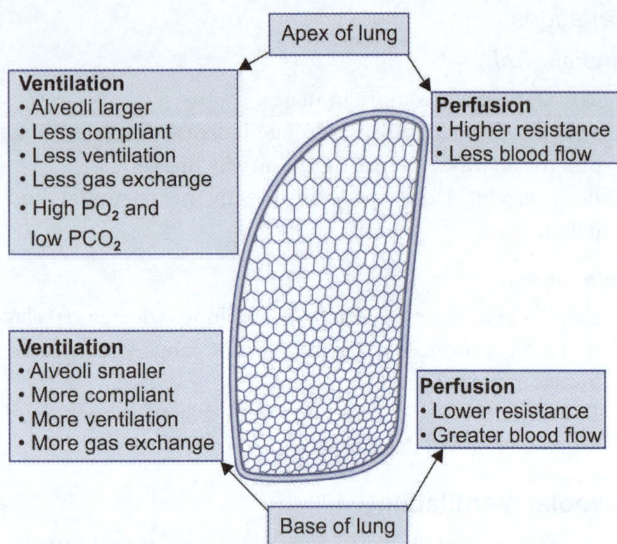

Fig. 3.14: Differences in ventilation—perfusion ratio in apex and base of lung

Ventilation-Perfusion (V/P) Ratio

The normal pulmonary blood flow (pulmonary perfusion) is the same as the right ventricular output, i.e. about 5.0 L/min. Considering that cardiac output is 5.0 L/min and alveolar ventilation is about 4.2 L/min, the overall ventilation—perfusion ratio is 0.8. This ratio of 0.8 is average for the entire lung. However, two different scenarios exist, one at the apex and another at the base.

It is very clear from the Figure 3.14 that both ventilation and perfusion are more in the base of lung than at the apex of lung. From apex to base, ventilation increases about 2.5 times but blood flow increases 4 times. That is the fall in perfusion at the apex is more than the fall in ventilation at the apex of lung. Perfusion is in denominator. Therefore, V/Q is maximum at apex (about 3.5) and least at base (about 0.5). Hence, apical alveoli are more underperfused than underventilated while the basal alveoli are more overperfused than overventilated.

- **At the apex:** Perfusion is low because heart has to pump against gravity toward apex of the lung. Hence the V/Q ratio is high (3.5). It means that the ventilation is not matched by enough perfusion; some of the ventilation is wasted due to inadequate blood flow. This is called 'physiologic dead space'.
- **At the base:** Perfusion is much greater compared to ventilation. The VA/Q ratio is low, about 0.5; this is called physiologic shunt. (There is blood flow but no adequate ventilation to match the blood flow. Hence some of the blood is 'shunted past the alveoli' without picking up oxygen.)

Since ventilation is far in excess of perfusion at apex, comparatively little oxygen is transferred from the alveoli to the blood and CO_2 transferred to the alveoli is also less. Hence, the gas tension at the apices are quiet close to those of inspired air, i.e. high PaO_2 and low $PaCO_2$. On the other hand, at the base of lung perfusion is better than ventilation; hence PaO_2 and $PaCO_2$ of basal alveoli are quiet close to those of pulmonary artery, i.e. low PaO_2 and high $PaCO_2$. In simple words, ventilation-perfusion mismatch is responsible for high PO_2 with low PCO_2 at apex and low PO_2 with high PCO_2 at base.

Factors Affecting V/P Ratio

Physiological causes

Effect of gravity—V/P ratio are high in the apical portions of the lung.

Pathological causes

All the factors which cause uneven alveolar ventilation or non-uniform blood flow to pulmonary circulation will alter the V/P ratio. For example:

- Bronchial asthma, pneumothorax, emphysema (causes of uneven alveolar ventilation).
- Fallot's tetrology, pulmonary embolism (causes of non-uniform pulmonary blood flow).

Clinical Note

It is said that the high V/P ratio at the apices account for the predilection of tuberculosis (TB) for this area because high alveolar pO_2 provides a favorable environment for the growth of tuberculosis bacteria.

Physiological Shunt and its Significance

When VA/Q, i.e. the ratio of alveolar ventilation to blood flow is below normal, there is inadequate ventilation to provide the O_2 needed to fully oxygenate the blood flowing through the alveolar capillaries. Therefore, a certain fraction of the venous blood passing through the pulmonary capillaries does not become oxygenated. This fraction is called shunted blood.

1. Although some of the bronchial vessels (bronchial arteries, branches of the thoracic aorta) enters the bronchial veins, some enters the pulmonary capillaries and veins, bypassing the right ventricle.
2. Blood that flows from the coronary arteries into the left side of the heart.

In this two exceptions, a physiological shunt is created and the blood in the systemic arteries has a pO_2 (Fig. 3.15) about 2 mm Hg lower than that of blood which has equalibrated with alveolar air. The greater the physiologic shunt, the greater the amount of blood that fails to be oxygenated as it passes through the lungs.

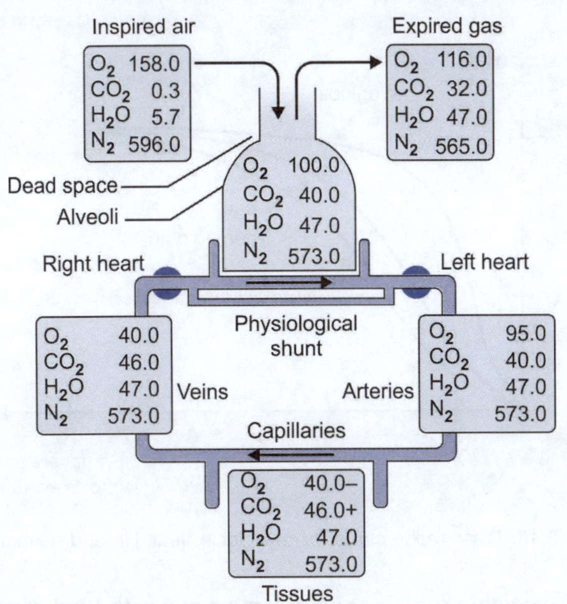

Fig. 3.15: Partial pressures of gases (mm Hg) in various parts of respiratory and in the circulatory system

TRANSPORT OF GASES

Oxygen Transport

Oxygen is transported in the blood in two forms.

1. *In dissolved form:* In dissolved form the amount of oxygen transported is 0.3 ml/100 ml of blood per 100 mm Hg pO_2. The dissolved O_2 obeys the Henry's law, i.e. amount dissolved is proportional to the pO_2. Dissolved O_2 asssumes its practical importance in case of hyperbaric O_2 therapy when this amount can be increased by giving O_2 at high pressure as in the treatment of CO poisoning, gas gangrene (here Hb gets denatured).
2. *In combination with hemoglobin:* Each Hb molecule has four heme groups which have an iron in ferrous form. The sixth valency bond of each Fe^{2+} combines with 1 mole (2 atoms) of O_2. Therefore, 4 moles (8 atoms) of O_2 combine with 1 mole of Hb. The O_2 carrying power of Hb is given by O_2-Hb dissociation curve (ODC curve). It is a curve relating percentage O_2 saturation of the Hb to the pO_2. The curve has a characteristic sigmoid shape due to shifting affinity of Hb for O_2.

In deoxy-Hb, the globin portion is tightly bound in a tense (T) configuration thereby reducing the affinity of the molecule for O_2. Combination of molecule with O_2 releases the bonds holding the globin units, producing a relaxed (R) configuration This results in the exposure of more O_2 binding sites and thereby the affinity of Hb molecule with O_2 increases. Since the 4 atoms of Fe^{2+} do not combine with O_2 simultaneously we do not get a vertical line. The combination is a step wise process and the affinity for O_2 is different at different steps.

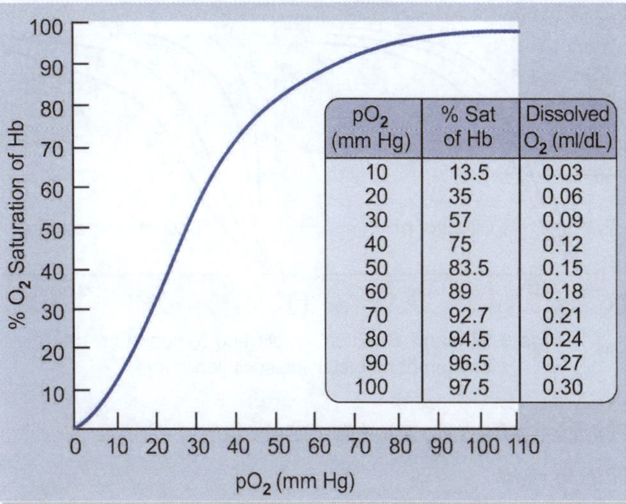

pO_2 (mm Hg)	% Sat of Hb	Dissolved O_2 (ml/dL)
10	13.5	0.03
20	35	0.06
30	57	0.09
40	75	0.12
50	83.5	0.15
60	89	0.18
70	92.7	0.21
80	94.5	0.24
90	96.5	0.27
100	97.5	0.30

Fig. 3.16: Oxygen-hemoglobin dissociation curve

The combination of 1st heme in the Hb molecule with O_2 increases the affinity of 2nd heme for O_2 and so on.

This shifting affinity of Hb for O_2 due to T-R interconversion produces the characteristic sigmoid curve (Fig. 3.16). This phenomenon is referred to as Heme-Heme Interaction.

Physiological Advantages of S-Shaped Curve

- It allows greater uptake of O_2 at lungs despite great variation in alveolar air pO_2 (from 95 to 60 mm Hg).
- When pO_2 is below 60 mm Hg, a small fall in pO_2 causes significant reduction in percent saturation of Hb. This means that peripheral tissue can withdraw large amount of O_2 for a small drop in tissue capillary pO_2. This behavior of Hb enables uptake of O_2 in lung where pO_2 is high and release of O_2 into tissue where pO_2 is low.

Note

1. *O_2 content:* It is the actual amount of O_2 present in the sample of blood (19.4 ml /100 ml, when 97.5% saturated).
2. *O_2 carrying capacity:* The maximum amount of O_2 that a particular amount of blood can combine with at full saturation. A 1 gm Hb can combine with 1.34 ml of O_2 (at max pO_2 of approx 120 mm Hg). Since the average Hb concentration is 15 gm%, therefore 100 ml of blood can carry, $1.34 \times 15 = 20.1$ ml (at full saturation).
3. Percentage saturation of Hb is given by the formulae = (O_2 content/O_2 capacity) × 100. Normally it is 97.5%.
4. *Utilization coefficient:* The percentage of the blood that gives up its O_2 as it passes through the tissue capillaries is called utilization coefficient. Normal value: 25%. During strenuous exercise, the utilization coefficient increases up to 75–80%. In some area where blood flow is extremely slow or metabolic rate is very high, utilization coefficient is approximately 100%.

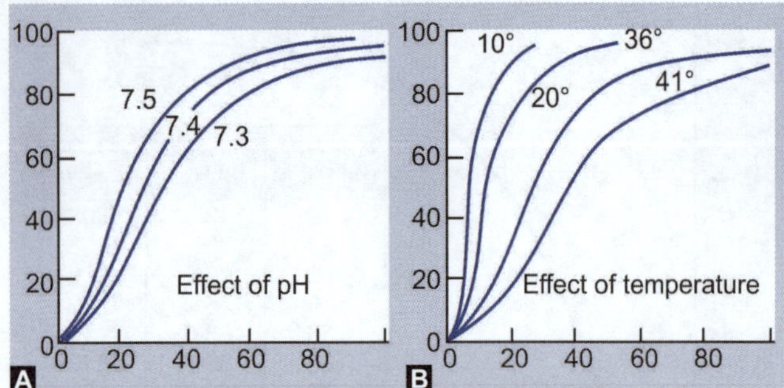

Figs 3.17A and B: Effect of pH and temperature on oxygen-hemoglobin dissociation curve

Factors Affecting O_2-Hb Dissociation Curve

Shift to right

A shift to right occurs if affinity of Hb for O_2 decreases.

Causes

1. Fall in blood pH/increase in H^+ (Fig. 3.17A).
2. Increase in CO_2 (respiratory/metabolic cause).
3. Increase in temperature (Fig. 3.17B).
4. Increase in the concentration of 2,3 DPG.

The 2,3 DPG is a product of glycolysis. It is a highly charged anion that binds to - β chains of deoxy-Hb. It competes with O_2 for the binding sites on the Hb molecule and therefore at a given pO_2 the percent saturation of Hb with O_2 will be reduced in the presence of 2,3 DPG.

Bohr effect

Increased CO_2 content of blood helps to release more O_2 from Hb. This is called Bohr effect. It can also be explained as the decrease in the O_2 affinity of Hb when the pH of blood falls. The Bohr effect is useful during physical exercise, when more CO_2 is produced and more O_2 is delivered to tissues, i.e. an active tissue gets more O_2.

Shift to left

A shift to left occurs when the affinity of Hb towards O_2 increases.

Causes

1. Decrease in body temperature.
2. Increase in blood pH (decrease in CO_2).
3. Fetal Hb (HbF).
4. Myoglobin.
5. Decrease in concentration of 2,3 DPG.
6. Carbon monoxide (CO).

Affinity of fetal Hb (HbF) for 2,3 DPG is considerably less than that of HbA (poor binding of 2,3 DPG by γ polypeptide chain). So HbF shifts the curve to the left, i.e. a lower pO_2 is required to bind a given amount of O_2. Thus, the affinity of HbF to combine with O_2 is more than that of HbA.

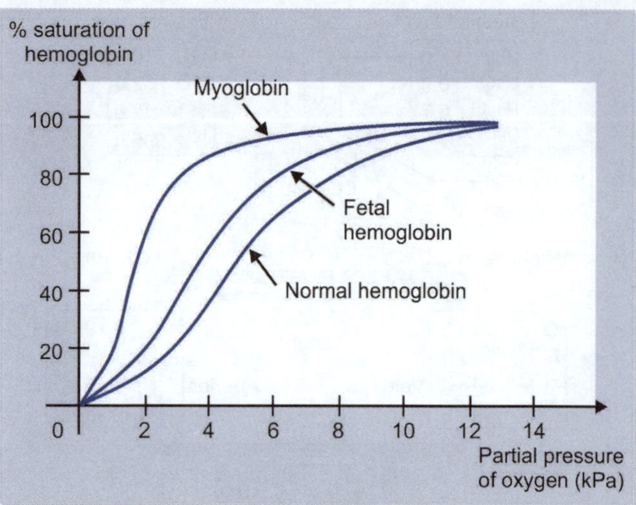

Fig. 3.18: Dissociation curve for myoglobin, fetal Hb and normal Hb

Myoglobin contains only 1 heme group with 1 polypeptide chain, i.e. 1 atom of iron per molecule (MW=1/4 MW of Hb). Its dissociation curve is rectangular hyperbola. It takes up O_2 from Hb in the blood and releases O_2 only at low pO_2 values, i.e. rate of association of myoglobin with O_2 is very fast. It does not show Bohr effect (Fig. 3.18).

CO shifts the curve to left due to inhibition of synthesis of 2, 3 DPG. Affinity of 'CO' to combine with Hb is 200 times more than that of O_2. Due to larger proportions of carboxyhemoglobin (COHb) formed Hb is unavailable for O_2 carriage.

Significance of P_{50}

P_{50} means the pO_2 at which the Hb is half (50%) saturated with O_2. Normal value is 26 mm Hg, at pCO_2 40 mm Hg, pH 7.4 and temperature 37°C. It helps to determine the Hb affinity for O_2. Hb affinity for O_2 is an inverse function of P_{50} value, i.e. the higher the P_{50}, the lower the affinity of Hb for O_2.

CO_2 Transport

CO_2 is produced due to tissue activity and it enters the blood due to:

- Difference in pCO_2 between arterial blood and tissues (arterial blood pCO_2 = 40 mm Hg, tissues pCO_2 = 46 mm Hg).
- High diffusion coefficient of CO_2 as compared to O_2 (20 times more than that of O_2).

CO_2 is carried in three forms:

1. In Dissolved Form (0.3 ml%)

CO_2 is transported as dissolved form in both plasma and RBC. The venous blood, with pCO_2 46 mm Hg contains about 2.7 ml/100 ml of CO_2 in dissolved form. The arterial blood with pCO_2 40 mm Hg contains 2.4 ml/100 ml of CO_2 in dissolved form. Thus only 0.3 ml of CO_2 is transported in dissolved state per 100 ml of blood from tissues to the lungs. This represents about 7% of all CO_2 that is transported.

2. As Carbamino Compounds (0.7 ml%)

After entering the blood, some of the CO_2 combines with proteins in blood, both in plasma and cells.

In plasma

CO_2 combines directly with plasma proteins to form carbamino proteins. This is a slow reaction and only 0.1 ml% of CO_2 is transported in this form.

$$CO_2 + PrNH_2 \longrightarrow PrNHCOOH$$

In RBC

CO_2 combines with amino group of Hb to form carbamino Hb. This is a fast reaction and 0.6 ml% of CO_2 is transported in this form.

$$CO_2 + HbNH_2 \longrightarrow HbNHCOOH$$

Approximately 23% of the total CO_2 (0.7 ml%) is transported in the blood in the form of carbamino compounds.

3. As Bicarbonates (3 ml%)

It accounts for about 70% of the total CO_2 (3 ml%) transported from the tissues to the lungs. These bicarbonates are formed in the RBC and then diffuse into plasma. This is because RBC has the required enzyme carbonic anhydrase (CA). After entering the blood most of the CO_2 enters the RBC, where in the presence of CA, it rapidly reacts with water to form carbonic acid. Carbonic acid dissociates into bicarbonate ions and hydrogen ions.

$$CO_2 + H_2O \xrightarrow{CA} H_2CO_3 \longrightarrow H^+ + HCO_3^-$$

RBC membrane is relatively impermeable to cations. So H^+ combine with Hb. This enables the reaction to proceed in the forward direction and prevent the backward reaction. The HCO_3^- (70%) diffuse out of RBCs into plasma. Some HCO_3^- remains in the RBCs as well.

Chloride shift (Fig. 3.19)

When the HCO_3^- diffuses out of RBCs into the plasma, the inside of the cell become less negatively charged. To maintain electrical neutrality Cl^- ions diffuse from plasma into the RBC to replace the HCO_3^-. The movement of Cl^- into the RBC is called chloride shift or **Hamburger phenomenon**. This process is mediated by a membrane protein called band 3 protein. As a result of chloride shift, the total number of ions inside the RBCs increases, so the osmotic pressure inside the RBCs becomes higher than that of plasma. This draws water and the RBCs become slightly larger. Thus PCV of venous blood is slightly higher (3%) than that of arterial blood.

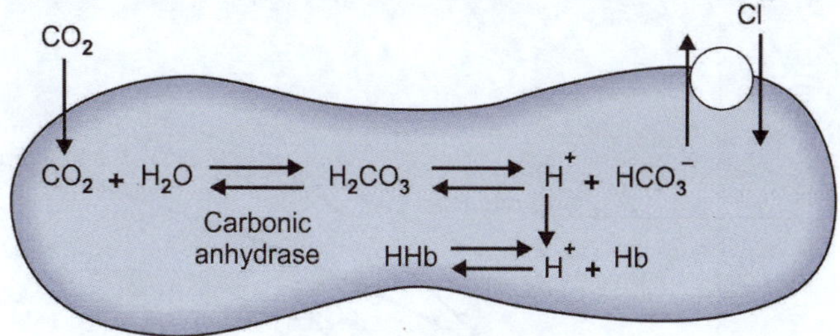

Fig. 3.19: Chloride shift

Summary of CO_2 Transport

Thus, out of about 52 ml% of CO_2 in venous blood, 4 ml% is given out in the lungs and the arterial blood contains about 48 ml%. Out of this 4 ml% 0.3 ml% is contributed by dissolved form, 0.7 ml% by carbamino compounds and 3 ml% by bicarbonate (Table 3.3).

Table 3.3: Amount of CO_2 held by different vehicles

Forms	Venous blood	Arterial blood
Dissolved form	2.7 ml%	2.4 ml%
Carbamino compound	3.7 ml%	3 ml%
Bicarbonate	45.6 ml%	42.6 ml%
Total	52 ml%	48 ml%

CO_2 Dissociation Curve (Fig. 3.20)

CO_2 dissociation curve is obtained by plotting the relationship between CO_2 and total CO_2 content of the blood. The graph shows that the relationship between the two is nearly linear over wider range of pCO_2 (compared to O_2-Hb dissociation curve which is sigmoid in shape). The pCO_2 of arterial and venous blood varies practically within a narrow range of

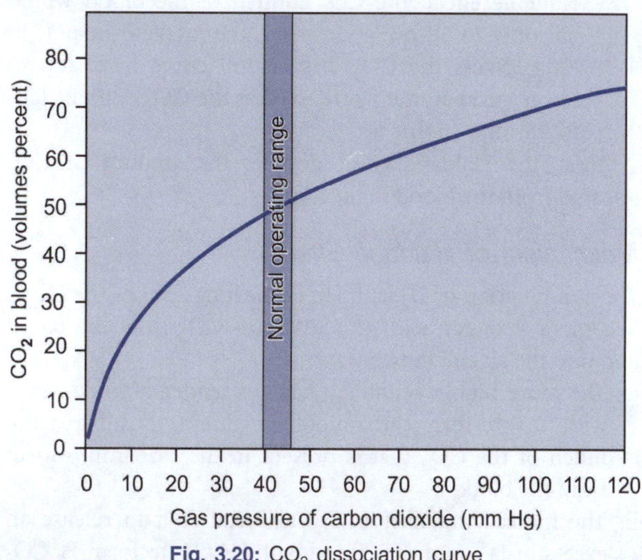

Fig. 3.20: CO_2 dissociation curve

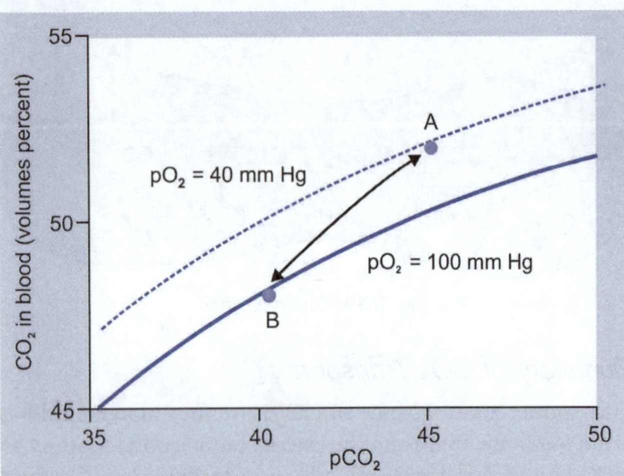

Fig. 3.21: Significance of Haldane effect on transport of CO_2 from tissue to the lungs

40–45 mm Hg. Binding of O_2 to Hb reduces its affinity for CO_2 from blood, shifting the CO_2 dissociation curve to right. This effect is called ***Haldane effect.***

Figure 3.21 demonstrates the significance of Haldane effect on the transport of CO_2 from the tissues to the lungs. Figure 3.21 shows small portions of two CO_2 dissociation curves.

1. When the pO_2 is 100 mm Hg, which is the case in blood capillaries of lungs.
2. When pO_2 is 40 mm Hg, which is the case in tissue capillaries.
   - Point A shows that the normal pCO_2 of 46 mm Hg in tissues causes 52 ml% of CO_2 to combine with the blood. On entering the lungs, pCO_2 falls to 40 mm Hg and the pO_2 rises to 100 mm Hg.
   - If the CO_2 dissociation curve did not shift because of Haldane effect, the CO_2 content of the blood would fall only to 50 ml%. However, the increase in pO_2 in lung lowers the CO_2 dissociation curve from top to lower curve in the figure, so that the CO_2 content falls to 48 ml% (point B).

Thus, the Haldane effect doubles the amount of CO_2 released from the blood in the lungs.

Mechanism of Haldane Effect

The combination of O_2 with Hb in the lungs causes the Hb to become a stronger acid. This displaces CO_2 from the blood and into the alveoli in two ways:

i. The more highly acidic Hb has less tendency to combine with CO_2 to form carbaminohemoglobin, thus displacing much of the CO_2 that is present in the carbamino form from the blood.
ii. The increased acidity of Hb also causes it to release an excess of H^+, and these bind with HCO_3^- to form H_2CO_3. Then this dissociates into H_2O and CO_2, and the CO_2 is released from the blood into the alveoli and finally into the air.

Clinical Note

Oxygen content is important in anemic patients. Oxygen content is more important than PO_2 and oxygen saturation for oxygenation of tissues, when the patient is anemic. A patient with Hb concentration 7g% or less may have a normal arterial PO_2 and Hb saturation but oxygen content will be grossly reduced. Oxygen saturation remains normal because oxygen content and capacity are proportionately reduced. Tissue suffers from hypoxia due to decreased oxygen content inspite of normal oxygen saturation.

REGULATION OF RESPIRATION

Spontaneous respiration is produced by rhythmic discharge of motor neurons that innervate the respiratory muscles. This discharge is totally dependent on nerve impulses from brain. During regulation of respiration, pulmonary ventilation is adjusted according to metabolic demands of the body. The metabolic demands are: (1) Supply of adequate O_2 to tissues, (2) Removal of CO_2 formed during metabolism and (3) Maintenance of optimum pH of blood.

Unlike all other organ system, respiration demonstrates automaticity as well as self modulation, i.e. we breath without thinking, but can willingly modify the breathing pattern. Rate, depth and rhythm of respiration is controlled by group of neurons situated reticular formation of brainstem. The collection of these neurons are called *respiratory center*. The rhythmic discharge from the brain that produces spontaneous respiration is regulated by two mechanisms: (1) Nervous regulatory mechanism and (2) Chemical regulatory mechanism.

Respiratory Centers

The rhythmic discharge is initiated by a group of pacemaker cells in the brainstem referred to as *Pre-Botzinger complex of neurons (PBZ)*. They are situated in either sides of medulla. These neurons discharge spontaneously and rhythmically. They produce rhythmic discharges in phrenic motor neurons. All the neurons regulating respiration project into PBZ (Fig. 3.22).

The respiratory centers are situated in the reticular formation of the brainstem and depending upon the situation in the brainstem, they are classified into medullary and pontine center. There are two centers in each group. Medullary centers include two group of neurons: the dorsal respiratory group (DRG), and ventral respiratory group (VRG) which generate the basic respiratory rhythm. The pontine centers include the apneustic center (APN) and pneumotaxic center (PNC), both of which modify the activity of medullary respiratory centers.

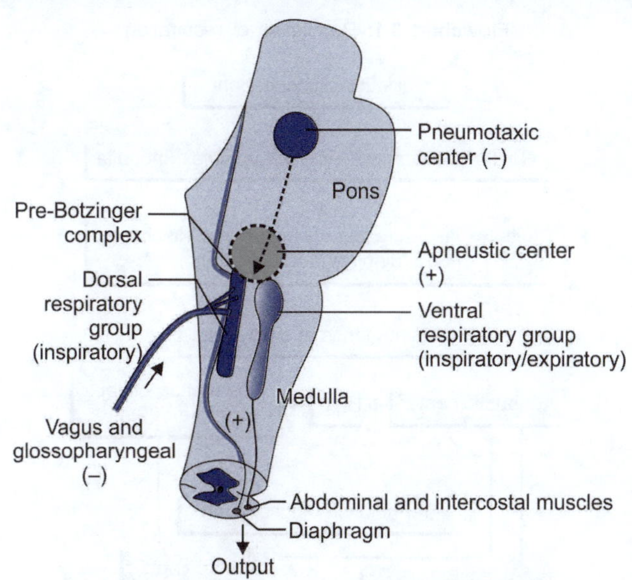

Fig. 3.22: Respiratory neurons in the brainstem

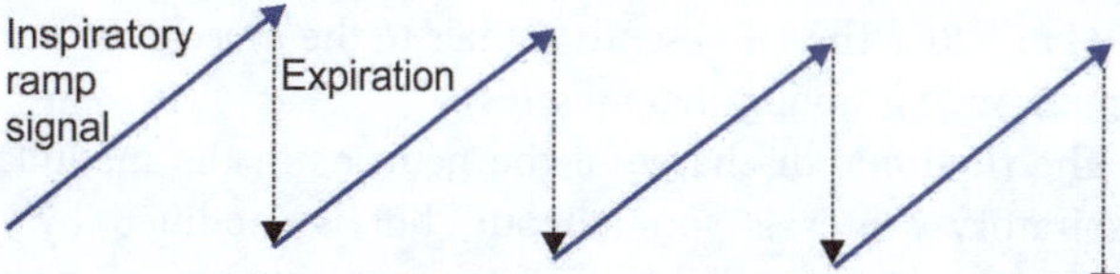

The diagrammatic representation of the inspiratory 'ramp' signal. The signal originating from DRG gradully becomes stronger, reaches speak and suddenly stops. As the signal abruptly falls to zero, the inspiration stops and the expiration follows automatically as a passive recoil process. Then, the next inspiratory signal generated by DRG causes the next respiratory cycle to occur.

Fig. 3.23: Inspiratory ramp signal

Pontomedullary respiratory center neurons are of two types—I and E neurons. I neurons are active during inspiration and E neurons are active only during forceful expiration (Table 3.4).

Dorsal Respiratory Group Neurons

Most of the neurons are located within the nucleus tractus solatarius (NTS) and some in the adjacent reticular substance. They are mainly concerned with inspiration. The basic pattern of spontaneous breathing is generated by the signals arising from dorsal respiratory group (DRG). They contain mainly I neurons. The signal generated by DRG is typically described as inspiratory ramp signal. DRG neurons project to Pre-Botzinger complex in medulla. This complex consists of pacemaker cells; spontaneous pattern of respiration is initiated by this complex.

DRG send fibers to phrenic motor neurons which innervate diaphragm. NTS is the sensory termination of both vagal and glossopharyngeal nerve (afferent) which transmit sensory signals into respiratory center from peripheral baroreceptors, chemoreceptors and pulmonary receptors. As inspiratory signals cause lungs to begin to distend, the stretch receptors in the lungs begin to be distorted. Impulses thereby initiated are sent via the afferent fibers to the medullary DRG neurons. When these feedback signals become strong enough, the inspiratory signal of DRG will be switched off, causing the inspiration to cease and expiration will follow. These signals affect inspiration in much the same way as signals from pneumotaxic center.

Inspiratory ramp signal (Fig. 3.23)

The nervous signal that is transmitted to the inspiratory muscles, mainly diaphragm is not an instantaneous burst of action potentials. It begins weakly and increases steadily in a ramp manner for about 2 sec. Then it ceases abruptly for the next 3 sec. During this period expiration occurs. At the end of 3 sec, the inspiratory ramp signals reappear in the same pattern and the cycle is repeated.

Ventral Respiratory Group Neurons

Ventral group is a long column of neurons that extends through nucleus ambiguus and nucleus retroambiguus in the ventrolateral medulla. They contain both I and E neurons. I neurons are situated in its midportion whereas E neurons at caudal and rostral end. Normally, this center is inactive during quiet breathing and it becomes active during forced breathing or when the inspiratory center is inhibited. They are mainly concerned with forceful expiration but also shows some activity during inspiration. In quite breathing, no signals are needed for expiration which occurs as a passive recoil process. With heavy breathing, there is spill over of impulses from

Table 3.4: Respiratory centers

Medullary respiratory group of neurons are	
• Dorsal respiratory group (DRG)	Concerned with inspiration
• Ventral respiratory group (VRG)	Mainly concerned with expiration, but also shows some activity during inspiration
• Pre-Botzinger complex	Responsible for generation of respiratory rhythm
Pontine respiratory centers are	
• Pneumotaxic center	The primary function is to limit inspiration, i.e. to control the switch off point of inspiratory ramp and control of inspiratory depth
• Apneustic center	Excites inspiratory center to prolongs inspiration

DRG to VRG. The VRG sends signals to the muscles of heavy expiration (e.g. abdominal muscles).

The rhythmic discharge of the neurons in the medullary respiratory center is spontaneous, but is modified by: (i) neurons in the pons and (ii) by afferents in the vagus nerves from receptors in the airways and lungs.

Pneumotaxic center

Situated in dorsal part of upper pons in nucleus parabrachialis and Kolliker-Fuse nuclei. It contains both I and E neurons. Main function of PNC is to switch off inspiratory ramp signal so that duration of inspiration is controlled. Indirectly PNC increases respiratory rate by limiting duration of inspiration, i.e. when the duration for inspiration is reduced, naturally the expiration time is also reduced so that respiratory rate increases. This results in shallow rapid breathing with decrease in tidal volume.

Apneustic center

Situated in the reticular formation of lower pons. It is made up of diffusely located neurons in the region of nucleus pontocaudalis and rostral part of nucleus gigantocellularis. This center is always excitatory to medullary inspiratory center and it increases the depth of inspiration. The respiration will be slow and deep. Collectively, pneumotaxic center in pons and vagus inhibits apneustic center to switch off inspiration. The pontine centers determine the rate and depth of breathing (Flowchart 3.1 and Fig. 3.24).

Flowchart 3.1: Regulation of respiration

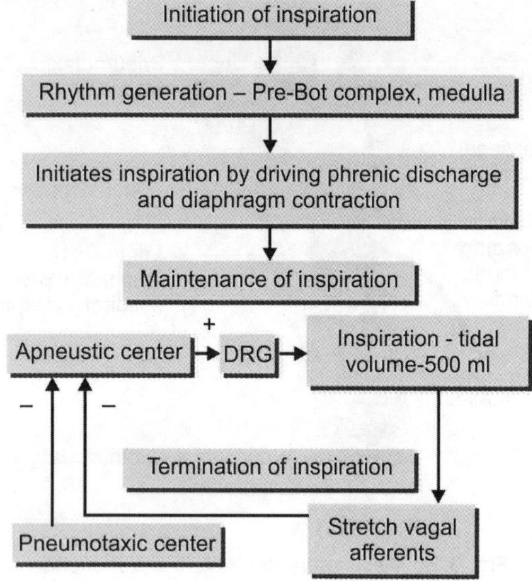

Neural Regulation

Two separate mechanisms: (i) Voluntary control and (ii) Automatic control.

Voluntary Control

Normally respiration is involuntary action. Voluntary control is possible, but only to a limited extent. Breathing can be

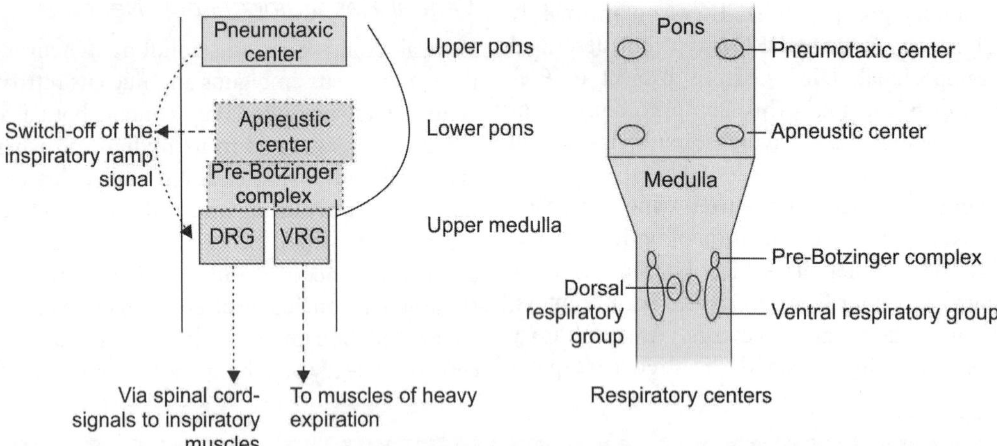

Diagrammatic presentation of the respiratory center. The inspiratory ramp signal to the respiratory muscles is initiated by the dorsal respiratory group (DRG), acting via the pre-Botzinger complex. The inspiratory signal is switched off by impulses from the pneumotaxic center (upper pons); inspiration will be shortened and respiratory rate will increase. The switch-off is inhibited by the apneustic center (lower pons); this will prolong the inspiration. Ventral respiratory group (VRG) neurons send signals to muscles of heavy expiration.

DRG: Dorsal respiratory group; **VRG:** Ventral respiratory group

Fig. 3.24: Diagrammatic representation of respiratory center

voluntary inhibited only for a short period of time. It becomes voluntary in spite of all our efforts to hold our breath. The point at which breathing can no longer be inhibited is called *breaking point*. Duration of breaking point is 40–80 sec. Breaking is due to rise in pCO_2 and fall in pO_2. Breaking point can be delayed by removing carotid body, breathing 100% O_2 before breath-holding, hyperventilation. Breathing point is reduced in exercise or CO_2 rich air.

Center of the pathway for voluntary control is in cerebral cortex. Impulses are sent to respiratory motor neuron via corticospinal tract. These nervous pathways bypass the medullary respiratory neurons. As automatic control is through neurons of pons and medulla, pathway for voluntary and automatic control are separate. Automatic control of respiration is sometimes destructed without loss of voluntary control. This clinical condition is called *Ondine's curse*.

Ondine's curse

In European folk tale, there is a mythical character of water nymph, called Ondine. She married a mortal human. When this human being becomes unfaithful toward her for the sake of his first fiancee, Ondine cursed him that he will breathe as long as he is awake and remembers to breathe. The fall out of the curse is - if he sleeps, he will die because the spontaneous automatic breathing will stop. Ondine's curse is associated with some congenital and acquired conditions.

This is seen in patients with poliomyelitis. Common to all those conditions is the underlying fact that respiration is regulated by voluntary mechanism (cortex) and involuntary mechanism (brainstem center); failure of the involuntary mechanism will cause the spontaneous automatic breathing to stop. Such a person will entirely depend on cortical conscious control of breathing, which can continue only so far as the person is awake. There will be stoppage of breathing when the person falls asleep.

Automatic Control

Automatic control of respiration is mainly through respiratory centers. The nerve fibers from the respiratory centers leave brainstem and descend in anterior part of lateral columns of spinal cord. These nerve fibers terminate in the motor neurons in the anterior horn cells of cervical and thoracic segments of spinal cord. From the motor neurons of spinal cord, two sets of nerve fibers arise which are:

a. Phrenic nerve fiber that supplies diaphragm.
b. The intercostals nerve fibers (supply intercostals). Impulses from higher centers and various reflexes influences respiratory centers.

Control from Higher Centers

Respiration is modified during deglutition, chewing, speaking, crying, singing, etc. This modification is done with the help of cerebral cortex, hypothalamus and limbic system.

Reflex Control

a. *Hering-Breuer reflex:* The impulses from the lungs bring about a respiratory reflex called *Hering-Breuer Reflex*. This reflex prevents over distention of lungs during inspiration and collapse of lungs during expiration. They represent a classic negative feedback loop between peripheral respiratory apparatus and the brainstem center for breathing. This is not important in the normal adults in the range of normal TV breathing. Important in neonates and infants.

   There are some stretch receptors on the muscular portions of the wall of bronchi and bronchioles of lungs. Overstretching of the lungs during inspiration stimulate the stretch receptors and impulses are carried by vagal afferent fibers to DRG and inspiration stops and expiration starts. This reflex is a protective reflex because, it restricts the inspiration and limits the overstreching of lung tissues. This is called *Hering-Breuer Inflation Reflex*. However, this reflex does not operate during quiet breathing. It operates, only when the tidal volume reaches above 1500 ml. Sometimes during exercise, with a very heavy breathing, a stage is reached when lungs just do not distend any further even with conscious effort.

   The reverse of this reflex is called Hering-Breuer Deflation Reflex. When peripheral alveoli are deflated, a prolonged and deep inspiratory is initiated. It creates a greater negative intrathoracic pressure and the alveoli are opened. That is reflex hyperpnea in response to deflation. Yawning may be considered as an example.

b. *J receptor mediated reflex:* 'J' receptors are juxtacapillary receptors. These receptors are the sensory nerve endings of the vagus. The fibers from these receptors are nonmyelinated and belong to C type. The 'J' receptors are situated in alveolar interstitium close to the pulmonary capillaries. The 'J' receptors are stimulated by certain chemicals released in the interstitium during pulmonary edema, pulmonary embolism, pulmonary congestion. The stimulation of the 'J' receptors produces a reflex response, which is characterized by a period of apnea followed by rapid breathing, bradycardia, hypotension and weakness of skeletal muscles.

   J receptors may have a physiological role in severe exercise. Severe muscular exercise $\rightarrow$ very mild degree collection of fluid in the alveoli $\rightarrow$ irritation of J receptors $\rightarrow$ muscle weakness $\rightarrow$ stoppage of exercise = breaking (compulsory stoppage) of exercise.

c. *Lung irritant reflex:* It is a protective reflex. Receptors are located in between epithelial cells of tracheobronchial tree. Stimulus is exposure to irritant fumes/dust. Stimulation of irritant receptors produces reflex bronchospasm (manifested as cough and sneeze) so that irritant fumes cannot reach the alveoli.

d. *Reflexes from muscle spindles of diaphragm and other inspiratory muscles:* In case of insufficient air entry in the lungs as in case of airway obstruction, the muscle spindle act in such a way that inspiratory muscles continue to contract more forcefully and this will help to overcome the obstruction.
e. *Reflexes from limbs, joints:* Movements of limbs cause stimulation of proprioreceptors (muscle spindle and golgitendon organ). This lead to increased rate and depth of respiration. The reflex is active during exercise.
f. *Baroreceptor reflex:* Rise in BP → arterial baroreceptors stimulated → afferent impulses teminates at VMC and respiratory center → the I neurons are inhibited → stoppage of inspiration.
g. *Chemoreceptor reflex*
h. *Cough reflex:* This is a protective reflex. Cough begins with deep inspiration followed by forced expiration against closed glottis. This increases intrapleural pressure above 100 mm Hg. The glottis is suddenly opened producing an explosive outflow of air.
i. *Sneezing reflex:* It is a similar expiratory effort with a continuously open glottis.
j. *Deglutition reflex:* During swallowing of the food, there is temporary arrest of respiration called deglutition apnea. This occurs during pharyngeal stage (2nd stage of respiration) and it prevents the entry of food particles into the respiratory tract. The nerve involved in this reflex is glossopharyngeal nerve.
k. *Others:* Rise in body temperature causes hyperventilation. Sharp acute pain increases the rate of respiration temporarily.

Chemical Regulation

The chemical mechanism of regulation of respiration is operated through the chemoreceptors. These receptors are stimulated by any change in the concentration of O_2, CO_2, H^+ and other drugs, chemical hormones. Chemoreceptors are of two types:

1. Central Chemoreceptors

Central chemoreceptors are situated in the ventral part of medulla. They are distinct and separate from pontomedullary respiratory center. Stimulus is increase in pCO_2.

Mechanism of stimulation of chemoreceptors

CO_2 from the arterial blood crosses blood-brain barrier and enters the CSF and brain interstitial fluid (Flowchart 3.2)

CO_2 cross the cell membrane, combine with H_2O to form H_2CO_3 which splits into H^+ and HCO_3^- (carbonic anhydrase mediated). It is this H^+ ion which stimulates respiration. Once stimulated sent impulse to pontomedullary respiratory center and influence rate and rhythm of respiration.

Flowchart 3.2: Chemical regulation of respiration

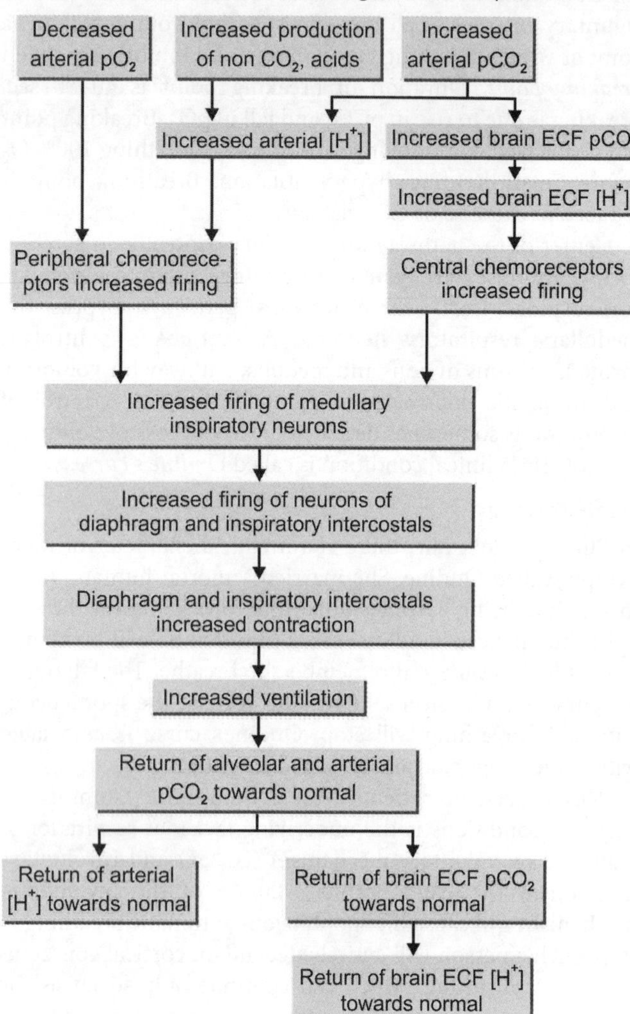

2. Peripheral Chemoreceptors

They are carotid body and aortic body. There are two carotid bodies, one on either side of midline near bifurcation of common carotid artery. These contain chemoreceptors which are sensors of arterial O_2 tension, CO_2 tension and blood pH. Usually two or more aortic bodies are present near the arch of aorta. From carotid body impulses are transmitted via Hering nerve and from aortic body through vagus. Each carotid and aortic body contains islands of two types of cells – Type I and Type II cells (Fig. 3.25).

Type I cells

Type I cells are also called glomus cells, these islands are surrounded by fenestrated sinusoidal capillaries. They are closely associated with cup-like endings of afferent nerve (glossopharyngeal). These cells have dense core granules. Granules contains catecholamine (dopamine). Neurotransmitter released at the junction of afferent nerve and receptor cell is dopamine.

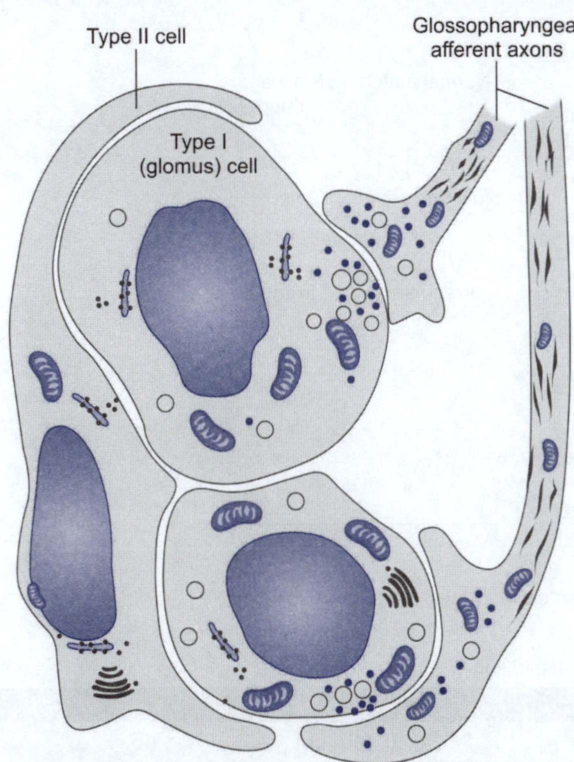

Fig. 3.25: Type 1 and type 2 cells seen in aortic and carotid bodies

Glomus cells are stimulated mainly by hypoxia, these cells have O_2 sensitive K^+ channels whose conductance is decreased proportionate to degree of hypoxia. This reduces K^+ efflux and depolarizes the cell → lead to Ca^{2+} influx → fusion of the released Ca^{2+} with neurotransmitter in receptor membrane → release of neurotransmitter into the synaptic cleft → dopamine bind with dopamine receptors on the postsynaptic membrane → AP in the afferent nerve (glossopharyngeal, vagus) → impulse transmitted to respiratory center.

Type II cells

They are also called glial/supporting cells.

Chemoreceptor Reflex

Afferent nerve: Glossopharyngeal and vagus.

Receptor: Carotid and aortic body.

Center: Respiratory center.

Efferent nerve: Nerves supplying muscles of respiration, diaphragm, intercostals.

Effector: Respiratory muscles causing increase in their activity (contraction).

Note

1. Anemic hypoxia will not stimulate chemoreceptors. Blood flow in each carotid body is 2000 ml/100 g tissue per min (highest and in brain only 54 ml/100 g/min; kidney 420 ml/100 g/ml). As the blood flow per unit area is enormous, O_2 needs can be met by dissolved O_2 alone. In anemia and CO poisoning, dissolved O_2 is normal and O_2 in combination with Hb varies.
2. Increase in H^+ ion concentration in blood cannot activate central chemoreceptors (H^+ cannot cross BBB).

Effects of Lesions in the Respiratory Centers and their Effect on Respiration (Fig. 3.26 and Table 3.5)

After reading neural regulation of respiration, one can easily understand the effects of transection at various levels.

- Transection above pons has no effect on respiration
- A midpontine transection (transection between upper and lower pans) or damage to pneumotaxic center
  - *When vagi are intact:* The inhibitory effect of pneumotaxic center on apneustic center is abolished. However, inhibitory effect of vagus is intact. Therefore, the activity of apneustic center is increased a little bit which results in prolongation of inspiratory ramp. Thus, breathing becomes deep and slow. But there is no change in rhythm.
  - *With bilateral vagotomy:* This eliminates the inhibitory influence of both pneumotaxic center and vagi on the apneustic center. The uninhibited effect of apneustic center results in sustained gasping inspiration which is interrupted by brief inefficient expiration, i.e. apneusis or inspiratory spasm.
- *Transection at pontomedullary junction:* Spontaneous respiration is maintained because the respiratory rhythm is generated in medulla which regulate the discharge of DRG and if required VRG. However, respiration is slight irregular and gasping.
- *Transection below the medulla:* Respiration is stopped completely.
- *Bilateral vagotomy (without any brain lesion):* No feedback signals from lungs to switch off inspiratory signal from DRG and apneustic center. Therefore, there is slight increase in activity of apneustic center; results in prolonged inspiration. However, inhibitory effect of pneumotaxic center remains intact. Breathing is deep and slow.

APPLIED PHYSIOLOGY

Hypoxia

Hypoxia is O_2 deficiency at the tissue level. It is a more relevant term than anoxia, where rarely no O_2 is left in the tissues.

Hypoxia is divided into four types (Table 3.6):

1. Hypoxic hypoxia (anoxic anoxia).
2. Anemic hypoxia.

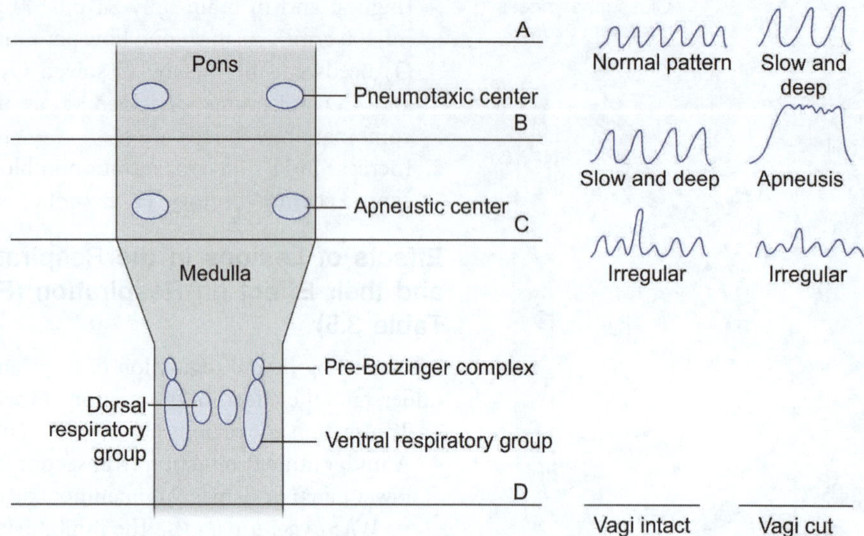

Fig. 3.26: Effect of lesions in the respiratory centers and their effect on respiration

Table 3.5: Effects of lesions in the respiratory centers and their effect on respiration

Lesion point	Lesion site	Inference	
		If vagi intact	**If vagi cut**
A	Above pons	• Normal breathing is seen since the respiratory neurons in pons and medulla are intact • Higher centers can no longer influence brainstem centers (loss of voluntary control)	• Breathing becomes slow, deep • This is because the stretch information from lung carried by vagus is missing
B	Mid pons—pneumotaxic center separated from apneustic center	• Breathing becomes slow, deep • This is because the inhibition of apneustic center by pneumotaxic center is lost	• Inspiration is markedly prolonged • This breathing pattern is called apneusis or inspiratory spasm
C	Pontomedullary junction—pons and medulla are separated	• Irregular respiration is seen • This is because the regularization of rhythm by pons is not there	• Irregular respiration is seen • This is because the regularization of rhythm by pons is not there
D	Below medulla	• Respiration stops	• Respiration stops

Table 3.6: Different types of hypoxia

Type	Example	PAO_2*	PaO_2†	O_2‡ content	A-V different
Hypoxic hypoxia	High altitude sickness	↓	↓	↓	±
Anemic hypoxia	Severe anemia	±	±	↓	±
Stagnant hypoxia	Left ventricular failure	±	±	±	↑
Histotoxic hypoxia	HCN poisoning	±	±	±	↑

*where $PAO_2 = pO_2$ of alveolar air
†$PaO_2 = pO_2$ of arterial blood
‡A-V difference = arterial and venous O_2 difference (O_2 utilization)

3. Stagnant/ischemic hypoxia (blood flow to the tissues is low, adequate O_2 not delivered).
4. Histotoxic hypoxia (because of the action of a toxic agent, tissue cells cannot make use of the O_2).

Hypoxic Hypoxia

It is characterized by a low arterial pO_2 when O_2 carrying capacity of blood and rate of blood flow to tissues are normal or elevated.

Hypoxic hypoxia is a problem in normal individuals at high altitude and is a complication of pneumonia and a variety of other diseases of respiratory system.

Causes for hypoxic hypoxia

a. *Low O_2 tension in the inspired air:* The O_2 tension in the inspired air reduces at high altitude or while breathing air in closed space and also breathing a gas mixture containing low pO_2.
b. *Decreased pulmonary ventilation:* Pulmonary ventilation decreases in the following conditions:
   i. Airway obstruction as in asthma
   ii. Depression of respiratory centers by drugs such as morphine.
   iii. Weakness/paralysis of respiratory muscles.
c. *Inadequate oxygenation of blood in lungs:* Oxygenation of blood in the lungs reduces by the following conditions:
   i. Impaired alveolar diffusion as in emphysema.
   ii. Presence of nonfunctioning alveoli as in fibrosis
d. *Cardiac disorders:*
   i. Venous arterial shunts (deoxygenated blood mixes with oxygenated blood)
   ii. Congestive heart failure.

Anemic Hypoxia

Here the arterial pO_2 normal, but amount of Hb to carry O_2 is reduced. It is a condition in which O_2 carrying capacity of blood is reduced. The O_2 availability is normal, but the blood is not able to take up sufficient amount of O_2 due to anemic condition.

Causes of anemic hypoxia

Anemic hypoxia can be due to two reasons:

a. *Quantitative deficiency of Hb:* For example: anemia, here the O_2 carrying capacity is decreased due to actual deficiency of Hb.
b. *Qualitative deficiency of Hb:* For example: altered Hb such as methemoglobin.
   Here the Hb content is normal, but due to its altered nature it cannot carry O_2. This also includes CO poisoning. The affinity of Hb for CO is 200 times its affinity for O_2 and COHb liberates CO very slowly. The difficulty is that when COHb is present the dissociation curve of the remaining HbO_2 shifts to the left, decreasing the amount of O_2 released. The characteristic feature of anemic hypoxia is that pO_2 of the arterial blood is normal, whereas the O_2 carrying capacity of blood is reduced.

Stagnant Hypoxia

In this type of hypoxia blood flow to the tissues is so low that adequate O_2 is not delivered to them despite a normal arterial pO_2 and Hb concentration. So A-V O_2 concentration difference increases, thereby the reduced Hb increases.

Hypoxia due to slow circulation is a problem in organs such as the kidneys and heart during shock. The liver and possibly the brain are damaged by stagnant hypoxia in congestive heart failure.

Causes of stagnant hypoxia

The velocity of blood flow decreases in the following conditions: Congestive cardiac failure, hemorrhage, surgical shock, vasospasm, thrombosis and embolism.

Histotoxic Hypoxia

Hypoxia in which the amount of oxygen delivered to the tissues is adequate, but because of the action of a toxic agent the tissue cells cannot make use of the O_2. It occurs due to inhibition of tissue oxidative processes and most commonly as a result of cyanide poisoning. Here the cyanide inhibits cytochrome-oxidase and possibly other enzymes. When cytochrome-oxidase enzymes are inhibited, oxidation stops in the tissues → O_2 from the capillary blood is not extracted → pO_2 of venous blood remains high. So A-V O_2 difference decreases. Methylene blue or nitrites are used to treat cyanide poisoning. They act by forming methemoglobin, which then reacts with cyanide to form cyanmethemoglobin (nontoxic compound).

Clinical Note

Histotoxic hypoxia cannot cause cyanosis as, reduced Hb is either not produced or produced in very small amount).

Effects of Hypoxia

On Blood

Hypoxia stimulates juxtaglomerular apparatus of kidney, increasing the secretion of erythropoietin. Erythropoietin stimulates the red bone marrow, RBC count increases with an increase in reticulocyte count (O_2 carrying capacity of blood is improved).

On CVS

Hypoxia (except anemic hypoxia) stimulates peripheral chemoreceptors which in turn stimulate cardiac and vasomotor centers, thereby there is an increase in the HR, force of contraction, CO and systemic arterial blood pressure.

On Respiration

All types of hypoxia except anemic hypoxia stimulate peripheral chemoreceptors to increase respiration. The rate of increase in ventilation is in proportion to the severity of the hypoxia of the peripheral chemoreceptors. Severe hypoxia causes direct inhibition of respiratory center and depress respiration.

On CNS

In mild hypoxia, the symptoms are similar to alcohol intoxication (depression, general loss of self control, headache, loss of time sense). In severe hypoxia, there is sudden loss of consciousness, if not treated immediately coma occurs which leads to death.

Treatment for Hypoxia (O_2 Therapy)

The best treatment for hypoxia is O_2 therapy, i.e. treating the affected person with O_2. Pure O_2 or O_2 combined with another gas is administered. Depending on the basic physiological principles of different types of hypoxia the valuability of oxygen therapy in various types can be understood.

Atmospheric Hypoxia (Hypoxic Hypoxia)

O_2 therapy can completely correct the depressed O_2 level in the inspired gases and therefore provide 100% effective therapy.

Hypoventilation Hypoxia

Here with O_2 therapy the amount of O_2 entering the alveoli with each breath can be increased. But this provides no benefit for the excess blood CO_2 also caused by hypoventilation.

In hypoxia caused by anemia, abnormal Hb, transport of O_2, circulatory deficiency or physiological shunt, oxygen therapy is of much less value because normal O_2 is already available in the alveoli.

In hypoxia caused by inadequate tissue use of O_2 (histotoxic hypoxia), O_2 therapy is of practically no value because:

- Here neither O_2 pick up by the lungs or transport to the tissues is deficient.
- The defect is in the tissue metabolic system so it cannot utilize the O_2 being delivered.

Dyspnea

Dyspnea is difficult or labored breathing in which the subject is conscious of shortness of breath or it is an abnormal uncomfortable awareness of breathing.

A normal individual is not conscious of respiration until ventilation is doubled and breathing becomes uncomfortable. Real dyspnea (uncomfortable breathing) occurs when pulmonary ventilation is tripled or quadrupled, i.e. when an imbalance between demand for ventilation and actual ventilation is achieved.

The basic mechanisms of dyspnea are:

1. Hypercapnea and hypoxia: Hypoxia and hypercapnea result in increased rate and depth of breathing regardless of the patient's subjective sensation.
2. Increased effort of breathing or increased work of breathing. For example, in bronchial asthma where airway resistance is increased and compliance is reduced.
3. Current hypothesis is that dyspnea occurs when there is a mismatch between incoming afferent information to the brain and outgoing motor signals from brain to respiratory muscles.

Causes

Diseases of respiratory system

a. Obstruction to any part of respiratory passage: Increase work of breathing. For example, bronchial asthma.
b. Diseases of lungs and pleura: Pneumonia, pulmonary-edema, fibrosis, pleural effusion and pneumothorax.
c. Interference with respiratory movement:
   - Weakness or paralysis of respiratory muscles
   - Pain due to injury to chest wall, ribs
   - Deformities of spine
   - Impaired movements of diaphragm.

Diseases of CVS

a. Chronic CCF: Initially dyspnea only on exertion, later even at rest.
b. Paroxysmal nocturnal dyspnea: Pulmonary edema of LVF.

Disorders of metabolism

a. Metabolic acidosis
b. Diabetic acidosis
c. Uremia.

Other causes: Anemia, cerebral hemorrhage and psychogenic.

Dyspneic Index/Breathing Reserve Percentage

It is the percentage of respiratory capacity not being used at a given RMV or pulmonary ventilation. Normal dyspneic index at rest is >90%.

Breathing reserve = MVV – RMV = 100 – 10 = 90 L

DI = MVV – RMV/MVV × 100

Where, MVV – Maximal voluntary ventilation

RMV – Residual minute volume

This means that breathing can be increased by 90 L, i.e. from 6–8 to 100 L or more. Dyspnea is there when this index is less than 70%, which is called *dyspneic point*. An example taken from a patient of emphysema will clarify it. The MVV has decreased from 100 L/min to 40 L/min, while RMV has increased 10 L/min to 20 L/min (due to respiratory stimulation by increased pCO_2 and low pO_2). DI = 40 – 20/40 × 100 = 50%.

This means that dyspneic point has been crossed, so that the patient is experiencing dyspnea.

Orthopnea

It refers to the dyspnea in lying position. Dyspnea increases when the person lies down and improves when the person sits up. This is usually seen in patients with cardiac failure. Improvements of dyspnea occurs in sitting position as the abdominal viscera do not press upon the diaphragm during sitting, so that the diaphragm can descend easily. Effect of gravity is that as the person lies down, the venous return to the heart increases and the symptoms of orthopnea flare up. When the person sits up, as a result of gravity the venous return to the heart decreases and the symptoms of orthopnea decreases.

Hypercapnia

Hypercapnia is retention of CO_2 in the body. In these patients pCO_2 is markedly elevated, there is severe respiratory acidosis and plasma HCO_3^- may be very high which partially compensates for the acidosis. Essential mechanisms underlying hypercapnia is inadequacy of alveolar ventilation for the amount of CO_2 produced.

Causes

1. Increased CO_2 production: In febrile patients 13% increase in CO_2 production for each 100°C rise in temperature. High carbohydrate diet increases CO_2 production.
2. Malfunction of respiratory pump: Hypercapnia is associated with hypoxia.
3. Inefficiency of gas exchange (Increased dead space or V/P mismatch).

In hypoxia due to poor diffusion through respiratory membrane, serious hypercapnia does not occur because CO_2 difuses 20 times rapidly as O_2.

Symptoms

1. Alveolar pCO_2 > 60–75 mm Hg; breathing becomes rapid and deep.
2. Alveolar pCO_2 > 80–100 mm Hg; symptoms due to depression of CNS, i.e. confusion, decreased sensory perception and eventually coma.
3. Alveolar pCO_2 > 120–150 mm Hg; anesthesia and death of the patient.

Hypocapnia

The chronic effects of hypocapnia are seen in neurotic patients who chronically hyperventilate themselves. Hypocapnia has a direct vasoconstrictor effect on cerebral vessels. So cerebral blood flow is reduced, thereby leading to cerebral ischemia that lead to dizziness and paresthesia.

If a person voluntarily hyperventilates, excess amount of CO_2 is washed out and pCO_2 decreases. This depresses respiration and leads to apnea. During this period of apnea CO_2 is accumulated and a fall in pO_2 occurs. This stimulates respiration and normal respiration is resumed.

If H^+ is normal and if there is prolonged hyperventilation, increased CO_2 is washed out and H^+ becomes less than normal and the condition is called respiratory alkalosis.

When H^+ is low or pH is high, the proteins are ionized. Ionised Ca^{2+} in blood combine with protein and Ca^{2+} gets converted to the bound form. When ECF concentration of Ca^{2+} falls below normal, the nervous system becomes progressively more excitable leading to increased permeability to Na^+ allowing easy initiation of action potentials. This may lead to symptoms of hypocalcemia and tetany.

Asphyxia

It is produced by occlusion of airways. This results in hypoxia (lack of O_2) and hypercapnia (excess of O_2). Asphyxia occurs in strangulation, acute tracheal obstruction due to foreign body in trachea or larynx, traumatic compression of chest by fall of heavy objects (trapped in building collapse). When a newborn does not begin to breath soon after birth, it develops asphyxia called asphyxia neonatorium.

Effects of asphyxia is described under three stages.

1. *Stage of exaggerated breathing*: Due to stimulation of respiratory centers by CO_2 breathing become deeper, more frequent and more labored.
2. *Stage of convulsion:* Due to spread of stimulation to centers in brain and spinal cord generalized convulsions appear. There is tachycardia, vasoconstriction, rise of BP and lack of consciousness.
3. *Stage of collapse:* Due to paralysis of respiratory centers convulsions cease abruptly and respiration becomes gasping in character. Pupils dilate, pulse becomes feeble, reflexes are absent. Finally death occurs by the failure of vital centers.

Note: In the earlier stages of asphyxia the knee-jerks are exaggerated, but when the third stage is reached they are entirely lost.

Cyanosis

It is a clinical condition characterized by bluish discoloration of skin and mucous membrane, best seen in people with white complexion. Cyanosis is caused when more than 5 gm of reduced Hb is present in the local blood. Thus in anemia where Hb is less than 5 gm%, no cyanosis is seen (enough reduced Hb is not formed to produce blue color). But in cases of polycythemia vera (excess RBC), the great excess of available Hb that can become deoxygenated leads frequently to cyanosis. Cyanosis does not occur in histotoxic hypoxia. Cyanosis is of two types:

1. *Central Cyanosis:* Central cyanosis is due to heart or lung disease and is associated with hyperkinetic circulation (tachycardia, increase in BP, warm periphery). It occurs mainly due to the shunting of blood from the right to left side of the heart, i.e. bypassing the lung. Therefore, the oxygenation of Hb is hampered resulting in the rise of reduced Hb on the blood. This condition is characterized by blue extremities which are warm due to hyperdynamic circulation. The site for central cyanosis is tongue and lip. It also occurs in different lung diseases where pulmonary gas exchange is affected.

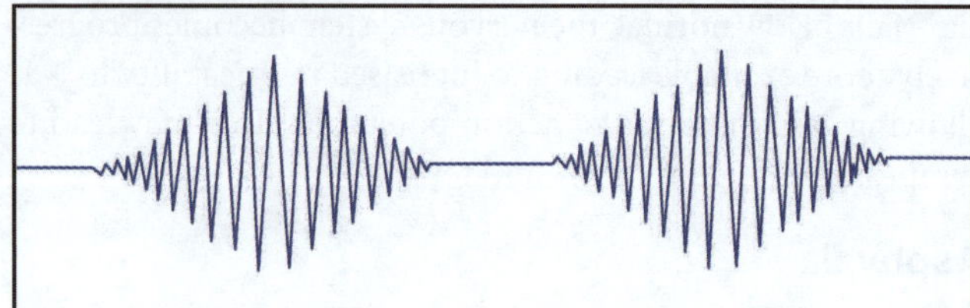

Fig. 3.27: Cheyne-Stokes breathing

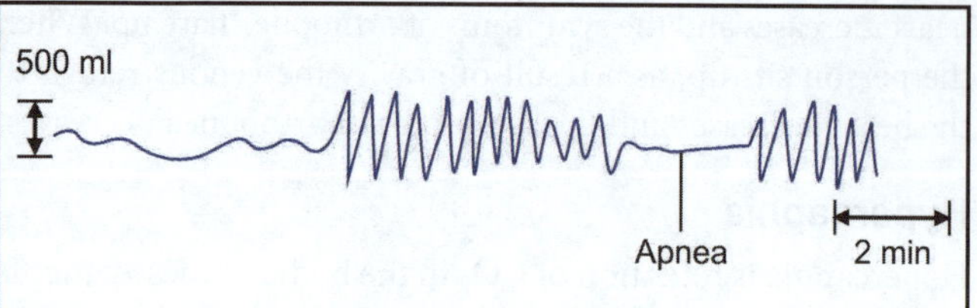

Fig. 3.28: Biot's breathing

2. *Peripheral cyanosis:* It is due to local causes. Here, there is severe vasoconstriction due to sympathetic stimulation. Vasoconstriction in the periphery leads to reduction of blood flow in the tissue while O_2 demand of the tissues remains the same, thus the concentration of reduced Hb rises. The site for peripheral cyanosis is toes and finger tips. This can occur in peripheral circulatory failure resulting in cold blue extremities.

Note: A discoloration of the skin and mucous membrane similar to cyanosis is produced by high circulating levels of methemoglobin.

Special Types of Respiration

Cheyne-Stoke's Breathing

When respiration shows alternate waxing and waning of tidal volume, it is called Cheyne-Stoke's breathing (Fig. 3.27). Physiological causes are voluntary hyperventilation, high altitude, during sleep in some normal individuals (especially infants). Pathological causes include chronic heart failure, brain damage, uremia and poisoning by narcotics.

Explanation

Voluntary hyperventilation: Voluntary hyperventilation for two minutes produces apnea followed by respiration. This cycle keeps on repeating but with a decreasing duration of apnea until the respiration comes to normal.

Mechanism: Hyperventilation cause increased alveolar pO_2 or decreased pCO_2. Decreased alveolar pCO_2 cause apnea. Apnea results in:

i. CO_2 accumulation in the body with gradual increase in alveolar pCO_2. As long as increase in alveolar pCO_2 remains below 40 mm Hg (threshold level) apneic spells are there.
ii. Fall in alveolar pO_2 to 60 mm Hg (hypoxia) via peripheral chemoreceptors stimulate the respiratory center producing hyperventilation.

Heart failure: It occurs mainly in left ventricular failure and is associated with pulmonary congestion producing hypoxia leading to the stimulation of respiratory center and thus ventilation increases. In heart failure, the circulation is slowed down from lungs to brain, therefore when such individuals hyperventilate, it takes longer than the normal time for the blood to reach the brain. When this blood reaches the brain, low pCO_2 inhibits the respiratory center producing 'apnea'.

Brain damage: If there is damage of supra medullary inhibitory pathway, the medullary chemoreceptor becomes more sensitive to the action of CO_2. Thus pulmonary ventilation increases, so CO_2 is washed out and alveolar pCO_2 falls, producing apnea. As a result, CO_2 accumulate, alveolar pCO_2 rises and respiration gets stimulated.

Effects of periodic breathing

a. Fall in arterial pCO_2 causes severe vasoconstriction of cerebral blood vessels, as a result, cerebral blood flow decreases producing dizziness.
b. Hyperventilation leads to respiratory alkalosis.

Biot's Respiration

This is a type of periodic breathing in which there are 3–4 cycles of normal respiration followed by abrupt onset of apnea and again abrupt onset of normal respiration (Fig. 3.28). It is seen in case of meningitis, severe brain damage, etc.

Kussmaul Breathing

It is also known as acidotic breathing/air hunger. It occurs in case of metabolic acidosis as in diabetic ketoacidosis, renal failure, etc. The respiration is characterized by rapid and deep breathing (due to stimulation of respiratory center by increased H^+). The main action of H^+ in the blood is via peripheral chemoreceptors. But H^+ ions can slowly cross the blood-brain barrier when the concentration is high and persistent, in that case the central chemoreceptors are also stimulated. It's aim is to wash out CO_2 and thereby to correct the acidosis. Here, the blood pCO_2 level is low.

Artificial Respiration

In acute asphyxia due to drowning, CO or other forms of gas poisoning, electrolution and anesthetic accidents, where breathing has ceased artificial respiration may be life saving. It should always be attempted, because respiration stops before the heart stops.

Mouth-to-mouth breathing (Figs 3.29A to C)

There are numerous methods of artificial respiration, but the method presently recommended to produce adequate

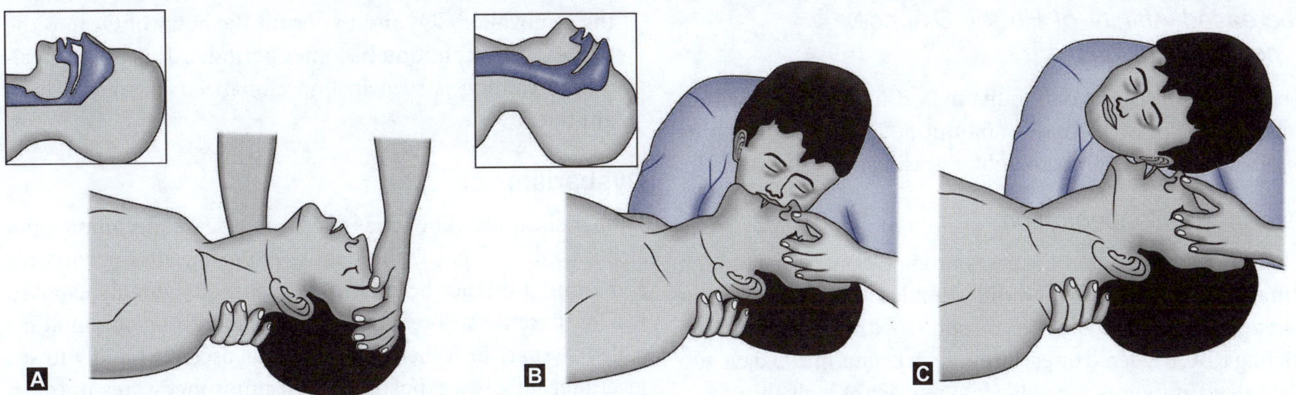

Figs 3.29A to C: Steps of mouth-to-mouth breathing

ventilation in all cases is mouth-to-mouth breathing. It works by expanding the lungs.

Method

1. In this form of resuscitation, the operator 1st places the victim in the supine position and opens the airway by placing a hand under the neck and lifting, while keeping pressure with the other hand on the victim's forehead. This extends the neck and lifts the tongue away from the back of the throat.
2. Now the victim's mouth is covered by the operator's mouth while the fingers of the hand already on the forehead occlude the nostrils.
3. About 12 times a minute, the operator blows into the victim's mouth a volume twice the tidal volume, then permits the elastic recoil of the victim's lungs to produce passive expiration (by unsealing mouth and nose). The victim's neck is kept extended. Rescuer should listen and feel for expiratory airflow.

Note

a. Any gas blown into the stomach can be expelled by applying upward pressure on the abdomen from time to time.
b. In apneic individuals in whom no heartbeat is detectable, mouth-to-mouth breathing should be alternated with cardiac massage.

Mechanical Ventilation

For treatment of chronic weakness of the respiratory muscles, airtight devices that cover the chest are available. By means of a motor, negative pressure is applied to the chest at intervals, drawing air into the lungs. In cases of acute respiratory failure and other conditions in which alveolar-capillary exchange is affected patients are intubated and pulses of air or mixtures of respiratory gases are delivered by machines. Various pressure adjustments are done to maintain a positive end-expiratory pressure (PEEP) to aid movement of O_2 into the blood and prevent atelectasis. However, excessive pressure can rupture the alveoli. For this and other reasons, mechanical ventilation should be discouraged as soon as possible.

HIGH ALTITUDE PHYSIOLOGY

The primary problem at high altitude is low atmospheric pressure, although a fall in environmental temperature is also associated with it. Since combination of air does not change with altitude, the partial pressure of oxygen forms about 21% of atmospheric pressure at any altitude. Hence, the PO_2 is low at high altitudes and therefore PO_2 of inspired air (PiO_2) is low.

The human body is designed to deliver adequate oxygen to tissues when supplied oxygen at a pressure closes to the sea level pressure. If the PO_2 falls much below the sea level tissue oxygenation suffers and consequently physiological functions are deranged. The earliest response to fall in PO_2 is hyperventilation which starts at an altitude of 3,000 meters above the sea level. Hypoxic symptoms starts at an altitude of 4,000 meters and become severe at 5,000 meters. Consciousness, is lost at about 6,000 meters.

Acclimatization

Various physiological readjustments and compensatory mechanisms in the body that reduce the effects of hypoxia in permanent residents at high altitude is called 'acclimatization' at high altitudes. Acclimatization is possible by the following compensatory mechanisms:

Increase in Pulmonary Ventilation

In acclimatized subjects, the sensitivity of respiratory center to 'hypoxia' increases. Therefore even with slight decrease of arterial pO_2, pulmonary ventilation increases and alveolar pCO_2 falls. This increase in pulmonary ventilation is maintained by active regulation of pH of CSF and blood to normal levels.

Decreased Affinity of Hb for O_2 under Hypoxic Conditions

When a person is exposed to hypoxia at high altitude within hours there will be increased amount of 2,3 DPG. This shifts O_2-Hb dissociation curve to right, releasing more O_2 from Hb.

Rise in Hb Concentration

Erythropoietin secretion increases promptly on ascent to high altitude. 'Hypoxia' is a powerful stimulus for erythropoietin secretion and thus activates erythropoiesis. This increase in circulating RBC triggered by erythropoietin begins in 2–3 days and is sustained as long as the individual remains at high altitude.

Changes at Tissue Level to Reduce the Effect of Hypoxia

Compensatory changes also occur in the tissues.

- Increase in the number of mitochondria which are the sites of oxidative reactions.
- Increase in cytochrome oxidase.
- Increase in myoglobin which facilitates the movement of O_2 in tissues.

Increased Vascularity of Hypoxic Tissues

Hypoxia increases tissue capillary density, i.e. more capillaries open up. Hypoxia also causes vasodilatation. Therefore, more O_2 can be supplied to tissues.

Increased Diffusion Capacity of Lungs for O_2

This occurs due to:

- Increase in the number of pulmonary capillaries secondary to increase in pulmonary artery pressure.
- Pulmonary vasodilatation.
- Increase in pulmonary blood flow.

Note

1. *Mountain sickness:* When a person ascends to high altitude he suffers from mountain sickness. It starts approx 8–12 hours after arrival at high altitude and lasts for about 4–8 days. It is characterized by nausea, vomiting, headache, insomnia, dyspnea and irritability. The exact cause of mountain sickness is not known, but it appears to be associated with cerebral edema or alkalosis.
2. When a person ascends to high altitude, the availability of O_2 in the inspired air decreases but the amount of CO_2 increases. So, in order to get adequate O_2 supply to the tissues, there is an increase in the rate of respiration. But consequently as the respiration rate increases, there is more entry of CO_2 with the inspired air. Therefore to facilitate the removal of CO_2 and to permit the entry of O_2 into the tissues, the respiration becomes periodic. This is why periodic breathing is seen in unacclimatized persons at high altitude.

Dysbarism

Dysbarism is also known as Caisson's disease, decompression sickness, divers' palsy, the bends. A person after staying for sometime in higher barometric pressure if suddenly exposed to a low barometric pressure, suffers from a group of symptoms called 'dysbarism'. When the individual ascends rapidly to sea level after sufficient exposure to high atmospheric pressure deep in the sea, N_2 is decompressed and escapes from the tissues at a faster rate. Being gas it forms bubbles while escaping rapidly from the tissues. The gases block the blood vessels producing tissue ischemia and sometimes the tissue death.

Caisson is an iron chamber used to lower individuals to work deep under the sea, they suffered from dysbarism and thus it is also called as Caisson's disease. This problem is also faced by professional divers and tunnel workers who are exposed to high barometric pressure.

Symptoms

1. Pain in joints and muscles of legs or arms. The joint pain accounts for the term 'bends' that is often applied to this condition.
2. *The chokes:* The chokes refers to serious shortness of breath which is often followed by severe pulmonary edema and, occasionally death.
3. Neurological symptoms like dizziness, paralysis of muscles, or collapse, paresthesia and unconsciousness may occur due to blockage of blood vessels of brain and spinal cord.
4. Paralysis of muscles may occur temporarily due to the presence of N_2 bubbles in the myelin sheath of motor nerves. This is called *diver's palsy*.
5. Coronary ischemia or MI may occur due to blockage of coronary capillaries by the N_2 bubbles.

Principle

When a person stays in a higher barometric pressure, his blood is equilibrated to the air of that pressure. So, all the gases dissolved in blood increase proportionately including N_2. Now when the person is suddenly exposed to low barometric pressure, these gases are liberated from the blood. CO_2 poses no problem as it can diffuse quickly and O_2 can be utilized by the tissues. But N_2 bubbles cannot be got rid of easily and they obstruct the blood vessel to produce the symptoms stated above.

Prevention

Diver or caisson workers should come to the surface slowly.

Treatment

Tank decompression is most important method in treating people in whom symptoms of decompression develops. In this case, the diver is recompressed immediately to a deep level. Then decompression is carried out over slowly to normal atmospheric pressure.

Note

1. Risk of decompression sickness can be reduced by breathing mixture of O_2 and helium during the dive.
2. N_2 bubbles may not appear for many minutes to hours because sometimes the gas can remain dissolved in the supersaturated state for hours before bubbling.
3. Recovery is often complete, but there may be residual neurologic sequele as a result of irreversible damage to the nervous system.

Hiccup

Hiccup is a spasmodic contraction of the diaphragm and other respiratory muscles that produces an inspiration during which the glottis closes suddenly. The glottic closure is responsible for the characteristic sensation and sound. Hiccups occur in the fetus *in utero* as well as throughout extrauterine life. Most attacks of hiccups are usually of short duration and they often respond to breath-holding or other measures that increases arterial pCO_2.

Oxygen Therapy and Oxygen Toxicity

100% oxygen is useful in hypoxia. Hyperbaric oxygen is given for treatment of CO poisoning, gas gangrene, and even for treating decompression sickness, radiation induced tissue injury. Aim of oxygen therapy is to increase the amount of dissolved O_2 content of arterial blood to 6 mL/100 mL. This amount is just enough to meet tissue needs without the functioning Hb. This will be achieved by 100% O_2 at 3 atmospheres, with an arterial PO_2 of 2000 mm Hg. (solubility coefficient = 0.003 mL/100 mL/mmHg.) 100% oxygen at 1 atmosphere may be tolerated up to 8 hours, without any symptoms.

Oxygen toxicity is due to formation of superoxide anion. 100% O_2 for more than 8 hours will cause substernal distress, nasal congestion, sore throat. 100% oxygen at 2-3 atmospheres may be tolerated, without any symptoms, for up to 5 hours. At 4 atmospheres, symptoms of toxicity may develop in 30 minutes; and at 6 atmospheres, convulsions develop in a few minutes. Thus, it should not be administered at a stretch for more than 5 hours and not more than 3 atmospheric pressure.

RESPIRATORY CHANGES IN EXERCISE

Many cardiovascular and respiratory mechanisms must operate in an integrated fashion if the O_2 needs of the active tissue are to be met and the extra CO_2 and heat removed from the body during exercise.

The circulatory changes maintains adequate circulation in the rest of the body while increased extraction of O_2 from the blood in exercising muscles ensures adequate ventilation This provides extra O_2 and eliminates extra CO_2 and some amount of heat.

Changes in Ventilation

During exercise, the amount of O_2 entering the blood in the lungs is increased because the amount of O_2 added to each unit of blood and the pulmonary blood flow per minute are increased. The pO_2 of blood flowing into the pulmonary capillaries falls 40–25 mm Hg and thereby an increased alveolar capillary pO_2 gradient is created and more O_2 enters the blood. Blood flow per minute is increased from 5.5 L/min to as much as 20–35 L/min and thereby the total amount of O_2 entering the blood and CO_2 extraction are increased markedly. The increase in O_2 uptake is proportional to the work load up to a maximum. Above this maximum, O_2 consumption level falls off and the blood lactate level continues to rise. The lactate comes from muscles where aerobic resynthesis of energy stores cannot keep pace with their utilization and an O_2 debt occurs.

Note

Oxygen debt

In any type of muscular exercises, O_2 requirement increases. Consumption of O_2 (VO_2) increase during 2–4 min of exercise and then reaches a plateau. So in the beginning (during adaptation phase), an O_2 deficit is established. This deficit is caused by the lag in circulatory adjustments during the start of exercise. During this period, muscles stores of ATP are used. This deficit is repaid in the form of O_2 debt (Fig. 3.30). Oxygen debt may be defined as the amount of excess O_2 that is consumed during recovery after an exercise. Physical performance is inversely related to O_2 deficit.

O_2 deficit is decreased by warm up and training. O_2 debt is meant for:

1. Reoxygenation of myoglobin.
2. Regeneration of depleted stores of ATP and creative phosphate.
3. Removal accumulated lactic acid from muscle tissues (lactic acid O_2 debt).
4. Resupply of dissolved O_2 in tissue fluids and blood.

Ventilation increases abruptly with the onset of exercise, followed after a brief pause by a further, more gradual

Table 3.7: Respiratory changes during exercise

	At rest	During exercise	Cause and control
Pulmonary ventilation (PV)	Frequency of breathing = 12/min TV = 500 ml PV = 6 l/min	Frequency of breathing = 40–45/min TV increases from 10–15% to 50% of VC PV = 100 l/min	PV increase in parallel to increase in O_2 consumption and increase in CO_2 output PV is increased due to: • Stimulation of respiratory center from motor cortex • Stimuli from proprioceptors of moving muscles, tendon and joints • Stimulation of carotid bodies • Increase in body temperature stimulates respiratory center • Increase in lactic acid and plasma K^+ level in blood *Note:* During heavy exercise, PV increase is not proportional to increase in O_2 consumption and increase in CO_2 output. This is due to anaerobiosis of working muscles, which contributes to the extra drive to respiratory center.
Diffusion capacity of O_2 (DO_2)	DO_2 = 20–30 ml/min/mm Hg	DO_2 increase above 3 times	DO_2 increase is due to: • Increase in blood perfusion around air sacs in the lungs • Opening of more capillaries. Both increase surface area of contact between alveoli and capillaries
Oxygen consumption	VO_2 = 250 ml/min	Increased to 15–20 times resting value	Due to: • Three times increase in A-V O_2 difference. • Five times increase in O_2 delivery to tissues Increased O_2 delivery to tissues is due to: increase in CO, alveolar ventilation, capillary density, RBC count

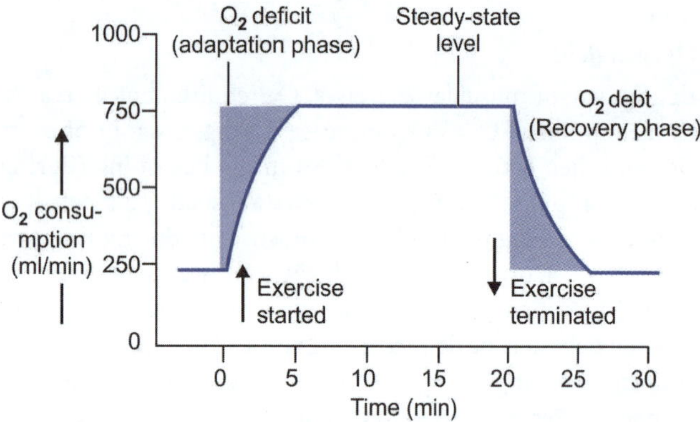

Fig. 3.30: Oxygen debt

increase. With moderate exercise, the increase is mostly due to an increase in the depth of respiration and when the exercise becomes more strenous this is accompanied by an increase in the respiratory rate.

Ventilation abruptly decreases when exercise ceases, followed after a brief pause by a more gradual decline to pre-exercise values. The abrupt increase in the ventilation at the start of exercise is presumably due to psychic stimuli and afferent impulses from proprioceptors in the muscles, tendons and joints. The increase in ventilation is proportionate to the increase in O_2 consumption. Exercise increases the plasma K^+ level and this increase may stimulate the peripheral chemoreceptors responsible for stimulation of respiration.

In addition, the sensitivity of the neurons controlling the response to CO_2 is increased and there will be increased fluctuations in the arterial pCO_2 therefore CO_2 is responsible for the increase in ventilation although O_2 seems to play some role.

When exercise becomes more vigorous, buffering of the increased amounts of lactic acid that are produced liberates more CO_2 and this further increases ventilation.

With respect to respiratory system, there are changes in (Table 3.7):

1. Pulmonary ventilation
2. Diffusion capacity of O_2 in lungs
3. Oxygen consumption.

CLINICAL QUESTIONS

1. **A diver after remaining in the sea for many hours came to the surface. He complained of pain in the joints and muscles, dizziness, breathlessness and then became unconscious.**
   a. What is the condition?
   b. What is the cause of pain in the joints and muscles?
   c. How can this condition be prevented?
2. **A trekker participating in a Himalayan expedition above the height of 3,000 meters suddenly developed nausea, vomiting, breathlessness and unconsciousness.**
   a. What is the probable condition?
   b. What is the cause?
   c. Give the physiological basis of treatment.
3. **Respiratory rate is – 20/ min. Tidal volume is – 500 ml. MVV is – 100 lit./mina)**
   a. Calculate breathing reserve and dyspnoeic index.
   b. What is its significance?
4. **Respiratory rate is 16/min, dead space volume is 150 ml and tidal volume is 400 ml. Oxygen consumption is 250 ml/min, arterial oxygen is 19 ml/min and venous oxygen is 14 ml/min.**
   a. Calculate alveolar ventilation.
   b. Calculate ventilation perfusion ratio.
   c. What is its significance?
5. **A doctor attending everest base camp expedition noticed mental irritability, incoordination of muscles and breathlessness in one of the expedition members.**
   a. Identify the condition with cause.
   b. Explain the features.
   c. Give physiological basis of treatment.

Answers for Clinical Questions are given in the Appendix

CHAPTER

4

Cardiovascular System

Cardiovascular system (Fig. 4.1) comprises of heart and blood vessels. The function of cardiovascular system is to supply O_2, nutrients and other essential substances to the tissues of the body and to remove CO_2 and other metabolic endproducts from tissues.

Some Important Characteristics of Cardiac Physiology

1. **Presence of intercalated discs:** These discs are present along the Z-lines of the cardiac sarcomeres. The myocardial fibers are tethered end-to-end on these discs. It provides a strong cell-to-cell cohesion, so that the contractile pull of one fiber is transmitted to the next one.
2. **Presence of 'gap junctions':** The myocardial cells are connected to each other by low resistance passages called gap junctions. These junctional regions allow free passage of ions from one cell to the next, and so on. Thus, the cells are electrically coupled. This arrangement creates a 'syncytium' of the cardiac muscle fibers. (Syncytium = mass of cytoplasm with numerous nuclei.) Benefit: When impulse reaches one point of a chamber, it quickly spreads through all cells. Thus, all cells excite almost together, and hence, all cells contract together as a single bundle. ('Syn' = together.). A simple example may explain syncytium. Think of an ice tray; water is poured from one end and it quickly spreads in all its cells.
3. **Long refractory period:** Due to the prolonged plateau phase, purkinje fibers and ventricular muscle have long refractory periods. The advantages of long refractory period is explained in page no 85.

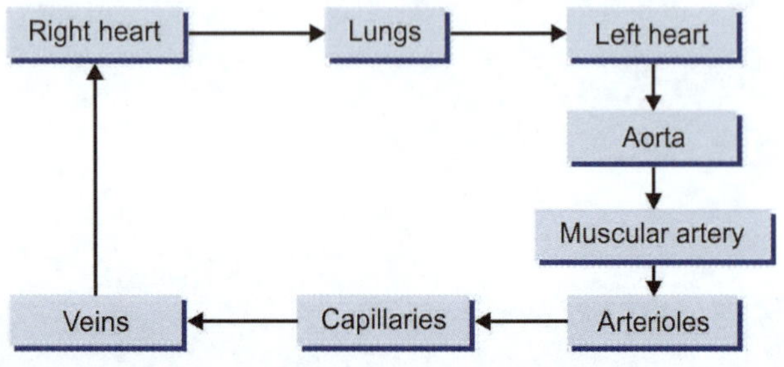

Fig. 4.1: Overview of cardiovascular system

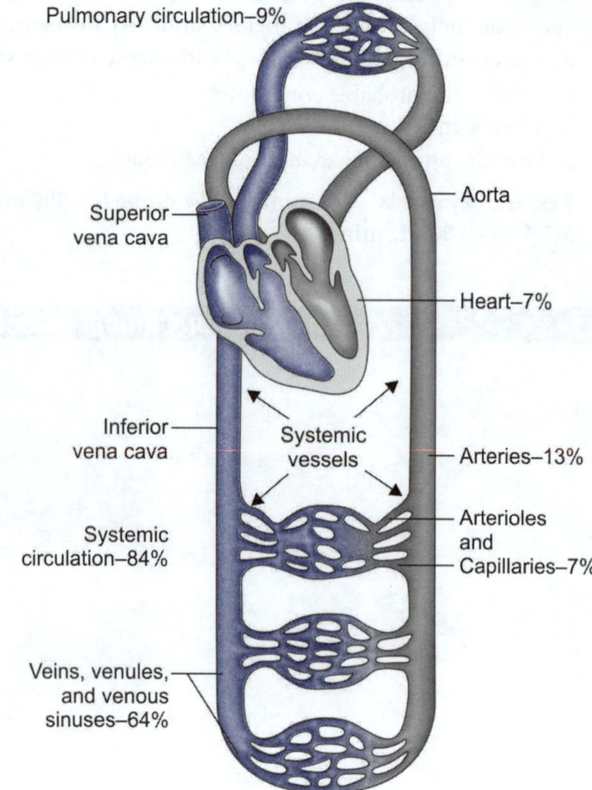

Fig. 4.2: Overview of cardiovascular system. Percentage represents volume of blood in different parts of the circulation

Note: CVS is a closed system that transports oxygenated blood from heart to tissues and returns deoxygenated blood from tissues to the heart. Pulmonary circulation is much smaller in comparison to systemic circulation. Volume of blood in different parts of the circulation (Fig. 4.2).

ORGANIZATION OF THE VASCULAR SYSTEM

Components of the Vasculature

Arteries

- Deliver oxygenated blood to the tissues.
- They are thick walled with extensive elastic tissue and smooth muscle.

- They are under high pressure.
- The blood volume contained in the arteries is called the stressed volume.

Arterioles

- They are the smallest branches of the arteries.
- They are the site of highest resistance in the cardiovascular system.
- They have a smooth muscle wall that is extensively innervated by autonomic nerve fibers.
- Arteriolar resistance is regulated by the autonomic nervous system (ANS).

Capillaries

- They have the largest total cross-sectional and surface area.
- They consist of a single layer of endothelial cells surrounded by basal lamina.
- They are thin walled.
- They are the site of exchange of nutrients, water and gases.

Venules

They are formed from merged capillaries.

Veins

- Progressively merge to form larger veins. The largest vein, the vena cava, returns blood to the heart.
- They are thin walled.
- They are under low pressure.
- They contain the highest proportion of the blood in the cardiovascular system.
- The blood volume contained in the veins is called the unstressed volume.

The functions of the circulation are achieved because the vascular system consists of the following type of blood vessels:

- *Windkessel vessels/distensible vessels:* These vessels are highly elastic (windkessel means elastic reservoir), e.g. aorta, pulmonary artery and their larger branches.
- *Resistance vessels:* These vessels contain less elastic tissue, but more smooth muscles. They can change the diameter by contraction or relaxation of smooth muscles. This changes the resistance and thus influences flow through these vessels. So these vessels are called resistance vessels, e.g. arterioles, metarterioles and precapillary sphincters.
- *Capacitance vessels:* These vessels are thin walled and highly distensible. So they have the ability to store large amount of blood and hence called capacitance vessels, e.g. veins.
- *Exchange vessels:* These vessels are thin walled and have fenestrations and helps in the exchange of materials between blood and interstitial fluid, e.g. capillaries.
- *Shunt (thoroughfare) vessels:* These are vessels which bypass the capillaries, e.g. arteriovenous anastomosis.

Blood flows along the following course:

- From the lungs to the left atrium via the pulmonary vein.
- From the left atrium to the left ventricle through the mitral valve.
- From the left ventricle to the aorta through the aortic valve.
- From the aorta to the systemic arteries and the systemic tissues (i.e. cerebral, coronary, renal, splanchnic, skeletal muscle and skin).
- From the tissues to the systemic veins and vena cava
- From the vena cava (mixed venous blood) to the right atrium.
- From the right atrium to the right ventricle through the tricuspid valve.
- From the right ventricle to the pulmonary artery through the pulmonic valve.
- From the pulmonary artery to the lungs for oxygenation.

Windkessel Effect (Figs 4.3A and B)

As the heart contracts intermittently, the pressure and blood flow in the large arteries is pulsatile (during systole volume of blood pumped is maximum and in diastole it is minimal). However the flow of blood through other blood vessels is continuous. It is because of the behavioral pattern of aorta and other large vessels.

During ventricular systole, blood enters large arteries with considerable force and this blood can be accommodated by distensible nature of blood vessels. During diastole, force is absent and volume of blood entering vessels is zero, but since vessels recoil due to elastic property, the BP is retained and the blood is pumped to periphery. This recoil effect is called

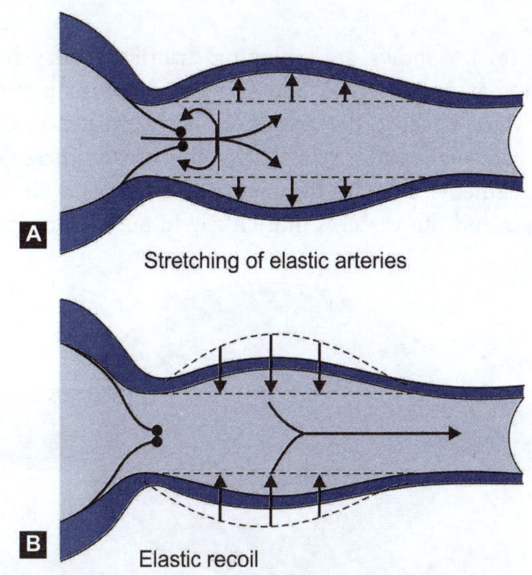

Figs 4.3A and B: Windkessel effect

PHYSICON—The Reliable Icon in Physiology

Windkessel effect and the vessels exerting this effect is called Windkessel vessels (aorta, pulmonary artery and their large branches).

HEMODYNAMICS

The flow of blood through the vascular system is governed by a group of physical laws.

Bernoulli's Principle

It states that, in a tube or blood vessel, the sum of the kinetic energy (KE) of flow and the pressure energy is constant. Therefore, when fluid flows through the narrow portion of tube, KE of flow increases as the velocity increases and the pressure energy is reduced (distending pressure decreases). Thus greater the velocity of flow in a vessel, the lesser will be the lateral pressure distending its walls.

Law of Laplace

It is the relationship between distending pressure and tension on the wall in a hollow viscous object. It states that distending pressure (P) in a distensible hollow object is equal to the tension in the wall (T) divided by two principal radii of curvature of object (R1 and R2). So, P = T/ R1 + T/ R2.

In a sphere, such as lung alveoli R1 = R2; therefore, P = 2T/R.

In a cylinder such as blood vessel, as one radius is infinite; therefore P = T/R.

Physiological Significance of Law of Laplace

Smaller the radius of blood vessel, lesser the tension in the wall necessary to balance the distending pressure. This is why the thin walled and delicate capillaries are less prone to rupture.

Figure 4.4 shows a developing arterial aneurysm. The pressures at points A, B, and C will be approximately the same. Thus, because the aneurysm has a greater radius, its wall tension is greater than that of the surrounding normal vessel segments. Also, as the aneurysm enlarges, wall tension increases and the vessel is more likely to burst. Examples are subarachnoid hemorrhage due to rupture of berry aneurysm, aortic aneurysm and diverticulitis.

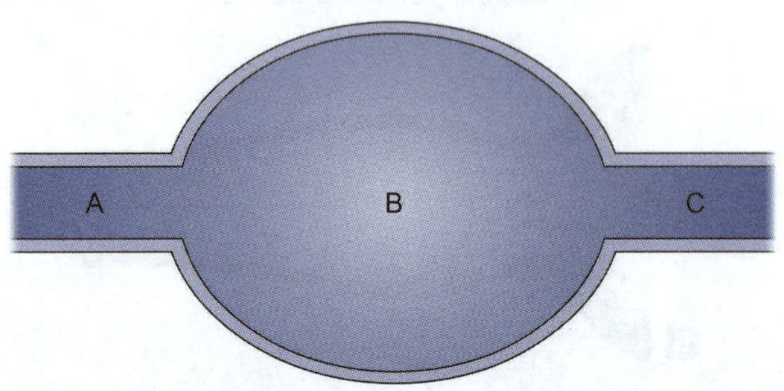

Fig. 4.4: Aortic enlargement

A dilated ventricle works more to pump the same amount of blood than the normal heart as explained by Laplace law (also see page no 124).

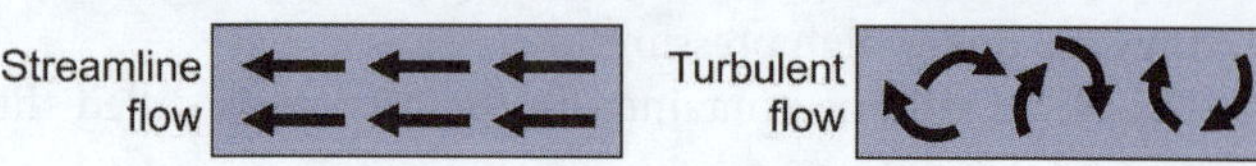

Fig. 4.5: Types of blood flow

Types of Blood Flow

There are two types of blood flow (Fig. 4.5):

1. *Laminar (streamline) blood flow:* In laminar flow, blood flows in large number of layers at a steady rate with each layer remaining at the same distance from the vessel wall. For example, characteristic of most part of the vascular system.
2. *Turbulent blood flow:* Here blood flows in all directions in the vessel and continuously mixing within the vessel. Thus there is a greater energy loss compared to laminar flow. For example, ventricles and aorta.

Laminar flow is silent; turbulent blood flow produces sounds that can be heard through stethoscope.

Reynolds Number

The probability for a blood flow to be turbulent is expressed as Reynolds number (Re),

$$Re = V\rho\, d/\eta$$

Where,

V = Velocity of flow in cm/sec

ρ = Density of blood

d = Diameter of blood vessel

η = Viscosity of blood in poise

When Re less than 1000, flow is always laminar. As the value increases the probability of turbulence also increases. Turbulence develops when Re exceeds 2000.

Constriction of an artery increases the velocity of blood flow through the constriction, producing turbulence and sounds (beyond constriction). Examples:

When arteries are constricted by atherosclerotic plaques, turbulence begins to develop in the systemic arteries and results in the vascular murmurs. The sound is called 'bruit'. When stethoscope is placed over brachial artery, there is no sound heard normally. However, while measuring BP by sphygmomanometer, artery is constricted (by BP cuff); upon release of cuff pressure, Korotkoff sounds can be heard via stethoscope. The sounds are produced by turbulence of blood created by constriction (and partial opening) of brachial artery.

Poiseuille-Hagen Formula

The Poiseuille equation represents the relationship of flow, pressure, and resistance. It can be applied to a single vessel (Fig. 4.6), an organ or an entire circuit.

R = 8 ηL/πr 4 (Where R = resistance, η= viscosity, L: length of the vessel and r = radius)

Since Flow = Pressure/Resistance

Flow = (P1 – P2) X πr 4/8ηL

The above formula is called the Poiseuille-Hagen formula. Resistance is directly proportional to viscosity and length of the vessel. It is inversely proportional to fourth power of radius of the tube. That is, if the radius of a vessel is increased by a factor of 'x', the resistance to blood flow through the vessel decreases by fourth power of 'x' (x^4); consequently, the blood flow increases by x^4.

For instance, if radius is doubled (increased by a factor of 2), the blood flow will increase by a 2^4, that is 16 times.

Series Versus Parallel Circuits (Figs 4.7A and B)

Series resistance is illustrated by the arrangement of blood vessels within a given organ. Each organ is supplied by a large artery, smaller arteries, arterioles, capillaries, and veins arranged in series. The total resistance is the sum of the individual resistances, as expressed by the following equation:

$$R_{(Total)} = R_{artery} + R_{arterioles} + R_{capillaries}$$

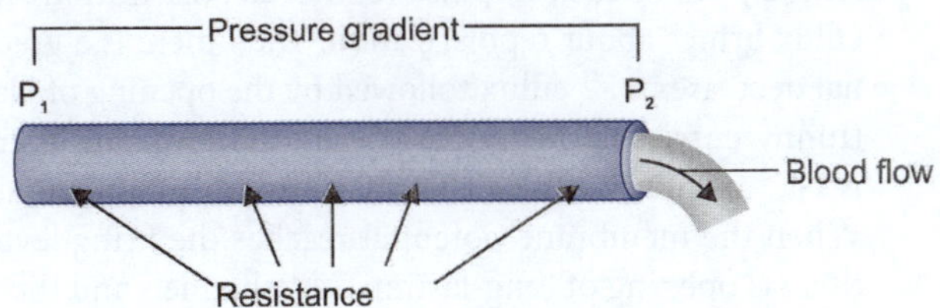

Fig. 4.6: Poiseuille-Hagen formula

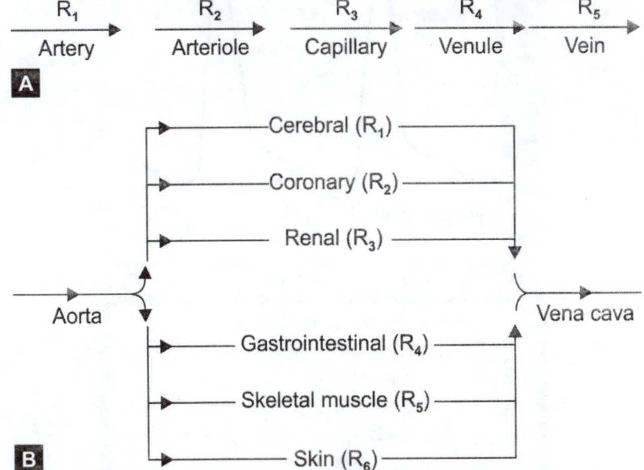

Figs 4.7A and B: A. Vascular resistance in series; **B.** Vascular resistance in parallel

The largest proportion of resistance in this series is contributed by the *arterioles*. Each blood vessel (e.g. the largest artery) or set of blood vessels (e.g. all of the capillaries) in series receives the same total blood flow. Thus, blood flow through the largest artery is the same as the total blood flow through all of the capillaries. As blood flows through the series of blood vessels, the pressure decreases.

Parallel resistance is illustrated by the systemic circulation. Each organ is supplied by an artery that branches off the aorta. The total resistance of this parallel arrangement is expressed by the following equation:

$$R_{(Total)} = 1/R_a + 1/R_b + 1/R_n$$

R_a, R_b, and R_n are the resistances of the renal, hepatic, and other circulations, respectively.

Each artery in parallel receives a fraction of the total blood flow. The total resistance is less than the resistance of any of the individual arteries. When an *artery is added in parallel, the total resistance decreases*. In each parallel artery, the pressure is the same.

Viscosity

As seen in the calculation of resistance, one of the factors on which resistance depends is the viscosity of the blood. Viscosity in turn depends mostly on hematocrit (details in page no 336). In large vessels, increase in hematocrit cause appreciable increases in viscosity. However, the change in viscosity with change in hematocrit is much less in smaller vessels, such as arterioles, capillaries and venules. This is due to the difference in the nature of flow through the small vessels. Therefore the net change in viscosity per unit change in hematocrit is much less in the body than *in vitro*. Viscosity also depends on composition of plasma (viscosity is high when immunoglobulins are markedly elevated), resistance of the cells to deformation (viscosity is high in hereditary spherocytosis).

PROPERTIES OF CARDIAC MUSCLE

Electrical Properties

- Excitability (Bathmotropism)
- Autorhythmicity (Chronotropism)
- Conductivity (Dromotropism).

Mechanical Properties

Contractility (Inotropism).

Other Properties

- Refractory period
- Frank-Starling law.

Excitability

The cardiac muscles are excitable and respond to proper stimuli with the production of action potentials. In heart two types of tissues are present.

a. *Conducting tissue:* They initiate and conduct impulses (SAN, AVN, internodal tract, bundle of His and Purkinje fibers).
b. *Contractile tissue:* They contracts in response to the impulse conducted (myocardial cells forming walls of cardiac chamber).

Action Potential

Action potential (AP) can be defined as sequence of changes in the membrane potential in an excitable cell due to opening and closure of different ion channels after the application of a threshold stimulus. Action potential in cardiac muscles is of two types:

1. *Fast response action potential:* This type of action potential is seen in working myocardium (atria, ventricles) and in Purkinje fibers (Fig. 4.8). It is characterized by:
   - *Rapid depolarization:* When the firing level is reached, there is a very rapid change of membrane potential producing a sharp upstroke called '0' (zero) phase. The resting membrane potential (RMP) of ventricular musculature is about –90 mV. In this phase the membrane potential crosses the zero line (positive overshoot). The inside of the cell becomes +ve with respect to outside and the cell is fully depolarized. The initial depolarization is due to Na^+ influx through rapidly opening Na^+ channels.
   - *Initial rapid repolarization:* After '0' phase there is a slight fall of membrane potential towards the zero potential line. This phase is named as phase '1'. This phase is due to closure of fast Na^+ channels and opening of K^+ channels (K^+ efflux begins).
   - *Plateau phase:* After phase '1', the membrane potential is maintained for sometime at that level, i.e. the repolarization is prolonged. This phase is named as phase '2'. It is due to opening of slow Ca^{2+} channels along with K^+ efflux. Thus, potential change due to K^+ efflux is neutralized.
   - *Late rapid repolarization:* Then there is a rapid repolarization at phase '3'. This is due to closure of slow Ca^{2+} channels and K^+ efflux.
   - *Baseline (polarized state):* In the last phase (phase '4') the RMP is restored by the activation of Na^+–K^+ pump (causing K^+ efflux).
2. *Slow response action potential:* This type of action potential is seen in the pacemaker tissues (Fig. 4.9). Before the sharp upstroke (seen in myocardial cells) there is a gradual slope. In sinoatrial node (SAN) and atrioventricular node (AVN) the depolarization in the beginning is gradual and RMP automatically approaches to –60 mV. This phase of gradual slope is called pacemaker potential.

   When this pacemaker potential reaches a value of –60 mV, firing occurs. Now there develops sharp upstroke. There is no plateau in the AP of SAN and AVN.

   The ionic basis of slow response AP:
   - At the peak of each impulse (end of depolarization) K^+ efflux brings about repolarization. Then there is a gradual decrease in K^+ efflux followed by the opening of Na^+ (funny current) and transient Ca^{2+} channels and there is Na^+ and Ca^{2+} influx. This accounts for prepotential.
   - When the membrane potential reaches the firing level, there is opening of long-lasting Ca^{2+} channels and there

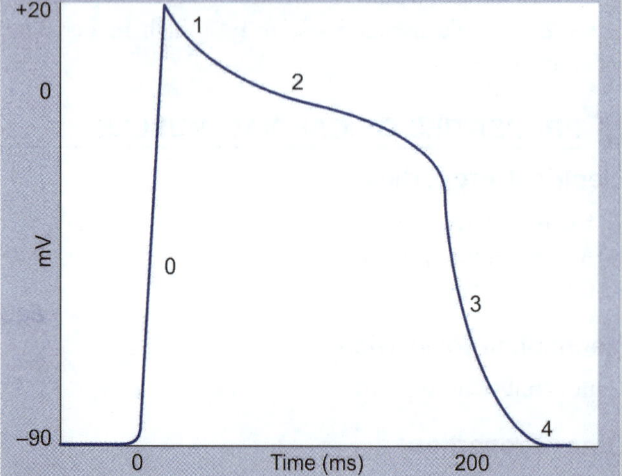

Fig. 4.8: Phases of action potential in a myocardial muscle fiber

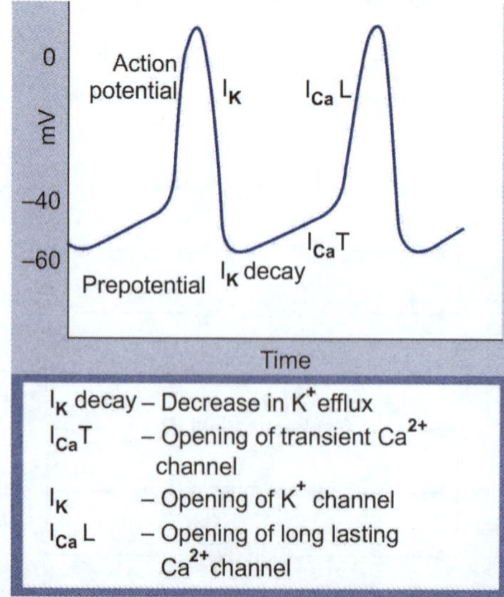

Fig. 4.9: Membrane potential of a pacemaker tissue

is Ca^{2+} influx. When the membrane potential reaches +35 mV, there is closing of Ca^{2+} channels and opening of K^+ channels.

Note: Electrical and mechanical response overlap in cardiac muscle in contrast to skeletal muscle (Fig. 4.10).

The summary of action potential and ionic basis is given in Table 4.1 and Figure 4.11.

Autorhythmicity

The property of spontaneous pre-potential followed by AP is called autorhythmicity. The RMP of working myocardial cells is about –90 mV and is stable. In conducting tissues, RMP is about –60 mV and it is unstable.

Because of continuous change in membrane permeability, their membrane potential declines towards the firing level spontaneously after each action potential. When the firing level is reached an action potential is triggered. This slow depolarization between action potential is called prepotential/ pacemaker potential/diastolic depolarization.

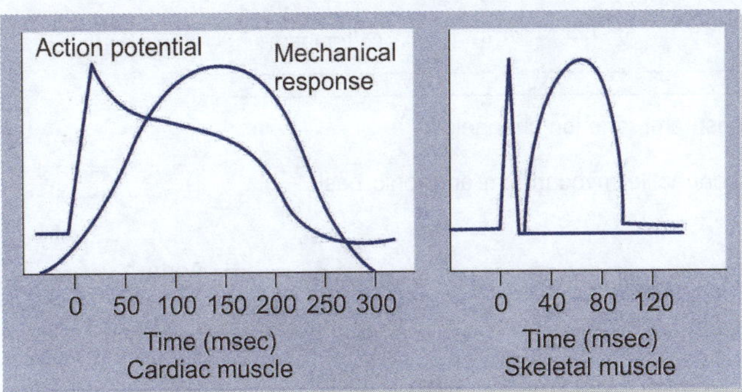

Fig. 4.10: Action potential in cardiac muscle and skeletal muscle compared

Table 4.1: Action potential in cardiac muscles

Phases	Ions responsible
Phase 0: Rapid depolarization	• Due to entry of sodium ions through voltage-gated, **fast Na^+** channels
Phase 1: Initial repolarization	• Due to inactivation of fast Na^+ channels • Also due to efflux of potassium ions through transient outward K^+ channels
Phase 2: Plateau phase	• Efflux of **potassium ions** continue • This is balanced by influx of **calcium ions** through (L-type) calcium channels • Since both are positively charged ions, membrane potential stays as plateau
Phase 3: Late repolarization	• Due to efflux of potassium ions through delayed rectifier potassium channels
Phase 4: Return to resting membrane potential	By Na K ATPase

The ionic basis of prepotential: At the peak of each impulse (at the end of depolarization) K^+ efflux brings about repolarization. Then there is a gradual decrease in K^+ efflux followed by the opening of Na^+ and transient Ca^{2+} channels.

Effect of Vagal (Cholinergic) Stimulation on Membrane Potential

When cholinergic fibers to nodal tissue are stimulated heart rate decreases (Fig. 4.12). ACh released at the nerve endings increases K^+ conductance at nodal tissues (mediated via M_2 muscarinic receptors).

There is an increase in K^+ efflux at nodal tissues resulting in hyperpolarization. In addition, activation of M_2 receptors slows the opening of Ca^{2+} channels. The result is a decrease in firing rate.

Effect of Sympathetic (Noradrenergic) Stimulation on Membrane Potential

When sympathetic cardiac nerves are stimulated heart rate increases (Fig. 4.13). Noradrenaline released makes membrane potential fall more rapidly (mediated via β_1 receptors). Noradrenaline facilitates the opening of Ca^{2+} channel and thus rapidity of depolarization is increased.

Note

1. The discharge frequency is increased when the temperature rises. This explains tachycardia associated with fever.
2. Digitalis depresses nodal tissue and exerts an effect like that of vagal stimulation, particularly on AV node.

Rate of impulse production

SA node	:	70 – 80/min
AV node	:	40 – 60/min
Bundle of His	:	30/min
Purkinje fibers	:	15 – 40/min
Atrial muscle	:	40 – 60/min
Ventricular muscle	:	20 – 30/min

Conductivity

The property which enables myocardium to conduct electrical impulse is called conductivity. Human heart has specialized conductive system through which the impulse from SA node are transmitted to all parts of the body.

The conductive system of human heart (Figs 4.14 and 4.15) comprises of as follows:

Sinoatrial Node

Sinoatrial node (SA node) is a small, flattened, ellipsoid strip of specialized cardiac muscle. It is about 3 mm wide, 15 mm long and 1 mm thick. It is located at the junction of the superior vena cava with the right atrium. The SA nodal fibers connect directly with atrial muscle fibers, so that AP from

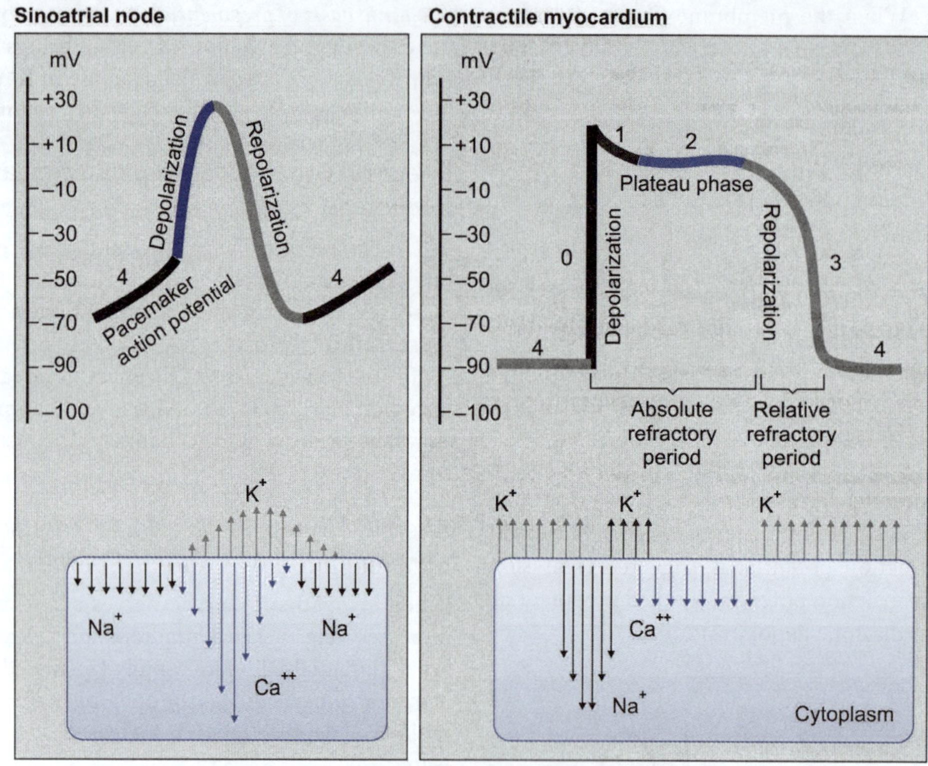

Fig. 4.11: Action potential of SA node and contractile myocardium and ionic basis

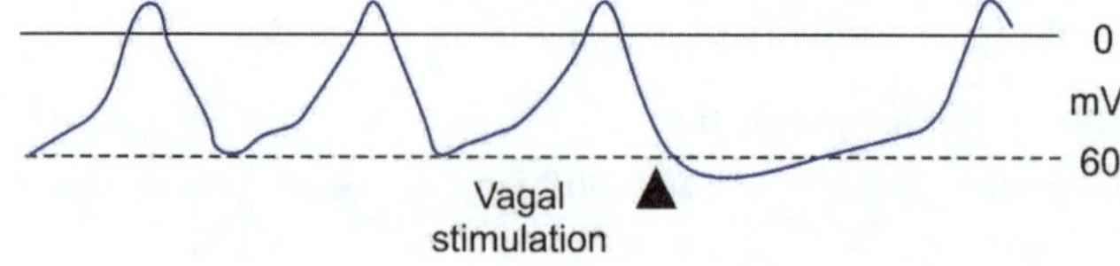

Fig. 4.12: Effect of vagal stimulation on membrane potential

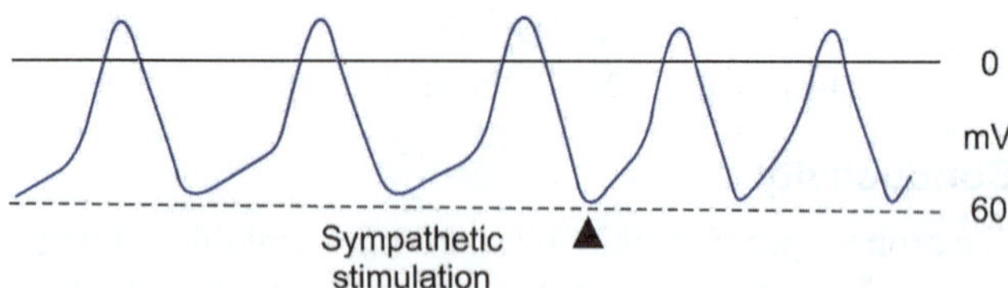

Fig. 4.13: Effect of sympathetic stimulation on membrane potential

the SA node immediately spreads to atrial wall. The SA node contains small round cells called P cells/pacemaker cells.

The action potential is largely due to Ca^{2+} with no contribution from Na^+ influx. Prepotential is most prominent in the SA node. Even though all parts of the conducting system can generate impulses, the rate of rhythmical discharge is faster than that of any other part of heart (70–80/min). The generated impulse spreads downwards and activates other parts of the heart. So depolarization of other parts of the conducting system occur before they discharge spontaneously and hence SA node is the pacemaker of normal heart.

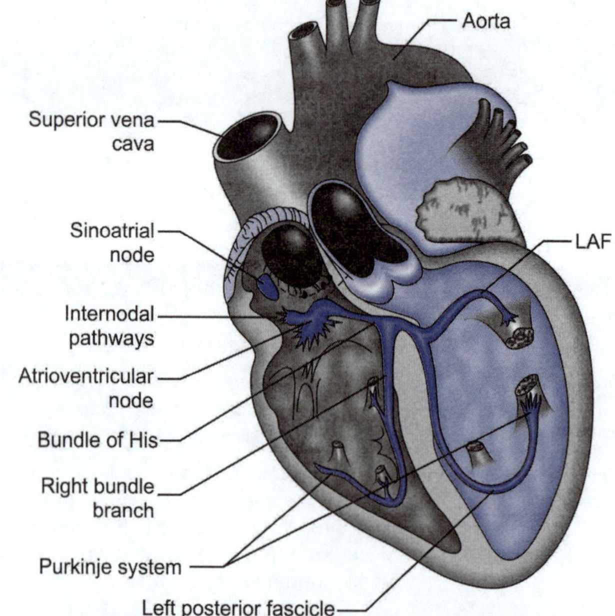

Fig. 4.14: Conduction system of heart

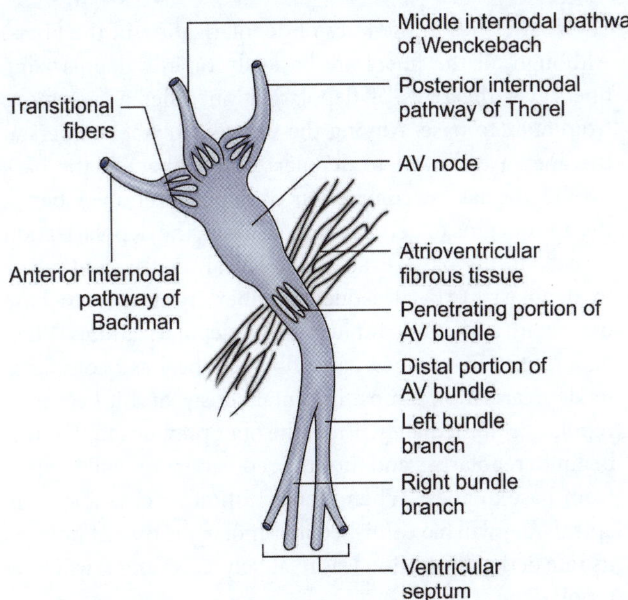

Fig. 4.15: Organization of atrioventricular node

Internodal Atrial Pathways

The ends of sinus nodal fibers connect directly with surrounding atrial fibers. But conduction is more rapid in some bands of atrial fibers. These bands of fibers are called internodal atrial pathways. There are three bundles of atrial fibers:

1. Anterior internodal tract of Bachman
2. Middle internodal tract of Wenckebach
3. Postinternodal tract of Thorel

The rapidity of conduction is because they contain a specialized fast conducting fibers of Purkinje type.

Atrioventricular Node

Atrioventricular node (AV node) is located in the right posterior portion of the interatrial septum. It is the only conducting pathway between atria and ventricles. This is because atrial muscle fibers are separated from the ventricular muscles by fibrous tissue ring (annuli fibrosii).

Atrioventricular node also contains P cells but fewer in number than SA node, so rate of impulse production is also less (40–60/min). Sometimes AV node can generate impulse when SA node is out of order or if the conduction from SA node is blocked. Other parts of the heart can generate this rhythm and they are called ectopic foci.

Atrioventricular Nodal Delay

On reaching AV node, the speed of impulse is slowed down and then it is transferred to the bundle of His. Thus transmission of impulse suffers a delay of about 0. 1 sec called AV nodal delay.

This is important because:

- Atria gets enough time to empty blood into ventricles.
- Efficiency of ventricular pumping is increased.
- It prevents entry of too rapid impulses from atria into the ventricles.

Causes

- Number of gap junctions is less between successive cells, so the velocity of conduction is decreased.
- Presence of multiple branching system in AV node.
- Cells of AV node are made up of small diameter fibers in which velocity of conduction is less.

Bundle of His (AV Bundle)

Atrioventricular node is continuous with bundle of His. Bundle of His originates from ventricular surface of AV node and runs along the right border of interventricular septum. It runs for a short distance and soon gives off a left bundle branch (at the top of interventricular septum) and continues as right bundle branch. The left bundle branch divides into an anterior fascicle and a posterior fascicle. All the branches run subendocardially on either side of septum. A special feature of AV bundle is one way conduction of impulse (except in abnormal states).

Purkinje System

It is an extensive network formed of the Purkinje cells present subendocardially, which transfer impulse to working myocardial cells. They are fast conducting, very large fibers with extensive gap junction. So the cardiac impulse is instantaneously transmitted to entire ventricular musculature. The ends of the Purkinje fibers penetrate into the muscle mass and finally become continuous with cardiac muscle fibers.

The conduction speeds in cardiac tissues are given in Table 4.2.

Spread of Electrical Activity (Figs 4.16A to E)

- Depolarization initiated in the SA node spreads radially through the atria. It then converges on the AV node. Atrial depolarization is completed in 0.1 sec.
- Conduction of AV node is slow and so there is a delay of 0.1 sec called AV nodal delay.

Table 4.2: Conduction speeds in cardiac tissue

Tissue	Conduction rate (m/sec)
SA node	0.05
Atrial pathways	1
AV node	0.05
Bundle of His	1
Purkinje system	4
Ventricular muscle	1

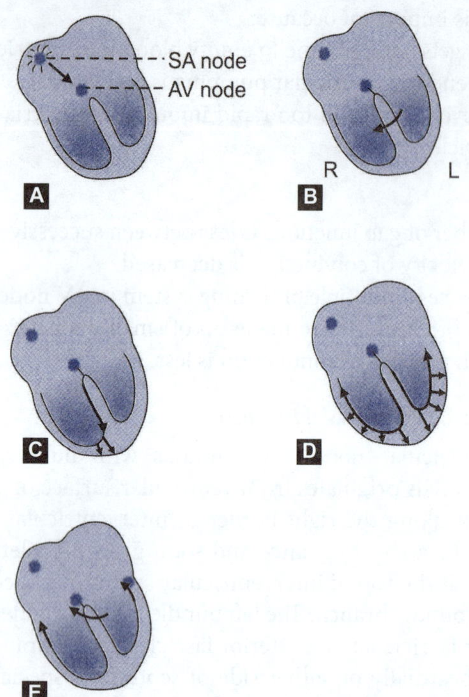

Figs 4.16A to E: Normal spread of electrical activity in the heart: **A.** Atrial activation; **B.** Septal activation from left to right; **C.** Activation of anteroseptal region of the ventricular myocardium; **D.** Activation of major portion of ventricular myocardium from endocardial surfaces; **E.** Late activation of posterobasal portion of the left ventricle and the pulmonary conus

- Impulse enters the bundle of His. From here, impulse first enters the left bundle branch first. Then, through interventricular septum it goes to the right branch. This spread of impulse from left to right is responsible for Q-wave on ECG.
- Impulse spreads toward the apex. And then, Purkinje fibers spread the impulse from apex to base; it is the fastest conducting part in the heart (4 m/sec). From the top of the septum, wave of depolarization spreads in the rapidly conducting Purkinje fibers to all parts of ventricle in 0.08-0.1 sec. Impulse spreads from apex to base, and from endocardium to epicardium. Last portions to be depolarized are base of left ventricle (LV), pulmonary conus, and uppermost part of interventricular septum. (LV has a thicker muscle mass compared to RV. Hence, LV takes little longer to depolarize, compared to RV.)
- Repolarization spreads in the opposite direction – from base to apex and from epicardium to endocardium. Last portion to be repolarized would be apical endocardium.
- How is it that the cell that is depolarized first (the cell at the apex) is repolarized last? And, the cell where depolarization reaches last (the cell at the base) is the first one to repolarize? The answer lies in the rates of depolarization of the fibers. Although all the fibers are basically rapidly depolarizing fibers, yet the rates of depolarization differ as we move from apex to base. Among the ventricular fibers, fibers at the apex are slowest to depolarize and fibers at the base exhibit the fastest completion of depolarization. Fiber at the apex begins to depolarize first. Then, the depolarization spreads to the base (even as the apical fiber is continuing to depolarize). Each sequential fiber from apex to base has rapid and more rapid rate of depolarization. When depolarization reaches base, fiber at the base completes its depolarization almost instantaneously, and it begins to repolarize immediately. Then, the fiber previous to that will begin to repolarize, and thus the repolarization will happen from base to apex. When repolarization reaches apex, the apical fiber will have finished its depolarization just now (as its rate of depolarization was relatively slow) and it will now repolarize.

Contractility

It is ability of the tissue to shorten in length (contraction) after receiving a stimulus. Isometric as well as isotonic contraction are seen in the heart.

Factors that Influence Contractility (Table 4.3)

V_{max}

Velocity of contraction is maximum when afterload is zero. The maximum velocity which will develop when afterload is zero is called V_{max} (Fig. 4.17). It is increased when contractility is increased and is reduced when contractility is decreased. It is not changed when the initial length of muscle fiber is changed.

Note

1. *Preload:* Degree to which myocardium is stretched before it contracts and it is equal to end-diastolic volume (EDV). Here the load acts before the muscle starts contracting.
2. *Afterload:* Resistance against which blood is expelled from the heart. Here the load acts on the muscle after it has started contracting.

Table 4.3: Factors that influence contractility

Increased contractility	Decreased contractility
Sympathetic stimulation	Parasympathetic stimulation
Increased Ca^{2+}	Hypercapnia
Xanthine	Quinidine, barbiturates
Glucagon	Myocardial damage
Thyroid hormones	Acidosis

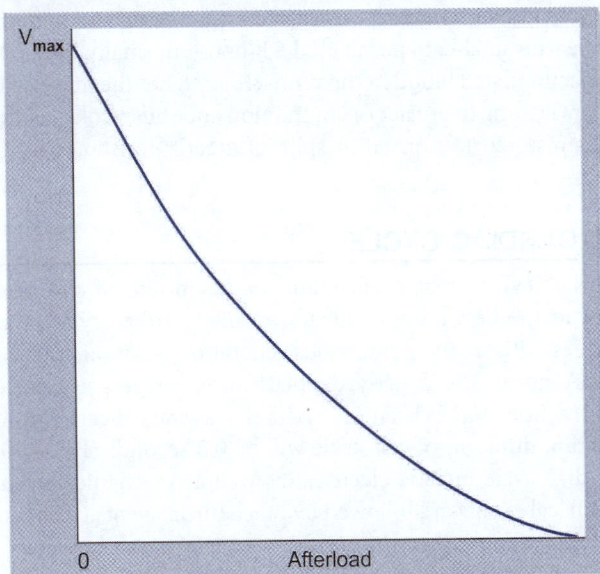

Fig. 4.17: Force velocity relationship

Extrasystole and Postextrasystolic Potentiation

- In a regularly beating heart if an extra stimulus is delivered so that it falls earlier than the usual timing, but after the refractory period then the heart responds to this stimulus by a weak extra contraction called *extrasystole.*
- Now the next regular impulse comes but it finds the heart refractory due to extrasystole, so there is no contraction and the gap produced is called *compensatory pause.*
- The subsequent regular impulse comes and the heart responds to it stronger than normal contraction due to postextrasystolic potentiation. The cause for this postextrasystolic is increased availability of intracellular Ca^{2+}.

Refractory Period

It is period in which the muscle does not show any response to a stimulus. Normal refractory period of ventricles is 250–300 msec and that of atria is 150 msec. Refractory period is of two types–absolute and relative (Fig. 4.18).

Absolute Refractory Period (180–200 msec)

Absolute refractory period is the period during which the muscle does not show any response at all, whatever may be the strength of the stimuli. During phases 0–2 and about half of phase 3 cardiac muscle is in its absolute refractory period.

Relative Refractory Period (50 msec)

The relative refractory period is the period during which muscle shows response, if the strength of the stimulus is increased to maximum. It remains relatively refractory until phase 4.

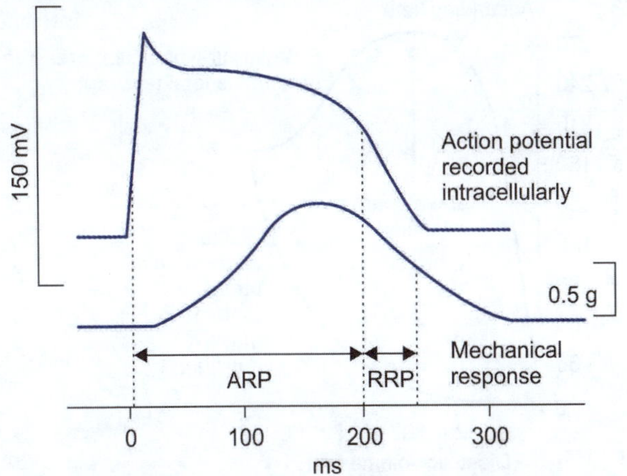

Fig. 4.18: Mechanical events in contractality (ARP: Absolute refractory period, RRP: Relative refractory period)

Significance

Due to the prolonged plateau phase, Purkinje fibers and ventricular muscle have long refractory periods. The long refractory period has following advantages:

- **Ventricular rate cannot be very high:** If SA node generates 200-250 impulses per minute, all those impulses will not cause ventricular excitation. Some of the impulses will be extinguished as they will find ventricles in refractory state. (If the ventricular rates were to be too high, cardiac cycle duration will be too short. Ventricular filling will suffer and cardiac output will be greatly diminished.)
- **Ventricles do not exhibit 'tetanus':** Tetanus is a sustained state of contraction, and failure to relax, occurring due to high frequency stimulation of a muscle. Due to long refractory periods, ventricles cannot be excited at high frequencies, and hence will not be tetanized. Also, heart muscle does not fatigue (even though it is continuously contracting). The long refractory period gives it sufficient time to maintain its blood supply and nutrition.

Frank-Starling Law (Fig. 4.19)

This law states that, the force of contraction of the heart is directly proportional to the initial length of cardiac muscle fiber within physiological limits. Initial length of the muscle fiber = length of the fiber at the end of diastole = end-diastolic fiber length. It may also be expressed as end-diastolic blood volume. When the ventricle is in early diastole, it is more compliant (it is more distensible). The blood at this stage, enters the ventricle, but the tension (this is called passive tension) of the ventricle (intraventricular pressure) does not rise appreciably. Only when the ventricle is reasonably filled, from then, the passive tension (intraventricular pressure) begins to rise steeply. The developed tension increases as the diastolic volume increases until it reaches a maximum

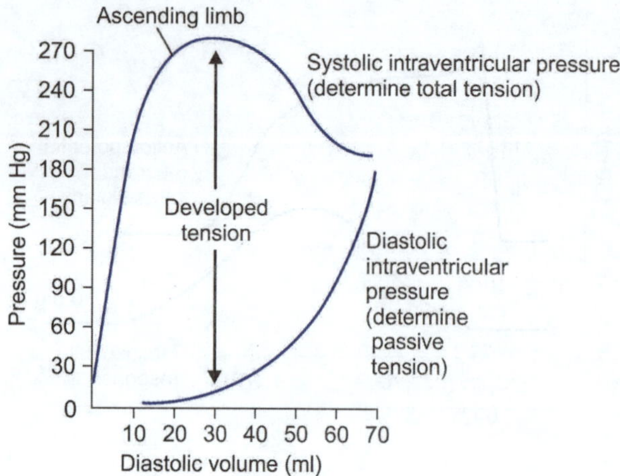

Fig. 4.19: Length-tension relationship in cardiac muscle

(ascending limb of Starlings curve), then tends to decrease (descending limb of Starling curve). The descending limb in human heart is seen only when cardiac muscles are ruptured. This law has an important role in the regulation of stroke volume and hence cardiac output.

Factors Affecting End-diastolic Volume (Table 4.4)

Physiological significance

- The law explains why blood ejected by each of the ventricle per heart beat is same. If RV output is more than the left, blood accumulates in the left side leading to greater force of contraction of left ventricle, thus increasing LV output.
- It serves as a life saving device in cardiac failure. LV failure causes accumulation of blood in the LV, thereby decreases blood supply to vital organs. Soon accumulation of blood in the LV increases the initial length of muscle fibers leading greater cardiac output according to Frank-Starling mechanism. If accumulation of blood exceeds physiological limit, the law fail to operate leading to death.

Table 4.4: Factors affecting end-diastolic volume

Factors increasing EDV		Factors decreasing EDV
Increased pumping action of skeletal muscle		Sitting and standing posture
Increased blood volume	Myocardial stretching (EDV)	Decreased total blood volume
Sympathetic discharge		Decreased ventricular compliance
Decreased intrathoracic pressure		Increased venous resistance (Pericardial effusion) Increased intrathoracic pressure

- When the peripheral resistance is increased, initially the heart is unable to pump all the blood it normally does. The accumulated blood in the ventricle stretches the muscle fibers leading to greater of contraction and thus stroke volume is restored to normal in spite of greater resistance to the flow.

CARDIAC CYCLE

Cardiac events that occur from the beginning of one heart beat to the beginning of next are called cardiac cycle. Each cycle is initiated by spontaneous generation of action potential in SA node. The orderly depolarization triggers a wave of contraction and relaxation. With an average heart rate of 75/min, duration of one cycle will be 0.8 seconds (Fig. 4.20). Cardiac cycle include electrical as well as mechanical event. Electrical events are followed by mechanical events.

The mechanical events are:

- Pressure changes in atria are ventricles.
- Pressure changes in aorta, pulmonary artery are jugular vein.
- Volume changes in atria are ventricles.
- Movements of heart and production of heart sounds.

Phases of Cardiac Cycle (Fig. 4.21)

1. Atrial systole (0.1 sec)
2. Ventricular systole (0.3 sec)
3. Ventricular diastole (0.5 sec)
4. Atrial diastole (0.7 sec)

Atrial Systole

Atrial systole can be taken as the initial phase of cardiac cycle. Before atrial contraction, AV valves are open, semilunar valves are closed and blood flows continuously from great

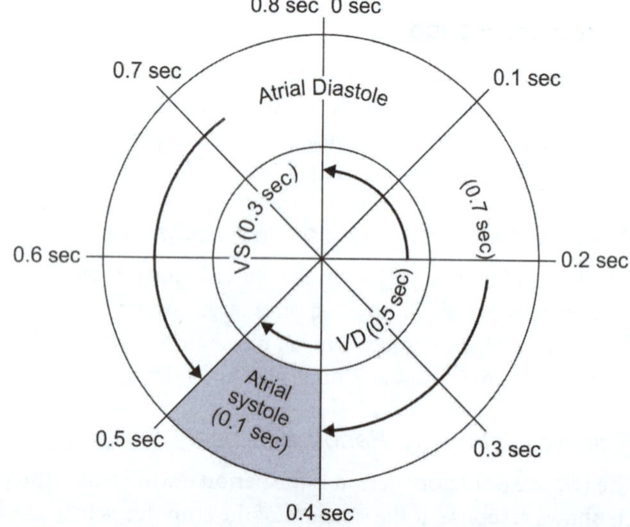

Fig. 4.20: Atrial and ventricular events of cardiac cycle

The phases of the cardiac cycle for a heart rate of 75 beats per minute

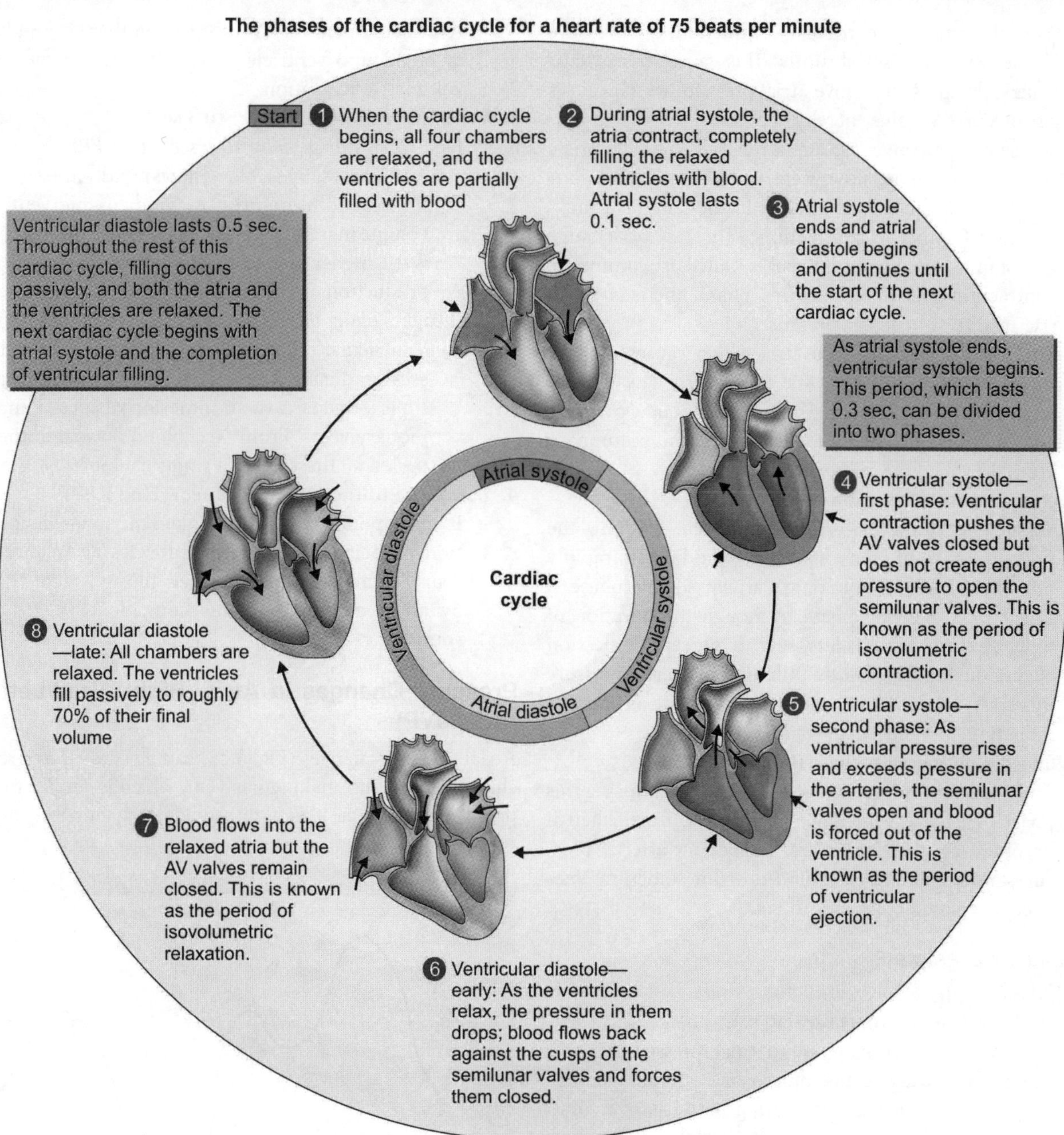

Fig. 4.21: Major changes in the cardiac chambers during cardiac cycle

veins to atria and from atria to ventricles. Seventy percent of ventricular filling occurs before atrial contraction. Atrial systole contributes only 30% of ventricular filling. Atria simply acts as booster pumps that increase the effectiveness of ventricular filling Atrial systole causes an elevation of atrial pressure which is recorded as 'a' wave in atrial pressure tracing. Here there is some regurgitation of blood into the great veins which is minimized by constriction of vena cava during contractrion of atrial muscles. Atrial systole starts after 'P' wave in ECG.

Ventricular Systole

Atrial systole is followed immediately by ventricular systole. It is divided into three phases:

1. **Isovolumetric (Isometric) ventricular contraction (0.05 sec) [ICP]**

- After the onset of ventricular contraction, the pressure in the ventricle rises abruptly. This causes increase in ventricular pressure above atrial pressure which causes closure of AV valve thereby the first heart sound.
- The semilunar valves are already closed so the ventricle is a closed chamber now. Ventricular muscles are contracting, but there is no change in the length of muscle fiber (isometric contraction). There is no change in volume also, so this phase is called isovolumetric contraction phase. During this phase, there is sharp rise in intraventricular pressure.
- The AV valves bulge into atria which causes a slight increase in atrial pressure and this recorded as 'c' wave in atrial pressure tracing. The intraventricular pressure rises sharply and when it exceeds aortic and pulmonary arterial pressure semilunar valves open.

2. **Maximum (rapid) ejection phase (0. 1 sec) (MEP)**
   - When the semilunar valves are open, initially the pressure gradient is more and the blood enters rapidly into the aorta and pulmonary artery, so this phase is called rapid ejection phase. Although the duration of rapid ejection phase is less, seventy percent of ejection occurs during this. Aortic pulmonary arterial pressure increases as the blood enters them. There is marked reduction in ventricular volume.
3. **Reduced/slow ejection phase (0. 15 sec) (REP)**
   - Thirty percent of ventricular ejection occurs during this phase. Ventricular pressure begins to fall are when it becomes less than aortic and pulmonary arterial pressure, momentum keeps blood flow for sometime ventricular volume continues to fall.

Ventricular Diastole

It includes four phases:

1. **Protodiastole phase (0.04 sec) (PDP)**
   - Ventricle starts relaxing, ventricular pressure reduces rapidly below aortic and pulmonary arterial pressure. When the momentum of flowing blood is overcome, semilunar valves close. So protodiastole is the short interval between ventricular diastole and closure of semilunar valves. The closure of valves is sharp and this leads to rebound of blood column, which is represented as a sharp deflection called incisura in aortic pressure tracing.
2. **Isovolumetric relaxation phase (0. 06 sec) (IRP)**
   - It starts from closure of semilunar valves. AV valves are already closed and ventricle is again a closed chamber. As there is no change in volume it is called isovolumetric relaxation. There is sudden reduction in pressure and when it becomes less than that of atrial pressure, AV valves open. As AV valves open there is rapid entry of blood into ventricles and it marks the end of isovolumetric relaxation.
3. **Ventricular diastole proper (0.3 sec)**
   - *First rapid filling phase (0.1 sec) (Ist RFP)*
     - As AV valves open, blood flows rapidly into ventricles. It is due to more pressure gradient and ventricular volume increases. Atrial pressure will decrease, but it is still higher than ventricular pressure (results in the production of 3rd heart sound).
   - *Reduced filling phase/Diastasis (0.2 sec)*
     - Ventricular inflow velocity decreases, volume increases gradually. Blood flows into the atria through superior vena cava and inferior vena cava and pulmonary veins. From atria blood flows into the ventricles, all these act as a single chamber.
4. **Last rapid filling phase (0.10 sec) (IInd RFP)**
   - It corresponds to atrial systole. Due to atrial contraction, velocity of flow into ventricles again increases. Thirty percent of ventricular filling is contributed by atrial contraction (this coincide with 4th heart sound).

Pressure Changes in Atria (Right Atrial/Left Atrial/JVP)

Atrial pressure changes (Fig. 4.22) can be studied by pressure changes in the internal jugular vein, which is similar to atrial pressure tracing as it is a retrograde transmission of atrial pressure changes.

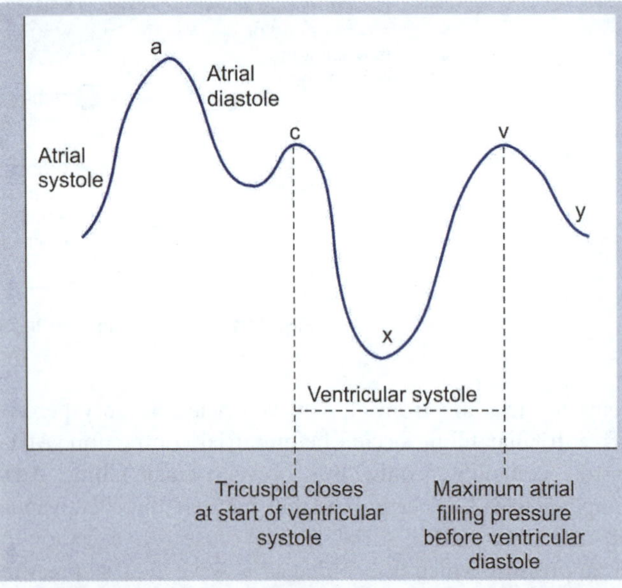

Fig. 4.22: Intra-atrial pressure changes during cardiac cycle/jugular venous pulse

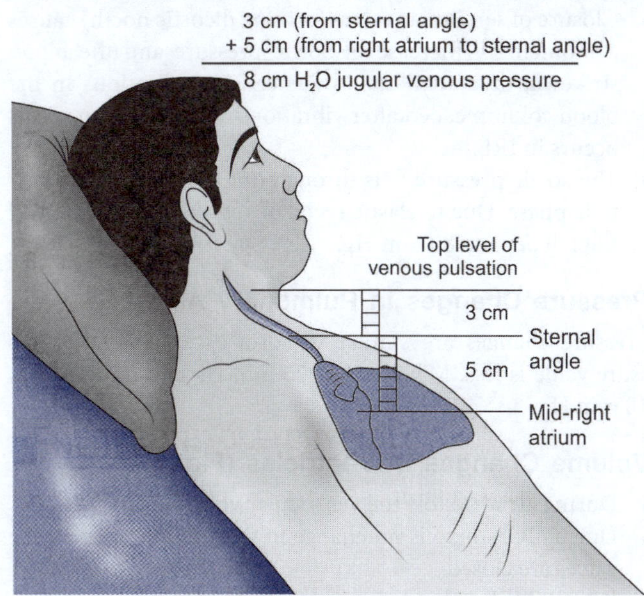

Fig. 4.23: Jugular venous pulsation

Normally, the center of right atrium is 5 cm below the sternal angle. Hence, add +5 cm to the above measurement to obtain the right atrial pressure. Normal JVP is 3 cm above sternal angle, i.e. 3 + 5 = 8 cm from right atrium (Fig. 4.23).

Atrial pressure rises during atrial systole and continue to rise during isovolumetric ventricular contraction when AV valve bulges into atria. When AV valves are pulled down by contrating ventricles during ejection phase, atrial pressure falls rapidly. The pressure then rises, until AV valves are again open. Then pressure in atria decreases. Atrial pressure changes are transmitted to great veins, producing three positive (a, c, v) and two negative waves (x, y).

'a' Wave

- It is due to atrial systole. Pressure in the jugular vein also increases as some blood regurgitates during atrial systole.
- In addition, venous inflow stops and the resultant rise in venous pressure contributes to a wave.

'c' Wave

It is manifested due to rise in atrial pressure produced by the bulging of AV valve into atria during isovolumetric contraction.

'x' Wave

- It is the 1st negative wave.
- Due to downward movement of AV ring during ejection.

'v' Wave

It is due to passive increase in pressure due to venous return.

'y' Wave

Due to emptying of atria as AV valve opens.

Jugular Venous Pulsation

Jugular venous pulsations is different from arterial pulsation in neck by following ways:

- Jugular venous pulsations is less sharp and less palpable and the pulsations 'c' and 'v' can be made out.
- There is slight change in JVP during respiratory cycle, but no such changes for arterial pulsation.
- Jugular venous pulsations can be abolished by slight pressure at the root of the neck.
- If pressure is applied in the abdomen the level of JVP rises.
- Jugular venous pulsations is better seen than felt.

Abnormalities of JVP

- Elevated in congestive heart failure.
- Large 'a' wave is seen when there is abnormal resistance to atrial contraction, also when there is narrowing (stenosis) of AV valves.
- Giant 'a' wave/Canon wave occurs when there is atrioventricular dissociation. Here atria contracts against closed ventricle and the condition is complete heart block.
- Giant 'c' wave is seen in tricuspid insufficiency.

Pressure Changes in Ventricles

Left Ventricular Pressure Changes (Fig. 4.24)

- A small rise in pressure (up to 10 mm Hg) is seen in the ventricle during atrial systole (AS).
- At the end of AS, pressure decreases to 2–3 mm Hg.
- In the ICP the pressure increases (80 mm Hg) and towards the end of this phase the semilunar valve opens. Further

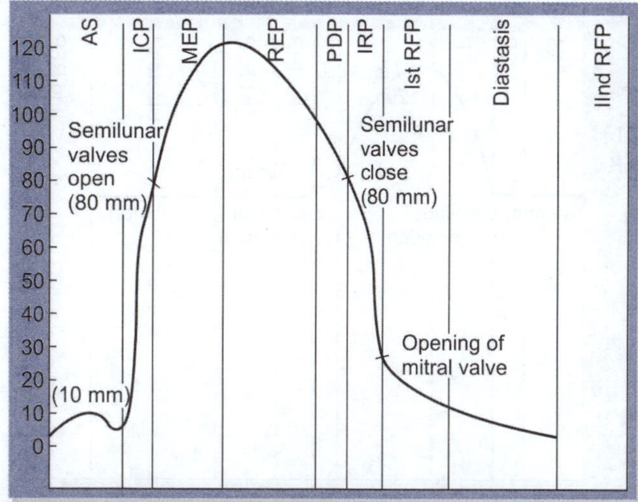

Fig. 4.24: Left ventricular pressure changes

PHYSICON—The Reliable Icon in Physiology

contraction is isotonic and the pressure reaches a maximum of 120–130 mm Hg.

- In the REP pressure starts decreasing, but it is higher than aortic pressure.
- In the PDP pressure again decreases and becomes less than aortic pressure resulting in closure of semilunar valves.
- In IRP there is a rapid fall in pressure. At the end of this phase pressure becomes less than that of atria, resulting in opening of AV valves.
- In the later stages, pressure falls to base line (1–3 mm Hg).

Right Ventricular Pressure Changes

- When compared to LV pressure changes, RV pressure is less in the different phases of cardiac cycle.
- In the ICP, the pressure in the RV is 10 mm Hg and in the MEP the pressure attained is 20–25 mm Hg.

Pressure Changes in Aorta (Fig. 4.25)

- Since pumping of blood by ventricle is intermittent, the aortic pressure fluctuates between systolic pressure of 120 mm Hg and diastolic pressure of 80 mm Hg.
- During AS and ICP there is no change in aortic pressure.
- In MEP blood is ejected into the aorta and the wall of aorta stretches due to elasticity. Aortic pressure reaches a peak of 120 mm Hg.
- In the REP amount of blood ejected into aorta becomes lesser and lesser. The peripheral run off into the smaller vessels become more and the aortic pressure starts to fall.
- During PDP ventricular pressure becomes less than that of aortic pressure. So there is a tendency of blood to flow back into left ventricle marked by a depression incisura. At the end of this phase semilunar valves close.
- Closure of semilunar valve (forming dicortic noch) causes a momentary increase in aortic pressure and the blood strikes against semilunar valve causing vibrations in the blood column called after vibrations in the recording. This occurs in IRP.
- The aortic pressure falls through out the ventricular diastolic phase. Due to elastic recoil of vessels the pressure will not fall beyond 80 mm Hg.

Pressure Changes in Pulmonary Artery

Pressure changes are similar to aorta except that the pressure value is less. Maximum is 25 mm Hg and minimum is 10 mm Hg.

Volume Changes in Ventricles (Fig. 4.26)

- During atrial systole the ventricular volume increases.
- During ICP there is no change in the volume since all the valves are closed.
- During MEP, volume decreases rapidly.
- During REP, decrease in volume is less.
- During IRP there is no change in volume.
- Rapid increase in volume occurs during RFP and a slow rise during diastasis.
- The rest of the filling is during AS.
- The amount of blood in the ventricle at the end of each diastole is called EDV (end diastolic volume) and is approximately 120–130 mL/each ventricle.

Pressure Volume Loop (Fig. 4.27)

The relationship between ventricular pressure and volume throughout the cardiac cycle can be represented in the pressure volume loop. This graph presents volume of blood in the ventricles on the X-axis and left ventricular pressure Y-axis.

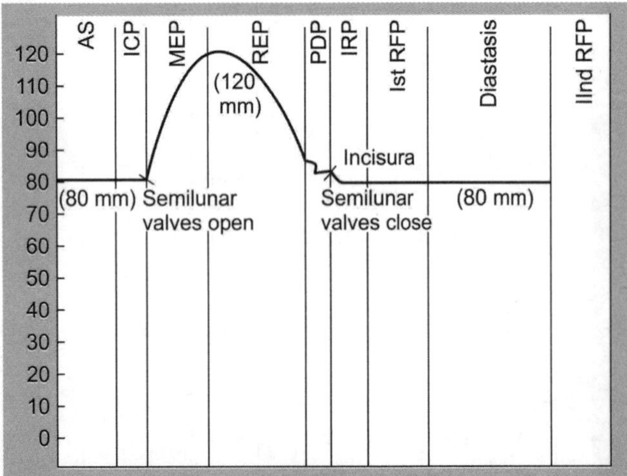

Fig. 4.25: Pressure changes in aorta

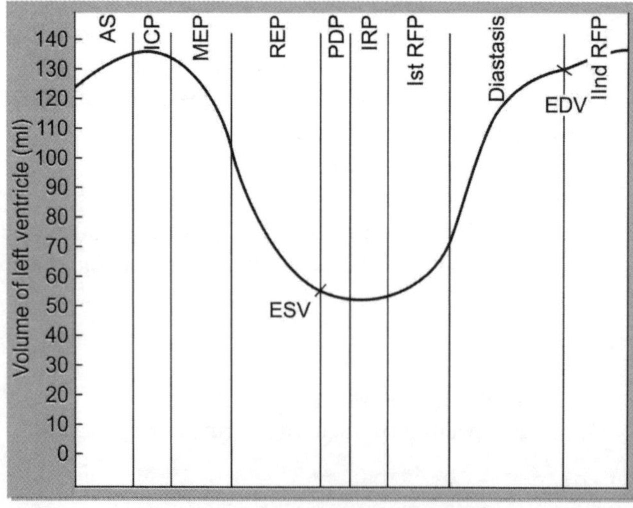

Fig. 4.26: Volume changes in ventricles

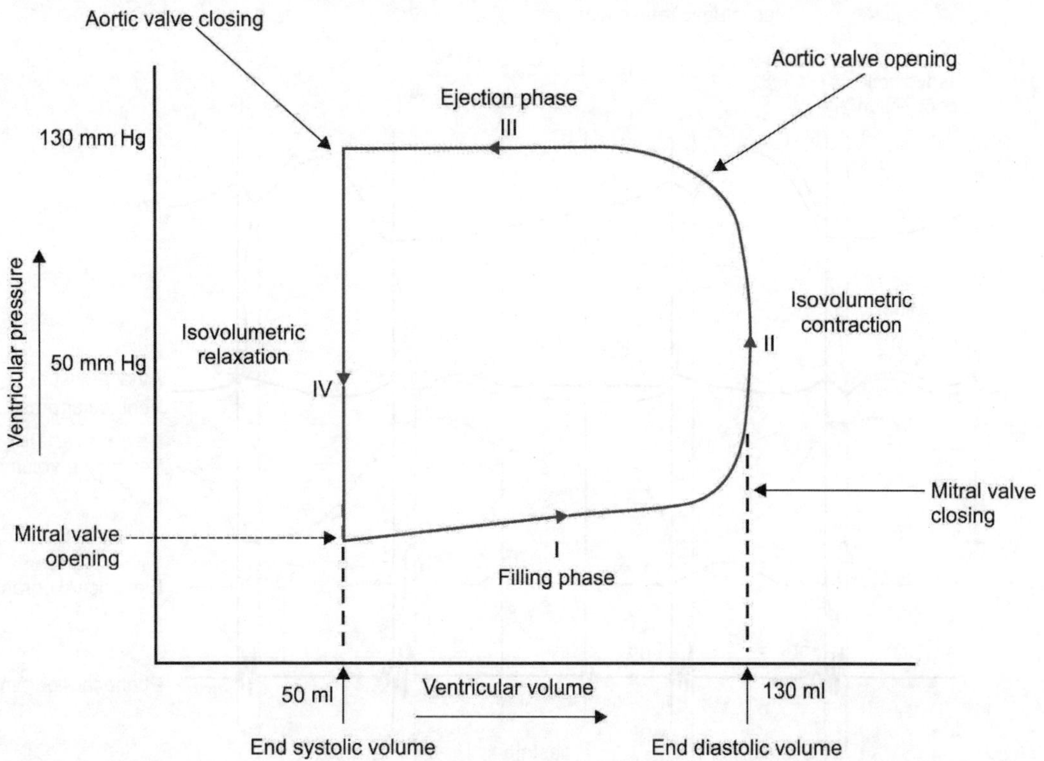

Fig. 4.27: Pressure volume loop: The ventricular pressure-volume changes during a cardiac cycle

The four periods of the cardiac cycle each represent one side of the closed loop. By following the directions of the arrows, one can read the graph.

- **Period of filling:** The ventricular volume increases from about 50 mL [end-systolic volume (EDV)] to about 130 mL (EDV). Note: Although the ventricles are filled with blood, the ventricular pressure does not rise.
- **Isovolumic contraction:** For the same volume (EDV), now the ventricular pressure rises. Volume remains the same; pressure rises.
- **Period of ejection:** Ventricular volume now decreases as blood is pumped out during ventricular systole. From 130 mL (EDV), about 80 mL (stroke volume) is pumped out. The remaining volume is end-systolic volume (ESV), about 50 mL.
- **Isovolumic relaxation:** For the same (end-systolic) volume, now the intraventricular pressure falls. Same volume; pressure falls.

Width of the PV loop indicates the stroke volume. Normally, EDV is about 130 mL, and the stroke volume is about 80 mL. End-systolic volume (ESV) is thus about 50 mL.

Height of the curve indicates the LV pressure. LV pressure, in turn, indicates the afterload on the LV. More the afterload on LV, greater is the rise of LV pressure during systole, increasing the height of the curve.

Also note that during ventricular filling, the blood is filled into ventricles; yet the ventricular pressure does not rise. This is due to 'receptive relaxation' and accommodation of blood into ventricles.

Cardiac Cycle Diagram (Wiggers Diagram)

Changes in the heart during cardiac cycle can be depicted in a diagram called cardiac cycle diagram.

The most important aspects of Figure 4.28 are the following:

- Contraction of ventricle → rise in ventricular pressure above atrial pressure → closure of mitral valve.
- It is always a pressure difference that causes the valves to open or close.
- Closure of the mitral valve terminates the ventricular filling phase and begins isovolumetric contraction.
- Isovolumetric contraction—No change in ventricular volume, and both valves (mitral, aortic) closed. Ventricular pressure increases, and volume is equivalent to end-diastolic volume.
- Opening of the aortic valve terminates isovolumetric contraction and begins the ejection phase. The aortic valve opens because pressure in the ventricle slightly exceeds aortic pressure.
- Ejection Phase—Ventricular volume decreases, but most rapidly in early stages. Ventricular and aortic pressures increase initially but decrease later in phase.

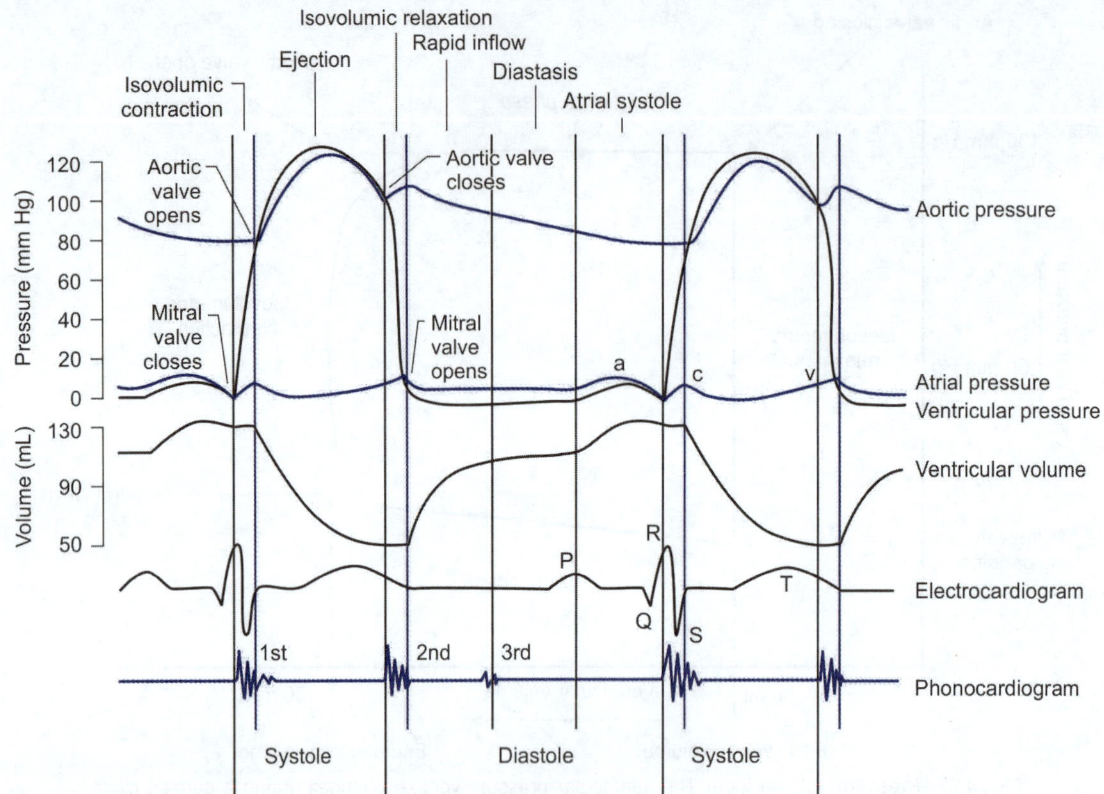

Fig. 4.28: Wiggers diagram, showing the cardiac cycle events occuring in the left ventricle

- Closure of the aortic valve terminates the ejection phase and begins isovolumetric relaxation. The aortic valve closes because pressure in the ventricle goes below aortic pressure. Closure of the aortic valve creates the dicrotic notch.
- Isovolumetric relaxation—No change in ventricular volume, and both valves (mitral, aortic) closed. Ventricular pressure decreases, and volume is equivalent to end-systolic volume.
- Opening of the mitral valve terminates isovolumetric relaxation and begins the filling phase. The mitral valve opens because pressure in the ventricle goes below atrial pressure.
- Filling Phase—The final relaxation of the ventricle occurs after the mitral valve opens and produces a rapid early filling of the ventricle. This rapid inflow will in some cases induce the third heart sound. The final increase in ventricular volume is due to atrial contraction, which is responsible for the fourth heart sound.

In a young, healthy individual, atrial contraction does not provide significant filling of the ventricle. However, the contribution of atrial contraction becomes more important when ventricular compliance is reduced.

ARTERIAL PULSE

As blood is forced into aorta during systole it sets up a pressure wave that travels along the artery with expansion of arterial wall and the expansion is palpable as a pulse. The rate at which the wave travels is 4 m/s in aorta, 8 m/s in small arteries and 16 m/s in arterioles. Pulse is felt in the radial artery at the wrist about 0.1 sec after the peak of systolic ejection into the aorta.

Arterial pulse can be measured by a sphygmograph and pulse recording is called sphygmogram. The normal pulse is called catacrotic pulse.

Arterial pulse tracing (Fig. 4.29) shows a sharp ascending limb (upstroke) – anacrotic limb and a slower downstroke – catacrotic limb with a dicrotic notch. Dicrotic notch is caused by vibrations set up when the aortic valve closes suddenly at the end of systole.

While examining pulse, the rate, rhythm, volume, character, condition of vessel wall, radiofemoral delay, other peripheral pulses, pulse deficit are observed. Arterial pulsation can be also felt in facial artery, common carotid artery, axillary artery, brachial artery, femoral artery popliteal artery, posterior tibial artery and dorsalis pedis artery (Fig. 4.30).

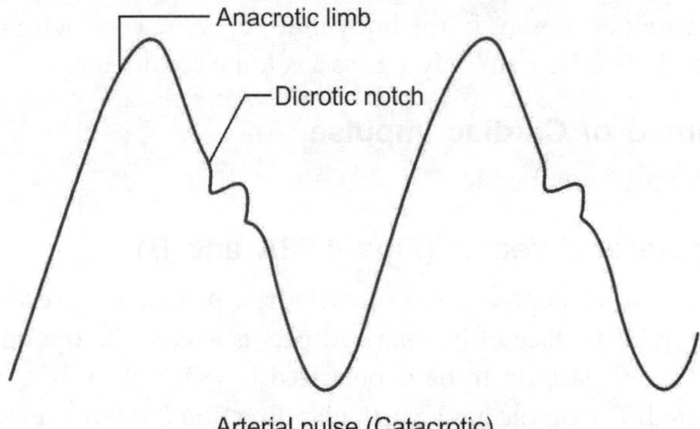

Fig. 4.29: Radial pulse tracing

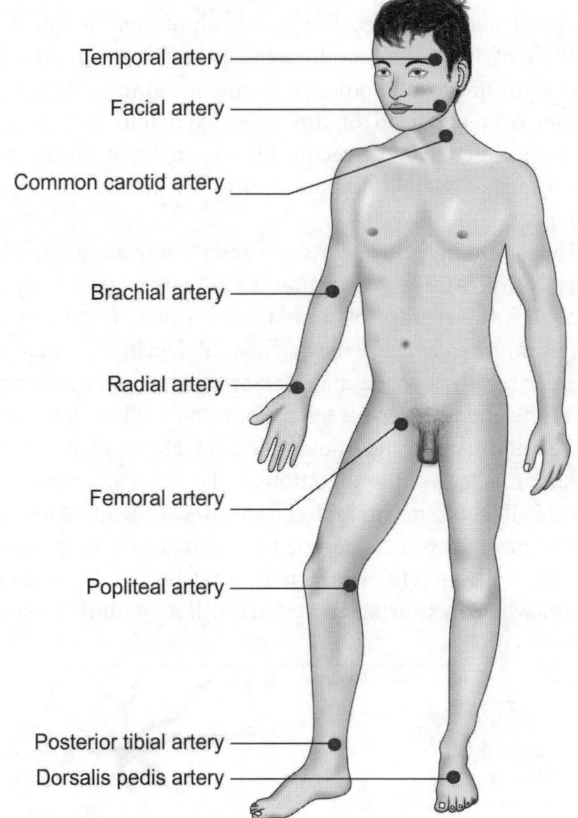

Fig. 4.30: Common sites to look for arterial pulse

Types of Pulse (Fig. 4.31)

- *Collapsing/water hammer pulse:* This is seen in aortic insufficiency. Here there is rapid upstroke and rapid downstroke without dicrotic notch. For example, aortic regurgitation.
- *Slow rising/hypokinetic/small volume pulse:* Here the volume ejected will be less. For example, aortic stenosis.
- *Pulsus alternans:* Here there will be alternate small and large volume pulse. For example, left ventricular failure.

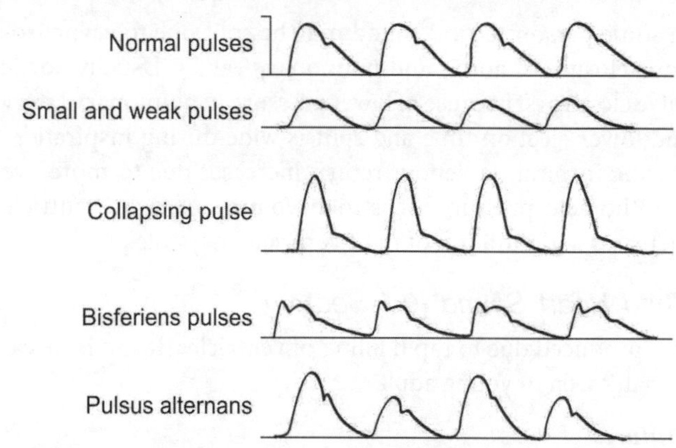

Fig. 4.31: Types of pulse

- *Bisferiens pulse:* It is a combination of slow rising and collapsing pulse. For example, aortic stenosis with aortic regurgitation.

HEART SOUNDS

When the valves open, no audible sounds are produced. Sounds are produced when the valves close. Two heart sounds are heard normally through a stethoscope. Closure of valves lead to vibration of valves, which causes vibration of adjacent column of blood and wall of heart which in turn is transmitted to chest wall.

First Heart Sound (0.15 sec)

It is produced due to closure of AV valves. It has two components–mitral and tricuspid.

It marks the beginning of ventricular systole. When the ventricles contract, the intraventricular pressure increases and becomes more than the atrial pressure. This will lead to AV valve closure.

Features

- Low pitched, soft (valves are thin and filmy)
- Prolonged lub sound
- Frequency: 25–45 Hz
- Heard in mitral and tricuspid area.

Second Heart Sound (0.12 Sec)

It is produced due to closure of semilunar valves. It has two components–aortic and pulmonary.

Features

- Short, high pitched
- Dup sound
- Frequency–50 Hz (high frequency is due to greater elasticity of semilunar valves)
- Heard over aortic and pulmonary areas.

In some person second sound may be split due to asynchronous closure of aortic and pulmonary valves. Usually aortic valve closes first because of lower pressure in pulmonary artery and lower ejection time and split is wide during inspiration. During inspiration venous return increases due to more –ve intrathoracic pressure. So stroke volume of right ventricle increases and duration of right ventricular systole prolongs.

Third Heart Sound (0.1 Sec)

It is produced due to rapid filling of ventricles. It can be occasionally seen in young adult.

Features

Soft, low pitched.

Fourth Heart Sound

Not heard normally and is heard best with the bell piece of stethoscope. It is heard just before 1st heart sound. It is produced due to rapid ventricular filling due to atrial contraction and occurs when atrial pressure is high.

Murmurs and Bruits

Murmurs are abnormal sounds heard over the heart and produced due to turbulence created at or near a valve or due to abnormal communication within the heart or between great vessels.

The major cause of cardiac murmur are diseases of heart valves. Bruits are abnormal sounds heard over vessels.

Normally the flow is streamline or laminar which is silent. When the flow exceeds a critical velocity the flow become turbulent and produce sound. When a valve is narrowed/stenosed, velocity of flow increases and the flow becomes turbulent. When a valve is incompetent, blood flows backward through this incompetent valve which is called regurgitation or insufficiency.

ECG

The electrical activities of myocardium is graphically recorded using surface electrodes. The biphasic recording thus obtained is called as electrocardiogram. It is possible because body acts as a volume conductor. Procedure is called electrocardiography and the equipment is called electrocardiograph (invented by William Einthoven). ECG provides useful information about: (a) heart rate, (b) cardiac rhythm, (c) cardiac hypertrophy, (d) conduction abnormalities, (e) ischemia and infarction, and (f) electrolyte changes.

Volume Conductor

The electrical activities of heart can be recorded from electrodes placed on various specific site, distant from the heart. Electrolytes present in the body fluids aids the conduction of electrical activity so body acts as a volume conductor.

Spread of Cardiac Impulse

Refer page number 84.

Dipole and Vector (Figs 4.32A and B)

The wave of depolarization travels in a particular direction. The outer surface of depolarized part is –ve, while the outer surface of part yet to be depolarized is +ve, thus a dipole is created. The dipole has a particular direction (–ve to +ve) and a particular magnitude. The magnitude and direction of dipole can be expressed by a vector known as dipole vector.

Heart is a functional syncytiun, many small dipoles form in a particular direction. The sum of all of them is called the resultant of dipole. The resultant of dipole changes in direction and magnitude from moment to moment. Summated resultant vectors over a period of time are taken into account and these are called average vector. ECG is analyzed on the basis of number of average vectors during the passage of cardiac impulse.

Thus, although tiny swirls of current may simultaneously be going off in every direction, each lead records only the instantaneous average of these forces. This concept is really quite simple; an analogy may be helpful. During the course of a soccer match, a goalie may kick or toss the ball many times to various members of his team. Some balls will go left, others right, still others straight down the field. However, by the end of the game, the average direction of all of the goalie's kicks and tosses is likely to be straight ahead, toward the opposing net. This average movement can be represented by a single arrow, or vector. This vector is precisely what our ECG electrodes record when measuring the electrical flow within the heart.

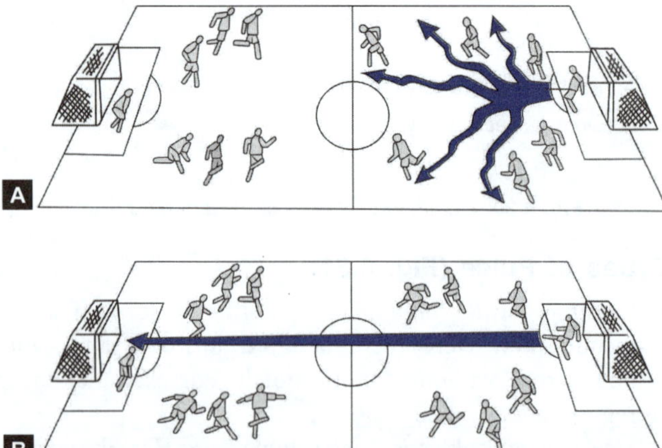

Figs 4.32A and B: A. The directions of each of the goalie's kicks during the course of the game; **B.** A single vector represents the average direction and distance of all of these kicks

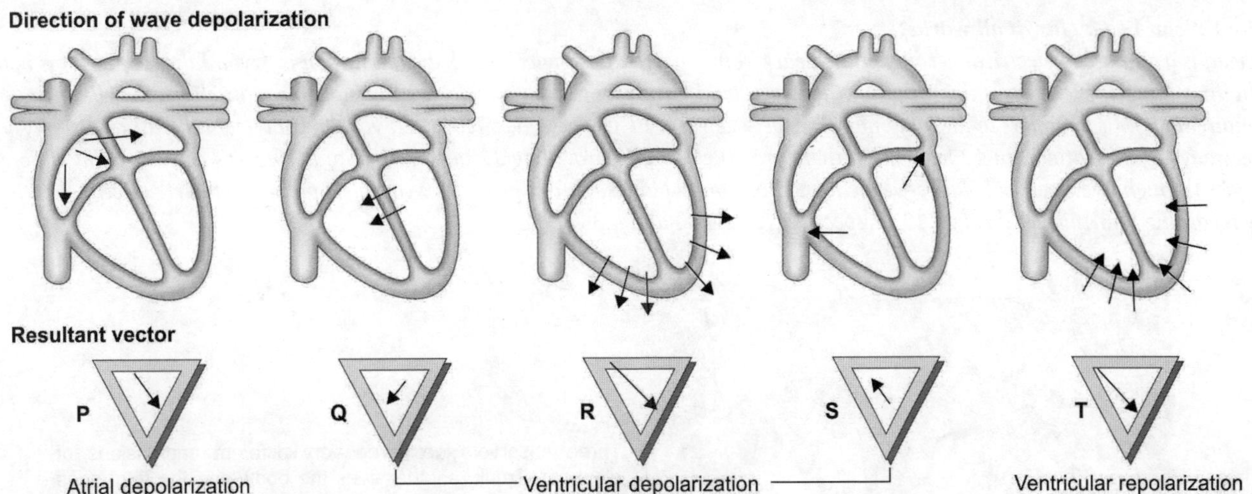

Fig. 4.33: Direction of wave of depolarization, the resultant vectors (only 3 ventricular vectors are shown) and corresponding ECG recording

The vector's angle of orientation represents the average direction of current flow, and its length represents the voltage (amplitude) attained. At any given moment, the electrical forces moving within the heart can be represented by a single vector, and this vector is translated by each of the 12 leads into the simple wave patterns that we see on the ECG. As the wave of depolarization spreads along the heart the following average vectors (Fig. 4.33) appears sequently.

- The vector of atrial depolarization is directed downwards and to the left.
- The ventricle has four main vectors.
  1. First ventricular vector (due to ventricular depolarization). It is directed obliquely downwards from left to right (as the left wall of interventricular septum is depolarized first and the wave of depolarization passes across the septum from left to right).
  2. Second ventricular vector (due to the passage of cardiac impulse towards apex). It is directed downwards.
  3. Third ventricular vector (due to depolarization of left ventricle). It is directed downwards and to the left because wave of depolarization proceeds from subendocardium to epicardium. It is largest because left ventricle has the largest muscle mass.
  4. Fourth ventricular vector (due to depolarization of the bases). It is directed upwards towards the base and small in size.

The resultant of all the four vectors is called mean electrical axis of heart. Normally, it is directed downwards and to the left and makes an angle of about 59° with the horizontal (angle may vary between –30 and +110).

Ventricular repolarization takes place from epicardium to endocardium. So T wave caused by ventricular repolarization is upright.

ECG Paper

ECG is recorded on a mm square graph paper, moving at a speed of 25 mm/sec. It is divided into 1 mm square by thin lines. Every 5th line is thick both horizontally and vertically.

Vertical lines are time calibration lines, 1 mm = 0.04 sec on X-axis. So time duration between two thick lines is 0.2 sec. Vertical amplitude of a wave is measured in mm, so a deflection of 10 mm represents 1 mV.

ECG Leads

The heart is a three-dimensional organ, and its electrical activity must be understood in three dimensions as well. A couple of electrodes are not adequate to do this, a fact that the original electrocardiographers recognized more than a century ago when they devised the first limb leads. Today, the standard ECG consists of 12 leads with each lead determined by the placement and orientation of various electrodes on the body. Each lead views the heart at a unique angle, enhancing its sensitivity to a particular region of the heart at the expense of others. The more views, the more information provided.

There are 12 leads in the ECG:

- Bipolar limb leads/Standard limb leads: Lead I, Lead II, Lead III.
- Augmented unipolar leads: aVR, aVL, aVF.
- Unipolar chest leads: V1 to V6.

Bipolar Limb Leads

When both the electrodes of a lead are active and a potential difference between them is recorded, the lead is then called bipolar lead. Each bipolar lead has one +ve and one –ve electrode.

The 12 lead ECG: How it all works

A lead is a glimpse of electrical activity of the heart from a particular angle. Detailed explanation is beyond the scope of this book. The first thing to clear up is definition of the word 'lead' in an ECG context (don't confuse leads with electrodes; both are not synonymous). Leads refers to an imaginary line between two ECG electrodes. However, you can only actually attach 10 physical electrodes to the patient. In 12 lead ECG, there are 10 electrodes providing 12 perspectives of the heart's activity using different angles through two electrical planes–vertical and horizontal planes. Thus it provides a complete picture of heart's electrical activity by recording information through 12 perspectives (Figs 4.34 and 4.35).

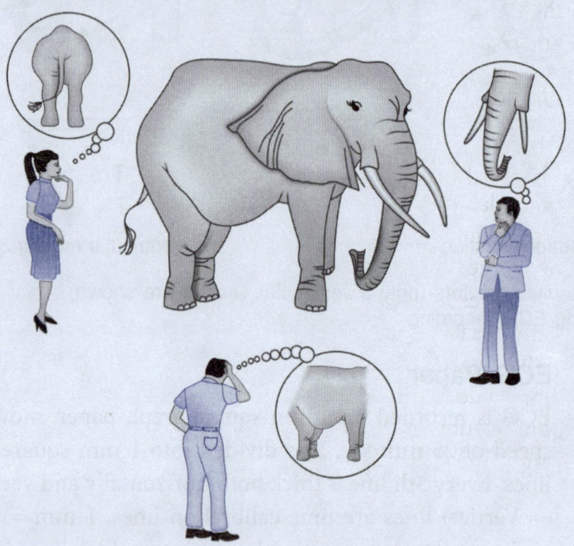

Three observers get three very different impressions of elephant. Trunk, another sees the body, and the third sees the tail. If you wanted the best description of the elephant, who would you ask? All three, of course. Similarly, different leads in ECG provides more information from different angles of the heart.

Fig. 4.34: Analogy to understand the need of different leads in an ECG

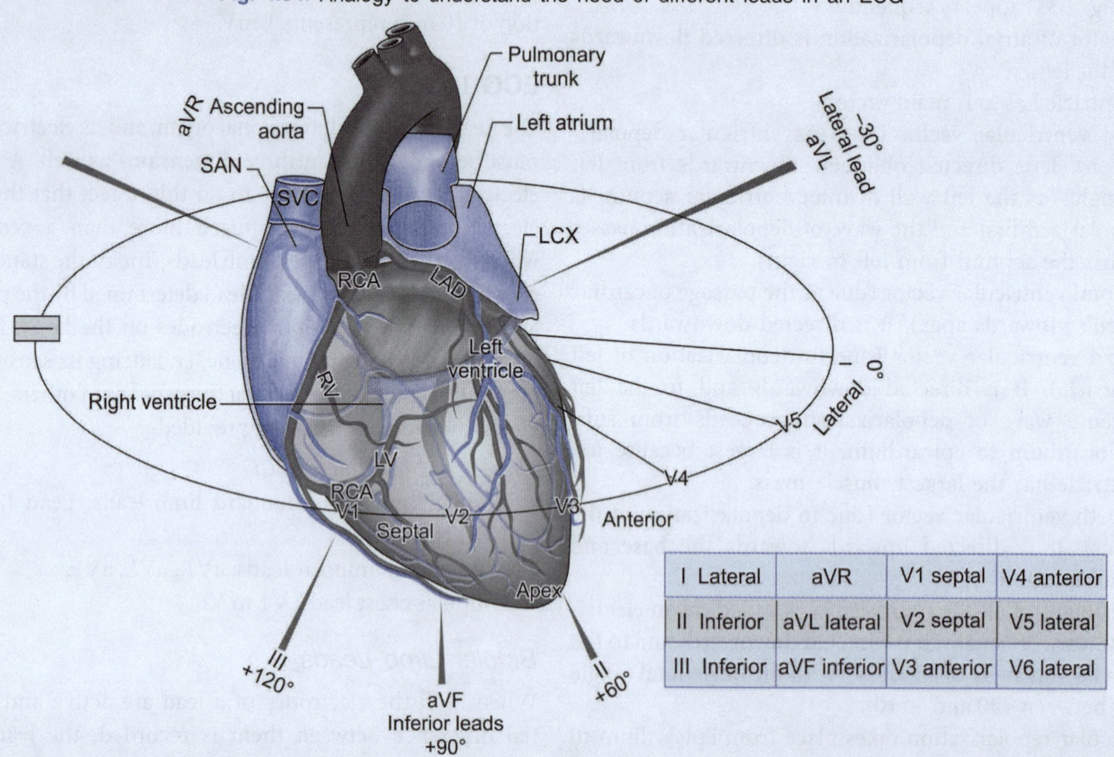

I Lateral	aVR	V1 septal	V4 anterior
II Inferior	aVL lateral	V2 septal	V5 lateral
III Inferior	aVF inferior	V3 anterior	V6 lateral

Fig. 4.35: ECG leads corresponding areas of heart

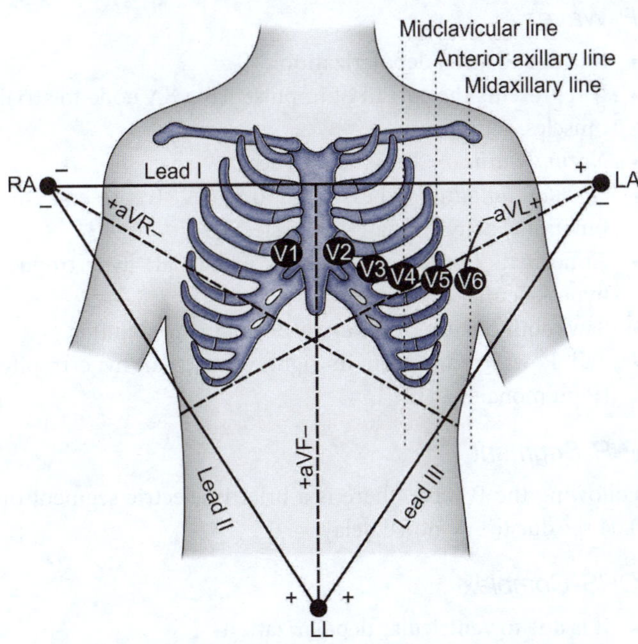

Fig. 4.36: Einthoven's triangle, position of various leads

When the vector is directed towards +ve electrode, positive/upward deflection is obtained and vice versa.

Einthoven selected three points in the body:

1. Left shoulder
2. Right shoulder
3. Left midinguinal point.

When the above points are joined together an equilateral triangle is obtained. Heart is assumed to be in its center and this triangle is called *Einthoven's triangle*. The positions of +ve and –ve electrodes of the bipolar leads are shown in the Figure 4.36.

If the electrical potential at left arm, right arm and left leg are designated as VL, VR, VF respectively, voltage recorded in:

LI = VL – VR

LII = VF – VR

LIII = VF – VL

LI + LII+ LIII = VL – VR+ VF – VR+ VF – VL ≠ 0

It would have been 0 if right arm is +ve and left foot is –ve. Einthoven deliberately changed the polarity of Lead II, in order to get upward deflection in all the three leads.

Then LII = VR – VF.

Now, VL – VR + VR – VF + VF – VL = 0

i.e. LI + LIII – LII = 0 (LI + LIII= LII)

At any given instant (moment), the sum of potentials in Lead I and Lead III equals the potential in lead II. This is called ***Einthoven's Law.*** So the maximum amplitude is obtained in LII.

Unipolar Leads

Unlike bipolar leads, unipolar lead has only one active electrode called exploring electrode. Other electrode is kept at zero potential and is called as indifferent electrode. So unipolar leads records the absolute electrical potential under the exploring electrode.

Depending on whether the lead is placed on the chest or the limbs, unipolar leads are classified as unipolar limb leads and unipolar chest leads.

Unipolar Limb Lead

An electrode is placed on the distal part of any limb (Rt arm, Lt arm, Lt foot) and the other electrode should be at zero potential. Indifferent electrode is designated as V. So the leads are designated as VL, VR, VF. Indifferent electrode is made by connecting the 3 limbs (Rt arm, Lt arm, Lt foot) through a high resistance of 5000 Ohm to a common terminal called Wilson's terminal.

These unipolar limb leads gives waves of very small amplitude, so these leads were augmented by removing the contribution of the respective limb to the central terminal (Fig. 4.37). This arrangement has increased amplitudes of the

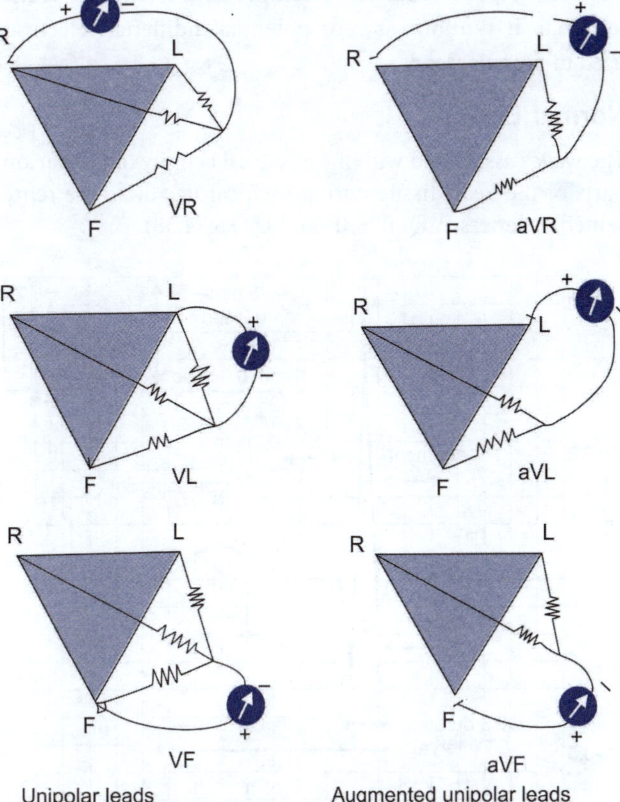

Fig. 4.37: Augmentation of leads

waves (aVR = 3/2 VR) and these are called augmented limb leads. The augmented limb leads are aVR, aVL, aVF.

Unipolar Chest Leads

These are named as V1, V2, V3, V4, V5, V6. The position of exploring electrodes of the various chest leads are as follows:

- V1 Right 4th intercostal space (ICS) near the sternal border
- V2 Left 4th ICS near the sternal border
- V3 In the midpoint between V2 and V4
- V4 Left 5th ICS on the midclavicular line
- V5 Left 5th ICS on the anterior axillary line
- V6 Left 5th ICS on the midaxillary line

Wilson Central Terminal

According to Kirchoff's law VR + VF + VL = 0. But it is not exactly zero as.

- Triangle is not exactly equilateral.
- Heart is not exactly at the center.

To tide over this problem three resistance of 5000 Ohm is connected to electrode placed at three apical points and they were connected to a common terminal called Wilson's central terminal. It funtions as zero potential indifferent electrode used in unipolar leads.

Normal ECG

The waves associated with the electrical activity of the various parts of the heart tissue during each cardiac cycle are represented by letters P, Q, R, S, T, and U (Fig. 4.38).

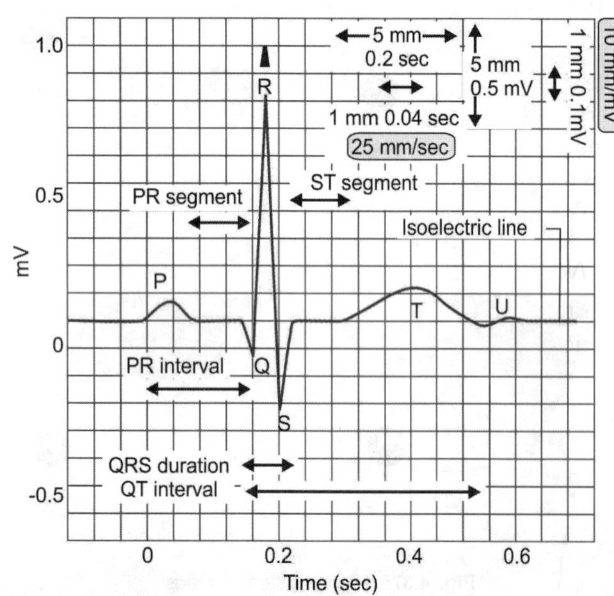

Fig. 4.38: Normal electrocardiogram; (lead II)

P Wave

- It is due to atrial depolarization.
- It represents the spread of impulse from SA node to atrial muscles.
- *Normal duration:* Less than 0.1 sec.
- *Normal amplitude:* Less than 0.5 mV (represents the functional activity of atrial muscles).
- Abnormal P waves are seen in atrial hypertrophy, hyperkalemia, etc.
- Saw tooth pattern of P wave are seen in atrial flutter.
- Tall P waves are seen in right ventricular hypertrophy (P pulmonale).

P-R Segment

Following the P wave, there is a brief isoelectric segment of 0.04 sec due to AV nodal delay.

QRS Complex

- It is due to ventricular depolarization
- *Normal duration:* 0.08–0.10 sec
- *Normal amplitude:* 1–1.5 mV
- It is a complex wave as it consist of an initial downward deflection – Q wave, an upward deflection – R wave and a downward deflection - S wave.

Q Wave

- It is the 1st wave of ventricular depolarization, which is always –ve.
- It is due to depolarization of interventricular septum from left to right.

R Wave

It is the 1st +ve wave of QRS complex. It is the main wave of ventricular depolarization and the tip of R wave is sharp and pointed.

S Wave

It is the –ve wave that follows R wave and ends at J point also marks the termination of QRS complex.

S-T Segment

- Following QRS complex there is a long isoelectrical segment.
- It represents the duration from end of ventricular depolarization to beginning of ventricular repolarization and its duration is 0.32 sec.
- In ventricular hypertrophy QRS amplitude increases.
- In MI, ST segment is elevated in leads overlying the area of infarct and ST segment is depressed in the reciprocal leads.

J Point

Junction between end of S wave and beginning of ST segment.

T Wave

- It is an upward deflection due to ventricular repolarization.
- Duration of T wave is longer as repolarization of ventricles takes longer time.

U Wave

- Rarely we get U wave after normal ECG.
- It denotes delayed repolarization of papillary muscle.

PR Interval

- It is the interval between beginning of P wave to the beginning of QRS complex.
- So this includes P wave and PR segment.
- Its normal duration is 0.12–0.2 sec.
- It indicates atrial depolarization and AV nodal delay.
- When Q wave is absent, it may be termed as PR interval and when Q wave is present it is termed as PQ interval.
- P-R interval is prolonged in heart block and hypokalemia.
- P-R interval is decreased in WPW syndrome and LGL syndrome.

QT Interval

- It is the interval between beginning of QRS complex and the end of T wave.
- This includes QRS complex, ST segment and T wave.
- This denotes the time taken for ventricular depolarization and repolarization.
- Normal duration is 0.35–0.43 sec.

ST Interval

- It denotes the duration between end of S wave and end of T wave.
- ST interval = ST segment + T wave.

Pattern of ECG in Other Leads

The pattern is same in LI, LII and LIII, but the amplitude is maximum in LII. In aVR – P, R, T waves are found to be inverted. This is because the depolarization curve is moving away from exploring electrode. In V1, small R and deep S wave is seen but as electrode position is changed from V1 to V5, height of R increases, but the depth of S decreases from V1 to V5. In V5 and V6 R wave is more prominent (Fig. 4.39).

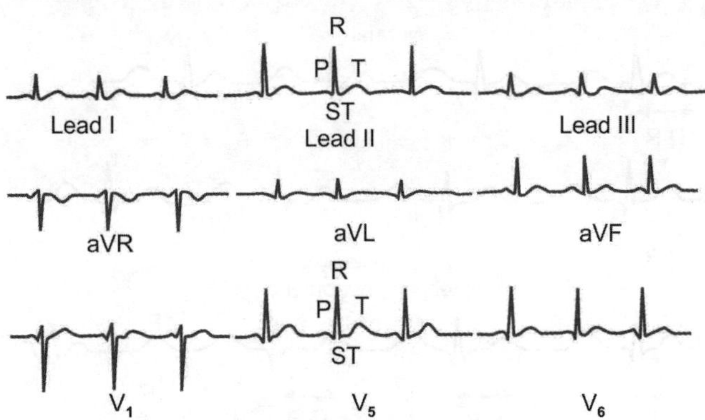

Fig. 4.39: Pattern of ECG in other leads

Examination of ECG

Heart rate =

$$\frac{1500}{\text{No. of small squares between two R waves}}$$

or

$$\frac{300}{\text{No. of big squares between two R waves}}$$

Rhythm can be assessed in the ECG by comparing length of R-R interval.

HEART BLOCK

Defined as the disturbance in the normal transmission of impulses generated in SAN. Normal P-R interval is 0.12 sec, when it exceeds 0.20 sec the condition is called heart block.

Causes

- MI
- Inflammation
- Excessive vagal stimulation.

Types

Sinoatrial Nodal Block

Here the level of block is within the substance of SAN. After an interval of approximately two cardiac cycle the heart resumes its normal action as some new pacemaker other than SAN takes over (Fig. 4.40). The impulse originate spontaneously in the AV node. Rate of QRS - T complex is altered.

AV Nodal Block (Fig. 4.41)

Here there is disturbance of conduction between atria and ventricles. It is of two types:

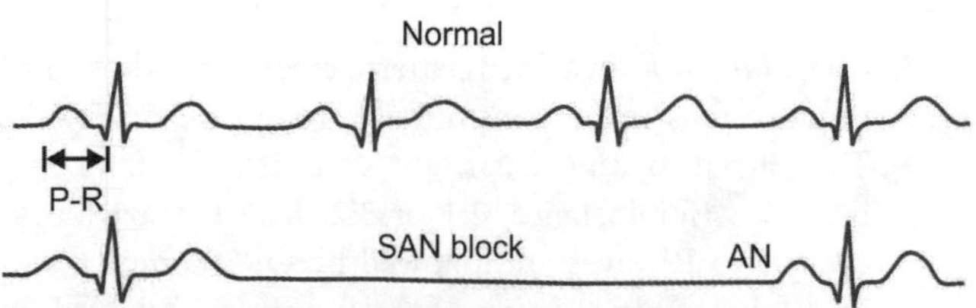

Fig. 4.40: Sinoatrial nodal block

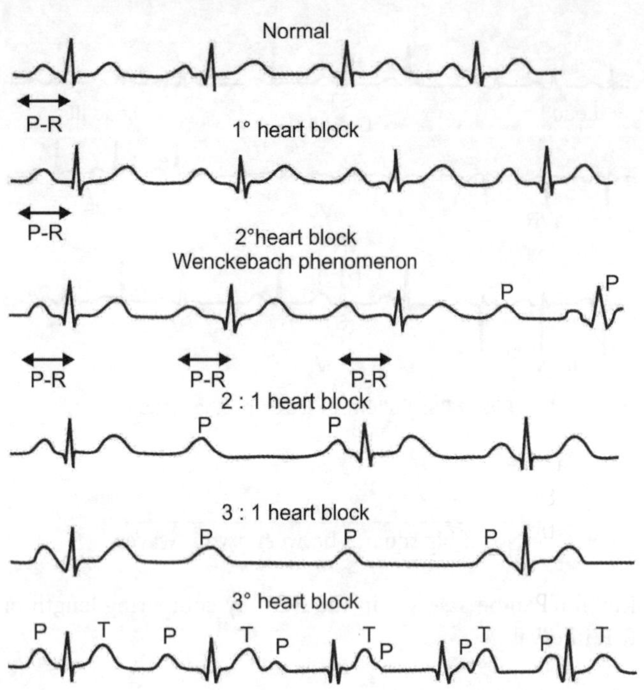

Fig. 4.41: AV nodal block

Incomplete (partial) heart block

It is of two types:

- *Ist degree:* In Ist degree block PR interval is prolonged (above 0.2 sec), but all atrial impulse reach ventricle. All P waves are followed by QRS complex.
- *IInd degree:* Characterized by the failure of the AV node to transmit all the atrial impulses to the ventricles; some impulses are transmitted, some are not – 'incomplete block'. Here also the PR interval is above 0.2 sec. All QRS complexes are preceded by P waves, but all the P waves are not followed by QRS complexes. It is of following types:
  1. *Mobitz type I block (or Wenckebach block):* There is progressive lengthening of the PR interval in successive beats and finally one impulse fails to be transmitted to the ventricles.
  2. *Mobitz type II block (or periodic block):* PR interval is constant from beat to beat; but there is occasional failure of transmission of an impulse through the AV node. Thus, in an inconsistent fashion, P wave will not be followed by QRS-complex and T wave in some beats.
  3. *Constant block:* In a fixed pattern, every second or third impulse fails to be transmitted through the AV node. Thus, atrial-to-ventricular rate is a constant small number ratio (for instance, 2:1 or 3:2. In 2:1 heart block, every two P waves are followed by QRS complex and in 3:1 heart block, every three P wave is followed by QRS complex).

Complete heart block (3rd degree heart block)

Here no impulse is transmitted from atria to ventricles. There is complete atrioventricular dissociation.

Atria contract at its own rate and ventricle contract independently at its own rate and rhythm (Idioventricular rhythm). When complete heart block occurs suddenly, the ventricles takes some time before it can beat at its own rhythm. During this time there is cerebral hypoxia (as there is no cardiac output). This will lead to syncope and fainting attack called **Stokes Adam's syndrome.**

Bundle Branch Block (BBB) (Fig. 4.42)

Here there is block of one of the branches of bundle of His. So excitation process passes normally down to bundle on the intact side and then sweeps back through the muscles to activate the ventricle on the blocked side. It may be right BBB, left BBB and hemiblock (fascicular block). When block occurs in the anterior or posterior fascicles of the left bundle branch, it produces hemiblock.

Note

- ***WPW syndrome (Wolff-Parkinson-White syndrome):*** Congenital anomaly where an accessory bundle of muscle fiber called *bundle of Kent* connects right atria to ventricles. As a result depolarization wave from the atria is transmitted to ventricle faster bypassing the AV node (So AV nodal delay absent and PR interval is shortened). Here wide, slurred QRS complex is obtained. Normally beat conducts down the AV node. But here impulse is transmitted retrograde to the atrium due aberrant bundle. A circus movement is thus established (Fig. 4.43).
- ***Lown-Ganong-Levine syndrome:*** Here depolarization passes from the atria to the ventricles via an aberrant bundle. The impulses bypasses the AV node, but enters the

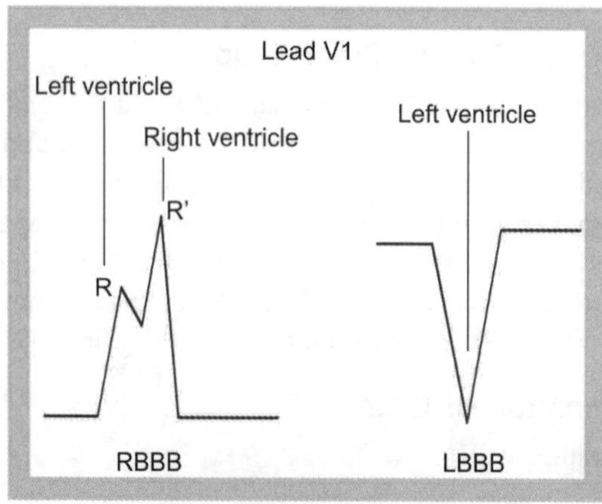

Fig. 4.42: Bundle branch blocks

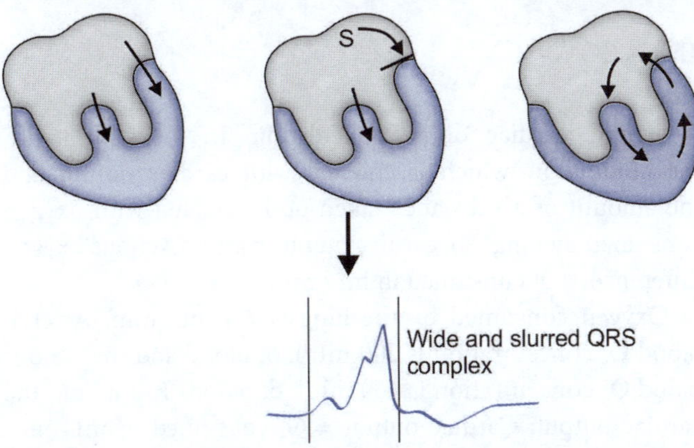

Fig. 4.43: Wolff-Parkinson-White syndrome

intraventricular conducting system distal to the node. QRS complex is normal and PR interval is shortened.

- ***Myocardial infarction (MI):*** Acute occlusion of a coronary artery most frequently occurs in a person who already has underlying atherosclerotic coronary heart disease. Immediately after an acute coronary occlusion, blood flow ceases in the coronary vessels beyond the occlusion except for small amounts of collateral flow from surrounding vessels. The area of muscle that has either zero flow or so little flow that it cannot sustain cardiac muscle function is said to be infarcted. The overall process is called a myocardial infarction.

Normally, a person cannot 'feel' his or her heart, but ischemic cardiac muscle often does cause pain sensation, sometimes severe. It is believed that ischemia causes the muscle to release acidic substances, such as lactic acid, or other pain-promoting products, such as histamine, kinins, or cellular proteolytic enzymes, that are not removed rapidly enough by the slowly moving coronary blood flow. The high concentrations of these abnormal products then stimulate pain nerve endings in the cardiac muscle, sending pain impulses through sensory afferent nerve fibers into the central nervous system. In most people who develop progressive constriction of their coronary arteries, cardiac pain called **angina pectoris**, begins to appear whenever the load on the heart becomes too great in relation to the available coronary blood flow.

This pain is usually felt beneath the upper sternum over the heart, and in addition it is often referred to distant surface areas of the body, most commonly to the left arm and left shoulder but also frequently to the neck and even to the side of the face. The reason for this distribution of pain is that the heart originates during embryonic life in the neck, as do the arms. Therefore, both the heart and these surface areas of the body receive pain nerve fibers from the same spinal cord segments.

Most people who have chronic angina pectoris feel pain when they exercise or when they experience emotions that increase metabolism of the heart or temporarily constrict the coronary vessels because of sympathetic vasoconstrictor nerve signals. Anginal pain is also exacerbated by cold temperatures or by having a full stomach, both of which increase the workload of the heart. The pain is frequently described as hot, pressing, and constricting. ECG is very useful for diagnosing ischemia and area of infarction.

Diagnosis of MI is based on specific electrocardiographic changes, elevation of enzymes specific for myocardial damage, and typical clinical presentation of the patient. ECG is very useful for diagnosing and locating areas of infarction. In acute infarction, the first change to occur is the ST segment elevation in the ECG leads recorded with electrodes placed over the chest representing the infarcted area. The leads placed on the opposite side of the infarction (reciprocal leads) record ST segment depression (Fig. 4.44). Other ECG changes includes pathological Q waves, T wave inversion. The damages myocardium releases enzymes into circulation. Detection of elevated level of these enzymes plays an important role in the diagnosis. The enzymes most commonly measured are troponins, creatine kinase.

Sick sinus syndrome: Disease processes affecting the sinus node lead to marked bradycardia accompanied by dizziness and syncope.

ECG Changes in Electrolyte Concentration

Hypokalemia (Fig. 4.45A)

Mild: Prominent U wave.

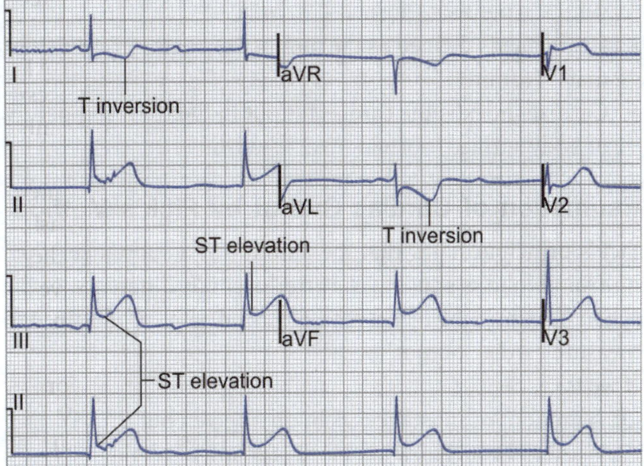

Fig. 4.44: ECG changes in MI. This ECG represents an inferior wall infarction as ST segment elevation can be seen in leads II, III, aVF. ST depression and T inversion can be seen in lead I, aVL (reciprocal leads).

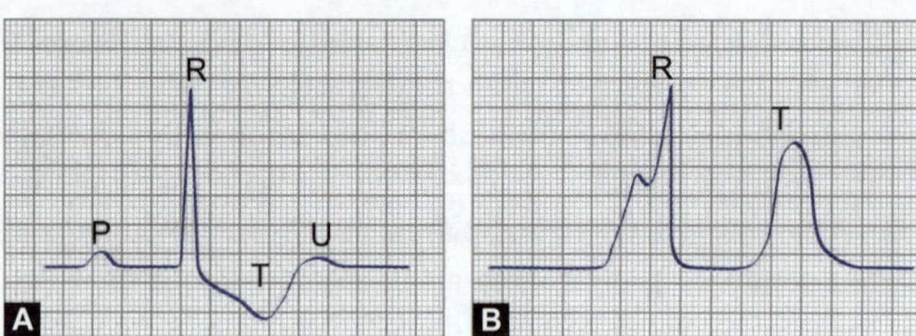

Figs 4.45A and B: A. Hypokalemia; **B.** Hyperkalemia

Severe:

- Prolongation of PR interval
- Prominent U wave
- Depression of ST wave
- Inversion of T wave.

Hyperkalemia (Fig. 4.45B)

Mild: Tall slender T wave.

Severe:

- Tall slender T wave
- Broad and slurred QRS complex.

Hypocalcemia

- Prolonged QT interval
- Ventricular fibrillation.

CARDIAC OUTPUT

Amount of blood pumped out of each ventricle per minute is called cardiac output (CO). Normal value – 5 liters in a normal adult.

- Cardiac output = Stroke volume × Heart rate.
- Stroke volume is the amount of blood pumped out of each ventricle per beat (normal – 70 mL).
- Heart rate is defined as the number of beats per min (normal – 75/min).
- Cardiac index is the cardiac output in liter per min per m^2 of body surface (normal – 3. 2 L/min/m^2).

Estimation of Cardiac Output by Fick's Method

Fick's principle states that the amount of a substance taken up from blood is equal to the arteriovenous difference of the substance times the blood flow. Fick's principle is modified to measure cardiac output.

If we take,

Qx = amount of substance taken up or given out

Ax = arterial concentration in mL/100 mL of blood

Vx = venous concentration in mL/100 mL of blood

CO = amount of substance taken up or given out by organ per unit time divided by arteriovenous concentration difference.

That is $CO = \dfrac{Qx}{Ax - Vx}$

Sample cardiac output calculation. In Ficks principle, the blood flow which is equated with cardiac output and the amount of a substance taken up is equated with oxygen consumed by lung. So, cardiac output x arteriovenous oxygen difference = O_2 consumed in mL/min.

Oxygen consumed by the lung is 200 mL/min. Arterial blood O_2 concentration is 200 mL/L of blood and the venous blood O_2 concentration is 160 mL/L of blood. To find out the cardiac output: Cardiac output = O_2 consumed in mL/min/ Arteriovenous oxygen difference

Cardiac output = 200 mL/min / 200 - 160 mL/L

So, Cardiac output = 5L/min

Variation in Cardiac Output

Physiological increase

- Exercise
- Anxiety
- Excitement
- Pregnancy

Physiological decrease

- Standing from lying position
- In females

Pathological increase

- Anemia
- Hyperthyroidism
- Hypoxia
- Fever
- Beriberi

Pathologically decrease

- Hypothyroidism
- MI
- Valvular heart disease
- Hemorrhage
- Cardiovascular shock

Regulation of Cardiac Output

Cardiac output is determined by stroke volume and heart rate (stroke volume × heart rate). Hence all the factors that regulate SV and HR regulates CO.

STROKE VOLUME

Stroke volume depends on three factors:

1. Preload
2. Afterload
3. Contractility.

PHYSICON—The Reliable Icon in Physiology

Regulation of Stroke Volume

By two important regulatory mechanism—heterometric and homometric regulation.

I. Heterometric Regulation

By factors that change the length of cardiac muscle fiber and this is affected by factors which act within the heart. So this is also called **intrinsic regulation.** This is based on Frank-Starling's law. Thus it is independent of chemical or nervous factors. As mentioned earlier, force of contraction is dependent on preloading and afterloading.

Preload

In the ventricle, the preload is the amount of blood present in it before it has started contracting (EDV). So within the physiological limit, more the EDV more will be the CO (Starling's law). Factors affecting EDV are:

- *Venous return:* When venous return increases EDV increases. Its turn depends on:
  - *Blood volume:* When BV increases, VR increases, EDV increases, SV increases, so CO increases.
  - *Venous tone:* Increase in venous tone leads to increased pooling of blood in periphery, VR increases, so EDV increases.
  - *Skeletal muscle pump:* Veins are surrounded by skeletal muscles and when they contract they reduce the capacity of venous reservoir by squeezing veins and diverting the blood to heart. EDV increases, so CO increases.
  - *Intrathoracic pressure:* An increase in the normal negative intrathoracic pressure increases the pressure gradient along which blood flows to heart; so more blood is sucked into the thorax, venous return increases. It is important during inspiration as intrapleural pressure falls.
  - *Posture of body:* Venous return is maximum in lying posture. During standing, there is venous pooling which in turn increases venous return.
- *Atrial contraction:* When atria contracts more effectively EDV increases.
- *Intrapericardial pressure:* As intrapericardial pressure increases, there is a limit for the ventricle to expand and so filling is increases.
- *Ventricular compliance:* If expansibility is less, EDV increases.

Afterload

For left ventricle, afterload is the blood pressure in the aorta. When afterload is more, ventricles have to work more. It is called as aortic impedence or aortic resistance. When afterload increases CO decreases.

II. Homometric Regulation

By changing the factors that change the contractility of myocardium and it is independent of cardiac muscle fiber length. It is regulated by factors which operate outside the heart like neural and chemical factors, so it is also called extrinsic regulation.

Neural

When there is sympathetic stimulation, there is an increase in the force of contraction (via β_1 adrenergic receptors–activation of adenylcyclase → increased cAMP → intracellular calcium channel remain open for more time). Parasympathetic stimulation produces –ve effect.

Chemical

- Xanthine like caffeine, theophiline inhibit the breakdown of cAMP. So more Ca^{2+} is available.
- Glucagon increases cAMP, so more Ca^{2+} available.
- Thyroid hormone increase cAMP.
- Drugs like barbiturates and quinidine decreases force of contraction.
- Hypoxia, hypercapnia, acidosis are the other chemical factors which decrease force of contraction.

HEART RATE

Normally ranges from 60–100/min. It is also called sinus rhythm as it originates from SA node.

Physiological Increase

- Muscular exercise
- Inspiration
- After a meal
- Excitement, anger and painful stimuli.

Physiological Decrease

- Expiration
- Sleep
- In trained athlete

Advantage of training: In strong athletes, the heart size increases due to physiological hypertrophy of the myocardium. In these individuals, cardiac output increases during exercise by mainly increasing the stroke volume rather than heart rate. The trained athletes have lower basal heart rate and greater stroke volume.

Pathological Increase

- Hyperthyroidism
- Circulatory shock
- Congestive cardiac failure
- Fever
- Sympathomimetic drugs (adrenaline, isoprenaline)

Pathologic Decrease

- Heart block
- Myxedema

Control of Heart Rate

Heart rate is not under voluntary control. Regulation of heart rate can be explained as neural, chemical and thermal regulation.

I. Neural Regulation

Neural control is by autonomic nervous system (ANS) and by medullary centers.

A. Autonomic Regulation (Role of Cardiac Innervation)

Sympathetic supply

Sympathetic fibers are cardioacceleratory nerves. They originate from lateral horn of upper thoracic spinal cord. Lateral horn is known as spinal center of sympathetic system. The neurons in the lateral horns are influenced by impulses from medulla, which inturn is influenced by impulses from cerebral cortex, hypothalamus, limbic system and various peripheral afferent.

Preganglionic fibers from spinal cord end in stellate ganglion. Postganglionic fibers arise from stellate ganglion and innervate heart and vascular smooth muscles in the heart. Sympathetic fibers supply atrial muscles, SA node, AV node, purkinje system and ventricular muscles. The transmitter released at the postganglionic sympathetic nerve ending is norepinephrine. It mediates its action through β receptors.

Effect of stimulation of sympathetic fibers

- Increase HR (+ve chronotropic effect)
- Increase force of contraction (+ve inotropic effect)
- Increase conductivity (+ve dromotropic effect)
- Increase excitability (+ve bathmotropic effect).

Note: Normally a moderate tonic discharge is present in cardiac muscle from sympathetic (sympathetic tone) but not as powerful as that of parasympathetic and this tone is responsible for maintaining normal heartbeat.

Parasympathetic supply

Parasympathetic supply to the heart is mainly through vagus nerve. It is cardioinhibitory. They arise from dorsal motor nucleus and nucleus ambiguus in medulla. From these nuclei fibers arise and descend through the main trunk of vagus till it reaches neck where the fibers of heart are separated and mixed with sympathetic fibers to form superficial and deep cardiac plexus. These give rise to superior and inferior cardiac nerves and these nerves supply nodal tissue and atrium.

Ventricles do not receive any parasympathetic innervations. Neurotransmitter released at postganglionic nerve endings is acetylchoine (ACh) (via nicotinic and muscarinic receptor). Right vagus innervate SA node and thus it controls heart rate. Left vagus innervate AV node, thus it controls conduction through AV node.

Effect of stimulation of parasympathetic fibers

- Decrease HR (-ve chronotropic effect)
- Decrease force of contraction (-ve inotropic effect)
- Decrease conductivity (-ve dromotropic effect)
- Decrease excitability (-ve bathmotropic effect).

Note: Normally, a constant stream of impulses pass through vagus, which is inhibitory to heart (vagal tone).

Stimulation of right vagus decreases heart rate, left vagus stimulation delay the conduction through AV node. Strong stimulation of vagus decreases heart rate and finally the heart stops and it is called *vagal inhibition.* But after a few seconds, heart escapes from the inhibitory effect of vagus, this is called *vagal escape* and starts producing impulses of its own at a rate of 1–90/min called *idioventricular rhythm.*

Clinical Note

Effect of denervation of heart: SA node, the natural pacemaker, has the intrinsic rhythmicity of 80-100/min. However, normal heart rate is 70-80 beats/min. The reason for this—Heart is predominantly under the influence of vagal tone. The vagus, being a parasympathetic nerve, is inhibitory to the heart. This slows down the intrinsic excitability of SA node and its impulse discharge frequency is decreased to about 70–80/min. If heart is denervated, this tonic inhibitory influence of vagus will be abolished and SA node will generate impulses at its natural intrinsic rhythmicity; heart rate will increase to about 100 beats per minute.

B. Medullary Regulation

By denervating both sympathetic and parasympathetic, HR is found to be 100/min. This shows that sympathetic and parasympathetic innervation of heart plays an important role in maintaining normal HR and this activity is modified by higher centers which include centers in medulla, mainly the vasomotor area, hypothalamus and limbic system.

Medullary cardiovascular centers include vasomotor center and cardiac vagal center. This medullary center is influenced by cerebral cortex, hypothalamus, limbic system, peripheral afferents or peripheral reflex.

Vasomotor center (VMC) consists of

- *Sensory area:* Nucleus tractus solitarius (NTS).
  This area receives impulse via IX and X nerve from periphery, particularly from the baroreceptors. In turn, this area sends impulses to control the vasoconstrictor and vasodilator areas.

- *Depressor area:* Caudal and intermediate ventrolateral nucleus of medulla (CVLM and IVLM).
  This area is otherwise called vasodilator area. This area suppresses the vasoconstrictor area and causes vasodilation. It is concerned with cardioinhibition.
- *Pressor area:* Rostral ventrolateral nucleus of medulla (RVLM).
  This area is otherwise called vasoconstrictor area. This area sends impulses to blood vessels through sympathetic vasoconstrictor fibers. So stimulation of this area causes vasoconstriction and rise in BP. This area is also concerned with acceleration of HR.

Cardiac inhibitory center (CIC) consist of

- Nucleus ambiguus (NA)
- Dorsal motor neuron/Dorsal motor nuclei.
  There is a constant discharge of impulses from CIC through the vagus to the heart. This is responsible for the vagal tone of the heart.

Factors Influencing VMC and CIC

1. Baroreceptor Reflex

Baroreceptors are stretch receptors located on the walls of heart and blood vessels, they are stimulated by distension or stretch. Different types of baroreceptors includes sinoaortic reflex, atrial stretch receptor, Bainbridge reflex, left ventricular receptors.

a. Sinoaortic Reflex

Receptors are mechanoreceptors and respond to pressure changes or stretch. They are free nerve endings and are located in carotid sinus and arch of aorta. They are also located in subclavian and other major arteries.

These receptors are stimulated when BP changes between 90–150 mm Hg. Baroreceptors of carotid sinus are supplied by Hering's nerve (branch of glossopharyngeal nerve). Baroreceptors of arch of aorta are supplied by aortic branch of vagus nerve (Fig. 4.46).

When there is rise in BP, baroreceptors are stimulated. The nerve fibers from baroreceptors end in NTS of same side and opposite side. Neurotransmitter released is glutamate. Neurons originating from NTS is stimulated and these neurons end in depressor area (CVLM and IVLM). The neurotransmitter released here is excitatory (glutamate). These stimulate neurons from depressor area and the neurons originating from depressor area end in pressor area (RVLM). Here, the neurotransmitter released is GABA which is inhibitory. So when depressor area is stimulated, pressor area is inhibited. From pressor area fibers are given to intermediolateral horn. Impulse transmission to spinal sympathetic center is thus inhibited. Inhibition of the pressor area reduces the normal sympathetic vasoconstrictor tone, leading to vasodilation.

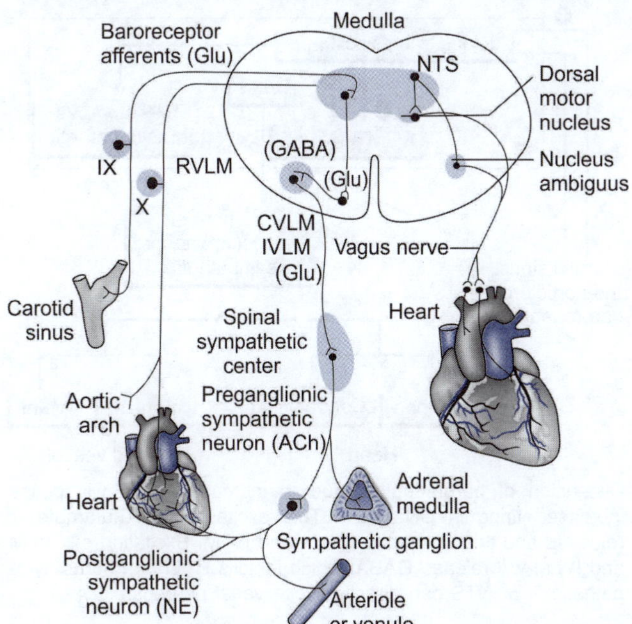

Fig. 4.46: Basic pathways involved in the medullary control of cardiovascular system

When NTS are stimulated impulses are also given to NA and dorsal motor neuron of vagus. That will lead to stimulation of vagus. When there is a rise in BP, there is increased parasympathetic and decreased sympathetic stimulation. The suppression of vasoconstrictor area reduces vasomotor tone (sympathetic tone). When vasomotor tone is reduced, there is vasodilatation which in turn leads to reduction in peripheral resistance. The simultaneous excitation of CIC reduces HR and force of contraction causing reduction in CO.

Both the factors, i.e. reduced peripheral resistance and reduced cardiac output ultimately decreases arterial BP. As the baroreceptor mechanism acts against the rise in arterial blood pressure it is called *pressure buffer mechanism* and the nerves from baroreceptors are called buffer nerves. When BP decreases, all the changes are reversed (Fig. 4.47).

Note

- From spinal sympathetic center sympathetic preganglionic fibers originate and these fibers end in sympathetic ganglia and adrenal medulla. When baroreceptors are not stimulated, spinal sympathetic center is not inhibited. Adrenal medulla is considered as a modified sympathetic ganglion. Adrenaline and noradrenaline are released from adrenal medulla. Adrenaline acts mainly on heart and nor adrenaline acts on smooth muscles or blood vessels to produce the pressor effects. From sympathetic ganglion postganglionic neurons originate and they innervate heart and blood vessels.

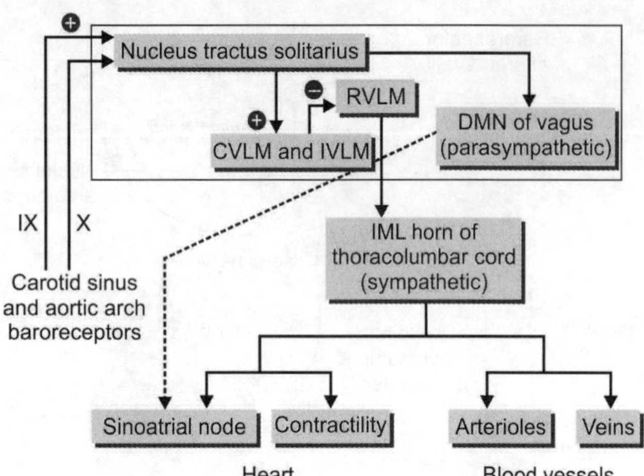

Distension of baroreceptors due to increase in BP will cause increased firing in CN IX, X. This excites NTS. Glutamate is released and this will excite CVLM and IVLM. Excitation of CVLM and IVLM will release GABA, which inhibits RVLM and thus sympathetic flow. NTS can directly excite vagal neurons.

Fig. 4.47: Schematic depiction of baroreceptor (negative) feedback regulation of BP

In simple terms, 'increased baroreceptor discharge inhibits the tonic discharge of sympathetic nerves and excites the vagal innervation of the heart. Effects of baroreceptor in response to increase in BP are vasodilation, venodilation, hypotension, bradycardia, decrease in cardiac output.

- *Mary's law:* It states that BP is inversely proportional to HR. This is mediated by baroreceptors, i.e. rise in BP will stimulate CIC and HR will decrease.

b. Cardiopulmonary Receptor

This includes atrial stretch receptors, Bainbridge reflex and left ventricular receptors.

- *Atrial stretch receptors (Flowchart 4.1):* These are stimulated by distension of atria. Increase in venous return leads to distension of atrial wall leading to increased discharge in receptors causing increase in HR. Increased HR causes vasodilatation which leads to fall in BP.

Flowchart 4.1: Atrial stretch reflex

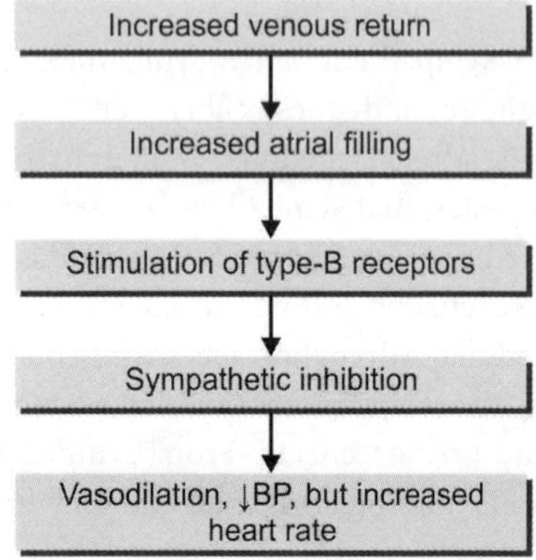

Flowchart 4.2: Bainbridge reflex

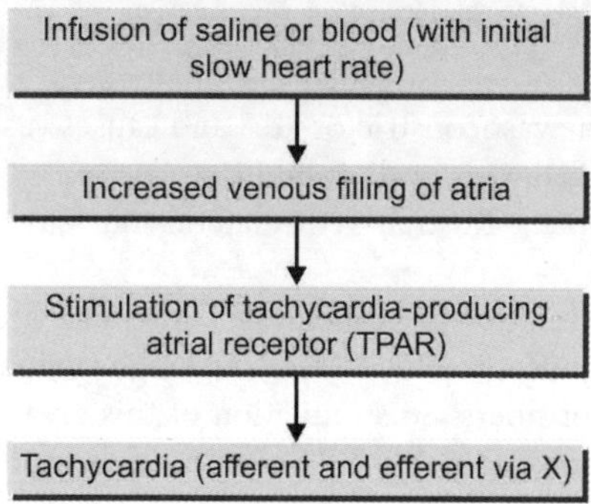

- *Bainbridge reflex (Flowchart 4.2):* Rapid infusion of blood or cold saline in anesthetized animals produces a rise in HR, if the initial HR is low. The receptors are tachycardia producing atrial receptors. The reflex competes with the baroreceptor mediated decrease in HR produced by volume expansion.

  Afferent and efferent are through vagus and the center is at medulla. It is diminished or absent when the initial HR is high.
- *Left ventricular receptors:* When the left ventricle is distended, there is fall in BP and HR. It takes considerable distention to produce this response and its physiological significance is uncertain. However, they may play a role in the maintenance of vagal tone that keeps HR low at rest.

2. Chemoreceptor

a. From carotid body and aortic body

Stimulated by fall in BP. Impulses are transmitted through IX and X cranial nerves. Impulses reach NTS and then it controls vasomotor center.

b. Coronary chemoreceptors (Bezold Jarish reflex)

In experimental animals, injection of serotonin, capsaicin, veratridine, etc. into the coronary artery supplying left ventricle cause apnea followed by rapid breathing, hypotension and bradycardia. The receptors are C fiber endings, the afferents are vagal and the center is medulla. They are also stimulated by occlusion of pulmonary artery or by substances released from damaged myocardium. In patients with MI, substances released from infarcted tissue stimulates C fiber ending of vagus and cause bradycardia, hypotension, apnea.

c. Pulmonary chemoreceptors (J receptor mediated)

The receptors are J receptors (juxtacapillary receptors). They are located in alveolar interstitium close to pulmonary capillaries. The effects are apnea followed by rapid breathing, hypotension and bradycardia.

d. Miscellaneous

Mild hypoxia and hypercapnia stimulate vasomotor center directly causing increased HR.

If hypoxia is severe it will depress the vasomotor center.

3. Cushing Reflex (Flowchart 4.3)

When intracranial pressure is increased, the blood supply to vasomotor area is decreased. This cause local hypoxia and hypercapnea. Vasomotor area is excited to increase BP which can increase blood supply to vasomotor area. When BP is increase there is reflex reduction in HR. This is the only condition in the body where we have increased BP associated with decreased HR.

Clinical Note

Bradycardia occurs in brain tumors. Increased ICP causes reflex bradycardia by activation of Cushing and baroreceptor reflexes.

Note: The heart rate varies with the phases of respiration. It increases during inspiration and decreases during expiration. This phenomenon is called *sinus arrhythmia*. During inspiration, impulses in the vagi from stretch receptors in the lungs inhibit the CIC in the medulla oblongata. Thus, the tonic vagal discharge that keeps HR low, decreases and HR rises.

4. Corticohypothalamic Pathways

Cerebral cortex and limbic system exerts strong influence on blood pressure and heart rate through medullary centers. Limbic system also influences through medullary center. Change in heart rate and BP during various emotional activities is due to influence of limbic system on medullary centers.

Flowchart 4.3: Cushings reflex

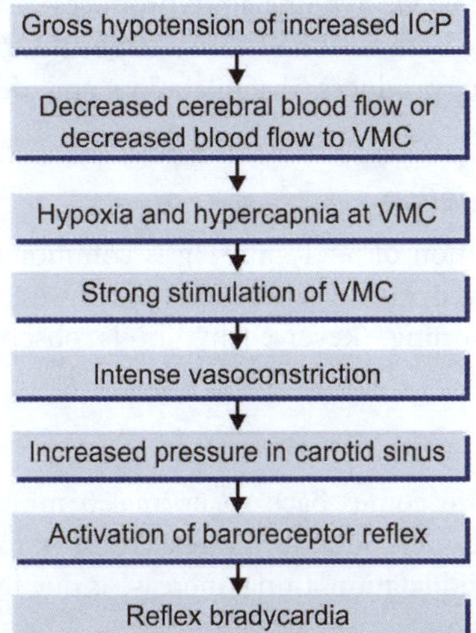

Note

Stimulation of baroreceptor → decreases BP
Stimulation of chemoreceptors → increases BP

II. Chemical Regulation

Norepinephrine has a direct chronotropic effect on heart, but its pressor action stimulates the baroreceptors leading to bradycardia. Thyroxine increases HR by increasing BMR and also by increasing the sensitivity of epinephrine and norepinephrine. Digitalis decreases HR.

III. Thermal Regulation

Increased body temperature increases HR and vice versa.

Summary of CO Regulation

CO = Stroke volume × Heart rate

Stroke Volume

Heterometric regulation

- EDV—as EDV increases, SV increases and it in turn depends on:
  - Venous return-blood volume, venous tone, skeletal muscle pump, intrathoracic pump, posture of body
  - Atrial contraction
  - Intrapericardial pressure
  - Ventricular compliance.
- Aortic resistance-if resistance is more SV is less.

Homometric regulation (Table 4.5)

Heart Rate

Neural regulation

- Autonomic regulation
- Medullary regulation, which is influenced by:
  - *Baroreceptors:* Sinoaortic reflex, atrial stretch reflex, Bainbridge reflex, LV receptors.
  - *Chemoreceptors:* From carotid body and aortic body, Bezold Jarish reflex, J receptor mediated, Cushings reflex.
  - Impulses from cerebral cortex, limbic system.

Table 4.5: Homometric regulation

Neural	Chemical
Sympathetic Parasympathetic	Xanthines Barbiturates Quinidine Digitalis Glucagon Hypoxia Hypercapnia Acidosis Calcium Thyroid hormones

Chemical regulation

Catecholamines, thyroxine, digitalis, hypercapnia, hypoxia.

Thermal Regulation

Temperature, exercise.

BLOOD PRESSURE

Arterial blood pressure is defined as the lateral pressure exerted by column of blood on the wall of arteries. Systolic pressure is defined as the maximum pressure exerted in the arteries during systole of heart (normal value: 100–140 mm Hg).

Diastolic pressure is the pressure exerted in the arteries during the diastole of heart. Systolic pressure is the pressure that is created when the ventricles contract. Diastolic pressure is the pressure that is created by the recoil of the aorta and the closure of the aortic semilunar valve (Fig. 4.48). Pulse pressure is the difference between the systolic pressure and diastolic pressure. Mean arterial blood pressure is the average pressure throughout the cardiac cycle (Fig. 4.49).

MAP = Diastolic pressure + 1/3 pulse pressure.

Let us consider the systolic BP = 120 mm Hg and diastolic BP = 80 mm Hg. The arithmetic average or mean value of 120 and 80 would be: (120 + 80)/2= (200/2) = 100. It would be equidistant between 120 and 80. However, MAP is actually calculated as: (diastolic BP) + one-third of pulse pressure. Pulse pressure for the given values is (120–80) = 40. One-third of 40 is approx 13. Hence, MAP of 120 and 80, by the given formula, is 93 mm Hg.

The conclusion is mean arterial pressure, i.e. the average pressure in the circulation, is closer to the diastolic BP and is not the arithmetic mean of systolic and diastolic pressures. Reason is that, in a cardiac cycle, diastole duration is longer (0.5 sec) than systole (0.3 sec). Hence, average pressure is closer to diastolic BP, rather than being the arithmetic mean.

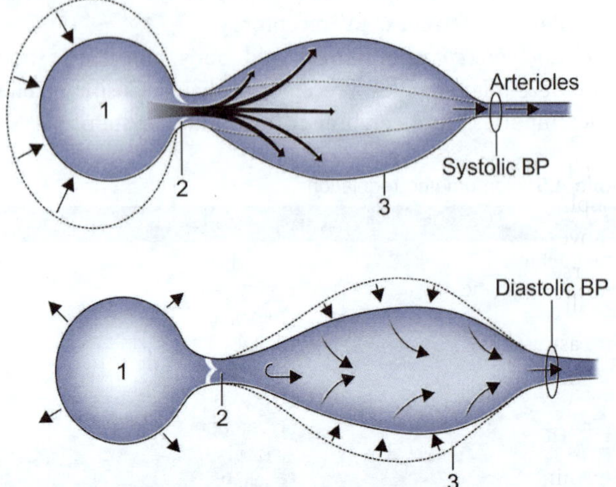

Fig. 4.48: Systolic and diastolic BP

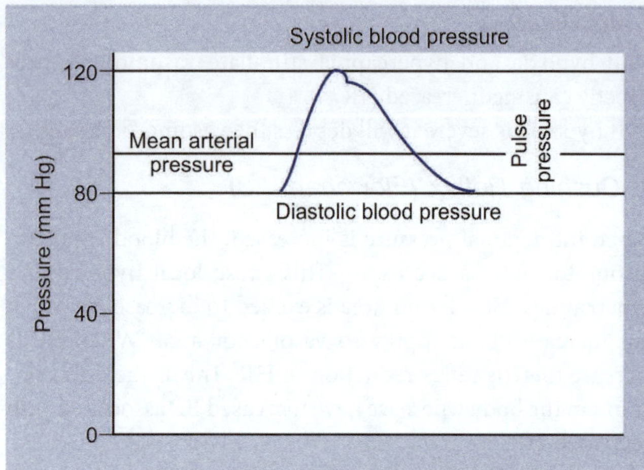

Fig. 4.49: Pulse pressure and mean pressure

Factors Affecting Arterial Blood Pressure

Age

Both systolic blood pressure (SBP) and diastolic blood pressure (DBP) increases with age. Systolic blood pressure (SBP) increases more than DBP due to decreased distensibility of arteries. The DBP decreases with age after 50–60 years.

Sex

In females before menopause SBP is 4–5 mm Hg less than males of same age. In females after menopause SBP is 4–5 Hg more than males. This effect is due to estrogen which prevents atherosclerosis.

Body Built

In obese individuals brachial arterial pressure gives high readings because there is more tissue between the cuff and artery.

Climate

Exposure to cold via hypothalamus produces vasoconstriction and increases both SBP and DBP. Exposure to warmth via hypothalamus produces vasodilatation and decreases both SBP and DBP.

Diurnal Variation

Diurnal variation of 5–10 mm Hg is common in SBP, peak values observed during afternoon and lowest during early hours of morning. Reverse rhythm is observed in night workers.

Exercise

Blood pressure comes back to normal 5 minutes after the stoppage of exercise due to the relaxation of muscles which produces vasodilatation. Initial increase is due to sympathetic vasoconstriction.

Emotions

Excitement, fear, worry increase SBP due to increase in CO secondary to increased sympathetic activity.

Gravity

Pressure in any vessel below the heart is increased by the effect of gravity. Pressure in any vessel above the heart is decreased by the effect of gravity. Magnitude of gravitational effect at normal density of blood is 0.77 mm Hg/cm vertical distance fron heart.

Hereditary

Familial tendencies of hypotension/hypertension with SBP are common.

Meals

Changes in systemic BP due to:

- Pressure over heart due to distended abdomen increases heart rate.
- Increase epinephrine release from adrenal medulla.

Therefore, SBP increases 5–6 mm Hg up to 1 hour after meals, DBP remains same/decreases slightly due to vasodilatation in digestive organs.

Sleep

Systolic blood pressure falls in early hours of sleep by 15–30 mm Hg, because of general vasodilatation of vessels in complete relaxed state. However, disturbed sleep increases SBP due to increased sympathetic discharge secondary to skeletal muscle tensioning.

Posture

Changes in DBP are more with the change of body posture. In standing posture DBP increases; in sitting remains normal and decreases in lying posture.

Mechanism

Upon standing

- Peripheral pooling of blood in dependent parts → decrease in VR → decreased CO → decrease in SBP → decrease in baroreceptor discharge → increase in DBP.
- Increase in peripheral resistance → increase in DBP

Therefore, sudden standing increases DBP, if recorded within 30–60 seconds of change in posture after that it comes to normal via the operation of baroreceptor reflexes.

Factors Determining BP

BP = Cardiac output × peripheral resistance.

Role of Cardiac Output

Pumping action of heart is the main factor for controlling CO. Therefore, alteration of CO will alter arterial BP. CO = HR × stroke volume. Systolic pressure depends mainly upon stroke volume. Stroke volume in turn depends on preload, afterload and contractility.

Role of Peripheral Resistance

This is the important factor which maintains diastolic pressure.

$$\text{Peripheral resistance} = \frac{8\eta l}{\pi r^4}$$

where,

η = viscosity of blood

l = length of vessel

r = radius of the vessel.

Peripheral Resistance

Peripheral resistance depends on:

- *Viscosity of blood:* Arterial pressure is directly proportional to viscosity of blood. When viscosity of blood is more, the frictional resistance is more and this increases blood pressure.
- *Radius of the vessel:* Peripheral resistance is inversely proportional to fourth power of radius. Even a slight change in diameter can produce great change in peripheral resistance. Changes in diameter is brought about by changes in sympathetic tone.
- *Elasticity of vessel wall:* Blood pressure is inversely related to the elasticity of blood vessel. It is due to the elastic properties, the arteries can dilate and accommodate considerable amount of blood with relative rise of BP. At lower pressure (less than 30–40 mm Hg) elasticity does not come to play and blood vessels behave like a rigid tube.
- *Velocity of blood flow:* The greater the velocity of flow in a vessel, the lower the lateral pressure distending its walls (according to Bernoulli's principle). When a vessel is narrowed, the velocity of flow in the narrowed portion increases and the distending pressure decreases.

Note: To take an accurate blood pressure (BP) reading, place the sphygmomanometer at the level of the heart. If the cuff is above the level of the heart, the reading will be falsely low; conversely, if the cuff is below the level of the heart, the reading will be falsely high.

Measurement of BP is discussed in page no 358 under practical section.

Regulation of Blood Pressure

Determinants can fix the level of BP, but when there is a fluctuation, it is brought back to normal level by various mechanisms available in our body. In short all the BP regulatory mechanisms are grouped under:

- Short-term regulatory mechanisms
- Intermediate regulatory mechanisms
- Long-term regulatory mechanisms.

Short-term Regulatory Mechanisms (sec-min)

The short-term regulation or nervous regulation is rapid among all mechanism involved in the regulation of BP. The ANS participate in the short-term regulation through different reflex mechanisms. They include baroreceptor reflexes, chemoreceptor reflexes and Cushing's reflex.

Baroreceptor reflexes

Sinoaortic reflex: Refer page no 105.

The sequence of events are given in Flowchart 4.4.

If we have such an efficient mechanism as the baroreceptor system, why do people suffer from hypertension?

The set point of baroreceptors, under normal circumstances, is around a mean BP of around 100 mm Hg (the average normal BP in adults). Any deviation from this BP and the baroreceptors will immediately bring it back toward the normal set point. However, if a person is consistently exposed to a situation that keeps the BP elevated, then after 48 hours, the baroreceptor set point is 'reset' to the new (elevated) level. Thus, it is not useful or efficient in long-term regulation or maintaining the BP normal/constant on a long-term basis.

Other reflexes: Atrial stretch receptors when stimulated will lead to fall in BP. Similarly, left ventricular stretch receptors when stimulated lead to fall in BP. Bainbridge reflex also have role in the regulation of BP but its main effect is on HR.

Flowchart 4.4: Regulation of blood pressure by baroreceptor mechanism

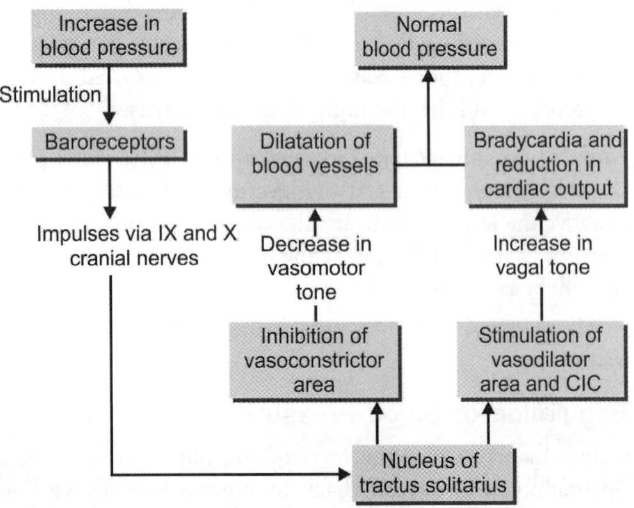

Chemoreceptor reflex

They give response to change in chemical constituents of blood. The receptors are carotid body and aortic body. They respond to hypoxia, hypercapnia, acidosis. When the mean pressure falls, it produces lack of O_2, excess of CO_2 and hydrogen ion concentration. When the arterial pressure falls below 80 mm Hg, chemoreceptors are stimulated. The chemoreceptors in the carotid body are supplied by glossopharygeal and those in the aortic body by vagal nerve fibers. The impulses reaches the medullary center, resulting in increased HR and BP.

Cushing reflex

This response is also called CNS ischemic response as this reflex is due to ischemia of brain. The mechanism is given under factors influencing VMC and CIC.

Intermediate Regulatory Mechanism (min-hrs)

They include stress relaxation of vasculature and capillary fluid shift mechanism.

Stress relaxation of vasculature

Whenever the smooth muscle is stretched for prolonged time it goes into relaxation.

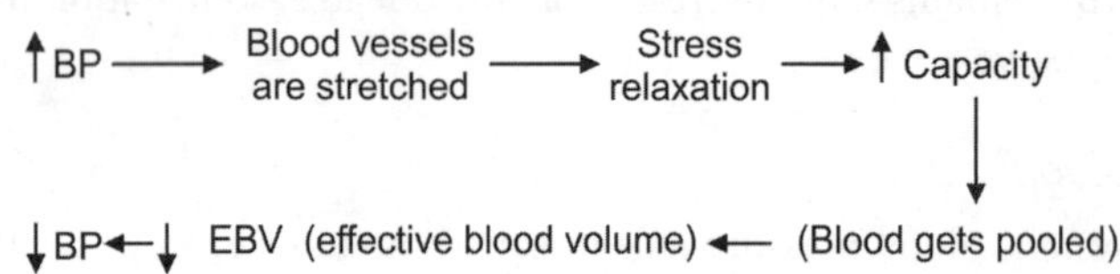

Reverse changes takes place when BP falls.

Capillary fluid shift mechanism

Whenever, there is an increase in BP more fluid is filtered through the capillary wall into the interstitial space. So blood volume decreases, resulting in decreased BP. Reverse changes takes place when BP falls.

Long-term Regulation (hrs-days)

All the mechanism that tend to alter the blood volume participate in long-term regulation. The kidneys play an important role in the long-term regulation of BP. These mechanisms include renin angiotensin mechanism, renal body fluid system and hormonal mechanism.

Renin-angiotensin mechanism

Whenever there is a fall in BP, there is decrease in blood flow to the kidney. This results in the release of renin from JG cells. It converts angiotensinogen to angiotensin I. This is converted to angiotensin II by angiotensin converting enzyme. Angiotensin II then acts to restore BP by:

- It acts directly on the kidneys to cause salt and water retention (by vasoconstriction).

- It causes adrenal glands to secrete aldosterone and the aldosterone in turn increases salt and water reabsorbtion by the kidney tubules.

  All these ultimately lead to restoration of BP.

Renal body fluid system (by regulation of ECF volume)

When the body contains too much extracellular fluid, the blood volume and arterial pressure rise. This rising pressure in turn has direct effect to cause the kidneys to excrete excess ECF, thus returning the pressure back to normal. Even a slight increase in BP can double water excretion, which is called *pressure diuresis.* Elevated BP can also leads to sodium excretion which is called pressure natriuresis. Reverse changes takes place when BP falls.

Hormonal mechanism

Hormones other than angiotensin also aids in the regulation of BP.

- *Aldosterone:* It causes the retention of water and Na^+ thereby increases ECF volume leading to increase in BP.
- *ADH (vasopressin):* Fall in BP causes increased production of ADH. It increases the reabsortion of water from renal tubules and collecting duct. ADH can also cause constriction of vascular smooth muscles.
- *Atrial natriuretic peptide:* ANP causes dilation of blood vessels and decreases blood pressure.
- *Catecholamines:* Released from adrenal medulla.
  - Epinephrine acts mainly on heart.
  - Norepinephrine acts on blood vessel.
- *Urotensin:* II-present in cardiac and vascular tissue. It is the one of the most potent vasoconstrictor.
- *Thyroid hormones:* Help in regulation of BP, mainly by their effect on metabolism. They also potentiate the effect on catecholamines on the vascular smooth muscle and the heart.
  - In hyperthyroidism - high BP
  - In hypothyroidism - low BP.

Hypertension

Hypertension (HTN) refers to a condition in which value of systolic blood pressure is persistently more than 140 mm Hg and/or that of diastolic blood pressure is above 90 mm Hg. If there is increase only in systolic blood pressure, it is called systolic hypertension in which pulse pressure is raised.

Types of Hypertension

It is of two types: primary and secondary hypertension:

1. Primary hypertension also known as essential hypertension is characterized by a raised blood pressure without any underlying disease. Risk factors for primary HTN include: heredity, obesity, mental tension and smoking.
2. Secondary hypertension refers to a condition in which blood pressure is raised due to some other underlying disease. Common causes of secondary hypertension are:
   - Cardiovascular diseases, e.g. atherosclerosis.
   - Renal diseases, e.g. glomerulonephritis and tumor of juxtaglomerular cells leading to formation of excess of angiotensin II.
   - Endocrinal disorders like hyperaldosteronism, phaeochromocytoma (tumor of adrenal medulla) and Cushing's syndrome (excessive secretion of glucocorticoids from adrenal cortex).
   - Neurologic disorders which may produce hypertension include raised intracranial pressure.
   - Pregnancy induced hypertension (PIH) is noticed in some of the pregnant women.

Complications of Hypertension

- *Cardiac conditions:* Left ventricular hypertrophy, cardiac failure, ischemia, myocardial infraction
- *CNS conditions:* Cerebral hemorrhage, stroke
- *Retinal conditions:* Hypertensive retinopathy, papilloedema
- *Renal conditions:* Renal failure.

Treatment of Hypertension

Primary HTN is treatable, but not curable.

- Salt, calorie, cholesterol and saturated fat restricted diet
- Avoid alcohol and smoking
- Exercise and lifestyle changes
- *Drugs:* There are different classes of drugs for treating HTN:
  1. Vasodilator drugs (decrease afterload)
  2. Natriuretic/diuretic drugs (decreases the tubular reabsorption of salt and H_2O). Other drugs used for the treatment of HTN include anti-adrenergic drugs, ACE inhibitors and Ca^{2+} channel blockers.

Secondary, HTN is not only treatable but sometimes also curable.

Distribution of Cardiac Output and Oxygen Consumption of Various Body Organs

Note the following points (Table 4.6):

- Blood flow (mL/min) is highest for liver. Blood flow per 100 g tissue per minute is highest for kidney. Arteriovenous Oxygen difference (AV O_2, mL/L) is highest for heart.
- Arteriovenous Oxygen difference (AV O_2, mL/L) is lowest for kidney.
- O_2 consumption (mL/min) is highest for liver. O_2 consumption per 100 g tissue per minute is highest for

Table 4.6: Blood flow and O_2 consumption of various tissues organs

Tissue/Organ	Blood flow (mL/min)	Blood flow (mL/100 g/min)	Oxygen consumption (mL/min)	% of cardiac output	% of body's total O_2 consumpton
Liver	1500	57.7	51	27.8	20.4
Kidneys	1260	420.0	18	23.3	7.2
Brain	750	54.0	46	13.9	18.4
Skeletal muscle	840	2.7	50	15.6	20.0
Skin	462	12.8	12	8.6	4.8

heart. Highest percentage of cardiac output goes to liver. Highest percentage of O_2 consumption is by liver.

Why is it that the heart is more prone to infarction?

Arteriovenous oxygen difference is about 25% for most other organs. When arteries bring 20 mL of O_2/100 mL blood into the tissues, only 5 mL out of that 20 mL is extracted by them, under basal conditions. (The remaining 15 mL oxygen goes into the venous blood. Hence, AV O_2 difference is [20–15 = 5 mL]. Thus, 5 mL/20 mL = 25%.) Thus, other tissues and organs have a good reserve of oxygen; they can extract more oxygen if the need arises.

In the case of heart, as coronary arteries bring 20 mL of O_2/100 mL blood, the myocardium extracts 15 mL out of the 20 mL oxygen. (Arteriovenous O_2 difference is 15 mL; i.e. 75%.) Thus, myocardium is already extracting maximum O_2 (75%), under basal conditions; it has a poor reserve of oxygen. Hence, if its need for oxygen increases (as with increasing heart rates), it can not increase its oxygen extraction beyond a certain limit. Myocardial oxygen delivery can be increased by coronary vasodilation. This too will have its limits. Eventually, the myocardium will suffer; there will be a lag between its oxygen demand and the oxygen availability to it. This may result in necrosis of myocardial cells and infarction of the myocardium.

CORONARY CIRCULATION

Coronary circulation means the circulation through the heart itself. Heart is supplied by two coronary arteries: left and right.

- In 50% of population right coronary artery carries major blood supply to heart.
- 20% individuals left coronary artery is dominant.
- In the rest 30% both arteries are dominant (equally dominant).

The coronary sinus and anterior cardiac veins drain the blood ultimately into right atrium. Some quantity of blood enters directly into cardiac chambers via arteriosinusoidal vessels, arteriolurninal vessels and the besian system of veins. Coronary blood flow in humans can be measured by Kety method or nitrous oxide technique (based on Fick's principle), radionuclides utilization technique, coronary angiography.

Special Features of Coronary Circulation

- It supplies the heart itself. Coronary blood flow at rest is 250 mL/min (5% of CO).
- In majority of people one artery is dominant to other.
- The vessels are subjected to force of myocardial contraction and are compressed during systole.
- Unlike other vascular bed it is mainly perfused during diastole. (During diastole cardiac muscle relaxes and it will not obstruct blood flow through LV muscle capillaries).
- O_2 extraction is highest in this bed. O_2 content of arterial blood is19 mL% and O_2 content of venous blood is 6.7 mL%. About 13 mL is utilized in heart (in other tissues 19–14 mL about 5 mL utilized).
- Coefficient of O_2 utilization is 70%, whereas it is about 20% in all other tissues. So increased blood flow is needed. This is a disadvantage for persons with any block in blood vessels. On exertion, the part with decreased blood flow will get necrosis and MI occurs.
- Collateral circulation is normally not very important but may develop in chronic CAD.
- Diameter of muscle less, so high capillary density.
- Change of blood flow in different phases of cardiac cycle (Figs 4.50 and 4.51).

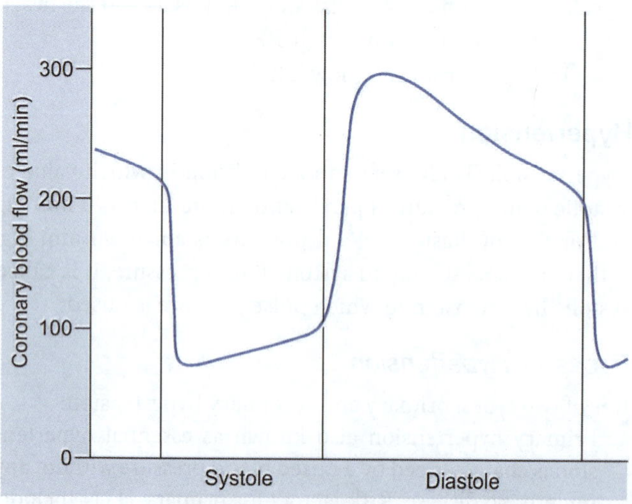

Fig. 4.50: Phasic changes in coronary blood flow

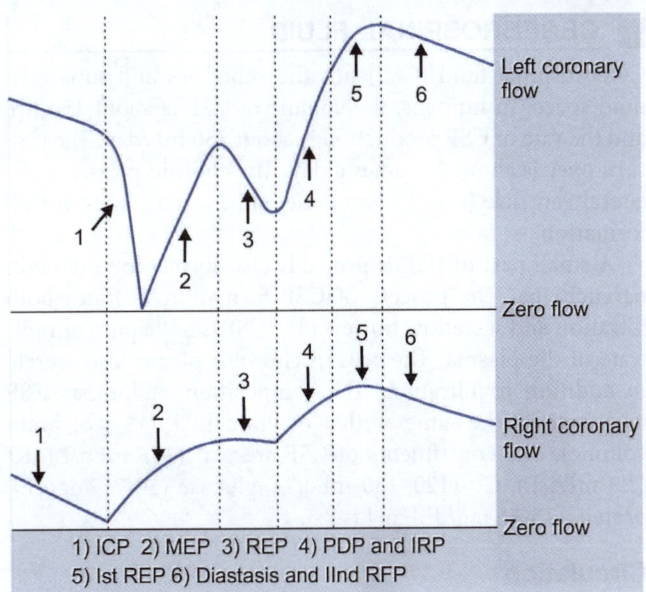

Fig. 4.51: Blood flow through coronary vessels during different phases of cardiac cycle

- Coronary circulation shows reactive hyperemia, which means increased blood flow to a part following a temporary obstruction of flow.
- Autoregulation: Even if there is change in pressure (60–160 mm Hg) there is no change in coronary blood flow. This is achieved through autoregulation.
- Metabolic factors are more important for controlling blood flow.

Factors Regulating Coronary Blood Flow

Rate of Metabolism

Local muscle metabolism (myocardium) is the primary controller of coronary flow. Higher the metabolic rate, higher is the O_2 demand and CBF increases. Due to increased metabolism there will be O_2 lack and increased concentration of CO_2, H^+, K^+, adenine, lactate, etc. and these produce vasodilation.

Perfusion Pressure

More the perfusion pressure, more is the blood flow, but up to a limit only (due to autoregulation in coronary circulation). In the systemic pressure range of 60–150 mm Hg, CBF remains constant if cardiac activity remains constant. Coronary perfusion pressure mainly depends on DBP in the aorta.

Effect of Ventricular Contraction

The vessels which are situated within the myocardium are compressed during myocardial contraction. During diastole, the cardiac muscle relaxes and no longer obstructs blood flow through the left ventricular muscle capillaries, so that blood flows rapidly during all of diastole.

Since, the blood pressure between aorta (120 mm Hg) and LV (121 mm Hg) is very small during systole, therefore, blood flows to subendocardial portion of LV only in diastole (0 mm Hg). However, pressure difference is more in superficial portion of LV to permit some flow in this region throught the cardiac cycle; while blood flow to RV (25 mm Hg in systole and 0 mm Hg in diastole) and atria occurs both during systole and diastole.

Note: Because there is no blood flow during systole in subendocardial portion of LV, this portion of LV is more prone to MI.

Neural Influence

The stimulation of autonomic nerves influence coronary blood flow both directly and indirectly. The direct effects result from the action of neurotransmitter acetylcholine (parasympathetic) and norepinephrine, epinephrine (sympathetic) on the coronary vessels themselves. The indirect effect (important role) results from secondary changes in coronary blood flow caused by increased or decreased activity of heart. ACh has a direct effect to dilate coronary arteries, thus increases CBF.

Norepinephrine and epinephrine can have vascular constrictor or vascular dilator effects [depending on the presence or absence of constrictor (α) or dilator (β) receptors]. Both the receptors are present in coronary vessels. The sympathetic stimulation due to α receptors leads to vasoconstriction and decreased CBF. Similarly, sympathetic stimulation due to β receptors leads to vasodilation and increased CBF.

CEREBRAL CIRCULATION

The principal arterial inflow to the brain in humans is via four arteries: Two internal carotid arteries and two vertebral arteries. The vertebral arteries unite to form the basilar artery. The basilar artery and the carotids form the circle of Willis. In human a relatively small fraction of the total arterial flow is carried by the vertebral arteries. Average blood flow rate in brain is about 750 mL/min of tissue.

Features of Cerebral Circulation

- The gray matter consumes a very high amount of O_2. It accounts for only 1% of total body weight but consumes about 20% of the total O_2 consumed in the body.
- The total quantity of blood flowing to the brain is remarkably constant (In other circulations of the body, quantity of blood flow varies sharply due to factors such as exercise).
- The brain keeps up its blood supply despite remarkable change in the perfusion pressure, as brain cannot survive anoxic assault.
- The brain is inside a rigid cranial box (except in infants before anterior fontanelle closure), i.e. neither the blood nor the CSF can be compressed, so if the volume of CSF expands, the brain blood flow has to be reduced.

Factors Determining the Blood Flow

Perfusion Pressure and Autoregulation

The brain blood flow will not increase as mean arterial BP increases. Between 60 to about 150 mm Hg of mean BP, the blood flow is not affected. This is autoregulation of brain blood flow. The principle factor in autoregulation is the accumulation of CO_2, although myogenic response to decreased distension may also have some role.

However, if the systemic BP falls very severely (below 60 mm Hg) as in severe cardiovascular shock there is an increased risk of cerebral anoxia.

CO_2 Concentration

When the CO_2 concentration of the local brain tissue rises, there is vasodilatation leading to increased blood flow.

O_2 Tension

High O_2 tension in the inspired air produces cerebral vasoconstriction so that the brain is protected from the dangers of O_2 poisoning.

Anesthetics

Majority of the anesthetics reduce the brain blood flow, e.g. halothane. They also decrease the cerebral metabolism.

Sympathetic Stimulation

Sympathetic stimulation produces cerebral vasoconstriction.

CEREBROSPINAL FLUID

Cerebrospinal fluid (CSF) fills the ventricles and subarachnoid space. In humans, the volume of CSF is about 150 mL and the rate of CSF production is about 550 mL/day. The CSF turn over is about 3.7 times a day. The choroid plexus of the lateral ventricle (also 3rd ventricle) are the main sites of CSF formation.

A small part of CSF is probably also formed by the brain parenchyma. The process of CSF formation includes both filtration and secretion, however the CSF is not a pure ultrafiltrate of the plasma. The cells of choroids plexus also secrete in addition to filtration. The composition of lumbar CSF is essentially the same as that of brain ECF (15% of brain volume). The constituents of CSF are Na^+ (148 mEq/L), K^+ (2.9 mEq/L), Cl^- (120–130 mEq/L), glucose (50-75 mg/dL), protein (15-45 mg/dL), pH is 7.3.

Circulation

The CSF, thus formed comes out of the lateral ventricle → enters the 3rd ventricle through the foramen of Monro → passes through the aqueduct of sylvius → enters the 4th ventricle → escapes mainly through the foramina of Luschka and Magendie → occupies the subarachnoid space and is distributed all over the brain. A small part of CSF enters the central canal (Fig. 4.52).

Absorption

At the sagittal sinus, finger like projections, called arachnoid villi, are seen to project from the arachnoid matter. These

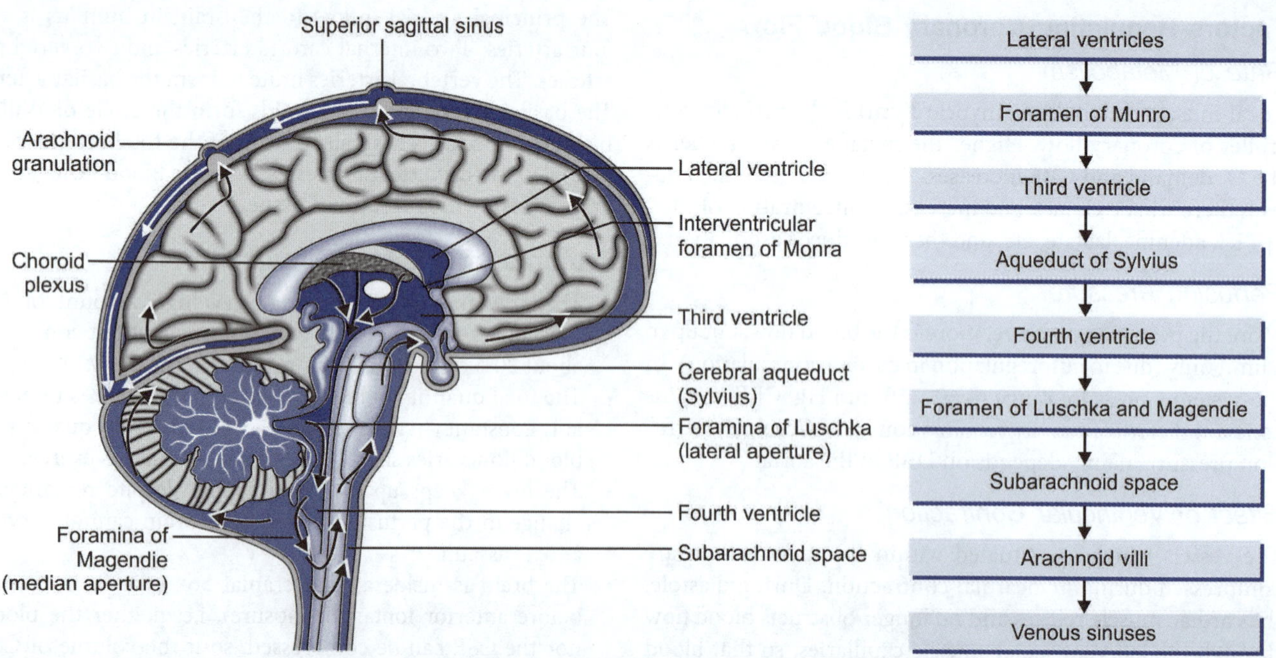

Fig. 4.52: Lateral view showing human ventricles and route of circulation of CSF within brain spaces

arachnoid villi come in contact with the venous blood of sagittal sinus. The membranous structure which separates the CSF within the arachnoid villi and the venous blood of sagittal sinus, consists of arachnoid mater plus the meningeal layer of the duramater. The epithelium of this membrane shows pores. When the pressure of the CSF (within the arachnoid villi) is high, the pores open up and the fluid escapes into the venous blood. But venous blood cannot enter the villi, because:

- Pressure within these sinuses are normally very low.
- If there is any rise of venous pressure within these sinuses the pores will close down. Further, colloidal osmotic tension of venous blood plasma is high (increased conc of plasma protein) whereas that in the CSF (of the villi) is very low which also aids in the transfer of CSF to the venous blood. A part of CSF is absorbed, via the arachnoid villi, into the venous blood of cranium and spinal cord.

Functions of CSF

- It forms a sort of cushion round the brain. If the head receives an injury, because of the presence of the CSF, the impact of injury is distributed all over the brain and thus no single area of the brain has to bear a high degree of impact.
- If there is an edema of the brain (as a result of brain injury/inflammation) the CSF escapes from the subarachnoid space into the venous sinuses and thus provides some room so that brain is not pressurized
- It may carry nutrients to the brain.

Applied Physiology

Lumbar Puncture

In some diseases it is necessary to examine the CSF for diagnostic purposes. For this a needle is passed in between the 3rd and 4th lumbar spinous processes into the subarachnoid space within the vertebral canal (spinal cord ends at the level of spinous process of L1 or L2 vertebra).

Other uses of lumbar puncture

- *Diagnostic:* For the diagnosis of meningitis, multiple sclerosis, subarachnoid hemorrhage.
- *Therapeutic:* To administrate antibiotics and antitumor agents.
- *Anesthetic:* To give spinal anesthesia.

Abnormal CSF

In cerebral/subarachnoid hemorrhage, the CSF contains blood. In purulent meningitis, the CSF is cloudy, cell count is high and consists of mainly neutrophils. Chemically sugar concentration falls, protein concentration rises. All these features are due to acute inflammation of meninges. In viral encephalitis, rise of the protein concentration may be the only abnormality.

Hydrocephalus

The aqueduct of Sylvius may be constricted (due to certain forms of neurosyphilis, tumor) and the CSF accumulates in the 3rd and lateral ventricle but fails to appear from 4th ventricle onwards. As a result of the accumulation, the intracranial tension rises, the brain matter is pressurized leading to considerable damage to the brain. The foramina of Luschka and Magendie may be obliterated (following inflammation to meninges) leading to similar conditions.

Blood-Brain Barrier

The tight junctions between capillary endothelial cells in the brain and between the epithelial cells in the choroids plexus effectively prevent proteins from entering the brain in adults and slows down the penetration of smaller molecules. For example, the slow penetration of urea. This uniquely limited exchange of substances into the brain is referred to as blood-brain barrier. Through the tight junctions in the endothelial cells of the brain capillaries, particles with molecular weight more than 2000 do not pass through. However at some sites the endothelial cells are covered by foot processes of astrocytes. This covering is, however incomplete and large enough to permit the substances with a molecular weight of 40,000. If any substance has to cross this wall, it has to penetrate the cell membrane of endothelial cells. So only lipid soluble materials cross this barrier, others do not. blood-brain barrier prevents the entry of many injurious substances to the brain as brain is more delicate and vital than other tissues.

PULMONARY CIRCULATION

Lungs have dual circulation: (a) Pulmonary circulation: that is for gas exchange with alveoli, (b) Bronchial circulation: to supply oxygen to airways and to the supporting tissue of the lung. Other than umbilical artery, pulmonary artery is the only artery that carries deoxygenated or venous blood. Pulmonary capillary bed is the largest vascular bed in the body. In the pulmonary artery, the average systolic and diastolic pressure values are 25/8 mm Hg. In contrast to 120/80 mm Hg in aorta. Mean pulmonary arterial pressure is 15 mm Hg.

The pulmonary blood volume is approximately 1 liter, which is located mostly in the pulmonary artery and veins. As compared to the systemic circulation, pulmonary circulation is a low pressure, low resistance system. The pulmonary vascular resistance is 10–15 fold lower than systemic vascular resistance. Pulmonary vessels are high-compliance vessels.

- **High compliance:** Pulmonary vessels are 24 times more compliant compared to their systemic counterparts. It is necessary as the same amount of blood that circulates through entire body has to circulate through this short path (RV to lungs to LV). Due to high compliance of the vessels, lungs accommodate large quantities of blood. Pulmonary vessels thus act as reservoir of blood. In situations where other tissues demand more blood flow, like standing or when there is hemorrhage, the extra blood from pulmonary circulation is shifted to systemic circulation, lungs divert their blood to those tissues.

- **Low resistance:** Pulmonary circulation is a low-pressure circulation.

Pulmonary blood flow is 15% of the circulating volume. Blood flow in all parts of the lung increases during exercise. This extra flow is made possible by opening up of inactive capillaries and the increase in the flow rate through each capillary. Most important regulatory factor for pulmonary circulation is hypoxia. Hypoxia causes vasoconstriction of lung vessels. This effect is different in systemic circulation where hypoxia causes vasodilatation. It is mediated by O_2-sensitive K^+ channels. Hypoxia is sensed by K^+ channels. This causes closure of the K^+ channels leading to accumulation of K^+ inside the membrane of the vascular smooth muscle cell (VSMC) resulting in depolarization of the VSMC. This will initiate contraction of the smooth muscle and constriction of the pulmonary vessel.

Like systemic blood vessels, gravity affects the pulmonary vessels also but the effect is more marked in the latter. In supine posture, pulmonary mean arterial pressure is same all over the lung. However, in erect posture, as compared to the pressure at heart level, the apical pressure is 15 mm Hg less and the based pressure 8 mm Hg greater. There are corresponding differences in regional blood flow which forms the basis of following lungs zones.

Zones of Blood Flow in the Lung (Fig. 4.53)

Due to hydrostatic factor, blood flow and pressure in the vessels at the base of lungs is greater than those at the apex. Due to this factor and surrounding alveolar pressures, there are zones of blood flow in the lungs. Blood flow is less and pressure is lower in the vessels at the apex of the lung. Reason: In upright posture, heart pumps the blood against gravity toward the apex of the lung. Vessels are surrounded by alveoli; alveoli have certain pressure in them. At the apex, the surrounding alveolar pressure is greater than the pressure in the pulmonary vessels.

- **Zone 1 (no blood flow):** No blood flows at all during any phase of cardiac cycle because capillary pressure never rises above alveolar pressure. Zone 1 is seen in the apex of lung. Zone 1 contributes to physiological dead space.
- **Zone 2 (intermittent blood flow):** It is upper half to third area of lung. It has intermittent blood flow, occurring only during the peaks of pulmonary arterial pressure. During systole, the pressure in the pulmonary artery becomes greater than the surrounding alveolar pressure (ventilated but not perfused).

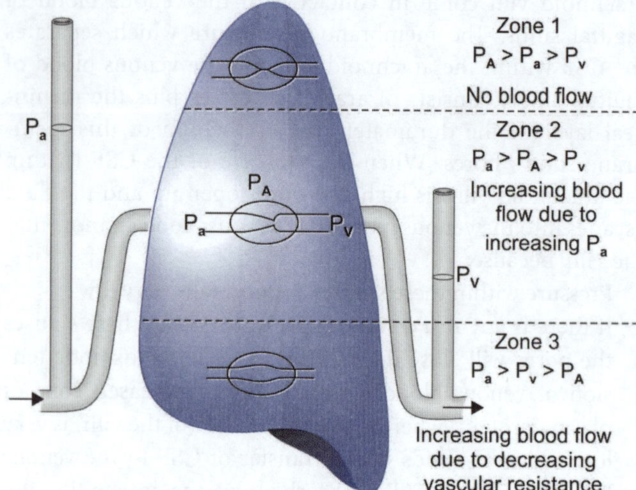

Fig. 4.53: Zone model of pulmonary perfusion

- **Zone 3 (continuous blood flow):** It is lower half to third area of lung. It has continuous blood low because pulmonary arterial pressure remains greater than alveolar air pressure throughout the cardiac cycle.

Zone 1: $P_{alv} > P_{art} > P_{vein}$ (no blood flow)
Zone 2: $P_{art} > P_{alv} > P_{vein}$ (intermittent flow)
Zone 3: $P_{art} > P_{vein} > P_{alv}$ (continuous flow)

Where, P_{-art} = pressure in pulmonary artery, P_{-vein} = pressure in pulmonary vein, P_{-alv} = alveolar pressure.

These zones are not fixed anatomic zones; they are functional zones or simply types of blood flow. With changes in alveolar pressure and alterations in the pulmonary vascular pressures, the zones can change. For instance, in lying down posture, zone 3 in entire lungs, in an upright person – zone 2 at the apex, and zone 3 in remaining lung. Explanation: In the recumbent posture, no part of the lung is above the level of heart. That is, heart does not have to pump against gravity to any part of the lung. Consequently, the pressure in the pulmonary vessels is good enough to overcome the surrounding alveolar pressure, resulting in a continuous flow.

Bronchial Circulation

About 2% of blood volume goes in bronchial circulation. It supplies oxygen to supporting structures. Bronchial venous blood is drained into pulmonary vein which goes to left side of heart (instead of right side). Hence, left ventricular output is about 2% greater than right ventricular output. The bronchial venous blood never goes to right side of heart; it mixes with oxygenated LV blood. Due to this 'venous admixture' of blood, PO_2 of the left ventricular blood is less than the alveolar PO_2.

Regulation of Pulmonary Circulation

Pulmonary blood vessels are richly innervated by sympathetic vasoconstrictor nerves. But these nerves show no resting tone (in contrast, systemic blood vessels have resting vasoconstrictor sympathetic tone), which means they can show only an increase in activity. This occurs during circulatory reflexes. Chemical control is more important than neural control. Local hypoxia (decrease in PO_2) produces vasoconstriction in pulmonary vessels, which is exactly opposite to systemic circulation where hypoxia (low PO_2) produces vasodilatation. The physiological significance of this phenomenon is to divert pulmonary blood flow from the alveoli that are poorly ventilated (low PO_2 in these alveoli causes vasoconstriction) to well ventilated alveoli (in these alveoli pulmonary, vessels are open due to normal PO_2). Increase in tissue PCO_2 (hypercarbia) and acidosis also produce pulmonary vasoconstriction, which is also an opposite response in comparison to systemic circulation where increased pCO_2 and acidosis cause vasodilatation.

FETAL CIRCULATION

The fetal circulation supplies the fetal tissues with oxygen and nutrients from the placenta. It bypasses the fetal lungs. Gas exchange occurs in placenta. The oxygenated blood enters the baby's umbilical vein from the placenta. The oxygenated blood in the umbilical vein by passes the hepatic sinusoids by passing through the ductus venosus. The ductus venosus, now carrying the oxygenated blood (passed on from the umbilical vein) joins the inferior vena cava (which is already carrying deoxygenated blood from the lower half of the fetus). This mixed blood in IVC is still having good oxygen saturation although less than that in umbilical vein. The presence of fetal hemoglobin (which has an oxygen dissociation curve shifted to the left compared with adult hemoglobin) ensures that oxygen delivery is maintained despite low oxygen partial pressures (Fig. 4.54).

The blood from IVC enters the right atrium, and through foramen ovale, gets directed to the left atrium. Some blood reaching the right atrium from IVC enters the right ventricle also. However, the major portion of blood entering the right ventricle is the blood reaching the right atrium via the superior vena cava which is blood returning from the myocardium and upper parts of body. This stream therefore is less oxygenated than that from IVC. The blood pumped by the right ventricle meets the resistance of pulmonary vasculature that is remaining coiled and almost closed (as the lungs are not expanded). Thus, blood takes the route of lesser resistance and gets shunted via ductus arteriosus to aorta and from there to the lower parts of the body via the descending aorta (right ventricular output passes into the aorta at a point distal to the origin of the arteries to the head and upper extremities). Blood flowing through the foramen ovale and into left atrium passes into the left ventricle where it is ejected into the ascending aorta. This relatively oxygen rich blood passes predominantly to the head and upper extremities. However, the umbilical artery, which arises from the aorta, transports blood to the placenta, where it is oxygenated and sent back to the fetus via fetal veins. Thus, placenta functions like lungs during fetal life.

At birth, the umbilical cord is clamped and so that blood enters the baby via the umbilical vein. So no blood goes via the ductus venosus and hence it closes (remains in later life as ligamentum venosum). Clamping of the umblical cord also obstructs the umbilical artery so as to increase the peripheral resistance against which the left ventricle has to pump. In the mean time, the baby has taken the breath and the pulmonary vessels have expanded. Thus now the pulmonary circulation becomes less resistant than the systemic circulation and thus flow in ductus arteriosus gets reversed—that is from the aorta to the pulmonary artery. The fall in resistance in pulmonary capillaries secondary to the expansion of the lung facilitates blood flow through the lungs and its oxygenation. Thus the blood reaching aorta now is oxygenated by the lungs and thus the blood getting shunted via the ductus arteriosus is highly oxygenated. Oxygen is the strongest stimulus for ductus contraction and hence the ductus contracts and closes (remains in later life as ligamentum arteriosum). Foramen ovale closes functionally soon after birth as the left atrial pressure becomes higher than the right atrial pressure, causing opposition of septum primum and septum secondum.

CUTANEOUS CIRCULATION AND TRIPLE RESPONSE

Circulation of blood through skin is called cutaneous circulation. Cutaneous vessels are innervated by sympathetic nerves. The vessels perform an important function of temperature regulation. Exposure to heat leads to cutaneous vasodilation, which increases heat loss from the body to the surrounding. Exposure to cold results in cutaneous vasoconstriction. Trauma produces the 'triple response' in skin (Figs 4.55A and B).

When skin is stroked firmly with a pointed object, it evokes a series of response classified as:

Red Reaction

Reddening appears over the line of stroke. Red reaction in 10 seconds, due to capillary dilatation and release of histamines.

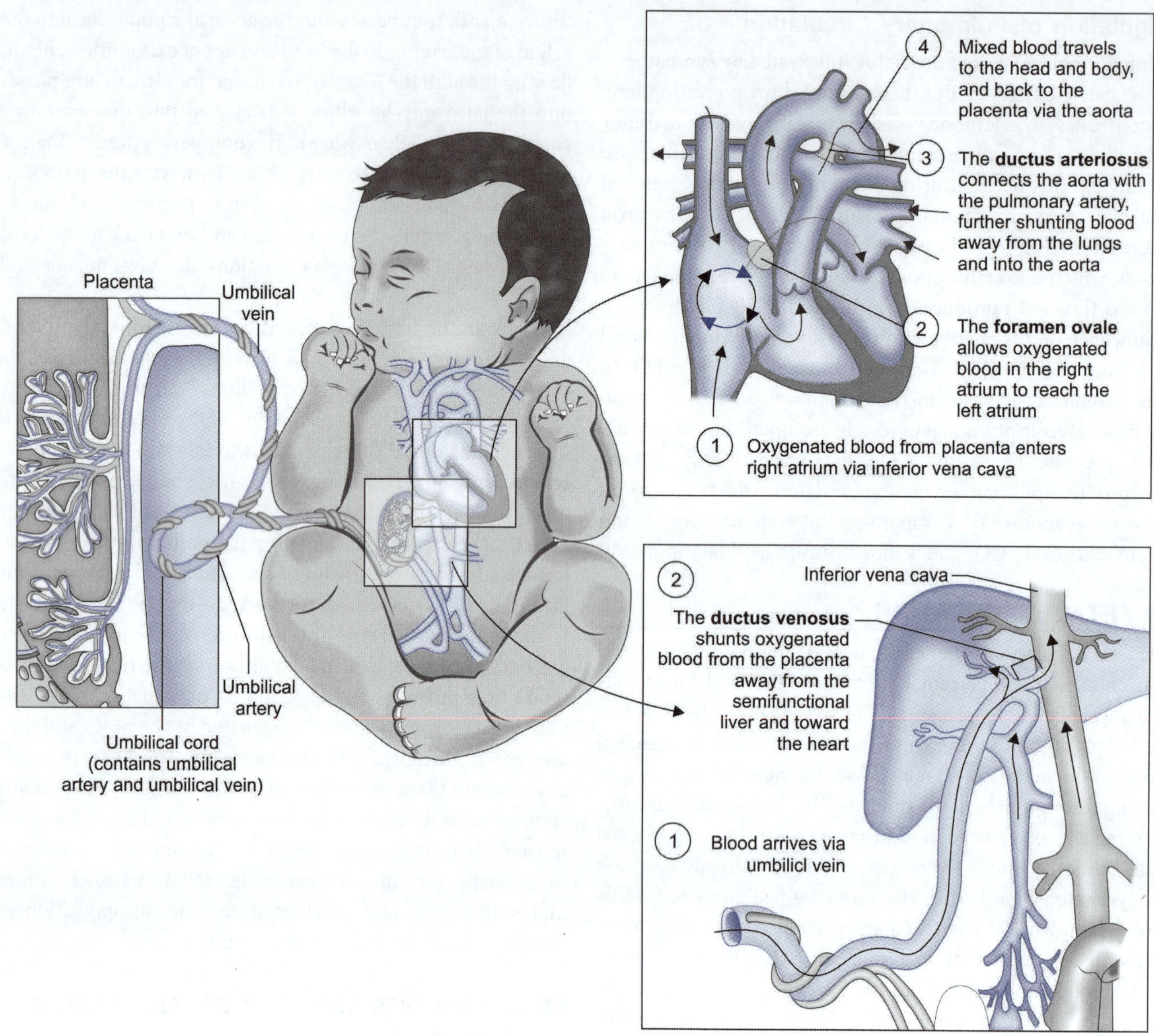

Fig. 4.54: Fetal circulation

Flare

Redness spreads out from the injury. Flare appears within 30 seconds after appearance of red line. It is due to dilatation of arterioles. Skin temperature overlying the area is raised.

The mechanism of arteriolar dilatation is due to axon reflex (Fig. 4.56) a response in which impulses initiated in sensory nerves by an injury are relayed antidromically down to other branches of sensory nerve fibers). The transmitter released at the central transmission of sensory C fiber neurons is substance P. Substance P, calcitonin gene related peptide (CGRP) dilates the arterioles. Flare is absent after a local anesthesia.

Wheal

If the stroke is strong enough, swelling is developed within the flare area. This localized edema is due to increased permeability of capillaries and postcapillary venules with consequent extravasations of fluid. Increase in permeability is produced by the release of histamine and related substances. Substance P cause extravasation of fluid. Wheal does not depend on nervous mechanism.

CIRCULATORY SHOCK

Circulatory shock is defined as inadequate tissue perfusion with a relative or absolute inadequacy of cardiac output. It is developed by cardiovascular dysfunction.

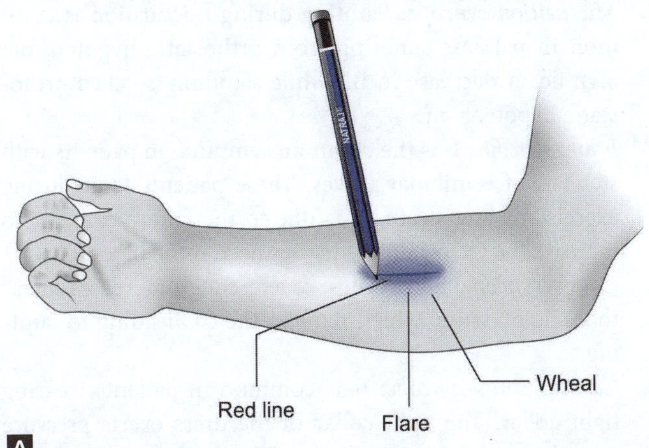

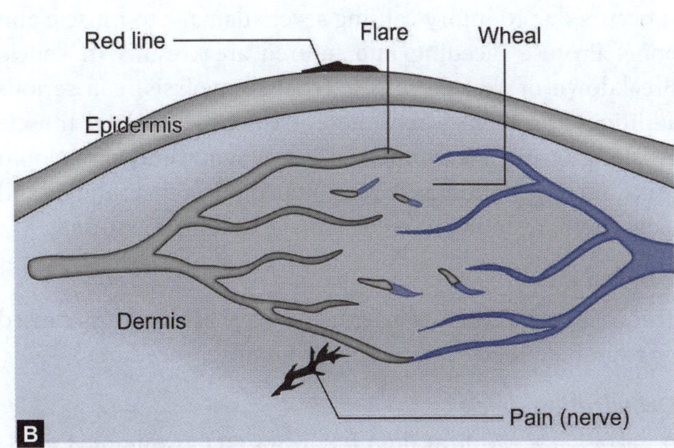

Figs 4.55A and B: Triple response. **A.** Note the redness of the area, flare and wheal; **B.** Vascular mechanisms of triple response

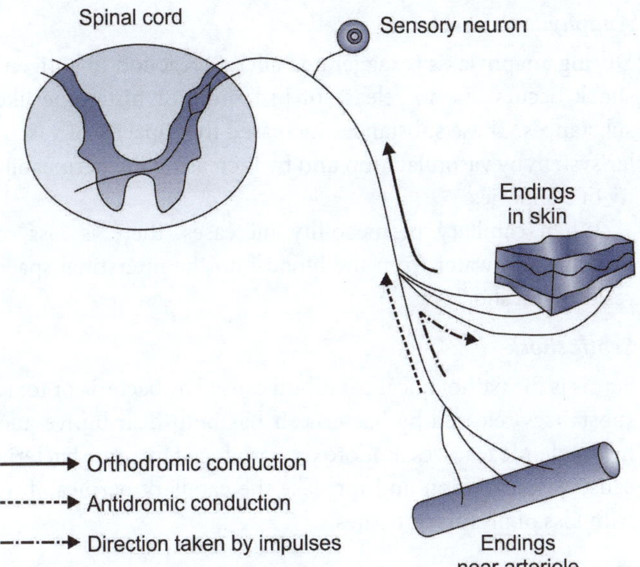

Fig. 4.56: Axon reflex pathway

Types of Shock (Table 4.7)

Hypovolemic Shock (Decrease in Blood Volume)

Here the amount of fluid in the vascular system is inadequate to fill it and this result in decreased circulating blood volume. Important hemodynamic changes are:

- Low cardiac output
- Low central venous pressure
- Increased systemic resistance (peripheral vasoconstriction).

Clinical features

- *Due to inadequate perfusion:* Cold, pale, cyanosed skin, oliguria, anuria, intense thirst.
- *Due to sympathetic stimulation:* Rapid thready pulse, increased sweating, hypotension.

Table 4.7: Causes of different types of circulatory shock

Types of shock	Causes
Shock due to decreased blood volume	• Hemorrhage-hemorrhagic shock • Trauma-traumatic shock • Surgery-surgical shock • Burns-burn shock • Dehydration-dehydration shock
Shock due to increased vascular capacity	• Sudden loss of vasomotor tone-neurogenic shock • Anaphylaxis-anaphylactic shock • Sepsis-septic shock
Shock due to cardiac disease	• Arrhythmia • Myocardial ischemia • Congestive heart failure
Shock due to obstruction of blood flow	• Tumor in myocardium • Cardiac tamponade • Obstruction of blood vessels in lungs

- *Due to metabolic acidosis:* Rapid respiration, lactic acid accumulation (due to anaerobic glycolysis), alertness and restlessness.

Hypovolemic shock is subdivided on the basis of cause into hemorrhagic, traumatic, surgical and dehydration shock.

Hemorrhagic shock/cold shock

Most important cause for hypovolemic shock. The decline in blood volume produced by bleeding results in reduced venous return and thus cardiac output falls. The heart rate is increased and with severe hemorrhage, a fall in BP occurs always. With moderate hemorrhage, pulse pressure is reduced but mean arterial pressure may be normal. BP changes vary from individual to individual even when exactly the same amount of blood is lost. The skin is cold and pale with a grayish tinge because of stasis in the capillaries and a small amount of cyanosis. Here, the inadequate tissue perfusion leads to increased anaerobic glycolysis resulting in lactic acidosis.

Traumatic shock

It occurs due to injury causing severe damage to muscle and bone. Profuse bleeding into injured area results in shock. Breakdown of skeletal muscle (rhabdomyolysis) is a serious additional problem where there is extensive skeletal muscle crushing (crush syndrome). In crush syndrome, myoglobin leaks into circulation, gets precipitated into renal tubules and clogs them, resulting in renal damage leading to anuria.

Surgical shock

This occurs as a result of external or internal blood loss caused by ruptured blood vessels (during surgical procedures).

Dehydration shock

It occurs as a result of fluid loss from GIT (prolonged vomiting, diarrhea), kidney (diabetes mellitus, diabetes insipidus). Fluid loss also occurs from the skin due to burns (burn shock) which is characterized by hemoconcentration. In burn shock, the most important abnormality is loss of plasma as exudate from the burned surfaces. Here the plasma is lost rather than the whole blood. So hematocrit rises and results in hemoconcentration.

Distributive (Vasogenic/Low Resistance Shock/ Warm Shock)

Here the blood supply to tissues is inadequate due to increased vascular capacity by extensive vasodilatation of blood vessels even though the blood volume is normal. The skin is not cold and clammy, hence called warm shock. The causes for vasodilation are:

- *Sudden loss of vasomotor tone:* Neurogenic shock
- *Anaphylaxis:* Anaphylactic shock
- *Sepsis:* Septic shock

Neurogenic shock

Neurogenic shock is characterized by sudden depression of nervous system due to loss of vasomotor tone which leads to vasodilatation. It is common in ischemia of brain, general anesthesia, spinal anesthesia and emotional conditions.

Fainting (syncope)

Fainting or syncope is the sudden and transient loss of consciousness and postural tone with spontaneous recovery. It occurs due to temporary inadequate cerebral blood flow. It is of different types:

- *Vasovagal syncope/emotional fainting:* It is also called neurocardiogenic syncope. It is due to extreme activation of parasympathetic system which leads to suppression of myocardium and severe vasodilatation. The cerebral blood flow also decreases.
- *Postural syncope:* It is due to pooling of blood in lower limbs because of prolonged standing.
- *Micturition syncope:* Fainting during micturition is common in patients suffering from orthostatic hypotension. Significant decrease in BP while standing is called orthostatic hypotension.
- *Effort syncope:* It is the common symptom in patients with stenosis of semilunar valves. These patients faint during exercise or any strain. It is due to the failure of heart to increase the CO when the tissues need more blood flow.
- *Cough syncope:* Sometimes, severe cough increases intrathoracic pressure, which reduces the CO leading to fainting.
- *Carotid sinus syncope:* It is common in patients wearing tight collar. The tight collar of the dress exerts pressure over the region of carotid sinus. This leads to reduction in heart rate, vasodilatation and fainting.

Anaphylactic shock

During anaphylaxis (exaggerated allergic reaction to antigen) shock occurs due to release of histamine or histamine like substances. These substances increased the capacity of vascular system by vasodilatation and by increasing the permeability of capillaries.

When capillary permeability increases, there is loss of proteins and water from the blood into the interstitial space resulting in shock.

Septic shock

Sepsis is the pathological condition caused by bacteria or toxic substances released by bacteria. It has both distributive and hypovolemic features. Endotoxins produced by some bacteria cause vasodilatation and increase the capillary permeability, with loss of plasma in tissues.

Cardiogenic shock/Congested Shock

When the pumping function of the heart is impaired, blood flow to the tissues is no longer adequate to meet resting metabolic demands, the condition that results is called cardiogenic shock. It is most commonly due to extensive infarction of the left ventricle, but it can also be caused by other diseases that severely compromise ventricular function.

Certain chemicals released by ischemic tissues stimulates ventricular receptors and cause reflex inhibition of vasomotor center producing bradycardia and hypotension (Bezold-Jarish reflex), making the shock worse. The symptoms are those of shock plus congestion of the lungs and viscera, because the heart fails to put out all the venous blood returned to it. This occurs mainly in MI, congestive heart failures, arrhythmias.

Obstructive Shock

Obstructive shock is due to obstruction of blood flow.

The conditions where obstructive shock occurs are pulmonary embolism, cardiac tumor, cardiac tamponade (bleeding into the pericardium with external pressure on the heart), tension, pneumothorax.

Stages of Shock

Shock is divided into the following three major stages:

Nonprogressive Stage/Compensated Stage

It is the stage from which the normal circulatory compensatory mechanism will eventually cause full recovery without help from outside therapy.

Progressive Stage

In this stage the shock becomes steadily worse until death. It is reversible with outside therapy.

Irreversible Stage (Refractory Shock)

Here the shock has progressed to such an extent that all forms of known therapy are inadequate to save the person's life. If not properly treated during 2nd stage, the person goes into this stage. If it becomes severe, cardiovascular tissues deteriorate. Refractory shock is the manifestation of late effects of sympathetic vasoconstriction, long sustained decrease of regional circulation and operation of positive feedback mechanisms.

The main causes which precipitate refractory shock and leading to death are:

Cardiac failure

Fall in BP and tachycardia → decreased coronary flow → myocardial depression → decreased cardiac output → decreased HR → decrease in coronary flow and myocardial depression.

Vasomotor failure

During initial stages of shock, vasomotor center is activated. If the abnormality is not corrected during 2nd stage; it will cause depression of vasomotor center.

Depression of vasomotor center → decrease in vasomotor center activity → fall in BP (both systolic and diastolic) → blood flow to vasomotor center decrease → progressive reduction in BP → finally vasomotor center fails.

Sluggish circulation

It causes blockage of minute vessels.

Blood supply to tissues affected → accumulation of lactic acid, carbonic acid, etc. → Severe acidosis → Depress the activities of myocardium, vasomotor and other tissues.

Note

Acute respiratory distress syndrome

Seen in septic and severe hypovolemic shock. It is due to hypoxia and accumulation of H^+ ions. There is damage to alveolar epithelium and endothelium and exudation of fluid into interstitial space.

Compensatory Mechanisms

It is divided into two groups.

Short-term Mechanisms

- Baroreceptor reflex
- *Chemoreceptor reflex:* Loss of blood causes anemia and stagnant hypoxia. It stimulates chemoreceptor reflex activities and activates vasomotor center.
- CNS ischemic reflex.
- Activation of renin-angiotensin system and formation of angiotensin II is increased. Angiotensin II acts on subfornical organ, which contain an osmoreceptor that increases the thirst.
- *Increased sympathetic activity:* It leads to generalized vasoconstriction except in brain and heart. In brain and heart, vasodilatation (by β_2 receptors.)
- *Venoconstriction:* Increased venous return, SV increases, CO increases.
- Intense constriction of splenic vessels lead to redistribution of blood to vital organs.
- Increases activity of reticular activating system, this increases muscle and thoracic pumping → increases venous return → increases cardiac output → increases BP.
- Increased ACTH and aldosterone secretion causes salt and water retention and cause increase in blood volume.
- In kidneys, there is constriction of afferent and efferent arterioles, GFR is decreased and prevents renal failure.

Long-term Mechanisms

It continues for hours to days to weeks.

- Increased thirst.
- Increased salt craving.
- Increased water absorption from renal tubules and water absorption from GIT.
- Conservation of salt and water by kidneys mediated by hormones.
- After moderate hemorrhage, circulating plasma volume is restored within 12–17 hours.
- Preformed albumin enters circulation from extravascular stores.
- Increased hepatic synthesis of albumin and other plasma proteins occurs in a period of 3–4 days.
- Increased formation of RBC. Formation of RBCs increases, reaches a peak in 10 days and RBC content restored to normal level within 4–48 weeks.
- Increased 2, 3 DPG content shifts O_2 dissociation curve to right side. It decreases the affinity of Hb for O_2. So more O_2 is released to tissues.

Physiological Basis of Treatment of Shock

- **Non-drug therapy**
  - **Head-low position:** The patient should be placed in horizontal/oblique position, with the head at least 12 inches lower than the feet. It promotes venous return and may help in increasing the cardiac output.
  - **Oxygen supplement:** Since the central problem of shock is the lack of oxygen supply to the tissues, giving the patient supplemental oxygen is logical. However, if the blood flow itself is badly affected, this oxygen supplementation may be of little use (as it may not be transported to the tissues as desired).
- **Replacement therapy:** (To replace the lost blood volume)
  - Intravenous fluids (saline, dextrose + saline, ringer lactate, etc.)
  - Plasma expanders: 'dextran' is a plasma expander. It is a large polysaccharide polymer of glucose. It exerts colloid osmotic pressure, so that fluid from out of the vessels can be pulled into the vessels. This will increase the circulating blood volume.
  - Blood/plasma transfusion.
- **Drug therapy:**
  - Most important life-saving drugs are sympathomimetic drugs. They have the actions similar to sympathetic stimulation ('mimic the sympathetic effects'), e.g. adrenaline.
  - Antihistaminic drugs and steroids may be useful in some types of shocks, particularly anaphylactic shock.

CARDIAC ARRHYTHMIAS

The heart normally beats at a regular rhythm set by SA node. Any deviation from this normal rhythm is called cardiac arrhythmia. When any irritable focus is capable of discharging repetitively at a rate more rapid than that of SAN, it can initiate and maintain heart beat for several seconds to few hours. This is called as ectopic cardiac beat. If an irritable ectopic focus discharges once, the result is a beat that occurs before the expected next normal beat and transiently interrupts the cardiac rhythm. This results in atrial, nodal or ventricular extrasystole or premature beat. If the focus discharges repetitively at a rate higher than that of the SA node, it produces rapid, regular tachycardia resulting in atrial, ventricular, or nodal paroxysmal tachycardia or atrial flutter. Cardiac arrhythmias are generally classified as follows:

- *Atrial arrhythmias:* If the excitation spreads from an independently discharging focus in the atria, it is called atrial arrhythmia. The impulses stimulate the AV node prematurely and is conducted to ventricles. Atrial arrhythmias are further classified into (Table 4.8):
  - *Atrial tachycardia:* This occurs when an atrial site (outside the SA node) become the dominant pacemaker. It is characterized by very regular rates ranging from 140–220 beats/min. Atrial tachycardia may be caused by overindulgence in caffeine, nicotine or alcohol and may also occur during anxiety attack. It is not associated with block.
  - *Atrial flutter:* If abnormal focus is in atria, it will lead to atrial flutter. Here the rate of impulse production is 200–350 beats/min. During atrial flutter AV node is unable to transmit all of the atrial impulses to the ventricles (max capacity to transmit impulse is 230 beats/min) and therefore the ventricular rate may be half, one-third or one-fourth of the atrial rates. This is associated with 2:1/3:1 heart block. In atrial flutter, QRS complex is normal.
  - *Atrial fibrillation:* Atrial fibrillation is characterized by a totally irregular, rapid rate (300 to 500 beats/min). In it, ventricular rate is completely irregular because only a fraction of the atrial impulses that reach the AV node are transmitted to the ventricles.
- *Ventricular arrhythmias:* Ventricular arrhythmias are more serious (particularly tachycardia) because, here cardiac output is affected. Ventricular arrhythmias are further classified into (Table 4.9):

Table 4.8: Atrial arrhythmias compared

	Atrial tachycardia	Atrial flutter	Atrial fibrillation
Atrial rate	Up to 220 bpm	Between 200–350 bpm	300–500 bpm
Atrial contractions	Normal, uniform	Alternate large and small contractions due to a partial refractory state in the atria	Irregular oscillations of the surface called fibrillations as length of refractory period further increases
Atrial (A) to ventricular (V) rate	A:V::1:1	A:V::2:1 (as AVN cannot transmit > 230 impulses/min)	A:V::2 or 3:1(due to irregular discharge from AVN)
ECG findings	All time intervals shorten	2° type of Hb	• Absence of 'P'wave • Appearance of fibrillation (f) wave • Irregular QRS complexes; no 'T'wave

Table 4.9: Ventricular arrhythmias compared

	Ventricular tachycardia	Ventricular flutter	Ventricular fibrillation
Ventricular rate	Up to 220 bpm	Between 500–350 bpm	300–500 bpm
ECG findings	QRS complexes: polymorphic	Hairpin curves where main and terminal deflection can no longer be differentiated	Irregular, fast, small potential fluctuations. Fibrillating ventricles cannot pump blood effectively. This can lead to sudden death

- *Ventricular tachycardia:* It is caused by abnormal automaticity or by re-entry within diseased ventricular tissue. This most often occurs in patients with coronary artery disease or cardiomyopathy. Here QRS complex is abnormal. It is broad and bizarre shaped.
- *Ventricular flutter:* If abnormal focus is in ventricle, it will lead to ventricular flutter. In ventricular flutter, the rate of ventricular contractions is between 200–350 beats/min. ECG shows large oscillations (hair pin curve) where main and terminal deflections can no longer be detected.
- *Ventricular fibrillation:* Here the rate of ventricular contractions is about 300–500 beats/min. It is a fatal condition, because fibrillating ventricles cannot pump blood effectively and circulation of blood stops causing sudden death.

Causes of Flutter and Fibrillations

Flutters and fibrillations occur due to a defect in conduction that permits a wave of excitation to propagate continuously within a closed circuit (circus movement). This is referred to as circus or re-entry phenomenon, i.e. formation of circuit around a ring of myocardial fibers by the excitation process. The common sites of occurrence of this phenomenon are:

- Tissues joining the opening of inferior and superior vena cava.
- Around the AV valves.

There are two mechanisms of development of circus movements:

1. *Depolarization of a ring of cardiac muscle:* Normally the excitation impulse spreads in both directions in the ring and the two impulses cancel when they meet on opposite side. If there is a transient block on one side due to slowed conduction, the impulse reaching here earlier via a shorter route will find this area refractory and die off. However, the impulse which goes around the ring and reaches here late, finds this area no longer refractory. It will pass this area and continue to circle indefinitely producing circus movement (Fig. 4.57).
2. *Retrograde conduction due to transient block in bundle of His:* Transient block due to slowed conduction in parts of conduction pathway prevents 'anterograde' conduction in a portion of bundle of His and then this area is invaded from below. The area above the block has had time to recover and is no longer refractory producing re-entry, i.e. retrograde conduction causing atrial depolarization resulting in atrial beat called as atrial echo beat.

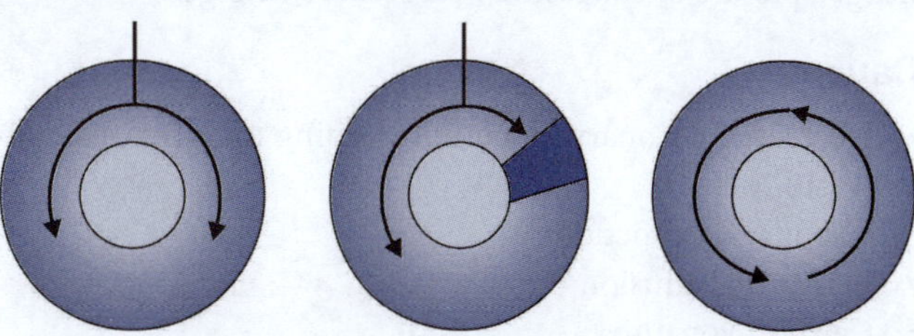

Fig. 4.57: Mechanism of development of circus movement; depolarization of a ring of cardiac tissue

Note

Arrhythmias can be also be broadly classified into:

- *Bradyarrhythmias:* Here the heart rate is reduced. It occurs in the following conditions:
  - Sick sinus syndrome (failure of SA node)
  - Heart block.
- *Tachyarrhythmias:* When heart rate is increased along with abnormal rhythm it is reffered to as tachyarrhythmias. The various tachyarrhythmias are:
  - Atrial and ventricular ectopic beat
  - Atrial and ventricular tachycardia
  - Atrial and ventricular flutter
  - Atrial and ventricular fibrillation

Paroxysmal tachycardia: If tachycardia appears and declines abruptly it is called as paroxysmal tachycardia. The attack may last from seconds or minutes to many days. It may be having focus either in the atria, i.e. paroxysmal atrial tachycardia (PAT) or in ventricles, i.e. paroxysmal ventricular tachycardia (PVT).

CARDIAC FAILURE

It can be defined as the inability of heart to pump blood in sufficient amount to meet the requirements of body. This disorder is characterized by the presence of cardiac enlargement, edema (prominent over the ankles or the sacrum), hepatic enlargement, dyspnea, distended neck veins (raised JVP), weakness and exercise intolerance. Weakness and exercise intolerance are due to inadequacy of the cardiac output (forward failure). Other symptoms and signs are the result of increased venous pressure and congestion (backward failure). Patients in early stages of heart failure have merely exercise intolerance as shown by shortness of breath and early fatigue. Later on, as the cardiac output decreases further, full-fledged picture of congestive heart failure emerges.

Causes

- Decreased coronary blood flow leading to decreased contractility (MI)
- Valvular dysfunction
- Pericardial effusion
- Cardiomyopathies
- Obstruction to outflow (in hypertension, coarctation of aorta)
- Thiamine deficiency, beriberi.

Types

- *Systolic/forward failure:* Due to weak pumping action of ventricle.
- *Diastolic/backward failure:* Due to decreased filling of ventricles.
- *High output failure:* This is the type in which, although the absolute value of cardiac output is more than normal, it cannot meet the requirements of body.

Compensatory Mechanisms

The compensatory mechanisms involve increased sympathetic discharge to the heart and the Starling mechanism, i.e. the heart operates at a greater end diastolic volume.

Baroreceptor Mechanism

Cardiac failure leads to decreased pumping action of heart. So cardiac output decreases and thus BP is decreased. This leads to the activation of baroreceptors. The activation of baroreceptor leads to the following changes.

- *Stimulation of the heart:* This results in increased contractility → stroke volume increases → heart rate increases → increase in CO → results in increase in BP.
- *Peripheral vasoconstriction:* This leads to increase in diastolic BP.
- *Peripheral venoconstriction:* This leads to increased VR → diastolic volume increases → stroke volume increases → CO increases.

Note: Adrenal medulla is a modified sympathetic ganglion, when stimulated leads to increased secretion of epinephrine and nonepinephrine in the circulation. Epinephrine acts on heart and blood vessels.

Decreased Cardiac Output Leads to Renal Hypoxia

Renin-angiotensin mechanism is activated. This will lead to vasoconstriction. There will be increased retention of salt and water by the action of aldosterone. This leads to increase in blood volume and there by CO increases.

Effect of Frank-Starling Law

In early stages of cardiac failure operation of Frank-Starling law helps in increasing CO.

(Decreased cardiac output → increased EDV → stretching of myocardium → increased force of contraction (Frank-Starling law) → increased stroke volume → increased CO).

Effect of Laplace Law

According to Laplace law.

Where, $P = \frac{2T}{R}$

P = Transmural pressure; Pressure across myocardium.
T = Tension of wall.
R = Radius.
Transmural pressure is responsible for pumping action.

Dilatation of chambers occurs during the later phases of cardiac failure. A dilated heart has to do more work and more energy is required to pump blood than a nondilated heart. This is because when the radius of a cardiac chamber is increased, greater tension must be developed in the myocardium to produce any given pressure.

Decompensated Heart Failure

In spite of compensatory mechanisms, if heart fails to pump adequately the blood after venous return, it is called decompensated heart failure. It can be a right sided or left sided or both sided heart failure.

In the treatment of heart failure, the primary aim is to lower the preload on the heart by administration of diuretic which decreases the blood volume. Further, the afterload can also be decreased by administration of vasodilator drugs. The contractility of the heart can be improved by administration of digoxin. Digoxin inhibits Na^+ - K^+ ATPase in the cardiac muscle. The consequent increase in Ca^{2+} in the myocytes improves myocardial contractility.

CARDIOVASCULAR CHANGES IN EXERCISE

CVS changes (Table 4.10) can be divided into:

Changes in Heart

This includes changes in heart rate, cardiac output and coronary blood flow.

Table 4.10: CVS changes during exercise

	Changes	Cause for the change
Heart rate (HR)	Increases proportional to severity of exercise. But in trained athletes, the increase is less than that in untrained individuals. In healthy individuals, HR will not exceed 180 beats/min. In advanced age there is less HR rise even with same weightage of work done	• Fall in vagal tone • Rise in sympathetic activity • Adrenaline secreted in early phases of exercise • Rise in body temperature in later phases (causing tachycardia)
Cardiac output	CO increases tremendously during exercise. The normal untrained persons can increase CO a little over 4-fold, and the well trained athlete can increase output about 6-fold	Increase in heart rate (mostly) with increase in stroke volume (mildly) together cause increase in CO (refer Frank-Starling law) As the HR increases, there is shortening of diastole (less time for cardiac inflow) but the venous return increases impressively compensating the decrease in diastole period In an untrained person in moderate exercise, stroke volume rises only mildly (10–30%), during severe exercise, in this person, stroke volume will rise further But in a trained athlete, the stroke volume rises sharply even in moderate exercise and in severe exercise it may be doubled
Coronary circulation	Coronary circulation increases with heaviness of exercise	This is primarily due to local hypoxia of myocardium Sympathetic activity also has some role in this
Systolic BP	SBP rises usually in moderate isotonic exercise	SBP depends more on CO and as the CO increases, SBP increases
Vessels of skeletal muscles	Severe vasodilatation of blood vessels occurs	This may be due to vasodilator cholinergic sympathetic activity or due to local metabolites and local hypoxia
A-V O_2 difference	Increases due to increased O_2 extraction as there will be raised coefficient of O_2 utilization. (from a resting value of 4 mL/100 mL to a max. of 16 mL/100 mL)	2, 3 DPG rise causes this difference. According to Bohr effect, this has to occur

Changes in Peripheral Circulatory System

This includes changes in systolic and diastolic blood pressure, blood vessels in skeletal muscles and capillary A-V O_2 difference.

Types of Muscular Exercises

There are two types of exercises: (1) Dynamic or isotonic (e.g. running, cycling, etc.) and (2) Static or isometric (e.g. weight training with pulleys). The cardiovascular changes are different for two types of exercises.

Dynamic/Isotonic Exercises

- **Skeletal muscle blood flow at the start of exercise:** Blood vessels within skeletal muscle have β_2-adrenergic receptors. These receptors mediate vasodilation in skeletal muscle, when sympathetic discharge increases. Blood vessels of skeletal muscle are innervated mainly by the sympathetic vasodilator fibers. During exercise, sympathetic outflow increases. Sympathetic discharge to the blood vessels of muscle causes vasodilatation in the skeletal muscle. This increases the blood flow to the exercising muscles at the start of exercise.
- **Moment-to-moment blood flow during dynamic exercise:** During dynamic exercise (e.g. running, swimming, etc.), there are alternate rhythmic contractions and relaxations of a group of muscles. As a muscle contracts, the blood vessel within the muscle will be compressed and the blood flow will decrease. Then the muscle relaxes, the blood vessel will open up and the blood flow will increase. In this fashion, the blood flow within a muscle oscillates during dynamic exercise.
- **Overall changes in muscle blood flow during the exercise:** As the muscles are contracting, their metabolism increases. The products of metabolism like CO_2, H^+, lactic acid, etc. are released into the circulation. These metabolic products will cause vasodilatation locally, and increase the blood flow in the muscle. This is called 'muscle chemoreflex'.

Cardiovascular changes during exercise

- Stroke volume increases (due to increased venous return and ventricular filling + increased sympathetic discharge to heart). Heart rate increases – tachycardia. Hence, cardiac output increases.

- Blood pressure during dynamic exercise:
  - Systolic BP increases.
  - **Diastolic BP:** It indicates peripheral resistance. The peripheral resistance to blood flow is encountered mainly in the skeletal muscle circulation. During dynamic exercise, there is vasodilatation in the skeletal muscle. This leads to decreased peripheral resistance. Consequently, the diastolic BP decreases. This is the reason why such exercises are prescribed to the hypertensive individuals.
  - Pulse pressure widens
  - Mean arterial pressure (MAP) decreases. It is determined mainly by the diastolic BP; hence, MAP decreases slightly (even though the pulse pressure increases, only one-third of its value is taken for MAP).

Static/Isometric Exercise

- **Muscle blood flow:** There may be a slight decrease in overall muscle blood flow. This is because, the group of muscles are mostly in a sustained state of compression. This will compress the vessels within those muscles.
- **Peripheral resistance:** The sustained contraction and consequent sustained compression of vessels will increase the peripheral resistance (as peripheral resistance is mainly contributed by skeletal muscle circulation).
- **Diastolic BP:** Increased peripheral resistance → increased diastolic BP. Hence, such exercises are contraindicated in hypertensives.
- Heart rate increases slightly.

CLINICAL QUESTIONS

1. **An elderly, obese male developed acute, retrosternal pain radiating to the left ulnar border. ECG showed ST segment elevation.**
   a. Identify the condition.
   b. What is the cause?
   c. Why is the pain referred to the left ulnar border?
2. **An elderly patient came to the clinic with breathlessness at rest and swelling over both the legs. On examination pitting edema was found and neck veins were prominent. P waves of ECG were tall.**
   a. Identify the condition.
   b. Why are the neck veins prominent?
   c. What is the cause of tall P wave?
3. **In an athlete, resting pulse rate was 50/min. Immediately after exercise his pulse rate became 120/min and blood pressure became 200/80 mm of Hg.**
   a. What is the cause of resting bradycardia?
   b. Explain the increment in pulse rate after exercise.
   c. Elaborate on the BP findings after exercise.
4. **During the first hematology practical, a 1st MBBS student suddenly collapsed after taking a bold prick for hemoglobin estimation. The teacher put her in horizontal position and she recovered within 5 minutes.**
   a. What is the probable diagnosis?
   b. What is the physiological basis of treatment?
5. **A patient had severe blood loss due to an accident and he went into hypovolemic shock.**
   a. What is the first line of treatment?
   b. What is replacement therapy?
   c. Name the drug of choice after replacement therapy.
6. **After giving a test dose of penicillin a patient collapsed. His pulse was feeble and BP was low.**
   a. Identify the condition.
   b. What is the cause?
   c. Give physiological basis of treatment.
7. **A patient was brought to the hospital after an accident. His extremities were cold. Pulse was feeble. Systolic BP was 60 mm Hg.**
   a. Identify the condition.
   b. Enumerate the compensatory mechanisms in body in this condition.
   c. Give physiological basis of treatment.
8. **A child aged 2 years was brought to the clinic with enlargement of the head. On examination, bulging of the fontanelle and widening of the sutures of the skull bones was revealed.**
   a. What is the condition?
   b. What is the probable cause?
   c. What is the physiological basis of treatment? (decrease the CSF production by acetazolamide; carbonic anhydrase inhibitor)

Answers for Clinical Questions are given in the Appendix

CHAPTER

5

Gastrointestinal System

To sustain life, the body needs a continual supply of water, electrolytes and nutrients. This function is served by the gastrointestinal system.

PHYSIOLOGICAL ANATOMY OF GIT

The different parts of gastrointestinal tract show certain common structural features. The wall of gastrointestinal system (GIT) from posterior pharynx to anus in general consists of three layers of smooth muscle, two longitudinal and one circular. Histologically four layers are identified, they are (Fig. 5.1).

- *Mucosa:* Consists of surface epithelium. Inner to that is the connective tissue layer called lamina propria containing glands, blood vessels, nerve fibers, lymphatics. External to the lamina propria is muscularis mucosa, a very thin layer of smooth muscle.
- *Submucosa:* Luminal surface is highly folded to increase the total surface area available for digestion and absorption. It contains Meissner's plexus (submucosal plexus), between the submucosa and middle circular layer.
- *Muscle Coat (Muscularis externa):* There are two layers of muscle, inner circular and outer longitudinal. In between the two layers Auerbach's (Myenteric) plexus is present. The contraction and relaxation of smooth muscle enables peristalsis.
- *Serosa:* Outermost layer.

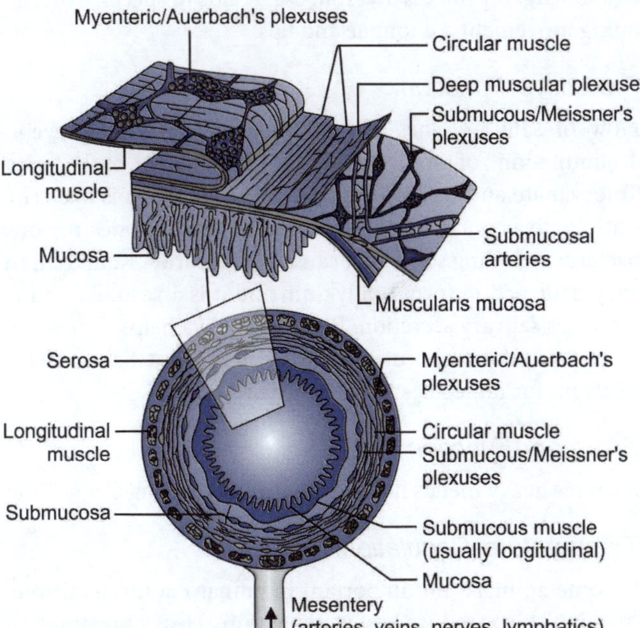

Fig. 5.1: Cross-section of GIT, showing the different layers of its wall

Nerve Supply of GIT

The gastrointestinal tract has a nervous all its own called the enteric nervous system. It lies entirely in the wall of the gut, beginning in the esophagus and extending all the way to the anus. Two types of innervation—they are enteric/intrinsic and extrinsic.

- *Extrinsic innervation:* Consists of parasympathetic and sympathetic components of ANS (Fig. 5.2). Parasympathetic fibers are through vagus (cranial out flow). Neurotransmitter is ACh. Fibers also originate from sacrum of spinal cord (sacral outflow). Stimulation increases the activity of intestinal smooth muscles, increases secretion and increases motility. It inhibits the sphincters. Sympathetic fibers arise from T8 to L2. Neurotransmitter is norepinephrine. They decreases motility and secretion.
- *Enteric nervous system:* It consists of the Auerbach/myenteric plexus and the submucous/Meissner's plexus.

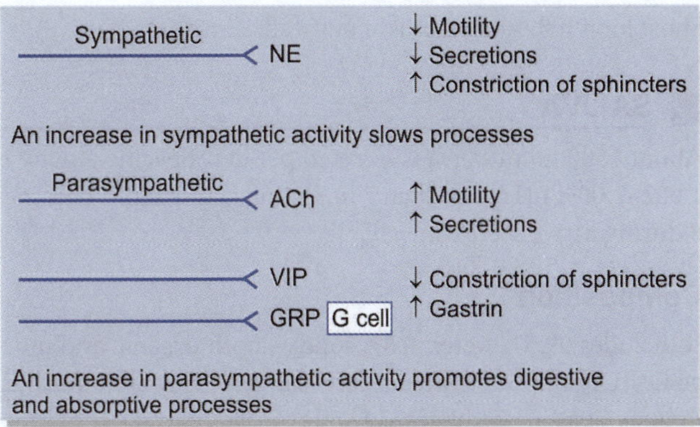

Fig. 5.2: The diagram illustrates how the synaptic junction at the end of a nerve fiber secretes norepinephrine (NE), ACh, VIP, GRP which then induces responses in the gastrointestinal (GI) system.

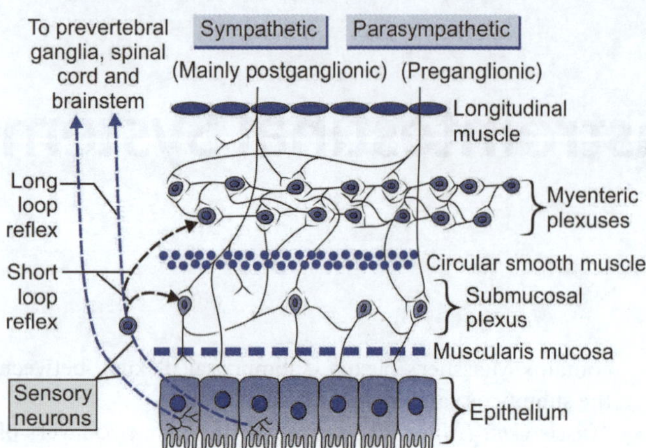

Fig. 5.3: Innervation of GIT

These two plexus are interconnected. It innervates the glandular epithelium, intestinal endocrine cells and submucosal blood vessels. It is involved in control of intestinal secretion. Neurotransmitter in the system include ACh, the amines norepinephrine and serotonin, the amino acid: glutamate, aspartate, D-serine, γ-aminobutyric acid (GABA), the purine ATP, the gases NO and CO and many peptides like enkephalin, gastrin releasing peptide (GRP), gelatin, neuropeptide-Y, neurotensin, substance P, vasoactive intestinal peptide (VIP), somatostatin. GI system contains about 100 million sensory neurons. Though enteric system is controlled by extrinsic nervous system, it can function autonomously. Sensory nerve fibers elicit local reflexes within the gut or other reflexes. They send afferents to (Fig. 5.3):

- Both plexus of enteric nervous system.
- Prevertebral ganglia of sympathetic nervous system.
- Spinal cord.

Note

Long loop reflex—center is at CNS.

Short loop reflex—center is at gut wall.

SALIVA

About 1500 ml of saliva is secreted per day. Specific gravity is 1.002–1.009. pH is less than 7 in resting gland and it becomes 8 during active secretion.

Composition

It includes 99.5% water, 0.5% solids—both organic and inorganic. Organic constituents are salivary amylase, mucous, lingual lipase, lysozymes, IgA, IgM, lactoferrin, epidermal growth factor, nerve growth factor, blood group substances, kallikrein, other substances like urea, uric acid, creatinine, thiocyanate, organisms like viruses (rabies) and bacteria. Inorganic constituents are Na^+, Cl^-, K^+ and HCO_3.

Salivary Glands

It inlcudes three pairs: Parotid, submandibular, sublingual (Table 5.1). The remaining 5% is contributed by minor glands in the oral cavity.

Table 5.1: Salivary glands—main features

Gland	Type	Secretion	% of total saliva
Parotid	Serous	Watery	20
Submandibular	Mixed	Moderatively	70
Sublingual	Mucous	Viscous	5

Functions of Saliva

Digestive Function

First digestive juice to which food is exposed. Enzymes present are lingual lipase and salivary amylase. Salivary amylase acts on cooked food. It is the 1st enzyme acting on carbohydrates. Starch is broken down into maltose plus maltotriose plus dextrin. Site of action is 1, 4 α-glycosidic linkage. Action is for short period in mouth and its action is continued in the stomach in the interior of bolus of food, stops when pH is less than 4. Lingual lipase, secreted by Ebner's gland is first enzyme acting on lipids. Action starts at acidic pH of stomach.

Lubricating Function

Mucin helps in lubrication of food. It assists mastication and swallowing. It protects oral mucosa. It aids in speech by facilitating movements of tongue and lips.

Protective Function

Flow of saliva washes away pathogenic bacteria, prevents accumulation of food and thus preventing oral caries. Thiocyanate and IgA are bactericidal. Lactoferrin is bacteriostatic. Saliva contains protein antibodies that can destroy oral bacteria including some that cause dental caries. Kallikrein by enzymatic action form bradykinin and it is a vasodilator and increases salivary secretion. Buffers in saliva helps to neutralize gastric juice and protect esophageal mucosa. Saliva acts as a solvent for molecules to reach taste receptors.

Excretory Function

Excretes heavy metals like Hg, penicillin, Pb drugs.

Temperature Regulation

In some animals (not important in human), a mechanism of "panting" helps reduce body temperature. Heavy breathing by a dog causes evaporation of saliva from the tongue, reducing the temperature in the oral region. Then, heat from the other parts of the body is carried via blood to the oral region and lost from there, thus reducing body temperature.

Role in Taste Sensation

Saliva acts as a solvent for various food stuffs. As taste is a chemical sense, the taste receptors respond only to dissolved substances.

Mechanism of Formation of Saliva

Primary Secretion of Saliva

The acinar cells of salivary glands secrete the initial saliva into the salivary ducts. The initial saliva is isotonic. The concentration of Na^+, Cl^-, K^+ and HCO_3^- is same as that of plasma (Fig. 5.4).

Modification of Saliva

Reabsorbtion of Na^+ and Cl^- occurs in the ductal cells that line the tubular portions of salivary glands. K^+ and HCO_3^- are secreted into the duct. The ducts are relatively impermeable to water and saliva becomes hypotonic and alkaline. Aldosterone acts on the ductal cells to increase the reabsorbtion of Na^+ and Cl^- from salivary ducts.

Note: K^+ content is highest in saliva.

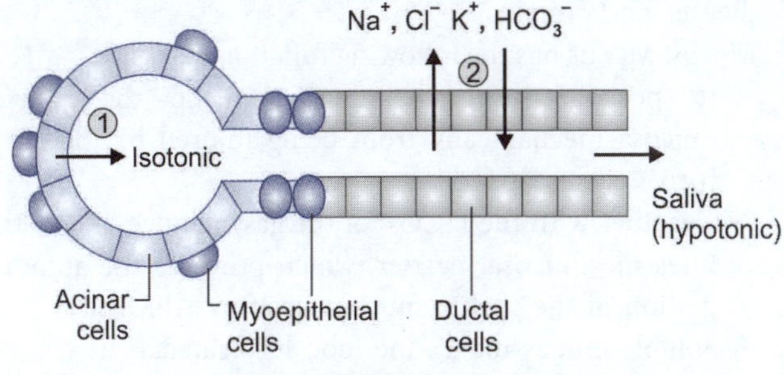

Fig. 5.4: Salivary secretion

Regulation of Salivary Secretion

It is under neural and vascular control. Neural consists of sympathetic and parasympathetic system.

Neural

Usual stimuli are taste, smell, tactile sensation from mouth, pharynx and reflexes from stomach and intestine. Parasympathetic stimulation increases water content and decreases organic constituents (associated with local release of VIP). Food in mouth control the secretion of saliva via following reflexes:

Conditioned

Conditioned reflex occurs only in previous experience. Sight, smell or even thought of palatable food increase the salivary secretion. Here, the parasympathetic supplying the salivary glands are stimulated by impulses coming from higher centers of brain.

Unconditioned

They are initiated by stimulation of receptors in the buccal cavity. Impulses are carried through vagus to medullary center. Efferent fibers are secretomotor fibers of 7th and 8th CN. Center is at superior (for submandibular and sublingual) and inferior (parotid) salivary nucleus.

Stimulation of sympathetic nerve supply causes vasoconstriction and secretion of small amounts of saliva rich in organic constituents.

Vascular

Increased blood supply increases nutrition which increases secretion.

Frey's/Chorda Tympani Syndrome

In cases of trauma or surgery, chorda tympani nerve will be affected. During regeneration, this nerve may join with nerve fibers innervating sweat gland in the submental region. This will result in increased sweating during salivation.

STOMACH AND ITS SECRETION

The muscle coat of stomach has three layers, an outer longitudinal, middle circular, and an inner oblique. The gastric epithelium surface shows a number of small openings called gastric pits. About 3–7 gastric glands open into a single gastric pit. Gastric glands are simple tubular glands located in mucosa. There are three types of glands: Fundic, pyloric and cardiac (Fig. 5.5A).

1. *Fundic:* Found in the fundus and over greater part of body of stomach. They contain four types of cells (Fig. 5.5B):
   a. *Chief cells (peptic):* Secrete pepsinogen and other proteolytic proenzyme.
   b. *Parietal cells (oxyntic):* Secrete HCl and intrinsic factor.
   c. *Enterochromaffin like (ECL) cells:* Histamine.
   d. *Neck mucous cells:* Secrete thin mucus.
2. *Pyloric:* Found in the antrum and pyloric region of the stomach. They contain two types of cells:
   a. *Neck mucous cells:* Secrete thin mucus
   b. *G-cells:* Responsible for the release of gastrin.
3. *Cardiac:* Found around the cardiac orifice and secrete thin mucus.

Functions of Stomach

- Reception of food
- Temporary storage of food
- Mechanical and chemical digestion
- Absorption of alcohol and drugs
- Intrinsic factor helps in absorption of vitamin B_{12}, thus helps in maturation of RBC
- Stomach empties its contents at a controlled rate to duodenum.

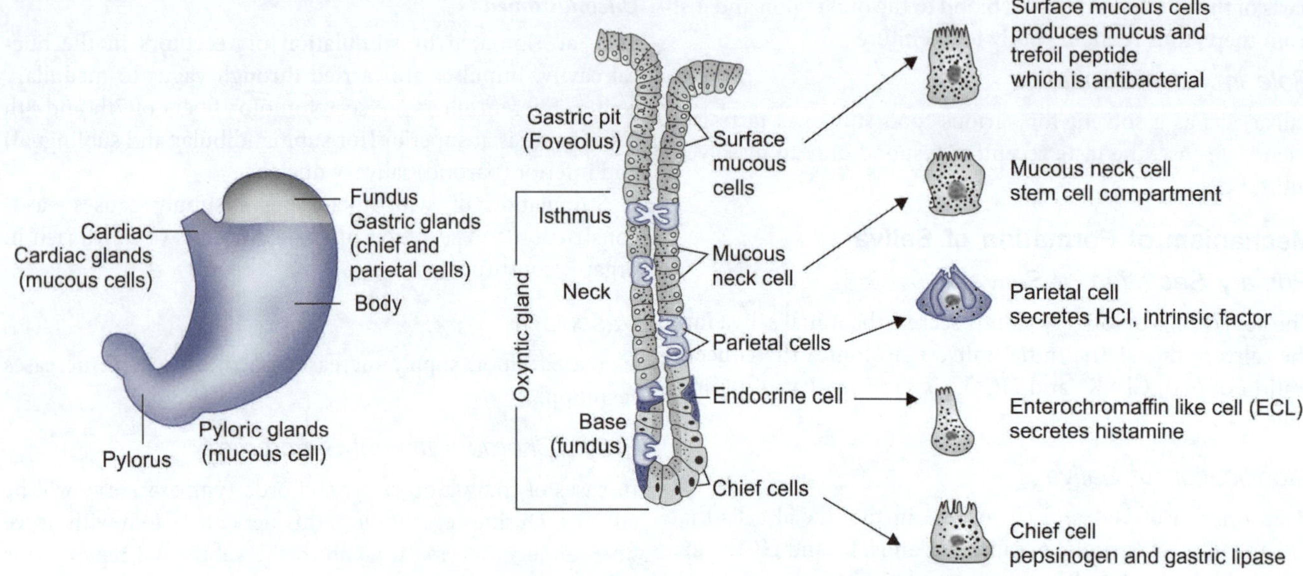

Figs 5.5A and B: A. Parts of stomach; B. Cells of gastric mucosa

Composition of Gastric Juice

About 2.5 liter of gastric juice is secreted per day pH~1. Composition is 99.5% water and 0.5% solids. Solids include both organic and inorganic.

Organic

Enzymes

Pepsinogen, gastric lipase, gelatinase.

Mucus

Two types: thick (insoluble) and thin (soluble).

1. Thick: Secreted by surface epithelial cells.
2. Thin: Secreted by neck mucous cells of pyloric and cardiac glands.

Intrinsic factor

Inorganic

HCl, SO_4^{2-}, HCO_3^-, Na^+, K^+.

Some further details about individual components:

- *HCl*: HCl is necessary for:
  - The conversion of pepsinogen to pepsin.
  - *Bacteriostatic action:* Food contains many bacteria, but they are killed by the gastric HCl, so that contents of the upper part of the small intestine are bacteriologically sterile.
  - It stimulates the secretion of some GI hormones.
  - HCl has a preventive role against gastric cancer. Person who suffer from achlorhydria are thus more susceptible to gastric cancer.
- *Pepsinogen:* In the presence of HCl, pepsin is very active and digests food protein. Thus, the combination of acid and the pepsin, called acid pepsin mixture (APM) powerfully digests food protein.
- *Mucus:* Mucus has the following functions:
  - It specially the thick mucus, protects the gastric mucosa mechanically from being injured by the corrosive effects of food.
  - Together with the HCO_3^- of the gastric juice, it constitutes the mucosal barrier, which prevents the autodigestion of the gastric mucosa itself by APM.
  - Soluble mucus makes the food lubricated.
- *Bicarbonates* act together with the gastric mucus to prevent the autodigestion of the stomach.
- *Intrinsic factor* is needed for the absorption of orally ingested vitamin B_{12}.
- *Gastric lipase* converts triglycerides into fatty acids and glycerols.
- *Gelatinase* liquefies gelatin (protein contained in connective tissue).

HCl Secretion

The acid is formed in the intracellular canaliculus of parietal cell (not within the cytoplasm so that the cell is not damaged due to high acidity). The intracellular canaliculi extend from apical surface of parietal cell into interior and contain H^+- K^+ ATPase and Cl^- channels on the walls. The basolateral membrane on parietal cell in contact with interstitial fluid contain Cl^--HCO_3^- exchangers and Na^+-K^+ ATPase (Fig. 5.6).

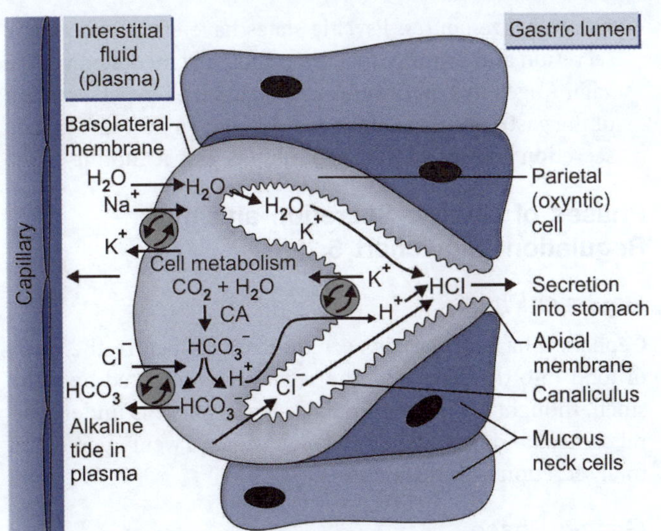

Fig. 5.6: HCl secretion by parietal cells in stomach

When parietal cells are stimulated, CO_2 and H_2O combine to form H_2CO_3 which splits to H^+ and HCO_3^- in presence of enzyme CA (carbonic unhydrase). H^+ is pumped into the lumen of canaliculus with the help of H^+-K^+ ATPase or proton pump (active transport). HCO_3^- leaves the parietal cell by an antiport in the basolateral membrane of parietal cells that exchange Cl^- for HCO_3^-. HCO_3^- binds with Na^+ to form $NaHCO_3$ in capillary blood.Cl^- in the cytoplasm diffuse into lumen of canaliculus. In the lumen of canaliculus, H^+ combines with this Cl^- to form HCl. This HCl reaches gastric lumen.

For each molecule of HCl formed in gastric lumen, one molecule of $NaHCO_3$ is formed in the blood. Hence, when HCl secretion is increased after a meal, pH of blood increases and this is called ***postprandial alkaline tide.***

Inhibitors of HCl Secretion

- Somatostatin
- Acid chyme
  - Direct action—inhibits parietal cell directly.
  - Indirect action—increases secretin secretion.
- Fatty food
  - Release GIP—inhibit G cells and parietal cell.
  - Enterogastrone—inhibit HCl.
- Hyperosmotic chyme-inhibit secretion and motility reflexly.
- Prostaglandins (particularly PGE).

Pepsinogen Secretion

Pepsinogen is an inactive precursor of pepsin. It is secreted by the chief cells. Pepsinogen has no digestive activity. However, as soon as it comes in contact with HCl, it is activated to form active pepsin. Pepsin functions as an active proteolytic enzyme in a high acid medium (optimum pH 1.8 – 3.5), but above a pH of about 5 it has no proteolytic activity and becomes completely inactivated in a short time.

Secretion of Intrinsic Factor

Intrinsic factor is secreted by parietal cells of gastric mucosa along with the secretion of HCl. The intrinsic factor is essential for absorption of vitamin B_{12}. It forms a complex with B_{12} which is carried to the terminal ileum where the vitamin is absorbed. When the acid-producing parietal cells of the stomach are destroyed (which frequently occurs in chronic gastritis), the person develops not only achlorhydria (lack of stomach acid secretion) but often also pernicious anemia because of failure of maturation of the red blood cells in the absence of vitamin B_{12} stimulation of the bone marrow.

Regulation of Secretion of Gastric Juice

Gastric secretion is accurately synchronized with the need for gastric juice. Mechanisms regulating the gastric secretion include neural control and chemical control.

Neural Control

Neural control over the gastric glands is exerted by local enteric plexus involving cholinergic neurons and impulses from CNS via vagal (extrinsic) innervations. Vagal stimulation increases the secretion of HCl by parietal cells and pepsin by chief cells.Vagal stimulation increases H^+ secretion by a direct and an indirect path.

In the direct path, the vagus nerve fibers innervating parietal cells stimulate H^+ secretion by releasing ACh which acts on through M_3 muscarinic receptors (to increase intracellular Ca^{2+}) on parietal cells it causes direct stimulation of secretion of gastric juice. In addition, ACh also potentiates the effects of histamine on H_2 receptors of parietal cells.

In the indirect pathway, the vagus innervates G cells and stimulates the release of gastrin into circulation through gastrin releasing peptide (GRP). The gastrin in turn stimulates H^+ secretion. ACh released on vagal stimulation also acts on enterochromaffin like (ECL) cells which release histamine. Histamine increases H^+ secretion by acting on H_2 receptors on the parietal cells, but the relative importance of ACh in stimulating their secretion is unsettled.

Peptic cells are stimulated by ACh released from vagus nerves or from gastric enteric nervous plexus.

Chemical Control

- *Role of gastrin:* It is a GI hormone produced by G cells located in the pyloric glands. Most known powerful stimulant of HCl secretion. Presence of products of protein digestion in the stomach acts on G cells to release gastrin. It stimulates secretory activity of parietal cell and chief cells.

Actions

- Gastrin stimulates the secretion of histamine from ECL cells. Histamine stimulates HCl secretion and this is the principal way by which gastrin stimulates acid secretion.
- Gastrin also stimulate HCl secretion by acting on the gastrin receptors in the parietal cell. This increases intracellular Ca^{2+}.
- To a lesser extent it stimulates chief cells to secrete pepsin.

- *Role of histamine:* Histamine is released from ECL cells. Enterochromaffin like cells bear both gastrin receptors and ACh receptors. They release histamine in response to both circulating gastrin as well as ACh released by vagal fibers. The histamine released stimulates HCl secretion from parietal cells by acting on H_2 receptors. Histamine bind to H_2 receptors and via G_s, this increases adenyl cyclase activity and intracellular cAMP (Fig. 5.7).

  Increase in intracellular cAMP and Ca^{2+} act via protein kinases to increase the transport of H^+ into the gastric lumen by H^+ - K^+ ATPase.
- *Role of somatostatin:* Somatostatin is secreted by D cells in the gastric glands. They inhibits gastric acid secretion.
- *PGE_2* acts via GI to decrease adenylyl cyclase activity and intracellular cAMP. This inhibits acid secretion.
- *Low pH* (< 3) in the stomach inhibits the secretion of H^+ by parietal cells by negative feedback mechanism.
- *Intestinal influences:* Fats, carbohydrates and acid in the duodenum inhibit gastric acid and pepsin secretion via neural and hormonal mechanisms.
- The rate of secretion of pepsinogen is strongly influenced by the *amount of acid* in the stomach. Acids elicits additional enteric nervous signals to the peptic cells.

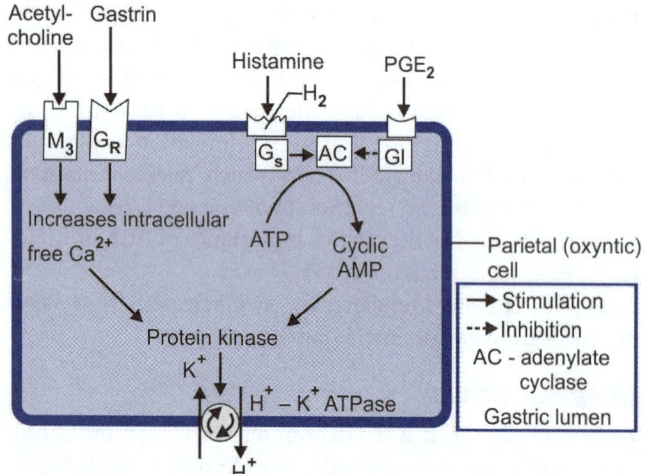

Fig. 5.7: Regulation of gastric acid secretion by the parietal cell

- *Emotional responses:* Psychic states have effects on gastric secretion and motility that are principally mediated via the vagi. Anger and motility are associated with hypersecretion of the gastric mucosa. Fear and depression decrease gastric secretion and blood flow and inhibits gastric motility.

Phases of Gastric Secretion and their Regulation (Flowchart 5.1)

Cephalic Phase

Cephalic phase of gastric secretion occurs before the entry of food into the stomach. The secretion is initiated by sight, smell, thought or taste of food. Cephalic phase is under neural control and is mediated through vagus. Twenty percent of total secretion is in this phase.

Gastric Phase

Gastric phase of gastric secretion occurs when food enters stomach. Seventy percent of total secretion occurs in this phase. It is mediated by neural and hormonal mechanism.

- *Neural:* Distension of stomach by food stimulates gastric juice secretion (through local myentric and vagovagal reflex).
- *Chemical/Hormonal:* Products of partial digestion stimulate the secretion of gastrin. Gastrin enters the circulation and stimulates gastric glands.

Flowchart 5.1: Phases of gastric acid secretion and their regulation

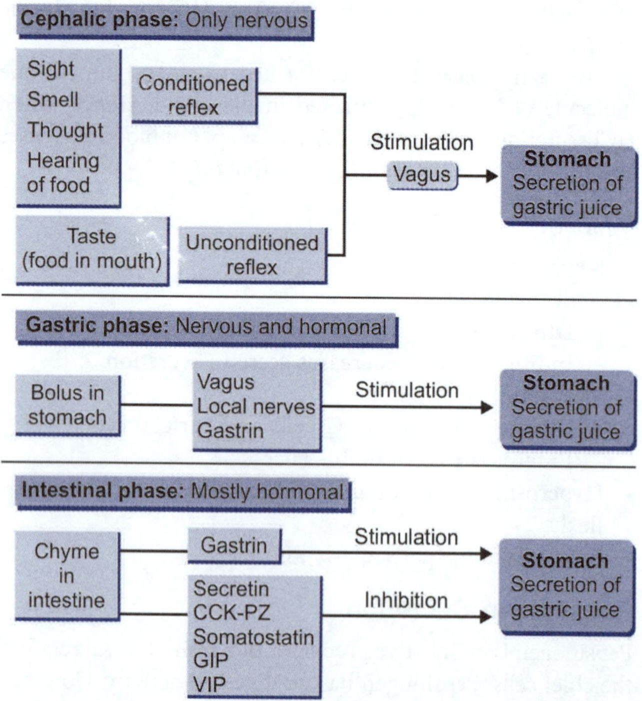

Intestinal Phase

Intestinal phase of gastric secretion begins as the chyme begins to empty from the stomach into duodenum. Accounts for 10% of gastric juice secretion. Initiatly (during the early intestinal phase) the secretion is increased and later it is inhibited. This inhibition results from the following influences.

- *Enterogastric reflex:* It is a reflex mechanism mediated through myentric nervous system as well as through extrinsic sympathetic system and vagus nerve. It is initiated by distension of small intestine in the presence of acids or protein breakdown products in the upper intestine and irritation of mucosa.
- *Hormonal mechanism:* Presence of acid, fat, protein break down products, hypoosmotic or hyperosmotic fluids and any irritating factors in the upper small intestine causes release of hormones like CCK, GIP, VIP and somatostatin which inhibit gastric secretion.

Sham Feeding

It is an experimental procedure devised by Pavlov to demonstrate the regulation of gastric secretion.

Procedure

- A hole is made in the neck of an anesthetized dog.
- The cut ends are drawn out through the hole in the neck.
- When the dog eats food, it comes out through the cut end of the esophagus.
- But the dog has the satisfaction of eating the food.

This experimental procedure is supported by the preparation of Pavlov's pouch with a fistula from the stomach. The fistula opens to the exterior and it is used to observe the gastric secretion. It is useful to demonstrate the secretion of gastric juice during cephalic phase. In the same animal after vagotomy, sham feeding does not induce gastric secretion (Fig. 5.8). It proves the role of vagus nerve during cephalic phase.

Peptic Ulcer

It is an excoriated area of stomach or intestinal mucosa caused principally by the digestive action of gastric juice or upper small intestinal secretion. It frequently occurs along the lesser curvature of the antral end, of the stomach. If peptic ulcer is found in stomach, it is called gastric ulcer and if found in duodenum it is called duodenal ulcer.

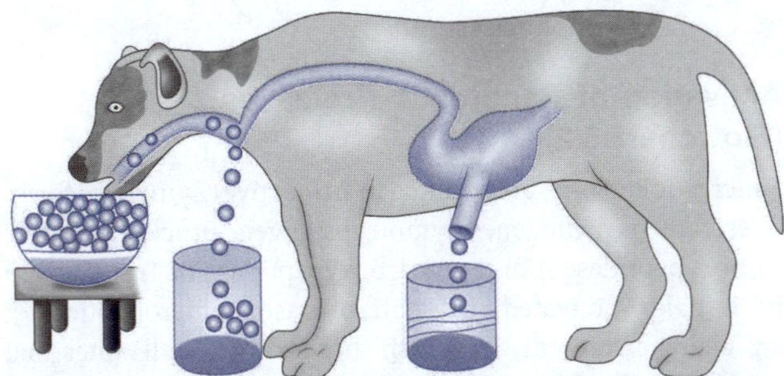

Fig. 5.8: Sham feeding

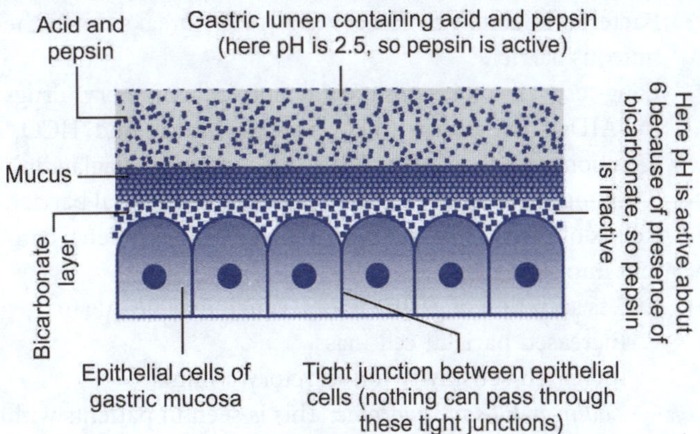

Fig. 5.9: Mucosal barrier

Mucosal Protective Mechanism

The autodigestion of mucosa is prevented by:

- *Mucosal barrier:* Gastric mucosal epithelium is covered by mucus. The mucus is primarily of the thick insoluble variety and does not flow or move easily. This is called 'unstirred layer'. But soluble mucus is also present. The acid and pepsin, after being secreted by the gastric glands reach the lumen to come in contact with the food. But it cannot come in contact with the mucosal epithelium, because mucus of the unstirred layer acts as a barrier (Fig. 5.9).
- *Bicarbonate secretion:* Between the mucus and the epithelium some bicarbonate rich fluid is present. Within the lumen, the pH is low (about 2.5), hence pepsin is very active (i.e. it can digest protein easily). But near the epithelium, because of the presence of HCO^{3-} ions, the pH is high, so that pepsin becomes inactive. This HCO^{3-} cannot move towards the lumen because of the presence of unstirred layer.
- *Epithelial barrier:* Intercellular tight junctions provide a barrier to back diffusion of H^+.
- *Trifoil peptides:* Trifoil peptides in the mucosa of stomach are acid resistant and protect stomach.
- *PGE_2:* Can help in the synthesis of mucus and formation of new mucosal cells. If there is injury in the gastric mucosa, the dead cells can be speedly replaced.

Causes of Peptic Ulcer

- The usual cause of peptic ulceration is an imbalance between the rate of secretion of gastric juice and the degree of protection offered by:
  - Gastroduodenal mucosal barrier
  - The neutralization of the gastric acid by bicarbonate.

- Bacterial infection by *Helicobacter pylori* breaks down the mucous barrier.
- Long-term use of nonsteroidal anti-inflammatory drugs (NSAIDs) like aspirin (they decrease mucus and HCO_3^- secretion since they inhibit the production of prostaglandin).
- Smoking, alcohol, etc. can also disrupt the mucosal barrier.
- Reflux of gastric content into esophagus and duodenal content into stomach.
- Excess secretion of gastric juices, which may be due to:
  - Increased parietal cell mass.
  - Increased sensitivity for secretory stimuli.
  - *Zollinger-Ellison syndrome*: This is seen in patients with gastrinomas (tumors secreting gastrin). These tumors can occur in stomach, duodenum and mostly in pancreas. Gastrin causes prolonged hypersecretion of acid and severe ulcers are produced.
- Poor blood supply.

The difference between duodenal and gastric ulcers is illustrated in Table 5.2.

Complications of Ulcer

- Perforations—ulcer burrows through all the coats of the stomach → gastric or duodenal lumen now communicates through this perforations with peritoneal cavity.
- Hemorrhage from the ulcer.

Physiology of Treatment

- Antacids (for example, Gelusil) neutralize the acid.
- Use of antibiotics along with other agents to kill infectious bacteria.

Table 5.2: Differences between duodenal and gastric ulcer

Duodenal ulcer	Gastric ulcer
It is seen in 2nd part of duodenum	More common curvature of stomach; esp at incisura angularis
More common	Less common
Incidence more in younger age group	More in older age group
More common in males	Equal in both sexes
Chronic duodenal ulcers are not associated with malignancy	Chronic gastric ulcers are associated with malignancy
Have higher gastric acid secretion because of back diffusion of H^+	Normal levels of gastric acid secretion
Pain relieved by food and antacids	No relief, food aggravate pain
Complication less	More severe
Superficial and smaller in size	Deep seated and larger in size

- Administration of an acid-suppressant drug such as ***cimetidine, ranitidine*** (both block H_2 histamine receptors on parietal cell), ***omeprazole*** (inhibits H^+- K^+ ATPase).
- NSAIDs induced ulcers can be treated by stopping the use of NSAIDs or by treatment with prostaglandin agonist ***misoprostol.***
- Gastrinomas can be removed surgically.
- Vagectomy, partial gastrectomy.
- Coating agents—sucralfate.
- Atropine—anticholinergic.

PANCREATIC JUICE

Pancreas is essentially two organs in one, an exocrine digestive gland and an endocrine gland. The endocrine part is discussed in endocrinology. Exocrine pancreas secrete pancreatic juice. The pancreatic juice is the most potent digestive secretion. The pancreatic juice is the major source of digestive enzymes that digest all components of the food, i.e. proteins, carbohydrate, fat and nucleic acid. About 1500 ml is secreted per day. It is alkaline and has high HCO_3^- content.

Composition

- *Cations:* Na^+, K^+, Ca^{2+}, Mg^{2+}
- *Anions:* HCO_3^-, Cl^-, SO_4^-, HPO_4^{2-}
- *Digestive enzymes*
  - Amylolytic enzymes
    Pancreatic amylase
  - Lipolytic enzymes
    - Pancreatic lipase
    - Cholesteryl ester hydrolase
    - Phospholipase A_2
    - Bile salt-acid lipase
    - Colipase
  - Proteolytic enzymes
    - Trypsin.
    - Chymotrypsin
    - Carboxypeptidase A and B
    - Elastase
    - Collagenase
    - Ribonuclease
    - Deoxyribonuclease

Activation of Pancreatic Proteases (Flowchart 5.2)

Pancreatic enzymes are secreted in an inactive (Zymogen) form. These are trypsinogen, chymotrypsinogen, proclastase, procarboxypeptidase A and procarboxypeptidase B. Trypsinogen is initially activated by enterokinase (enteropeptidase), an enzyme present in brush border of small intestinal epithelial cells. The conversion of inactive trypsinogen into

Flowchart 5.2: Activation of pancreatic proteases in the duodenal lumen

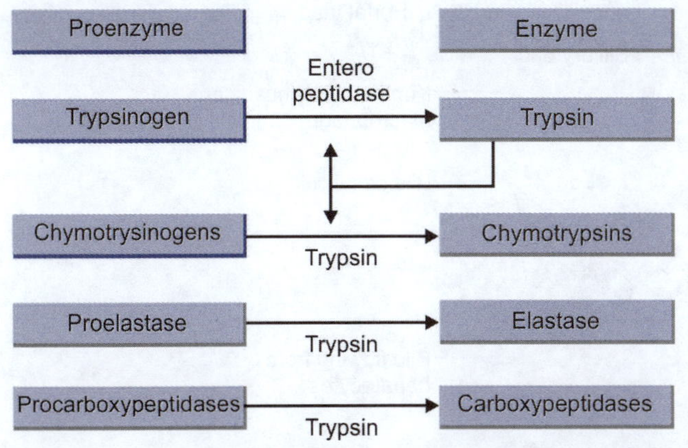

active trypsin requires removal of an N-terminal peptide by enteropeptidase (enterokinase). Trypsin is a powerful proteolytic enzyme which can digest the pancreatic cells itself. However, normally this does not occur as pancreas secretes its exocrine products as enzymatically inert proenzyme (with exception of amylase and lipase). This also helps to efficiently utilize the enzymes within the lumen of duodenum. Once some trypsin has been generated by enterokinase, it can activate more trypsinogen as well as other inactive enzymes.

Functions

- It contains large amount of bicarbonate ions, which helps in neutralizing the acidity of the chyme emptied from stomach.
- Trypsin and chymotrypsin splits digested proteins into peptides of various sizes.
- Carboxypeptidase split some peptides into individual amino acids.
- Amylase splits polysaccharides into disaccharides and trisaccharides
- Lipase is capable of hydrolyzing neutral fat into fatty acids and monoglycerides.
- Cholesterol esterase hydrolyzes cholesterol esters.
- Phospholipase splits fatty acids from phospholipids.

Regulation of Secretion

Secretion of pancreatic juice is regulated by both nervous and hormonal factors, with the later playing the predominant role. Neural regulation is through vagal efferents supplying the exocrine gland of pancreas and hormonal regulation is through secretin, CCK-PZ, gastrin and somatostatin.

Regulation of Cephalic Phase

Cephalic phase of pancreatic secretion like that of gastric secretion, occurs before the entry of food into the stomach. Regulation of this phase is mainly through the reflex vagal stimulation which occurs:

- By conditioned reflexes, initiated by sight, smell and thought of food.
- Unconditioned reflexes initiated by stimulation of taste buds by food in the oral cavity, the act of chewing and swallowing.

Regulation of Gastric Phase

Gastric phase of pancreatic secretion occurs when stomach is distended by the food. This phase is regulated by neural control exerted through vagus and hormonal control executed through the hormone gastrin.

Regulation of Intestinal Secretion

The intestinal phase of pancreatic secretion begins when the chyme enters the duodenum and jejunum. It is characterized by marked increase in the secretion of both enzymes and aqueous component of pancreatic juice. This phase is regulated by hormones secretin and CCK-PZ.

Role of secretin

Secretin enters the blood circulation and after reaching the pancreas it acts on the duct cells and produces large amount of watery juice with high concentration of HCO_3^- and poor in enzymes. The effect is due to increase in intracellular cAMP.

Role of CCK-PZ

CCK-PZ acts on the acinar cells to cause the release of zymogen granules and production of pancreatic juice rich in enzymes but low in volume. Effect is mediated by phospholipase C.

Steatorrhea

Pancreatectomized animals and patients with diseases that destroy the exocrine portion of pancreas have fatty, bulky, clay colored stools, because of the impaired digestion and absorption of fat. It is mostly due to lipase deficiency. Lack of alkaline secretion from pancreas also contributes by lowering the pH of intesine contents as acid inhibits lipase. Hyper secretion of gastric acid and defective reabsortion of bile salts in the distal ileum can also cause this.

LIVER

Basic structural unit of liver is lobule. Each hepatic lobule is made of ramifying columns of hepatic cells. It is polyhedral in shape with central vein at the center. Liver cells are arranged in radial manner from the central vein in rows of 2 to 3 layers thickness. These hepatic cell are tunneled by a communicating system of lacunae called blood sinusoids. Sinusoids are lined by fenestrated endothelial cells. Endothelium contains Kupffer cells. Portal vein and hepatic artery both empties into the sinusoids. Sinusoids open into central vein. Bile canaliculi are formed or they are spaced between hepatocytes. No separate lining cells for canaliculi. Canaliculi start from central

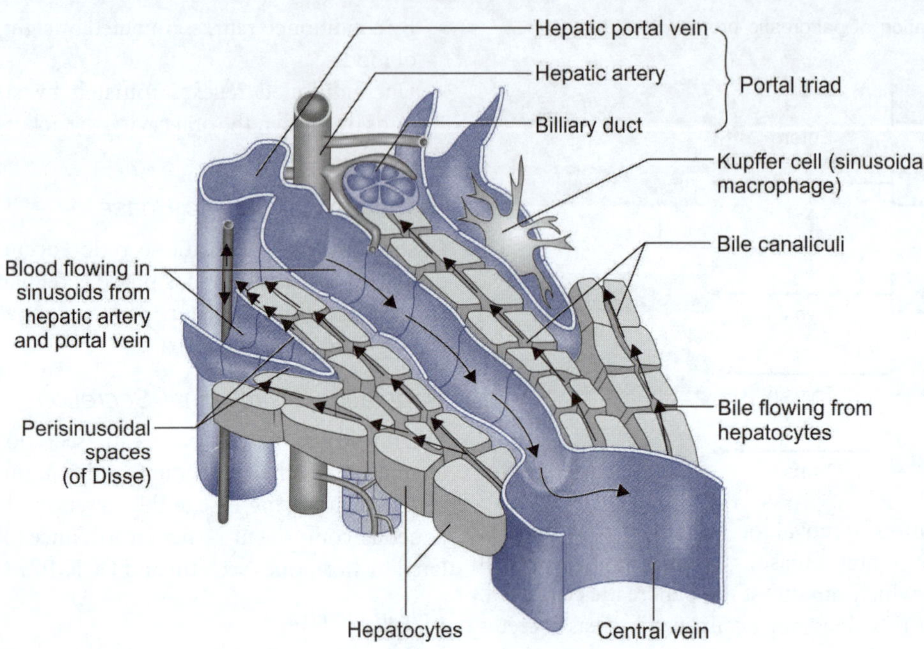

Fig. 5.10: Cross-section of a liver lobule

vein region. Along the periphery of each lobule are present portal triads consisting of one branch each of hepatic artery, portal vein and an interlobular bile duct. This concept of liver lobule is classic lobule (Fig. 5.10).

Another concept is acinus. Acinus is considered as basic functional unit of liver. According to this concept, individual acinus is diamond shaped, central vein occupies two corners and portal triad occupies other two corners. The region of cells near the equatorial zone is called zone-1. The cells in this zone are provided with more O_2 and nutrients. The zone near central vein region is called zone-3 and is least supplied by O_2 and nutrients. Zone between 1 and 3 is called zone-3 (Fig. 5.11).

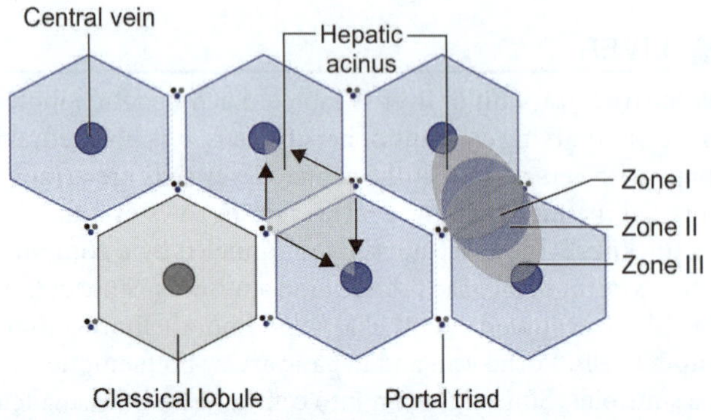

Fig. 5.11: Schematic of liver operational unit: The classic and the acinus

Blood Supply

From two sources—Portal vein and hepatic artery. Venous drainage is by hepatic vien. Portal vein carries blood from small intestine, large intestine, spleen and pancreas. It is rich in nutrients and poor in O_2. Inside the liver, portal vein divides, redivides and ultimately give rise to sinusoids. Sinusoids run with hepatic cells in liver lobules. Hepatic artery also divides and redivides and finally empties into sinusoids. It is rich in O_2. In the sinusoids, hepatic arterial and portal venous blood mixes. Sinusoids → central vein → unite to form large vein → hepatic vein → inferior venacava. Large gaps in endothelial cells helps in easy transport of nutrients to hepatocytes for nutriton. Kupffer cells provide immunity, they are macrophages.

Functions

Synthetic Functions

Liver synthesize

- Most of plasma proteins especially, albumin.
- Synthesis of clotting factors 5, 7, 9, 10, fibrinogen, prothrombin.
- Enzymes like alkaline phosphatase, serum glutamate oxaloacetate transaminase (SGOT), serum glutamate pyruvate transaminase (SGPT), serum isocitrate dehydrogenase (SICD).
- Urea.

Metabolic functions

- *Carbohydrates:* Helps in synthesis, storage and release of glucose, i.e. glycogenolysis, glucogenesis, gluconeogenesis.
- *Proteins:* Synthesis enzymes, glycoproteins, clotting factor, plasma proteins.
- *Lipids:* Both degradation and synthesis of fat takes place in liver. Oxidation in mitochondria to form fatty acids. (Non esterified fatty acids → esterified fatty acids → triglycerides).

  Synthesize lipoproteins, i.e. HDL, LDL, VLDL, chylomicrons.

  Synthesis of saturated fatty acids, cholesterol, phospholipids for cell membrane.

Bile Secretion

Components of bile (bile salts, bile acids) are formed by hepatocytes. Conjugation of bilirubin occurs in hepatocytes.

Detoxification and Protective Functions

Many drugs and toxins are detoxified by liver and excreted.

Miscellaneous

- *Storage function:* Glycogen, protein, fat, vitamin B_{12} and vitamin A.
- *Hormonal inactivation:* Cortisol, aldosterone, insulin, glucagon, testosterone.
- Liver is the site of erythropoiesis in intrauterine life.
- Reservoir of blood.

Biliary System

Small amount of bile is continuously synthesized in the liver. It is transfered to the gallbladder through the cystic duct because during the interdigestive period, tone of sphincter of Oddi is so high that the bile cannot enter the duodenum.

Bile is formed in tiny vacuoles in hepatocytes. It is discharged into bile canaliculus. Canaliculi → bile duct at portal triad (interlobular duct) → interlobar duct → right and left hepatic duct → common hepatic duct → joins cystic duct from gallbladder → joins pancreatic duct → opens at 2nd part of duodenum at ampulla of Vater or opening of sphincter of Oddi.

GALLBLADDER

It is a sac like structure where bile is stored in between meals. Bile ducts can hold certain amount of bile and when pressure of common bile duct is about 70 mm of H_2O bile begins to pass to gallbladder. After meals, the pressure again increases and it is released to duodenum by contraction of gallbladder and relaxation of spincter of Oddi. Gallbladder has capacity to absorb H_2O and HCO_3^-, i.e. it has concentrating function and alkalinity is slightly decreased. Gallbladder can concentrate bile up to 50 times.

Functions

- Storage of bile
- Concentration of bile by absorbing water and bicarbonate.
- Secrete mucus.
- Releases bile to duodenum at a controlled rate or according to the need, thus equalizing pressure in biliary system.

Formation and Composition of Bile

Bile is made up of bile salts, bile pigments and other substances dissolved in alkaline electrolyte solution. The bile salts are synthesized and secreted by hepatocytes. Bile pigments are picked up from blood sinusoids. Secretion is about 500 ml/day. Of all the constituents, only bile salts are of importance to the digestive system. The amphipathic (molecules that contain both hydrophilic and hydrophobic regions) property of bile salts are important for fat emulsification and micelle formation. They also have choleretic function.

Color—yellow

Taste—bitter.

So bile is an alkaline juice comprised of water and solids.

Organic: Bile salts, bile acids, bile pigments, lecithin, fatty acids, mucous, proteins, (lysosomal enzymes, Ig, glycoproteins, bacteria, virus.

Inorganic: Na^+, K^+, HCO_3^-

Bile secreted by hepatocytes (called hepatic bile) is concentrated in the gallbladder (called gallbladder bile).

Comparison of hepatic duct bile and gallbladder bile are shown in Table 5.3 and composition of bile is shown in Table 5.4.

Table 5.3: Comparison of liver bile and gallbladder bile

	Hepatic bile	Gallbladder bile
Percentage of solids	2–4	10–12
Bile salts (mmol/L)	10–20	50–200
pH	7.8–8.6	7.0–7.4

Table 5.4: Composition of bile

	Liver bile	Gallbladder bile
Water	97.5 g/dl	92 g/d
Bile salts	1.1 g/dl	6 g/dl
Bilirubin	0.04 g/dl	0.3 g/dl
Cholesterol	0.1 g/dl	0.3 to 0.9 g/dl
Fatty acids	0.12 g/dl	0.3 to 1.2 g/dl
Lecithin	0.04 g/dl	0.3 g/dl
Na^+	145.04 mEq/L	130 mEq/L
K^+	5 mEq/L	12 mEq/L
Ca^{2+}	5 mEq/L	23 mEq/L
Cl^-	100 mEq/L	25 mEq/L

Bile Acids

Primary bile acids are produced by hepatocytes from cholesterol. They includes cholic acid and chenodeoxycholic acids. Primary bile acids contains steroid nucleus with cyclopentano perhydro phenanthrene ring. They reach duodenum through bile. In the small intestine and colon, it is converted into secondary bile acids by bacterial action. Secondary bile acids include deoxycholic acid and lithocholic acid.

Bile Salts

Bile salts are the most important constituents of the bile. They are the sodium and potassium salts of bile acids conjugated to amino acids, e.g. glycine or taurine. The important bile acids are cholic acid and chenodeoxycholic acid. Bile acids are derived from cholesterol. Bile salts = Sodium or potassium + Amino acid (glycine or taurine) + Bile acids (cholic acid or chenodeoxycholic acid). So bile salts are:

Sodium + glycine + cholic acid = Sodium glycocholic acid (sodium glycocholate)

Sodium + taurine + cholic acid = Sodium taurocholic acid (sodium taurocholate)

Sodium + glycine + chenodeoxycholic acid = Sodium glycochenodeoxycholic acid

Sodium + taurine + chenodeoxycholic acid = Sodium taurochenodeoxycholic acid

Similarly potassium salts bile salts are potassium glycocholate, potassium taurocholate, potassium glycochenodeoxycholate, and potassium taurochenodeoxycholate. Bile salts act as detergents, i.e. they have surface tension lowering action. Detergent action is due to amphipathic nature of bile salts.

Functions

- Emulsification and digestion of fat
- Absorption of fat
- Stimulate formation of bile by hepatocyte called choleretic action
- Stimulate release of bile from gallbladder called cholagogue action
- Laxative action helps in easily bowel movements, stimulate peristalsis
- Form route for removal of cholesterol as they are formed from cholesterol.

Bile Pigments

These are the excretory products in bile. They are formed by breakdown of hemoglobin in RES. Bilirubin is transported to liver along with plasma proteins (this is called unconjugated bilirubin).This bilirubin is broken down by hepatocytes. Proteins separates and bilirubin conjugate with glucuronic acid and form conjugated bilirubin. In intestine, bacteria act upon bilirubin and 50% of bilirubin is converted to bilinogen. Most of bilinogen enters liver through enterohepatic circulation and is re-excreted through bile. About 5% of urobilinogen is excreted by kidney through urine. Some unabsorbed part is excreted through feces as stercobilinogen. This gives yellow color to urine and feces.

Functions of Bile

- Required for digestion and absorption of fat by two mechanisms:
  - Active pancreatic lipase helps in digestion.
  - Emulsification of fat and formation of micelle helps in absorption.
- Absorption of fat soluble vitamins.
- *Choleretic and cholagogue action:* Choleretics are substances that increase hepatic bile secretion. The most important choleretics are bile salt themselves. Other choleretic is secretin. Cholagogues are substance that cause gallbladder contraction to pour its bile. The most important cholagogue is cholecystokinin (CCK), fatty acids and amino acids in the duodenum stimulate the release of CCK which causes gallbladder contraction.
- Endogenous synthesis of bile salts.
- Bacteriostatic action.
- Major route for loss of cholesterol from body.
- Lubricating function due to mucous.
- Alkaline helps in neutralizing acidic chyme.

Enterohepatic Circulation

About 94% of the bile salts are reabsorbed into the blood from the small intestine, (about one-half of this by diffusion through the mucosa in the early portions of the small intestine and the remainder by an active transport process through the intestinal mucosa in the distal ileum) (Fig. 5.12). They then enter the portal blood and pass back to the liver. On reaching the liver these salts are absorbed almost entirely back into the hepatic cells and are resecreted into the bile.

In this way, about 94% of all the bile salts are recirculated into the bile, so that on the average these salts make the entire circuit some 17 times before being carried out in the feces. The small quantities of bile salts lost into the feces are replaced by new amounts formed continually by the liver cells. This recirculation of the bile salts is called the enterohepatic circulation of bile. This circulation is necessary because of limited pool of bile salts.

Jaundice

Jaundice or icterus refers to the yellowish discoloration of skin, sclera, mucous membrane due to increased amount of bilirubin in body fluids. Nervous and collagen tissues

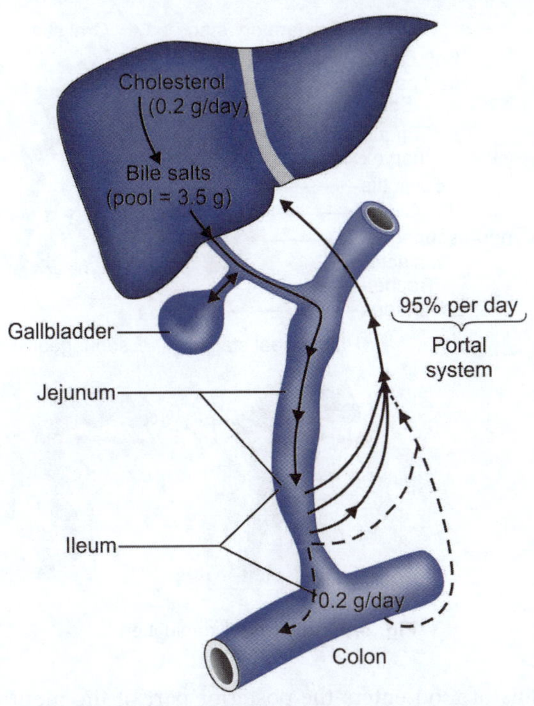

Fig. 5.12: Enterohepatic circulation of bile salts

have higher affinity towards bile pigments. The yellowish discoloration will be 1st detected in sclera. Different types of jaundice and their causes are mentioned in Table 5.5.

Total bilirubin is 1 mg%. When it exceeds 2-3 mg%, it is clinically detected. When it is between 1-2 mg%, it is subclinical jaundice. Other causes of yellow discoloration are: (1) Hypercarotenemia, (2) Hypothyroidism, (3) Drug mepacrine.

SMALL INTESTINE

Small intestine is the major site of digestion and absorbtion of carbohydrates, proteins and fats. The intestinal juice also called succus entericus. It is secreted by cells present in the crypts of Lieberkuhn. It comprises of:

- Aqueous component (water and electrolytes)
- Intestinal enzymes
- Mucus

  Daily secretion: Three liters. It is isotonic with plasma. pH = 7.6

Electrolytes includes Na^+, K^+, Ca^{2+}, Mg^{2+}, Cl^-, HCO_3^-, PO_4^{3-}

Intestinal Enzymes

They are located in the brush border of epithelial cells.

- Peptidases
- Disaccharidases—sucrase, maltase, lactase and limiting α-dextrinase.
- Intestinal lipase
- Enterokinase (enteropeptidase)—it activates trypsinogen.

Mucus

It is secreted by Brunner's gland (in duodenum) and globlet cells. They protect the intestinal wall from acid chyme. The mucus lubricates the food and hold immunoglobulins in place. Its secretion is accelerated by cholinergic stimulation and by chemical and physical irritation.

Table 5.5: Different types of jaundice and their causes

Type	Hemolytic/Prehepatic	Hepatocellular/Hepatic	Hepatocellular/Hepatic
Reason	Due to hemolysis resulting in increased destruction of RBC	Due to liver disease, there is impaired uptake and release of bilirubin	Obstruction of flow of bile
Causes	**Intracorpuscular defect** • Defect in RBC, e.g. hereditary spherocytosis (due to deficiency of protein spectrin). • Hemoglobinopathies, e.g. sickle cell anemia, thalassemia **Extracorpuscular defect** • Infection—malarial parasite • Radiation—treatment for malignancy • Immunological anti-Ab	• Viral infection—hepatitis, Wiel's disease, malaria • Septicemia • Drugs—anesthesia and anti-TB • Liver cirrhosis	**Intrahepatic** • Drugs causing edema • Alcohol **Extrahepatic** • Stones • Strictures—narrowing of opening due to infection or congenital • Parasites (worm infection • Malignant growth (benign and malignant)
Bilirubin in blood	Unconjugated bilirubin	Conjugated and unconjugated bilirubin	Conjugated bilirubin
Bile pigments in urine	Nil	Present	Present
Urobilinogen in blood and urine	Present	Present	Absent
Stercobilinogen in feces	Present	Present	Absent (gray-colored stools)
van den Bergh reaction	Indirect +ve	Biphasic	Direct +ve

PHYSICON—The Reliable Icon in Physiology

LARGE INTESTINE

There is no villi in large intestine. Large intestine plays an important role in the absorbtion of water, electrolytes, drugs, etc. Large intestine secretions mainly comprise mucus secreted by globlet cell. It also contains some amount of HCO_3^-. The mucus has got lubricating activity and movement of bowel is facilitated. Alkaline nature of large intestine juice neutralize the acids formed by bacterial action on the fecal matter.

MOVEMENTS OF GIT

Mastication

Process of grinding of food into smaller particles with the help of teeth and jaw muscles. It helps in mixing with secretions of salivary glands. This wetting and homogenizing action aids swallowing and subsequent digestion. It is a voluntary reflex with center in medulla oblongata. Nerve involved is 5th cranial nerve. Hypothalamus, cerebral cortex and amygdala are also involved.

Presence of bolus in the mouth → sensory areas stimulated → reflex inhibition of muscles of mastication → lower jaw drops → initiation of stretch reflex → rebound contraction of jaw muscles → raises the jaw to cause the closure of teeth → compression of bolus against sensory areas in mouth.

Functions

- Food is made fit for swallowing.
- Breaks undigestable cellulose in fruits and raw vegetables.
- Increases surface area and rate of digestion.
- Damage caused by the mucosal lining can be prevented.
- Facilitates lubrication and initiates digestion of starch by enzymes.
- Chewing brings food in contact with taste receptors.
- Olfactory receptors are able to detect odor of food particles.

Deglutition

Deglutition refers to the passage of food from oral cavity into the stomach. It is a reflex response that is triggered by afferent impulses in the 5th, 9th, and 10th cranial nerve. These impulses are integrated in the nucleus of tractus solitarius and nucleus ambiguous. The efferent fibers pass to pharyngeal musculature and the tongue via 5th, 7th and 12th cranial nerve. It has three stages (Fig. 5.13):

1. *Oral phase:* It is a voluntary stage. Food passes from mouth to pharynx. Includes voluntary placing of food and rolling of tongue. This backward and upward movement of tongue presses food against palate and bolus moves from mouth to pharynx.
2. *Pharyngeal phase:* It constitutes passage of food through pharynx into esophagus. It is an involuntary phase. As the bolus of food enters the posterior part of the mouth and pharynx, it stimulates sensory receptors located in these areas. This will initiates reflex contraction of pharyngeal muscles. Once the food is in oropharynx, there are four possible outlets for food:

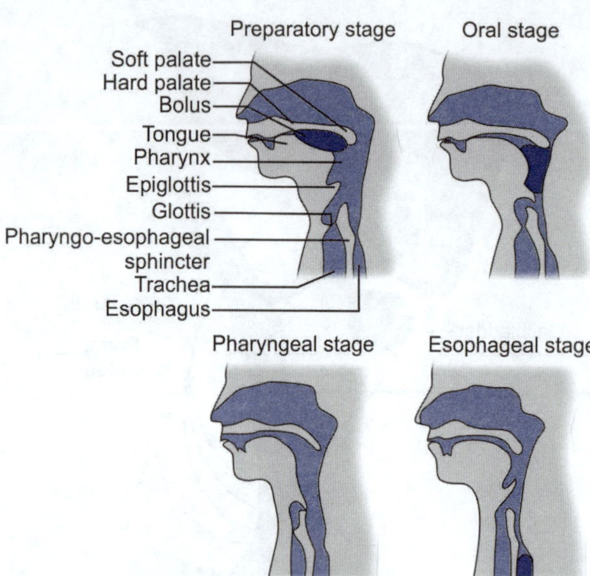

Fig. 5.13: Stages of deglutition

a. Back to mouth
b. To nasal cavity
c. Into respiratory tract
d. Into esophagus.

Entry of food into mouth is prevented by approximation of tongue against roof of mouth. Soft palate is pulled upward to close the posterior nares, to prevent reflux of food into nasal cavities. Palatopharyngeal folds are pulled medially to make a slit like opening, through which food must pass into posterior pharynx. This slit performs selective action, allowing only properly masticated food to pass through. Vocal cords are strongly approximated (stopping the breathing temporarily called *deglutition apnea*) and the larynx is pulled upward and anteriorly by the neck muscles. Epiglottis swings backwards to close the laryngeal opening. All these guides the food towards the esophagus and prevent its entry into trachea. The upward movement of the larynx also pulls up and enlarges the opening to the esophagus and upper esophageal sphincter relaxes, thus allowing the food to move easily from the posterior pharynx into the upper esophagus. This spintcher remains strongly contracted in between swallows to prevent entry of air into esophagus during respiration. Entire muscular wall of pharynx contracts (beginning in the superior part, then spreading downward over the middle and inferior pharyngeal areas) which propels the food by *peristalsis* (*it is a reflex response that is initiated when the gut wall is stretched by the contents of the lumen and it occurs in all parts of GIT from esophagus to the rectum*) into the esophagus. The entire process of this stage occurs in less than 2 seconds.

3. *Esophageal phase:* During this phase food bolus is propelled from upper part of esophagus to stomach. It is an involuntary stage and exhibits two types of peristalsis: Primary and secondary peristalsis.
   a. *Primary peristalsis:* It is the continuation of peristaltic wave that begins in the pharynx and spreads to esophagus during pharyngeal stage. This wave passes from pharynx to stomach in 8-10 seconds.
   b. *Secondary peristalsis:* When primary peristalsis fails to empty the bolus into the stomach, the retained food initiates secondary peristaltic waves due to the distention of esophagus. The 2nd waves are initiated partly by intrinsic neural circuits (in the myentric plexus) and partly by reflexes that begin in the pharynx. They are transmitted upward through afferent fibers of vagus to medulla and back again to esophagus through IX and X cranial nerve.

      When the peristaltic wave reaches lower esophageal sphincter it relaxes and allows the food to enter the stomach. This relaxation is mediated via neurons that release NO and VIP.

Disorders of Swallowing

Dysphagia

Difficulty in swallowing.

Achalasia

It is a condition in which food accumulates in the esophagus. Esophagus is massively dilated.

It is due to increased resting lower esophageal sphincter (LES) tone and incomplete relaxation upon swallowing. The myenteric plexus of the esophagus is deficient at the LES in this condition, and the release of NO and VIP is defective. It can be treated by pneumatic dilation of the sphincter or incision of the esophageal muscle (myotomy). Inhibition of acetylcholine release by injection of botulinum toxin into the LES is also effective and produces relief that lasts for several months.

Gastroesophageal Reflux Disease

- It refers to a condition in which there is a reflux of gastric contents into the esophagus.
- It is due to the incompetence of LES.
- This reflux causes heart burn and esophagitis and can lead to ulceration of esophagus.

Aerophagia

Some people (especially in nervous people) swallow large amounts of air. Some air is regurgitated by bleaching, some of it is absorbed and the rest reaches colon and is expelled as flatus. In some individuals, gas in intestine causes cramps, *borborygmi* (rumbling noises) and abdominal discomfort.

GASTRIC MOVEMENTS

Initiation of Gastric Motility

Basic Electrical Rhythm

Basic electrical rhythm (BER)/Gastric slow waves are initiated due to spontaneous rhythmic fluctuation in membrane potential (between –65 and –45 mV) of smooth muscle of GIT (except in esophagus and proximal portion of stomach). The function of BER is to cordinate peristalitic and other motor activities in GIT. They originate from interstitial cells of Cajal, which has stellate mesenchymal pacemaker cells. (These are situated in the outer circular muscle layer near the myenteric plexus in the stomach and small intestine. In the colon, they are at the submucosal border of circular muscle layer). These cells send long multiple branched processes into the smooth muscles. Slow waves include waves of depolarization and repolarization.

Spike potentials occur superimposed on most of the depolarized portion of BER waves, which will increase the tension of smooth muscle (Fig. 5.14). The depolarization portion of the spike is due to Ca^{2+} influx and repolarization is due to K^+ efflux. The rate of BER varies in different parts of GIT.

- Stomach – 4/min
- Duodenum – 12/min
- Distal ileum – 8/min
- Cecum – 9/min
- Sigmoid colon – 16/min

The degree of spike potential and tension of smooth muscle is increased by ACh released by vagal ending, gastric distension, gastrin. They are inhibited by release of epinephrine when sympathetic nervous system is stimulated, duodenal distension, presence of fat, acidic chyme and hypertonicity.

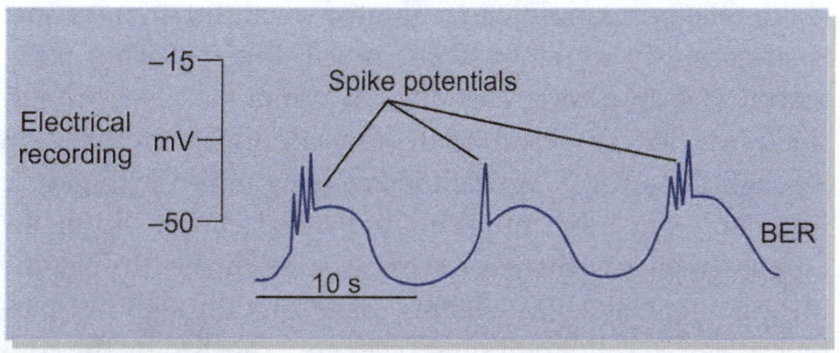

Fig. 5.14: Basic electrical rhythm or gastric slow waves

Motility of Empty Stomach/During Interdigestive Period

Migrating motor complex

During the interdigestive period, the pattern of electrical and motor activity in the gastrointestinal smooth muscles are modified. The cycles of motor activity will be conducted from the stomach to the distal ileum. Each cycle or MMC starts with quiescent period called phase-1. Phase-1 is continuous with period of irregular pattern of electrical and motor activity called phase-2. Then motor activity drives towards aboral end at the rate of 5 cm/sec and they occur at an interval of approx 90 minutes. Migrating motor complex (MMC) clear contents from stomach and small intestine in preparation for next meal. MMC stops with intake of food and with return of other movements like BER and peristalsis.

Hunger Contractions

When stomach is empty for several hours, rhythmic persistant contraction occur in the body of stomach. These are associated with hunger and considered to regulate the appetite. Sometimes, when these contractions occur successively and becomes stronger, fusion of these contractions occur to cause tetanic contraction of smooth muscle which will last for 2 to 3 minutes. These are intense in healthy normal young people but also seen in people whose blood sugar is lower than normal.

The hunger contractions which cause mild pain in the width of stomach is called hunger pangs.

These hunger pangs don't occur unless 12–24 hours of starvation is present. The intensity of hunger pangs increases in 3 to 4 days and then subsides.

Gastric Motility Related to Meals/During Digestive Period

Receptive relaxation

When food enters the stomach, the fundus and the greater curvature relaxes to accommodate the food. Receptive relaxation is a vagovagal reflex initiated by distention of stomach. Its significance is to accommodate the food easily without much increase in pressure (until a capacity of 1.5 L).

Peristalsis

It is a reflex response that is initiated when the stomach wall is stretched by contents of the lumen. Initiated from pacemaker zone in greater curvature of stomach. It is a propulsive wave that propels food in stomach into the duodenum through the pylorus. As the food is being mixed with gastric juice and converted into semifluid called chyme. From the incisura angularis, intense waves carry the chyme through the pylorus in small squirts. Fluids easily pass through but partially digested solid food substances are propelled by the contraction of pyloric sphincter. This action is called retropulsion so that chyme is further mixed with gastric juice. Peristalsis is controlled by BER. Peristalsis in stomach occurs at 3–4 times/min. Peristalsis is due to the integrated activity of the enteric nervous system and it is independent of extrinsic innervation. Local stretch releases serotonin, which activates myenteric plexus.

Gastric Emptying

Duration the chyme remains in the stomach and empties itself into the small intestine is called gastric emptying time. It takes 3–4 hours for emptying of chyme from stomach into small intestine.

Factors influencing are:

- **Consistency of the food:** Liquid food empties faster than solids because solids depends on mixing movements to convert it to semisolid chyme.
- **Gastric factors (promotes emptying)**
  - *Volume of gastric content:* Greater the volume of food in the stomach, greater is the stretching of stomach wall leading to strong peristaltic waves and increased rate of gastric emptying.
  - *Gastrin hormone:* It promote gastric emptying.
  - *Type of food ingested:* Rate of emptying - carbohydrates > proteins > fats.
- **Duodenal factors (inhibit gastrc emptying)**

  Enterogastric reflex (reflex initiated in duodenum).

  Stimulated by:
  - Acidity of chyme
  - Osmolarity of food
  - Partially digested proteins
  - Distention of duodenum with partially digested food.

  Hormones
  - CCK-PZ
  - Secretin
  - Gastroinhibitory peptide (GIP).

Vomiting

It refers to the force full expulsion of contents from stomach and intestine. It is a visceral reflex action integrated in the medulla oblongata. Vomiting can be activated by two ways:

Activation of Vomiting Center

Vomiting center is situated in the reticular formation of medulla. It may be activated directly or through afferents.

- Direct activation of vomiting center in medulla oblongata, e.g. increased intracranial pressure, cerebral tumor, etc. causing projectile vomiting without nausea.
- Afferent impulses activating vomiting center includes:
  - Impulses from GIT due to the irritation of mucosa.
  - Impulses from the vestibular nuclei mediate nausea and vomiting of motion sickness.

- Afferents from higher centers due to emotional stimuli like nauseating smell, sickening sight, noise, etc.
- *Pregnancy:* Due to distention of uterus, it is also associated with nausea.

Due to Activation of Chemoreceptor Trigger Zone

Chemoreceptor trigger zone (CTZ) in medulla contains chemoreceptor cells that initiate vomiting when they are stimulated. These cells are located in the area prostema. This area can be stimulated by:

- Circulating emetic substances in patients with uremia and radiation sickness.
- Circulating emetic agents like morphine, apomorphine, etc.

Vomiting reflex

Vomiting is a reflex act. The sensory impulses for vomiting arise from the irritated or distended part of GI tract or other organs and are transmitted to the vomiting center through vagus and sympathetic afferent fibers. Pathway of vomiting reflex in case of irritation of GI tract is given below (Flowchart 5.3).

Flowchart 5.3: Vomiting reflex

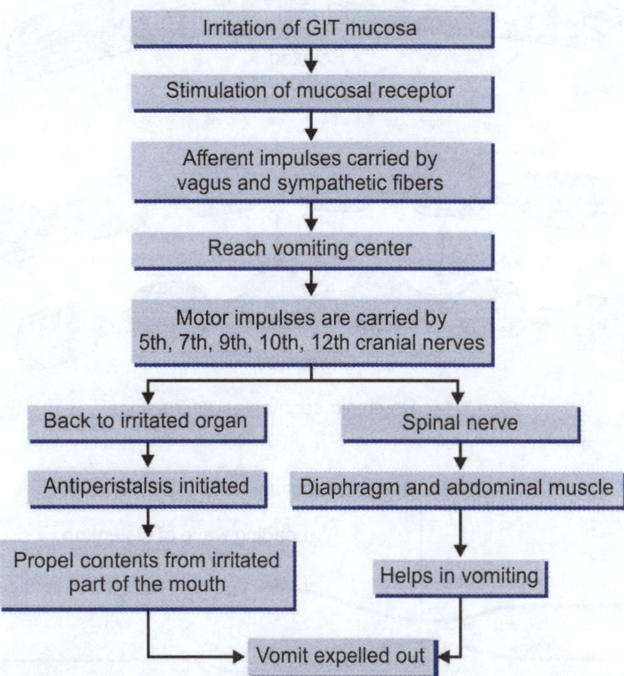

Vomiting act

Vomiting starts with salivation and sensation of nausea. Reverse peristalsis empties material from upper part of SI into the stomach. The glottis closes (to prevent the entry of vomitus into trachea). The breath is held in mid inspiration. The muscles of abdominal wall contracts and thus intra-abdominal pressure is increased. The LES and esophagus relax and the gastric contents are ejected.

Note: Strong involuntary movements in the GI tract start even before actual vomiting and intensify the feeling of vomiting. This condition is called retching. Vomiting occurs few minutes after this.

MOVEMENTS OF SMALL INTESTINE

In the SI there are an average of 12 BER /min in the proximal jejunum, declining to 8/min in the distal ileum.

Motility of SI During Interdigestive Period

Migrating Motor Complexes (MMC)

The MMC pass along the small intestine at regular intervals during inter digestive period. The MMC sweep out the chyme remaining in the SI.

Motility of SI During Digestive Period

They are mixing movements and include:

Pendular Movement

When there is distention of a portion of small intestine with chyme, then there will be lengthening and shortening of smooth muscles of that portion, particularly longitudinal muscles. This will result in contraction and relaxation of those muscles and because of this, chyme move to and fro or side to side movements in pendular fashion. Purpose is to mix chyme with intestinal juice.

Rhythmic Segmentation Contraction

They are ring like contraction that appear at regular intervals along the segments of small intestine when they are loaded with chyme. These ring like contractions then disappear and are replaced by another set of ring like contractions in the segments between the previous contractions (i.e. areas of relaxation become areas of constriction and vice versa) (Fig. 5.15). They move to and fro and increases its exposure to the mucosal surface. They are initiated by focal increase in Ca^{2+} influx with waves of increased Ca^{2+} concentration spread from each focus. It is purely myogenic than neurogenic.

Propulsive Movements

Peristalsis

It is a propulsive wave which propels intestinal contents towards large intestine. Peristaltic contraction involves contraction of a segment behind the bolus and simultaneous relaxation of the segment in front of the bolus (Fig. 5.16). The stimulus for peristalsis is distension. Each contraction travels for a short distance and then dies out. A new contraction is then initiated from a site little distal to the site of origin of the

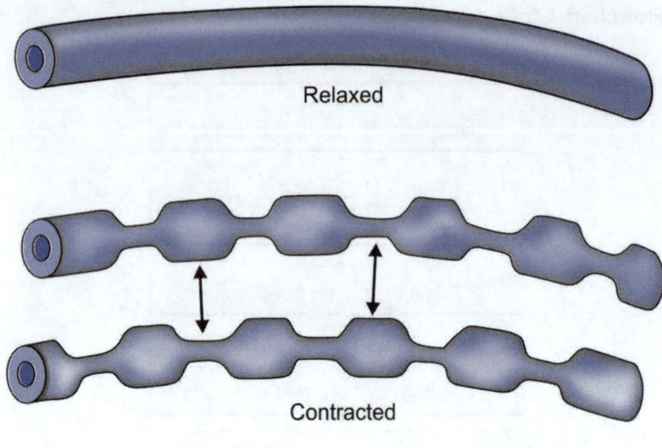

Fig. 5.15: Rhythmic segmental contractions

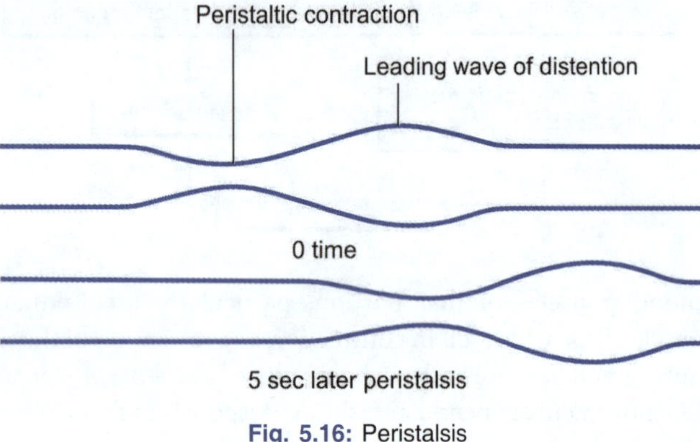

Fig. 5.16: Peristalsis

previous contraction. In this way, a continous peristaltic wave is set in the intestine.

The peristaltic waves always travel from oral end towards the aboral end of intestine. This is called Starlings law of gut.

Peristaltic Rush

Peristaltic rush refers to a very powerful peristaltic waves. It is not seen normally, but they occur when the intestine is obstructed.

Movements of Villi

Movements of villi consists of alternate shortening and elongation of villi. Movements of villi helps in emptying lymph from central lacteal into the lymphatic system. The surface area of villi is increased during elongation. This helps in absorption of digested food particles from the lumen of intestine.

MOVEMENTS OF LARGE INTESTINE/COLON

The movements of the colon are co-ordinated by BER of the colon. The frequency of this wave increases along the colon from about 2/min at ileocecal valve to 6/min at the sigmoid. The movements include:

Haustrations

Large circular constrictions occurs along the colon. At each constriction, about 2.5 cm of circular muscle contracts and this contraction can cause obliteration of lumen in the colon. When circular muscles are contracting, simultaneously the longitudinal muscles called *taenia coli* contracts. Because of the combined action, the portion of the colon wall bulges outward like a sac where fecal matter is present. Each hostile movement reaches peak intensity in 30 seconds and disappears during next 60 seconds and then appears again. This movement helps the fecal matter to be dugged and rolled over so that it is exposed to mucosal surface of colon. Because of this, fluid and electrolytes can be absorbed and it is converted into semisolid form.

Mass Peristalsis

Mass peristalsis are forceful peristaltic contractions that can propel the fecal matter into the rectum from the splenic flexure of colon. It is a propulsive type of movement.

Mass Action Contractions

This is observed only in the colon. There is a simultaneous contraction of the smooth muscles over large confluent areas. These contractions move fecal material from one portion of the colon to another. They also move material into the rectum and rectal distension initiates they defecation reflex.

Defecation

Distention of the rectum with feces initiates reflex contractions of its musculature and the desire to defecate. Defecation involves both voluntary and reflex activity. The urge to defecate 1st occurs when the rectal pressure increases to about 18 mm Hg. When this pressure reaches 55 mm Hg, the external as well as the internal anal sphincter relaxes and there is reflex expulsion of contents of the rectum. Continual dribbling of fecal matter through the anus is prevented by tonic constriction of:

- *Internal anal sphincter (involuntary):* This sphincter relaxes reflexly in response to strech receptors when the rectum is distended. Sympathetic supply is excitatory and parasympathetic is inhibitory.
  - **Sympathetic:** Presacral nerve fibers from T12, L1, L2
  - **Parasympathetic:** Through pelvic splanchnic nerve
- *External anal sphincter (voluntary):* The nerve supply is through pudendal nerve. It is maintained in a state of tonic contraction. Mild-to-moderate distention of the rectum

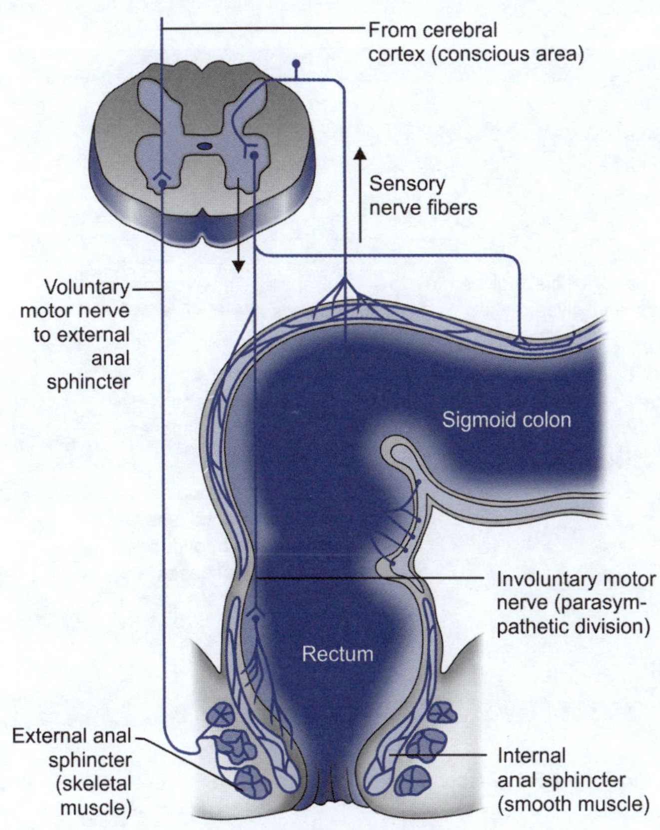

Fig. 5.17: Defecation reflex

increases its force of contraction whereas moderately severe distension of rectum relaxes it.

Defecation Reflexes (Fig. 5.17)

Defecation is a spinal reflex initiated by the distension of the rectum with feces. The distension is sensed by mechanoreceptors located in the wall of rectum. It brings about activation of defecation reflex which leads to a propulsive wave extending from descending colon.

Intrinsic reflex

It is mediated by intrinsic nerve plexus. Distension of rectum initiates afferent signals that spreads through myenteric plexus and initiates mass peristaltic waves in the descending colon, sigmoid colon and rectum that propel fecal matter towards the anus. The intrinsic defecation reflex functioning by itself is relatively weak. To be effective this reflex is fortified by parasympathetic defecation reflex.

Parasympathetic defecation reflex

Distension of rectum by feces causes transmission of afferent impulses through pelvic nerve to sacral segments of spinal cord. This induces reflex parasympathetic discharge (mainly from S2) over the pelvic splanchnic nerve to cause:

- Inhibition of internal anal sphincter.
- When the rectal pressure reaches 55 mm Hg, discharge in the pudendal nerve is inhibited.

  This relaxes external anal sphincter and fecal matter is expelled out.

Note: Gastrocolic and duodenocolic reflexes also aid in defecation.

Voluntary defecation

Before the pressure that relaxes the external anal sphincter is reached (55 mm Hg), voluntary defecation can be initiated by straining. Defecation can be voluntarily facilitated by relaxing the external anal sphincter and contracting the abdominal muscles or inhibited by keeping the external anal sphincter contracted.

Hirschsprung's Disease

Hirschsprung's disease or aganglionic megacolon refers to the congenital absence of ganglion cells in both the myenteric and submucosal plexus. The site of involvement is distal colon. This leads to the blockage of both peristalsis and mass contractions at the aganglionic segment. Therefore, the feces pass the aganglionic region with difficulty and accumulate in large intestine. The disease can be treated by cutting the aganglionic portion of the colon and anastomosing the cut ends.

DIGESTION AND ABSORPTION

Protein, fats and carbohydrates of the food cannot be absorbed as such. Therefore in the gastrointestinal tract proteins, fats and complex carbohydrates are broken down into absorbable units. This process is called digestion. The products of digestion and the vitamins, minerals, and water cross the mucosa and enter the lymph or the blood; a process called absorption. Digestion and absorption of most of the nutrients takes place mostly in the small intestine (Table 5.6).

Carbohydrates

The most abundant carbohydrate in our food is starch. The other forms of carbohydrate which are consumes in substantial amounts are sucrose and lactose.

Digestion

In mouth

Ptyalin (salivary amylase) acts on cooked food. The products of digestion are maltose, maltotriose and α-dextrins.

In stomach

No amylytic enzyme is secreted by stomach. Salivary amylase action continues in the stomach till the highly acidic gastric juice mixes with the food and makes it inactive. The products of digestion are maltose, maltotriose and α-dextrins.

Table 5.6: Digestion of carbohydrate, lipids and protein

	Digestion		
Parts of GIT	**Carbohydrates**	**Lipids**	**Proteins**
Mouth	Saliva contains salivary amylase or ptyalin hydrolyses α(1 → 4) glycoside bonds of starch products formed are α-limit dextrins, maltotriose, and maltose	No enzyme	No enzyme
Stomach	No enzyme for carbohydrate digestion	Gastric lipase—splits triglycerides to fatty acids and glycerol	Pepsins—cleaves peptide bonds
Exocrine pancreas	Pancreatic amylase hydrolyses α(1 → 4) glycoside bonds of starch	• Pancreatic lipase—splits triglycerides to fatty acids and monoglycerides. • Colipase—aids the function of lipase • Cholesteryl ester hydrolase—splits cholesteryl esters to cholesterol	• Trypsin • Chymotrypsin • Carboxypeptidase A • Carboxypeptidases B • Elastase
Intestine	Brush border enzymes namely Disaccharidases like, • Maltase—converts maltose to glucose • Lactase—converts lactose to glucose and galactose • Sucrase—converts sucrose to glucose and fructose • Isomaltase—converts maltose to glucose	No enzyme	• Enteropeptidases • Aminopeptidases • Carboxypeptidases • Endopeptidases • Dipeptidases

In upper SI (duodenum)

Pancreatic amylase acts both on cooked and uncooked food at α 1,4 glycosidic. The products of digestion are maltose, maltotriose and α dextrins.

Lower part of small intestine

Final digestion of carbohydrates takes place here. Enzymes used are brush border enzymes. It includes disaccharidases like maltase, lactase, sucrase. The end product of the digestions are glucose, galactose, and fructose (Flowchart 5.4).

Flowchart 5.4: Carbohydrate digestion

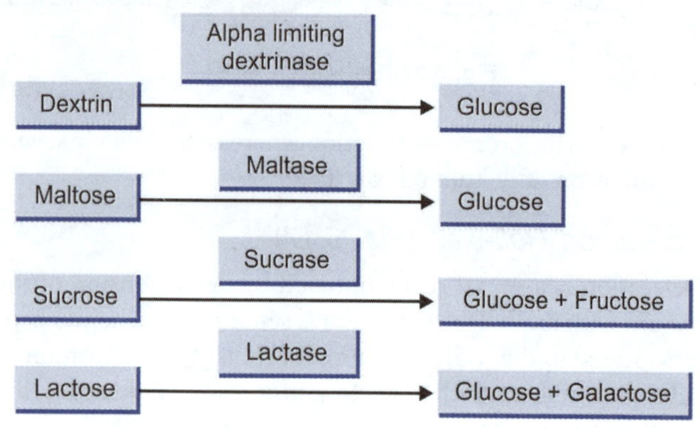

Absorption

Carbohydrates are absorbed in the form of monosaccharides.

- Glucose and galactose—Common Na^+ dependent active transport system.
- Fructose—Facilitated diffusion.
- Pentoses—Simple diffusion.

Glucose and galactose are absorbed by sodium co-transport mechanism. The carrier protein is called SGLT-1 (sodium dependant glucose transporter). Glucose and Na^+ combines with SGLT-1 and is released inside the intestinal cell. The Na^+ is transported into the lateral intercellular spaces and the glucose is transported by glucose transporter 2 (GLUT-2) into the interstitial space and thence to blood capillaries (Fig. 5.18).

Proteins

The digestion of proteins begins in the stomach.

Digestion (Table 5.6)

In mouth

Digestion of proteins does not occur in the mouth, as there are no proteolytic enzymes in the saliva.

In stomach

Pepsin, the important peptic enzyme of the stomach, is secreted by chief cells of gastric glands in an inactive form. Pepsinogen is converted into pepsin by HCl. Pepsin is most active at a pH of 2.0 to 3.0 and is inactive at a pH above 5, therefore HCl secretion by stomach is essential for the digestion of proteins.

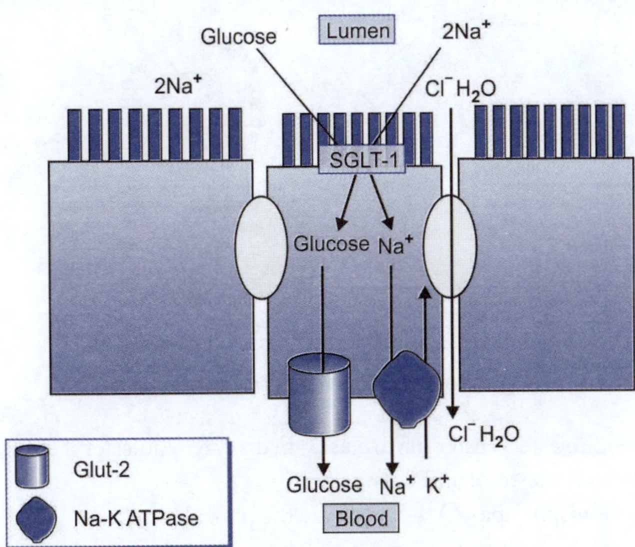

Fig. 5.18: Mechanism of glucose absorption across intestinal epithelium

- Pepsin acts on proteins and splits it into proteoses, peptones and polypeptides. This splitting of proteins occurs as a result of hydrolysis at the peptide linkages between amino acids.
- Gelatinase liquefies gelatin.
- Rennin is absent in adult human.
- Optimum pH in stomach is 1.6–3.2.

In small intestine

Most protein digestion occurs in the upper small intestine, in the duodenum and jejunum, under the influence of proteolytic enzymes from pancreatic secretion. Immediately on entering the small intestine from the stomach, the partial breakdown products of the protein foods are attacked by major proteolytic pancreatic enzymes: trypsin, chymotrypsin, carboxypolypeptidase and proelastase.

- Trypsin, chymotrypsin and elastase ***(endopeptidases)*** act on interior of peptide chain and form small peptides. Elastase digests elastin fibers.
- Carboxy peptidases ***(exopeptidases)*** act on terminal amino acids and produce small peptidases and amino acids.
- Only a small percentage of the proteins are digested all the way to their constituent amino acids by the pancreatic juices. Most remain as dipeptides and tripeptides.

The last digestive stage of the proteins in the intestinal lumen is achieved by the enterocytes that line the villi of the small intestine, mainly in the duodenum and jejunum. These cells have a brush border that consists of hundreds of microvilli projecting from the surface of each cell. In the membrane of each of these microvilli, there are multiple peptidases that protrude through the membranes to the exterior, where they come in contact with the intestinal fluids.

Two types of peptidase enzymes are especially important, aminopolypeptidase and several dipeptidases. They succeed in splitting the remaining larger polypeptides into tripeptides and dipeptides and a few into amino acids. Both the amino acids plus the dipeptides and tripeptides are easily transported through the microvillar membrane to the interior of the enterocyte.

Finally, inside the cytosol of the enterocyte there are intracellular peptidases that are specific for the remaining types of linkages between amino acids. Within minutes, virtually all the last dipeptides and tripeptides are digested to the final stage to form single amino acids. Thus, the final digestion into amino acids occurs in three locations: (1) Intestinal lumen, (2) Brush border, (3) Cytoplasm of enterocyte.

Digestion of Nucleic Acids

Nucleic acids are split into nucleotides in the intestine by the pancreatic nucleases and the nucleotides are split into the nucleosides and phosphoric acid by enzymes that appear to be located on the luminal surfaces of the mucosal cells. The nucleosides are then split into their constituent sugar, purine and pyrimidine bases. The bases are absorbed by active transport.

Transport and Absorption

Most proteins after digestion are absorbed through the luminal membranes of the intestinal epithelial cells in the form of dipeptides, tripeptides and a few free amino acids. At least seven different systems transport amino acids into enterocyte. This multiplicity of transport proteins is required because of the diverse binding properties of different amino acids and peptides. Five of these require Na^+ and co-transport amino acids and Na^+ in a fashion similar to the co-transport of Na^+ and glucose. Two of these five also require Cl^-. In two systems, transport is independent of Na^+. Dipeptides and tripeptides are transported into the enterocyte by a system that requires H^+ instead of Na^+.

In the enterocytes, amino acids released from the peptides by intracellular hydrolysis plus the amino acids absorbed from the intestinal lumen and brush border are transported out of the enterocytes along their basolateral borders by five transport systems. Two of these systems are dependent on Na^+, and three are not. From there via, hepatic portal blood they reach the liver and general circulation. Significant amounts of small peptides also enter the portal blood.

Fats

Fat digestion essentially begins in the duodenum with entry of pancreatic and biliary secretions.

Digestion (Table 5.6)

In mouth

Lingual lipase is secreted by Ebener's gland on the dorsal surface of tongue. But it has no action in the mouth.

In stomach

Lingual lipase is active in stomach (action starts in acidic pH).
- Digests 30% of dietary triglyceride.
- Gastric lipase is secreted in stomach, but has little importance except in pancreatic insufficiency.

In small intestine

Most of the fat digestion begins in the duodenum, pancreatic lipase being one of the most important enzymes involved. The digestion of fat includes three steps:
1. Emulsification of fat by bile salts.
2. Hydrolysis of fat by pancreatic and enteric lipolytic enzymes.
3. Acceleration of fat digestion by micelle formation.

Emulsification of Fat by Bile Salts

The first step in fat digestion is physically to break the fat globules into very small sizes so that the water-soluble digestive enzymes can act on the globule surfaces. This process is called emulsification of the fat (Fig. 5.19).

Emulsification of fat mostly occurs in the duodenum under the influence of bile. Bile contains large quantity of bile salts as well as the phospholipid lecithin. Both of these, but especially the lecithin, are extremely important for emulsification of the fat. The polar parts of the bile salts and lecithin molecules are highly soluble in water, whereas the lipophilic non polar portions of their molecules are highly soluble in fat. Therefore, the fat-soluble portions of these liver secretions dissolve in the surface layer of the fat globules, with the polar portions projecting. The polar projections, in turn, are soluble in the surrounding watery fluids, which greatly decreases the surface tension of the fat and makes it soluble as well.

With the lowered surface tension of fats, segmentation movements of small intestine break up large fat globules into fine droplets. The surface area available for action of lipase is increased many thousand times by the emulsification of fat.

Hydrolysis of Fat by Pancreatic and Enteric Lipolytic Enzymes

Pancreatic lipolytic enzymes

- Pancreatic lipase—hydrolyzes triglycerides (triglycerides $\rightarrow$ free fatty acids + 2 monoglycerides).
- Colipase-binds with pancreatic lipase and increases its lipolytic activity.
- Bile salt activated lipase—catalyzes the hydrolysis of cholesterol esters, esters of fat soluble vitamins, phospholipids and triglycerides.

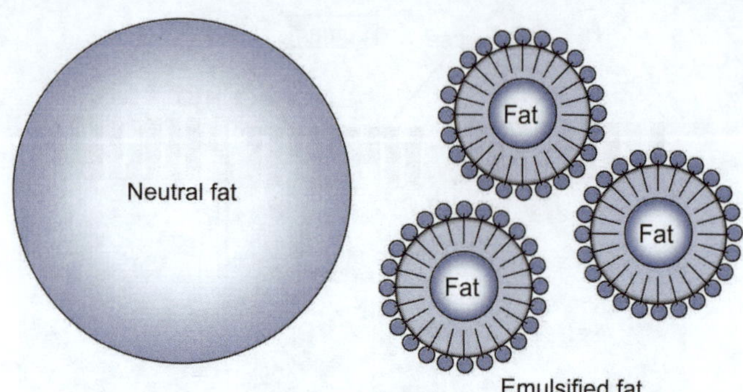

Fig. 5.19: Emulsification of fats by bile salts

- Cholesteryl ester hrydrolase—hydrolyzes cholesteryl esters to cholesterol and fatty acids.
- Phospholipase A_2—hydrolyze the phospholipids.

Enteric lipase

The enterocytes of the small intestine contain small amount of lipase, known as enteric lipase, but this is usually not needed.

Acceleration of Fat Digestion by Micelle Formation

The hydrolysis of triglycerides is a highly reversible process; therefore, accumulation of monoglycerides and free fatty acids in the vicinity of digesting fats quickly blocks further digestion. But the bile salts play the additional important role of removing the monoglycerides and free fatty acids from the vicinity of the digesting fat globules almost as rapidly as these end products of digestion are formed.

Bile salts, when in high concentration (the concentration is called critical micellar concentration), have the tendency to form micelles. They are small spherical, cylindrical globules 3 to 6 nanometers in diameter composed of 20 to 40 molecules of bile salt in such a way that their lipid soluble non polar ends are in the central fat globule and water soluble polar ends fan out to form the outer covering of micelle. The monoglycerides and fatty acids released from the digestion of fat are quickly incorporated into the central fatty portions of micelles forming, what is known as mixed micelles (Fig. 5.20). In this way bile salts accelerate the fat digestion by allowing the lipolytic action to continue.

The bile salt micelles also act as a transport medium to carry the monoglycerides and free fatty acids, both of which would otherwise be relatively insoluble, to the brush borders of the intestinal epithelial cells. There the monoglycerides and free fatty acids are absorbed into the blood, but the bile salts themselves are released back into the chyme to be used again and again.

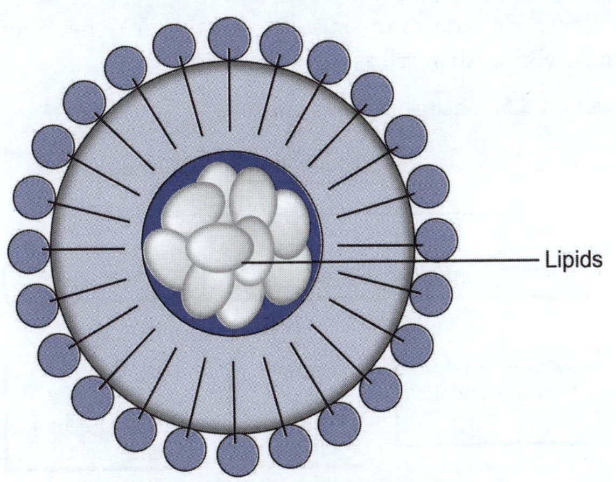

Fig. 5.20: Mixed micelle

Absorption of Fat

Normally though lipids are thought to enter the enterocyte by passive diffusion, evidences are there regarding the involvement of carriers. In the enterocytes, the fate of fatty acids is as follows:

- Fatty acids with less than 10 to 12 carbon atoms are water soluble and they pass through the enterocyte unmodified and are actively transported into the portal blood. They circulate as free (unesterified) fatty acids.
- Fatty acids with more than 10 to 12 carbon atoms are re-esterified into triglycerides. The absorbed cholesterol is also esterified. Triglycerides and cholesteryl esters are then coated with a layer of proteins, cholesterol, phospholipids to form chylomicrons. They leave the cells and enter lymphatics [In mucosal cells, triglycerides are formed from 2-monoglycerides (in smooth ER). Some are formed from glycerophosphate (product of glucose catabolism). Glycerophospholipids formed from glycerophosphates (in rough ER) also participate in chylomicron formation] (Fig. 5.21).
- Finished chylomicrons are extruded by exocytosis from the basal or lateral aspects of the cell. The free fatty acids are diffused into portal blood while the lipids from chylomicrons are diffused into lacteal and then through the thoracic duct into circulation.
- Absorption of long chain fatty acids is greatest in the upper part of the small intestine, but appreciable amounts are also absorbed in the ileum.

Note: Short chain fatty acids and medium chain fatty acids are directly absorbed from the intestinal lumen into the portal vein and is taken to the liver. Short chain fatty acids have 2 to 5 carbon atoms. They are formed by the action of colonic bacteria on complex carbohydrates, resistant starches and other components of the dietary fibers. Thus, short chain fatty acid is produced in the colon and absorbed from it.

Dietary Fibers (Roughage or Ruffage)

Dietary fiber consists of unabsorbable cell wall and other constituents of vegetable food like cellulose, lignin, hemicellulose, gums, pectins, alginates and other polysaccharides. In herbivorous animals, intestinal microorganism breakdown these polysaccharides into acetate, propionate and butyrate. These polysaccharides contain beta-glycosidic linkages. Therefore, they cannot be digested by alpha-amylase present in human saliva and pancreatic juice because alpha-amylase breaks alpha-glycosidic bond (especially 1–4 alpha linkage). So, dietary fibers are not digested or hydrolyzed but are fermented by colonic bacteria except for lignin, which is neither digested nor fermented by intestinal microorganisms. Therefore, ingested cellulose passes out unchanged and substances which are enclosed in cellulose wall escape digestion and absorption. Dietary fiber absorbes water in the intestine, swells, increase bulk of stool by increasing water content of feces and soften it, decreases transit time by facilitating colonic transit. The presence of fiber shortens the transit times and increases the stool bulk.

Physiological Significance of Dietary Fibers

- Increased bulk of this undigested residue stimulates intestinal peristalsis which in turn increases passage of food through intestine.
- Increased cellulose content of food increases the bulk of feces and thus high fiber content has role in prevention and treatment of constipation.

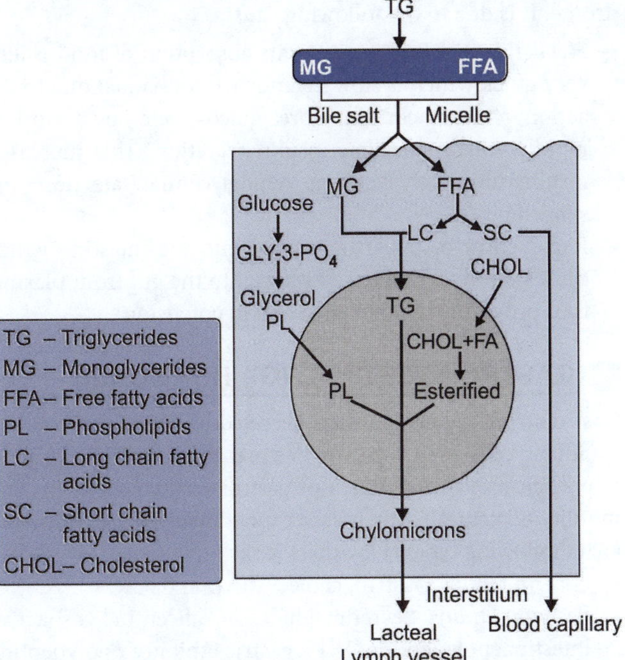

Fig. 5.21: Intraluminal events during fat digestion and absorption

- Reduces efficacy of absorption of digested food stuffs by forming mechanical barrier between nutrients and absorptive surfaces, thus reduces sudden increase in blood glucose level after a meal (postprandial hyperglycemia) This also reduces requirements of insulin during postprandial phase. This is why a high fiber diet helps in the prevention and treatment of an individual from diabetes mellitus.
- Decreases blood cholestrol level by binding the bile salts. Binding of bile salt by dietary fibers → increases excretion of bile salts in feces → decreased amount of bile salt available for enterohepatic circulation → increases synthesis of fresh bile salt in the liver → increases cholesterol utilization → decreases the blood cholesterol; thus help to control metabolic disorders associated with over nutrition such as obesity, atherosclerosis, hypercholesterolemia and diabetes mellitus.
- Decreases incidence of colon cancer by:
  - Dilution of carcinogens by the water held by dietary fibers.
  - Decreases duration of contact between carcinogen and mucous membrane of colon (as fibers increases colon mobility).
  - Carcinogen binds to dietary fibers.

Note

Dumping syndrome: A condition characterized by development of weakness, dizziness and sweating after meals. It may be seen in patients who have undergone complete removal of stomach or gastrojejunostomy. In these cases, food enters directly and rapidly into the intestine and leads to this syndrome. It is due to the following causes:

- *Hypoglycemia:* In these patients absorption of food is also very quick which is slow in a normal individual due to the action of stomach. Therefore, glucose, etc. are absorbed rapidly which stimulate insulin secretion. This increased insulin ultimately leads to hypoglycemia (late dumping syndrome).
- Rapid entry of hypertonic meal into the intestine which causes rapid movement of water into the gut from plasma, thus providing hypovolemia and hypotension.

GASTROINTESTINAL (GI) HORMONES

Gastrointestinal hormones are secreted by nerve endings and glandular cells in the gastrointestinal mucosa. They play an important role in regulation of gastrointestinal secretion and motility. Structurally and to lesser functionally, these hormones are of following types (Flowchart 5.5):

- *Gastrin family:* Gastrin, cholecystokinin (CCK)
- *Secretin family:* Secretin, glucagon, glicentin, vasoactive intestinal polypeptide (VIP), gastric inhibitory polypeptide (GIP)
- *Others:* Somatostatin, motilin, peptide YY, neurotensin, guanylin, gastrin releasing polypeptide.

Flowchart 5.5: Gastrointestinal hormones

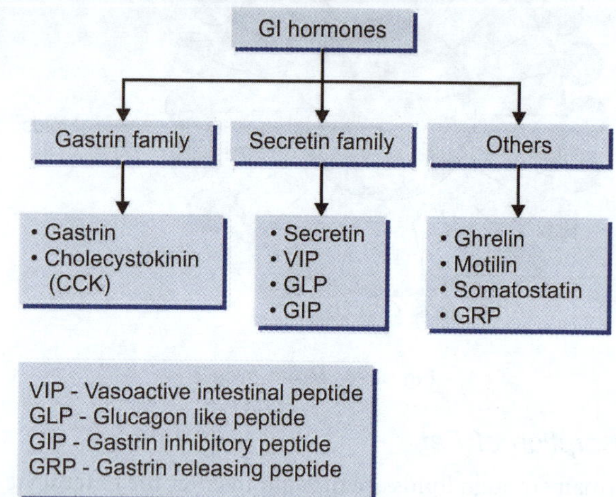

Gastrin

It is a GI hormone produced by G cells located in the pyloric glands. Most known powerful stimulant of HCl secretion. It reaches the stomach through arterial circulation (it is secreted into venous blood, enters right heart, then reaches pulmonary circulation, passes to left side of heart and then to aorta and finally through gastric vessels it reaches stomach). Presence of products of protein digestion in the stomach acts on G cells to release gastrin. It stimulates secretory activity of parietal cell and chief cells.

Actions

- Gastrin stimulates the secretion of histamine from ECL cells. Histamine stimulates HCl secretion and this is the principal way by which gastrin stimulates acid secretion.
- Gastrin also stimulate HCl secretion by acting on the gastrin receptors in the parietal cell. This increases intracellular Ca^{2+}.
- To a lesser extent it stimulates chief cells to secrete pepsin.
- Stimulates insulin secretion after a protein meal.
- Stimulation of the growth of the mucosa of the stomach, small and large intestine.

Stimuli that increase gastrin secretion

Luminal

- Peptides and amino acids
- Distention.

Neural

Increased vagal discharge via gastrin releasing peptide (GRP) rather than ACh

Blood borne
- Calcium
- Epinephrine

Stimuli that inhibit gastric secretion
Luminal
- Acid
- Somastatin

Blood borne
- Secretin
- GIP
- VIP
- Glucogen
- Calcitonin

Clinical Box

Gastrin release though vagally mediated is not blocked by atropine. This is because, the transmitter secreted by the postganglionic vagal fibers that innervate the gastrin cells is GRP and not ACh.

CCK-PZ

It is a polypeptide containing 33 amino acids with 5 terminal amino acids as those of gastrin, which account for some stimulant properties that they have in common. It is produced by granular mucosal cells of upper part of small intestine, duodenum and jejunum.

Actions

- The hormone causes contraction of gallbladder to release bile and causes secretion of pancreatic juice rich in enzymes by causing discharge of zymogen granules from the pancreatic acinar cells and the effect is mediated by activation of phospholipase C.
- It also increases the secretion of enterokinase (enteropeptidase) from the duodenum and may also increase the motility of small and large intestine.
- It produces trophic effect (i.e. increased growth) on pancreas.
- It is found in neurons in the brain where it helps in the regulation of food intake and is related to the production of anxiety and analgesia.

Secretin

It was the first hormone discovered. It is a polypeptide and consists of 27 amino acids. It is produced by argentaffin cells in the crypts of the mucosa of upper part of small intestine, duodenum and jejunum. It is secreted as prosecetin which gets converted by gastric HCl and salts of fatty acids (soap) into secretin (active).

Actions

- It acts on the duct cells of pancreas to produce a flow of alkaline watery pancreatic juice, but poor in enzymes. The effect is mediated by increase in intracellular cAMP. As volume of pancreatic secretion increases, its Cl^- concentration falls and HCO_3^- concentration rises. Although, HCO_3^- are secreted in small ducts, it is reabsorbed in the large ducts in exchange for Cl^-. The magnitude of the exchange is inversely proportional to the rate of flow.
- It also stimulates bile secretion and potentiates the effect of CCK-PZ on the pancreas.
- It along with CCK-PZ causes contraction of pyloric sphincter and delays gastric emptying and thus, preventing the efflux of duodenal contents into the stomach.

Note: Secretin and CCK-PZ potentiates the action of other. Factors which increase secretin and CCK-PZ release:
- Acid in the duodenum causes more of secretin liberation and feeble stimulation of CCK-PZ.
- Products of carbohydrates, fats and protein digestion in small intestine, cause more of CCK-PZ release.

Motilin

Motilin is a polypeptide containing 22 amino acid residues that is secreted by 'M' cells of the duodenal mucosa. It is also secreted by enterochromaffin cells of the intestine. Motilin causes contraction of GI smooth muscle and increases intestinal motility. It seems to be involved in regulation of gastrointestinal motility during the interdigestive phase. Conversely, when a meal is ingested, secretion of motilin is suppressed until digestion and absorption are complete.

Other GIT Hormones

- Gastric inhibitory polypeptide (GIP): It is a glucose dependent insulinotropic polypeptide
- Vasoactive intestinal peptide (VIP)
- Glucagon
- Glucagon like immunoreactivity (GLI), Glicentin
- Motilin
- Neurotensin
- Substance P
- Gastrin releasing peptide (GRP)
- Somatostatin
- Ghrelin

CLINICAL QUESTIONS

1. **A 45-year-old executive who was a heavy smoker, complained of burning pain in the abdomen, 2 to 3 hours after a meal, which was relieved by taking a glass of cold milk.**
   a. What is the condition?
   b. What is the cause?
   c. What is the physiological basis of treatment?
2. **A patient came to the doctor with the complaints of mild fever, nausea and vomiting. On examination icterus was present, liver was palpable-one finger, soft and tender.**
   a. Identify the condition?
   b. Which investigations will you do?
3. **A fat, fertile, female aged 50 years came with the complaints of colicky pain in the abdomen and fever. Examination revealed icterus. Conjugated bilirubin levels were elevated.**
   a. Identify the condition.
   b. Which other investigations would you advice to confirm your diagnosis?
   c. Why are the levels of conjugated bilirubin elevated?
4. **A cachexia person came to the clinic with complaints of burning pain in the epigastric region immediately after taking meals.**
   a. Identify the condition.
   b. Give physiological basis of treatment.

Answers for Clinical Questions are given in the Appendix

CHAPTER

6

Renal Physiology

INTRODUCTION

Renal system consists of a pair of kidneys, ureters, urinary bladder and urethra.

The structural and functional unit of kidney is called nephron. Each kidney contains approximately 1–1.3 million nephron. Each kidney has two distinct zone: the outer cortex and the inner medulla. The medulla comprises renal pyramids. The medullary pyramid shows striations, which extend some distance upward in the cortex where they are called the medullary rays. The medulla is further subdivided into outer and inner strips; and inner medulla (papillary zone). Thus from superficial to deep, kidney shows following layer: cortical layer (cortex), medullary rays, outer medullar stripe, inner medullar stripe, inner medulla (papillary zone). The apex of medullary pyramid is called papillae. The tip of papilla has visible pores which are the opening of the collecting ducts into the minor calyx (Fig. 6.1).

Functions of Kidney

1. *Excretory:* Formation of urine by three mechanisms: Glomerular filtration, tubular reabsorption, tubular secretion. Excretion of urea, uric acid, creatinine, etc.

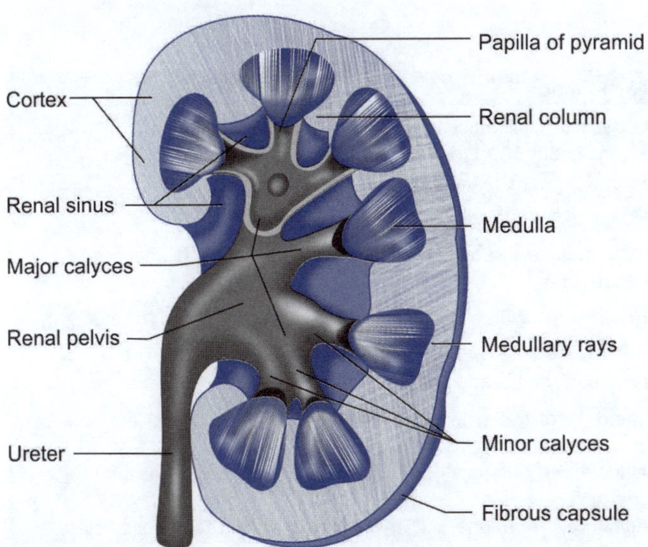

Fig. 6.1: Cross-section of kidney

2. *Homeostatic:* It maintains constant internal environment by maintaining water and electrolyte balance and through buffering actions.
3. *Endocrine*
   - Renin secretion during renal ischemia
   - Release of renal erythropoietic factor during hypoxia
   - Release of local hormones, kininogens, etc. to regulate renal blood flow.
4. Formation of vitamin D_3.
5. Regulation of normal arterial blood pressure.
6. Hydroxylation of 25-hydroxycholecalciferol to 1, 25 dihydroxycholecalciferol (active form of vitamin D).

NEPHRON

The functional unit of kidney are nephrons (1.3 millions/kidney). Each nephron is formed by two parts—renal corpuscle and renal tubules (Fig. 6.2 and Table 6.1).

Renal Corpuscle

It is formed by two portions:

1. *Glomerulus (200 μm diameter):* Glomerulus is a tuft of capillaries enclosed by Bowman's capsule. Blood enters glomerulus through afferent arteriole and leaves through an efferent arteriole.
2. *Bowman's capsule:* Dilated portion of a nephron.

Renal Tubules

1. *Proximal convoluted tubule (PCT):* Parts-Pars convoluta (convoluted portion) and Pars recta (straight portion). Its wall is made up of single layer of cells whose luminal edges have striate brush border due to the presence of microvilli. This increases surface area for resorption. Tubular cells are rich in mitochondria to support active transport processes. The tubular cells are connected by tight junctions at their luminal edges, but there is space between the cells along the rest of their lateral borders called as lateral intercellular spaces.
2. *Loop of Henle:* It consists of a descending and ascending limb. The descending portion of loop and proximal portion of the ascending limb is made up of thin and permeable

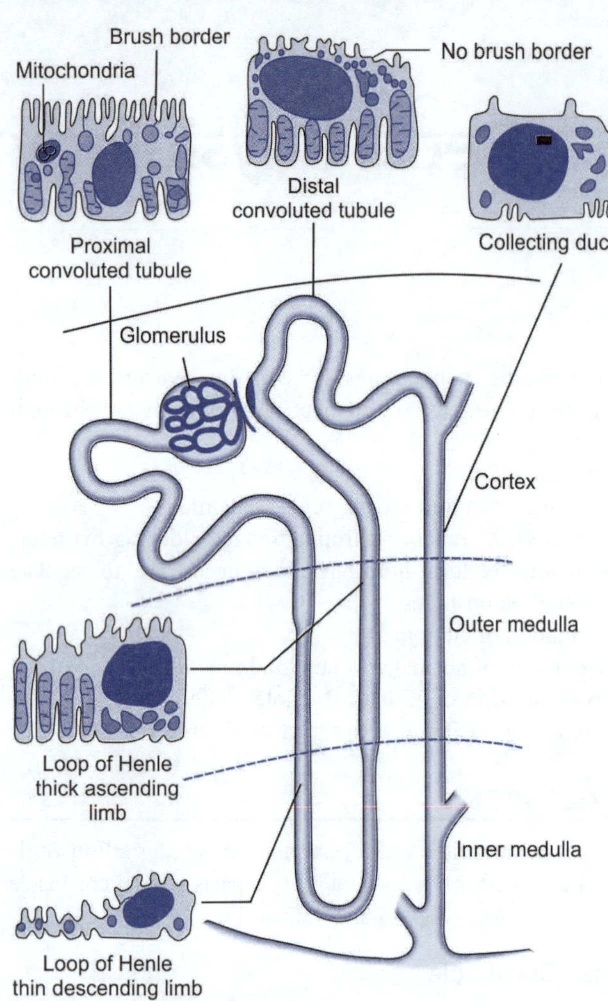

Fig. 6.2: Histology of a typical nephron

cells, whereas the thick portion of ascending limb is made up of thick cells containing many mitochondria.

3. *Distal convoluted tubule (DCT):* Few microvilli present; no distinct brush border.
4. *Collecting duct:* The distal convoluted tubule opens into collecting duct. Epithelium is made up of principal cells (P cells) and intercalated cells (I cells). P cells are involved in Na^+ reabsorption and vasopressin stimulated water reabsorption. I cells are concerned with acid excretion and HCO_3^-.

Based on the situation of renal corpuscle, nephrons are classified as cortical and juxtamedullary nephrons (Table 6.2).

Ultrastructure of Glomerular Membrane

Ultrastructure of glomerular membrane refers to the membrane that separates blood of glomerular capillaries from the glomerular filtrate in the Bowman's capsule. It consists of three layers (Fig. 6.3).

Capillary Endothelium

It is perforated with thousands of small pores called fenestrae (pores have diameter of 70–90 nm). Endothelial cells have fixed negative charges that hinder the passage of plasma proteins (negatively charged).

Basement Membrane

It consists of meshwork of collagen and proteoglycan fibrillae that have large spaces through which water and small solutes are permeable. They effectively prevent filtration of plasma proteins because of strong negative charges associated with proteoglycans.

Table 6.1: Parts of a nephron

Parts of a nephron	Lining epithelium	Major function
Glomerulus	Simple squamous	• Is the site of filtration • Filters about 180 L/day
Proximal convoluted tubule	Cuboidal cells with brush border	• Reabsorbs about 2/3rd of the filtered water, sodium, and chloride • Reabsorbs 100% glucose and amino acids
Descending limb of loop of Henle (thin)	Simple squamous	• Impermeable to solutes but permeable to water (Concentrating segment)
Ascending limb of loop of Henle (thick)	Cuboidal epithelium	Permeable to solutes but impermeable to water (Diluting segment)
Distal convoluted tubule	Cuboidal epithelium	• Reabsorb some additional salt and water (5%)
Collecting tubule	Cuboidal epithelium	• Made up of two types of cell: principal cells (P cells) and intercalated cells (I cells) • Aldosterone enhances sodium reabsorption and potassium secretion here • Antidiuretic hormone (ADH) enhances water reabsorption here

Table 6.2: Differences between cortical and juxtamedullary nephron

Cortical nephron (85%)	Juxtamedullary nephrone (15%)
Occupies 2/3rd of cortex and a very small portion of medulla	Occupies 1/3rd of cortex and most other parts in medulla
Loop of Henle is short	Loop of Henle is long
Descending limb of loop of Henle contains a thin segment where as ascending limb contain thin and thick segment	Both descending and ascending limb contains thin segment
Efferent arteriole continues as peritubular capillaries	Efferent arteriole continues as vasa recta
Associated with formation of urine	Associated with concentration of urine
Efferent arteriole is smaller than afferent	Efferent arteriole has same diameter as afferent

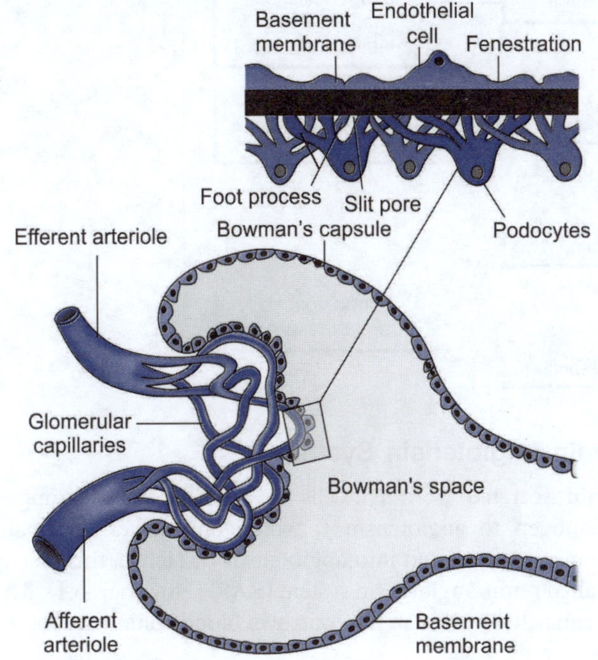

Fig. 6.3: Filtering membrane in renal corpuscle

Layer of Epithelial Cells

Visceral epithelium of Bowman's capsule is constituting the epithelial layer. It is formed of special cells called podocytes. They have foot-like processes (pseudopodia) towards the basement membrane that encircle the outer surface of the capillaries. The foot processes are separated by gaps called slit pores (25 nm wide) through which the glomerular filtrate moves. The epithelial cells, which also have negative charges provide additional restriction to movement of plasma proteins.

Net diameter of a pore in glomerular membrane is 8 nm. The pore allows passage of neutral substances up to 4 nm. Around 4 to 8 nm particles can pass based on charge and size. For example, albumin (6 nm) due to its negative charge is not filtered through the glomerular membrane. Particles greater than 8 nm are completely withheld.

Clinical Note

- The negativity of epithelial cells are lost in some renal diseases. Then negatively charged substances like albumin is filtered. Hence proteinuria occurs.
- Nephrotic syndrome is characterized by loss of podocyte structure, abnormal or absent slit diaphragms, and a resultant increase in permeability of the glomerular capillaries to proteins. Proteins are filtered out and lost in the urine (proteinuria).

JUXTAGLOMERULAR APPARATUS

Juxtaglomerular apparatus (JGA) is a complex specialized structure found at the region where the tubule lies in contact with its own glomerulus forming specialized cells of varying functions.

The JGA plays an important role in the feedback mechanism called tubuloglomerular feedback mechanism which regulates glomerular filtration rate and blood flow through glomerular capillaries.

Specialized cells are (Fig. 6.4):

1. *Macula densa:* Macula densa are tightly packed specialized group of epithelial cells in the distal tubules that comes in

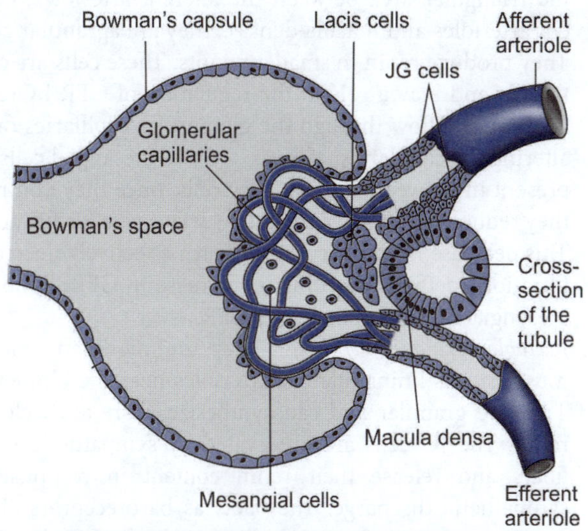

Fig. 6.4: Structure of juxtaglomerular apparatus

Flowchart 6.1: Release and actions of Renin-Angiotensin System

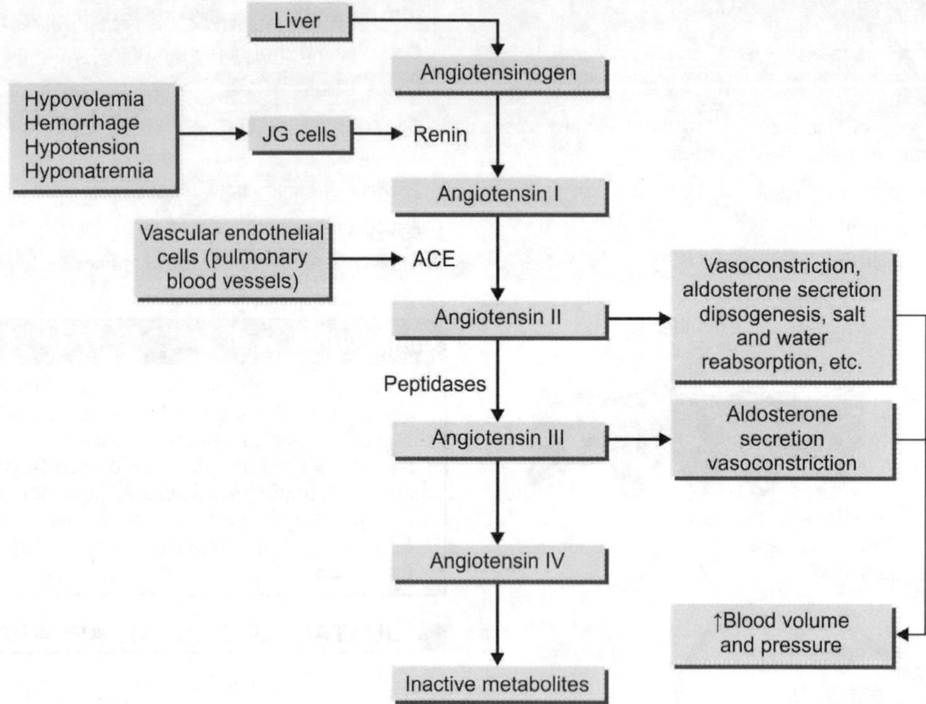

contact with afferent and efferent arterioles of its own glomerules. These cells can detect the Na^+ load in the filtrate and can regulate secretion of renin. It is likely that macula densa mediated renin secretion helps to maintain systemic arterial pressure under conditions of reduced vascular volume.

2. *Lacis cell/Extraglomerular mesangial cells:* Lacis cells are mesangial cells located outside the glomerulus (found in the triangular area between the afferent arterioles, efferent arterioles and macula densa). They are agranular cells. They produce renin in small amounts. These cells are contractile and play a role in the regulation of GFR by regulating blood flow through the glomerular capillaries or by altering the capillary surface area. Since mesangial cells are present in between two capillary cells, once they contract, they reduce the effective capillary surface area for filtration. This decrease in capillary surface area effectively decreases filtration coefficient leading to decrease in GFR. Similarly mesangial relaxation increases GFR.
3. *Juxtaglomerular (JG) Cells:* They are modified smooth muscles cells lining afferent arterioles near the glomeruli. They are granular and can synthesize, store and releases renin. The JG cells are innervated by sympathetic nerve fibers and release their renin content in response to sympathetic discharge. They acts as baroreceptors. They monitor renal perfusion pressure and are stimulated by hypovolemia or decreased renal perfusion pressure.

Renin-Angiotensin System

Renin secreted from JG cells of kidneys activates angiotensinogen to angiotensin I, which on further enzymatic action gets converted into angiotensin II. Hence, this system is called renin-angiotensin system (RAS) (Flowchart 6.1). RAS is primarily involved in the control of blood volume and blood pressure.

Cells in the afferent arterioles (JG cells) are the sites of synthesis, storage and release of the proteolytic enzyme renin.

Stimulants for Renin Secretion

1. Fall in arterial BP.
2. Reduction in ECF volume.
3. Increased sympathetic activity.
4. Decreased load of Na^+ and Cl^- in macula densa.
5. Prostaglandins.

Inhibitors for Renin Secretion

1. Increased load of Na^+ and Cl^- in macula densa.
2. Increased afferent arteriolar pressure.
3. Angiotensin II (via negative feedback).
4. Vasopressin.

Renin alone does not have a physiological function, it functions solely as a proteolytic enzyme. Its substrate is a circulating protein angiotensinogen which is produced by the liver. Angiotensinogen is cleaved by renin to yield a decapeptide, angiotensin I. Angiotensin I also has no physiological function, and it is further cleaved to an octapeptide, angiotensin II by a converting enzyme (ACE) secreted from the lungs. Various peptidases converts angiotensin II to angiotensin III (heptapeptide) and angiotensin IV (hexapeptide).

Actions of Angiotensin II

1. Causes vasoconstriction leading to increase in arterial BP.
2. Increases BP indirectly by increasing release of norepinephrine from postganglionic sympathetic fibers (norepinephrine is a vasoconstrictor).
3. Acts directly on adrenal cortex to increase the secretion of aldosterone (aldosterone increases retention of Na).
4. It acts on brain to decrease response of baroreceptor reflex.
5. It increases water intake by stimulating thirst center.
6. It increase the secretion of ADH and ACTH.

Angiotensin III has pressor activity and aldosterone stimulating activity.

Clinical Note

Angiotensin converting enzyme inhibitors are drugs (e.g. ramipril) used in the treatment of hypertension and congestive cardiac failure. They inhibits the formation of angiotensin II and thus decrease Na+ and water retention.

RENAL CIRCULATION

The renal artery enters the kidney through the hilum and then branches progressively to form the interlobar arteries, arcuate arteries, interlobular arteries and finally afferent arterioles. Afferent arteriole divides into network of capillaries to form glomerulus. Glomerular capillaries reunite to form efferent arteriole. Efferent arteriole divides to form a second capillary network, the peritubular capillaries that surrounds the renal tubules. The renal circulation is unique in having two capillary beds, the glomerulus (arise from afferent arteriole) and peritubular capillaries (arise from efferent arteriole). In the cortical nephrons, efferent arteriole drains into peritubular capillaries, whereas in juxtamedullary nephrons, efferent arteriole not only drains into peritubular capillaries but also in vasa recta. Vasa recta are long and straight capillaries that follow the course of the loop of Henle. Normal renal blood flow is 1100 ml/min, i.e. 22% of cardiac output.

Special Features of Renal Circulation

1. Renal blood flow is maximum when compared to other circulations in the body, i.e. 25% of total cardiac output.
2. *Double portal system:* Two types of blood vessels are present. They are glomerular capillaries (for filtration) and peritubular capillaries (for reabsorption).
3. *Regional blood flow:* There is a variation in the blood flow through various parts of the kidney, i.e. flow to cortex is greater than flow to medulla. Renal cortex has 4–5 ml/g/min where as medulla has only 1–2 ml/g/min (outer) and 0.3 ml/g/min (inner).
4. *O_2 consumption:* Kidney is the 2nd highest O_2 consumer next to heart, i.e. 6 ml/100g/min.
5. *Renal arterial blood pressure:* Highest as it originates directly from abdominal aorta.
6. *Vasa recta:* Presence of vasa recta, the longest capillary, for concentrating the urine.
7. Shows autoregulation.

Why blood flow in cortex is greater than in medulla?

Cortex contains major components of the nephron. In inner medulla, long vasa recta and high interstitial osmotic pressure causes slower blood flow. This is one of the reason for production of hypertonic urine.

Renal Blood Vessels

The following is the order of flow of blood in the kidney.

Renal artery → interlobar artery → arcuate artery → interlobular artery → afferent arterioles → glomerular capillaries → efferent arterioles → stellate vein → interlobular vein arcuate vein → interlobar vein → renal vein (Fig. 6.5).

Increased blood flow to kidney increases the delivery of blood to glomerulus that promotes filtration and conversely decreased flow decreases filtration. Afferent arteriolar dilation (decreased resistance) or efferent arteriolar constriction (increased resistance) increases capillary hydrostatic pressure and therefore, increases GFR. This is because more blood is delivered to the glomerulus. Conversely, afferent arteriolar constriction (increased resistance) or efferent arteriolar dilation (decresed resistance) decreases GFR (Fig. 6.6).

Regulation of Renal Blood Flow

Regulatory mechanism of renal blood flow (RBF) include autoregulation, neural regulation and hormonal regulation. Autoregulation is also called as intrinsic mechanism. Extrinsic mechanism include both neural and hormonal mechanisms.

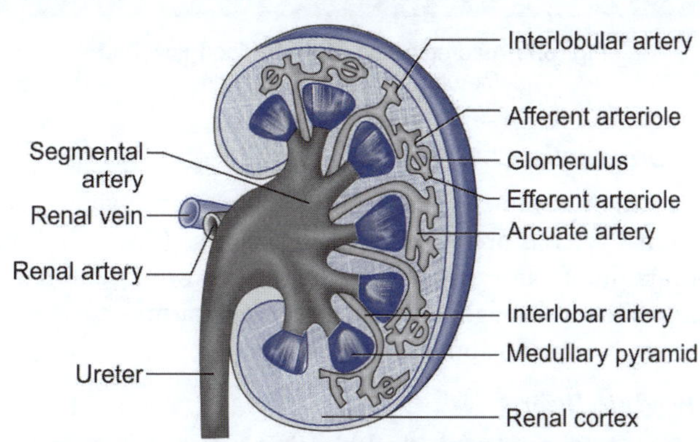

Fig. 6.5: Renal circulation

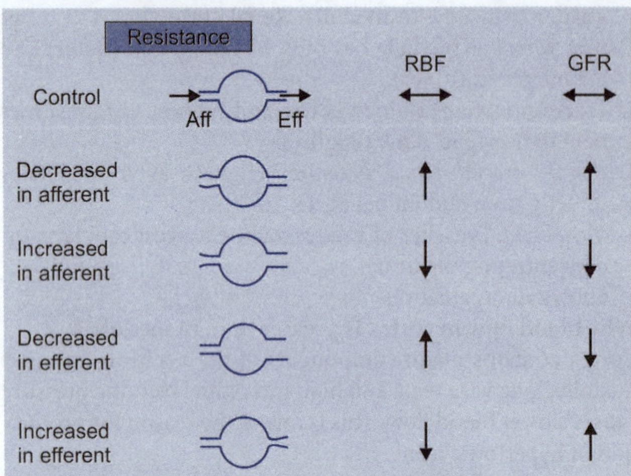

Fig. 6.6: Effects of changes in renal vascular resistance with constant renal perfusion

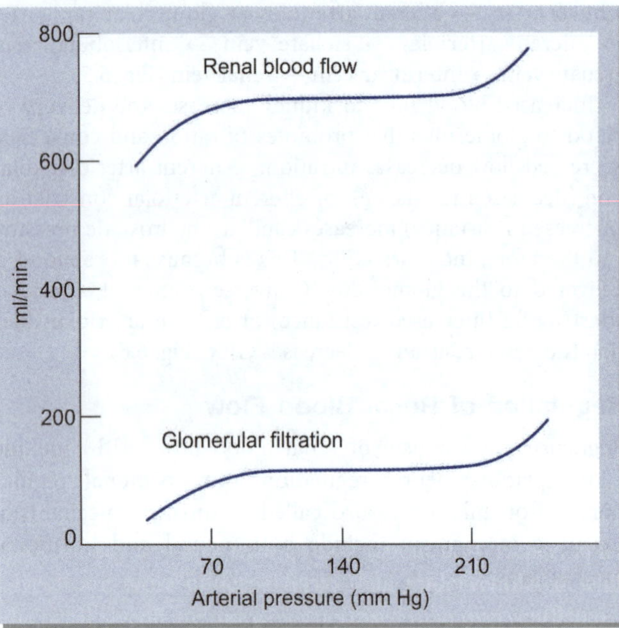

Fig. 6.7: Autoregulation of renal blood flow and glomerular filtration rate in kidney

Autoregulation by Kidney

The RBF and thus GFR remain constant over a wide range of renal arterial pressures (90–220 mm Hg) (Fig. 6.7). This occurs due to an intrarenal mechanism known as autoregulation. This is brought about by two mechanisms—myogenic theory and tubuloglomerular feedback.

Myogenic Theory

It is the ability of individual blood vessels to resist stretching during increased arterial pressure. This phenomenon is referred to as myogenic mechanism of autoregulation of RBF. When the blood flow to the kidneys increases (BP increases), it stretches the elastic wall of the afferent arteriole. The stretch of the vessel wall increases the flow of calcium ions from extracellular fluid into the cells. The influx of calcium ions lead to the contraction of smooth muscles in afferent arteriole which causes constriction and increase in resistance in afferent arteriole. There by the blood flow is controlled.

Tubuloglomerular Feedback

This mechanism is based on NaCl concentration of tubular fluid. Tubuloglomerular feedback mechanism maintains a constant RBF and GFR when there is a fluctuation in arterial BP between 90–220 mm Hg.

The signals from the renal tubules in each nephron feedback to affect filtration in it's glomerulus. The tubuloglomerular feedback mechanism has two components that act together to control GFR (Fig. 6.8):

1. An afferent arteriolar feedback mechanism
2. An efferent arteriolar feedback mechanism.

When GFR is decreased NaCl load reaching the macula densa is decreased (due to increased NaCl reabsorption at PCT). Macula densa senses NaCl concentration in the tubular fluid. Decrease in NaCl concentration initiates a signal from the macula densa that has two effects:

1. It decreases resistance to blood flow in afferent arterioles which raises glomerular hydrostatic pressure and thus GFR is brought back to normal.

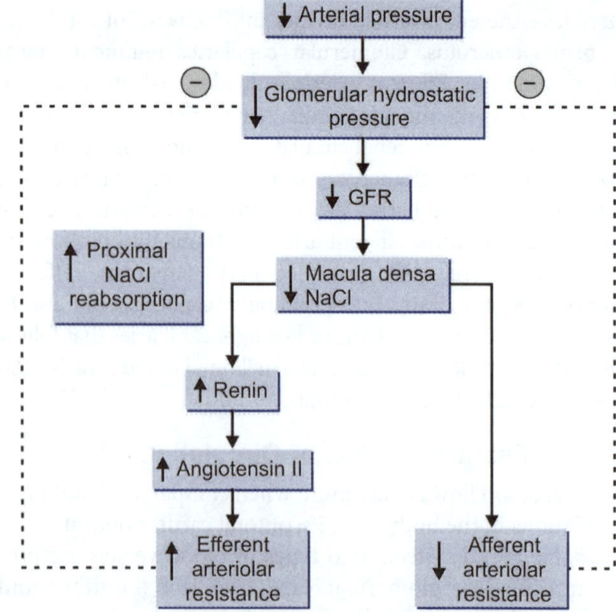

Fig. 6.8: Macula densa feedback mechanism for autoregulation of glomerular hydrostatic pressure and GFR during decreased renal arterial pressure

2. It increases renin release from JG cells of afferent and efferent arterioles.

Renin increases efferent arteriolar resistance by increasing the concentration of angiotensin I, which is converted to angiotensin II. Thus GFR and RBF are brought back to normal.

Neural Regulation

Afferent and efferent arteriolar lining smooth muscles are supplied by sympathetic nervous system. Here, slight to moderate sympathetic stimulation will not affect GFR and RBF much as autoregulation overrides nervous regulation. But very strong sympathetic stimulation causes constriction of renal arterioles resulting in decreased RBF and GFR.

If strong sympathetic stimulation is continued, RBF and GFR increases within 20–30 min. This may be due to decay of neurotransmitter at nerve endings. There are some nerves innervating renal tubular cells and JG cells. If they are stimulated, JG cells secrete renin. Then RBF increases.

Hormonal Regulation

a. *Catecholamines*
   i. Norepinephrine: Renal vasoconstriction, increased resistance, decreased RBF.
   ii. *Dopamine:* Renal vasodilatation increased RBF.
b. *Angiotensin II:* Vasoconstriction, decreased RBF.
c. *Prostaglandins:* Renal vasodilatation, increased RBF.
d. *Ach:* Renal vasodilatation, increased RBF.
e. *ADH:* Vasoconstriction, decreased RBF, so decreased urine output.
f. *ANP:* Renal vasodilation, increased RBF.

Other Factors

a. *Hypoxia:* When arterial O_2 becomes <50% normal → chemo receptor are stimulated → vasomotor center activated leading to renal vasoconstriction and decreased RBF.
b. *Hemorrhage:* When blood loss occurs, RBF decreases.
c. *Renal arterial blood pressure:* When BP increases sympathetic tone decreases reflexly → renal vasodilatation → RBF increases.
d. *High protein diet:* RBF increases as a result of increased glomerular capillary pressure.
e. *Postural changes and in muscular exercise:* A change in position from supine to standing posture causes decrease in RBF, due to increased sympathetic activity.
f. *Bacterial pyrogens:* Renal vasodilatation, increased RBF.
g. *Fever due to other reasons:* Vasoconstriction, decreased RBF.

MECHANISM OF URINE FORMATION

The formation of urine include four processes (Fig. 6.9):

1. **Glomerular filtration:** It is the process by which water and solutes in the blood leave plasma through the filtration barrier and enter Bowman's space.

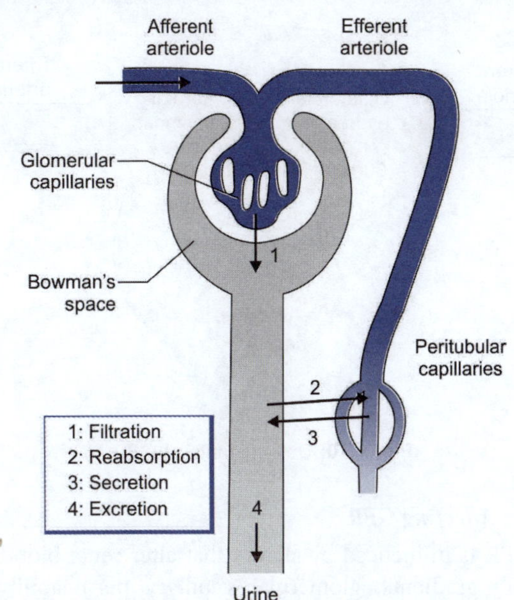

Fig. 6.9: Renal processes

2. **Tubular reabsorption:** It is the process of moving substances from the lumen across the epithelial layer into the surrounding interstitium and finally to the peritubular capillaries.
3. **Tubular secretion:** It is the process of moving substances into the tubular lumen from the tubular epithelial cells.
4. **Excretion:** It means exit of the substance from the body.

The substances to be excreted are removed by glomerular filtration and renal tubular secretion and passed into the urine. The substances that the body needs are retained by tubular reabsorption, e.g. Na^+, HCO_3^-.

Glomerular Filtration

Glomerular filtration is the initial step in urine formation. The plasma that traverses the glomerular capillaries is filtered by the highly permeable glomerular membrane and the resultant fluid, the glomerular filtrate is passed in to Bowman's capsule. Glomerular filtrate is identical with the plasma in respect of osmolality, pH, electrical conductivity, concentration of electrolytes except that it contains no proteins and no cells. Therefore glomerular filtrate is called the ultrafiltrate of plasma.

Glomerular Filtration Rate

Glomerular filtration rate (GFR) refers to the volume of the glomerular filtrate formed each minute by all the nephrons in both the kidneys. Normal value -125 mL/min =180 L/day. Note that 180 L of filtrate is formed every day. But the final urine volume per day is only about 1 to 1.5 L. It means, almost 178.5 L of the filtered volume is reabsorbed by the tubules.

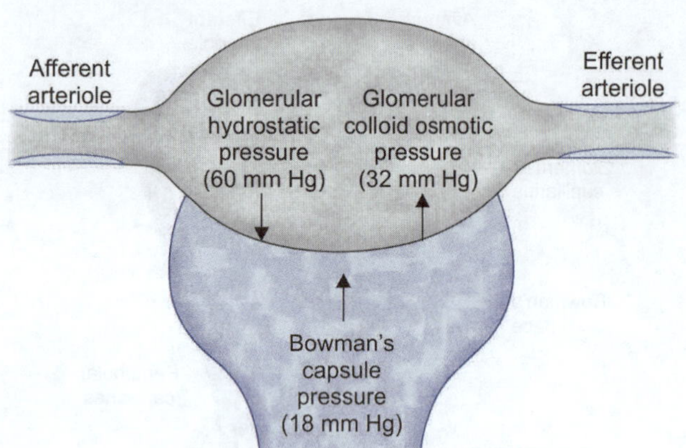

Fig. 6.10: Determinants of GFR

Factors Affecting GFR

The GFR is influenced by factors that alter renal blood flow, pressure gradients, glomerular capillary permeability and surface area for filtration. Factors favoring filtration at the glomerular capillaries includes hydrostatic pressure in glomerular capillary. It tends to push the plasma fluid out of the glomerular capillaries, into the Bowman's capsule. This pressure is about 60 mm Hg (Fig. 6.10).

Factors opposing filtration at the glomerular capillaries includes:

a. *Colloid osmotic pressure of glomerular capillary:* It is exerted by the plasma proteins (in the glomerular capillaries). It tends to pull the fluid back into the capillaries; thus it works in the opposite direction (that is, against filtration). It is about 32 mm Hg.
b. *Hydrostatic pressure in Bowman's capsule:* It is exerted by the filtrate accumulated in the Bowman's capsule. It tends to push the fluid back into the glomerular capillaries, thus opposing filtration. It is about 18 mm Hg.

$$GFR = K_f [(P_G - P_B) - (\pi_G - \pi_B)$$

So GFR depends on P_G, P_B, π_G, π_B and K_f

Where,

P_G= Hydrostatic pressure in the glomerular capillaries (60 mm Hg)

P_B= Hydrostatic pressure in Bowman's capsule (18 mm Hg)

π_G= Colloidal osmotic pressure of glomerular capillary (32 mm Hg)

π_B= Colloidal osmotic pressure of Bowman's capsule (negligible)

K_f= Filtration coefficient (permeability of capillaries × effective capillary surface area).

1. *Hydrostatic pressure in the glomerular capillaries (P_G)*
   - GFR is directly proportional to P_G.
   - Increased arterial pressure causes increase in P_G, so GFR increases.
   - Increase in afferent arteriolar resistance decreases P_G then GFR decreases.
   - Increase in efferent arteriolar resistance increases PG, but renal blood flow decreases therefore GFR increases slightly but if there is severe constriction, GFR decreases.
2. *Hydrostatic pressure in Bowman's capsule (P_B)*
   - GFR is inversely proportional to P_B.
   - P_B increases in case of obstruction of urinary tract. Then GFR decreases, e.g. kidney stones.
3. *Colloidal osmotic pressure in glomerular capillary (π_G)*
   GFR is inversely proportional to π_G.
   - In hypoprotienemia π_G decreases, so GFR increases.
   - During dehydration : π_G increases, then GFR decreases.
   - Increase in arterial plasma COP: increases π_G; so decrease in GFR.
   - Increase in filtration fraction (fraction of plasma filtered by glomerular capillary) causes increase in π_G and so decrease in GFR.
   - Filtration fraction = GFR/RPF
     = 125/700
     = 19% of RPF
4. *Colloidal osmotic pressure in Bowman's capsule (π_B):* It favors filtration. But the colloid osmotic pressure in Bowman's capsule is negligible. Proteins do not get filtered from the glomerular capillaries; thus no proteins in the Bowman's capsule to exert this pressure.
5. *Filtration coefficient (K_f)*
   It is the rate at which the filtrate is formed per unit time across the capillaries per unit time.
   It is a function of the membrane permeability and capillary surface area.
   - *Permeability of capillaries-depends on:*
     - Size of particle
     - Charge of particle
       All neutral substances having diameter less than 4 nm can pass through. Around 4–8 nm particles can pass based on charge and size. Particles greater than 8 nm are completely withheld. Glomerular membrane contain proteoglycans which are negatively charged. So they repel negatively charged albumin.
   - *Capillary surface area:* Contraction of mesangial cells decreases surface area available for filtration. This decreases filtration coefficient (K_f). Angiotensin II is an important regulator of mesangial contraction.

Note: In chronic uncontrolled diabetes mellitus and hypertension, K_f decreases due to thickness of glomerular capillary membrane.

Table 6.3: Hormones and autocoids that influence GFR

Hormone or autocoid	Effect on GFR
Norepinephrine	Decrease
Epinephrine	Decrease
Endothelium	Decrease
Angiotensin II	Do change, but prevents decrease
Endothelial derived nitric oxide	Increase
Prostaglandins	Increase

6. *Renal blood flow (RBF):* GFR is directly proportional to the RBF.
7. *Age:* GFR decreases with increasing age due to decrease in the renal plasma flow (RPF), cardiac output (CO) and renal tissue mass.

Regulation of Glomerular Filtration Rate (Table 6.3)

1. Autoregulation: Refer from regulation of RBF.
2. Neural: Write from regulation of RBF.
3. Hormonal

Note

1. ***Net filtration pressure (NFP)***
   It is the balance between the pressure favoring filtration and pressure opposing filtration.
   $NFP = (P_G - P_B) - (\pi_G - \pi_B)$
   Pressure favoring filtration = 60 mm Hg
   Pressure opposing filtration = (32 + 18) = 50 mm Hg.
   Thus, net filtration pressure = (60 – 50) = 10 mm Hg.
   The net filtration pressure (or "effective" filtration pressure) determines the rate of formation of filtrate at the glomerulus.
   $GFR = K_f \times NFP$
   K_f = Filtration coefficient of the glomerular membrane is 12.5 ml/min/mm Hg. It is the GFR at 1 mm Hg NFP. That is for every 1 mm Hg filtration pressure, the capillaries filter out 12.5 mL of fluid per minute.
2. ***Filtration fraction***
   The fraction of the renal plasma which becomes the filtrate.

$$\text{Filtration fraction} = \frac{\text{GFR}}{\text{Renal plasma flow}} \times 100$$

Normal value = 0.16 – 0.2

Tubular Reabsorption

Tubular reabsorption is selective. There are two routes (Fig. 6.11) for the substances to be reabsorbed from tubular lumen into peritubular capillary called transcellular and paracellular routes. Substances in the tubular lumen eventually reach peritubular capillaries by one of these two routes.

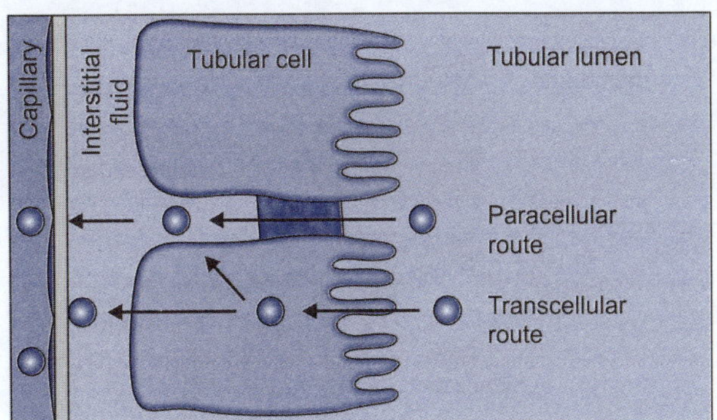

Fig. 6.11: Routes of reabsorption

In transcellular pathway, substances enter PCT through its apical side, transported out through its basolateral side. In paracellular pathway it is through tight junctions between PCT cells.

Reabsorption of Sodium in Proximal Convoluted Tubule

Sixty seven percent of sodium is reabsorbed in PCT. The process of Na^+ reabsorption in PCT is iso-osmotic, i.e. the reabsorption of Na^+ and water are exactly proportional. Mechanism of Na^+ reabsorption in the early proximal tubule and late proximal tubule is different.

In the Early Proximal Tubule

The Na^+ absorption is a three step process:

1. Transport from tubular lumen into tubular cell. Na^+ is transported from tubular lumen into tubular cell by:
   - *Unidirectional Na^+ transport/symport:* Na^+ moves out of tubular lumen along with glucose (and other solutes like aminoacids, lactate) through the apical membrane of the tubule.
   - *Na^+ - H^+ exchange/antiport:* Here Na^+ is reabsorbed in exchange of H^+. Na^+-H^+ antiporter couples entry of Na^+ with extrusion of H^+ from the cell. H^+ secretion results in reabsorption of $NaHCO_3$.
2. Transport from tubular cell into interstitial fluid and lateral intercellular spaces.
   Most of the Na^+ are actively pumped into the lateral intercellular spaces by Na^+ - K^+ ATPase. The rest of the Na are pumped into the interstitial fluid by Na^+ - K^+ pump situated at the basal part of the cell membrane (Fig. 6.12).
   Note: A small amount of Na^+ re-enters the tubular lumen by passive transport through the tight junctions.
3. Transport from interstitial fluid and lateral intercellular spaces to peritubular capillaries.
   From the lateral intercellular spaces and interstitial fluid, Na^+ enters the peritubular capillaries by concentration gradient.

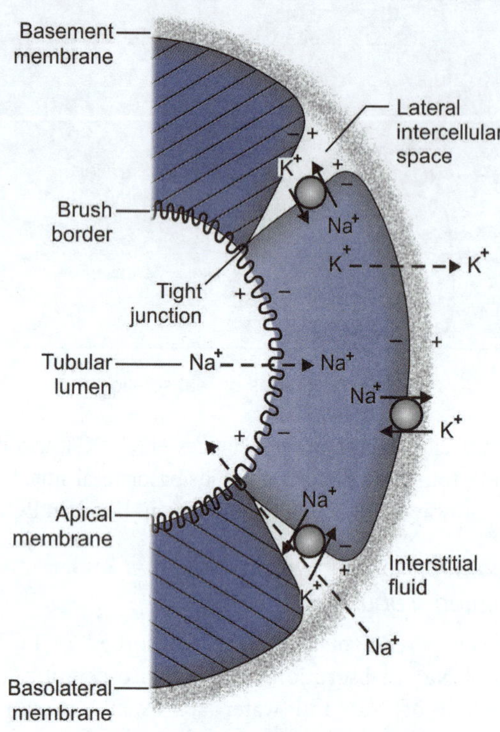

Fig. 6.12: Sodium reabsorption from early proximal convoluted tubule

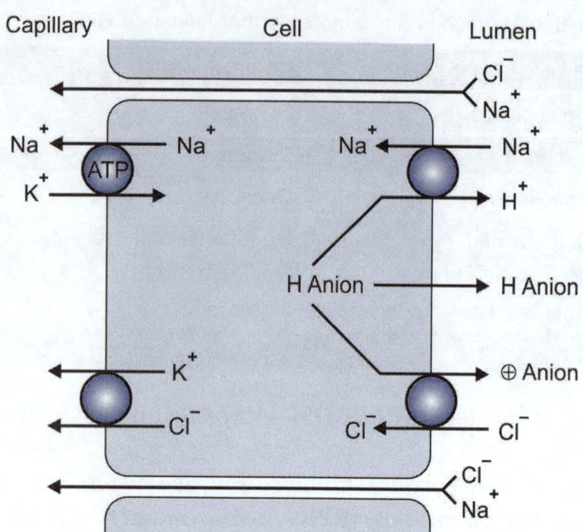

Fig. 6.13: Sodium reabsorption from late PCT

In the Late Proximal Tubule

In the 2nd half of the proximal tubule, Na^+ is mainly reabsorbed with Cl^- across both the transcellular and paracellular pathways.

- *Paracellular pathways:* Na^+ is primarily reabsorbed with Cl^- rather than organic solutes or HCO_3^- as the accompanying anion because the Na^+ transport mechanisms in the 2nd half of the proximal tubule differ from those in the 1st half. Further more, the tubular fluid that enters the 2nd half contains very little glucose and amino acids, but the high concentration of Cl^- (140 mEq/L) in tubule fluid exceeds that in the 1st half (105 mEq/L). The high $[Cl^-]$ is due to the preferential reabsorption of Na^+ with HCO_3^- and organic solutes in the first half of the proximal tubule. This concentration gradient favors diffusion of Cl^- from the tubular lumen across the tight junction into the lateral intercellular space. Movement of the negatively charged Cl^- results in the tubular fluid becoming positively charged relative to blood cell.
- *Transcellular pathways:* Na^+ and Cl^- enter the cell across the apical membrane via the operation of parallel Na^+-H^+ and Cl^- - anion antiporters. The secreted H^+ and anion combine in the tubular fluid to form an H^+-anion complex that can recycle across the plasma membrane.

Accumulation of the H^+-anion complex in tubular fluid establishes an H^+-anion concentration gradient that favors H^+-anion recycling across apical plasma membrane into the cell. Inside the cell, H^+ and the anion dissociate and recycle back across the apical plasma membrane. The net result is the uptake of NaCl across the apical membrane. The anion may be hydroxide ions, formate, oxalate, bicarbonate or sulfate (Fig. 6.13).

In Loop of Henle

Twenty-five percent of Na is reabsorbed. Ascending limb is permeable to solutes and impermeable to water. Descending limb is permeable to water and impermeable to solutes. When the filtrate enters loop, it is isotonic. But in descending limb, H_2O is reabsorbed thus filtrate becomes hypertonic. In the ascending limb it becomes hypotonic. Here $1Na^+$, $1K^+$, $2Cl^-$ are reabsorbed into the tubular cell (by Na^+-K^+-$2Cl^-$ transporter). From the cell Na is reabsorbed into the peritubular capillaries by Na^+ - K^+ pump. One K^+ and one Cl^- are co-transported out of the cell; another Cl^- passes out passively by diffusion. The other K^+ is secreted back into the lumen (Fig. 6.14 and Table 6.4).

An Na^+- H^+ antiport in apical cell membrane also mediates Na^+ reabsorption, as well as H^+ secretion. Paracellular passive reabsorption of Na^+, K^+, Ca^{2+} and Mg^{2+} also occurs in the thick ascending limb.

Note

Because thick ascending limb does not reabsorb water, reabsorption of NaCl and other solutes reduces the osmolarity to 150 mOsm/L. Thus because the thick ascending limb produces a fluid that is dilute relative to plasma, the ascending limb of Henle's loop is called the ***'diluting segment'***.

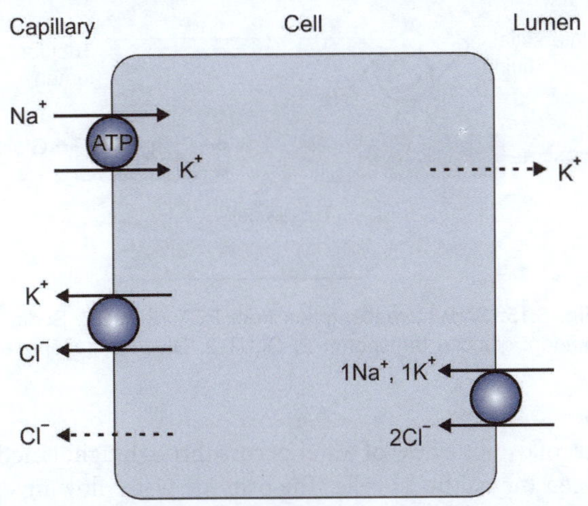

Fig. 6.14: Sodium reabsorption in loop of Henle

Table 6.4: NaCl transport along the nephron

Segment	Percentage of filtrate reabsorbed	Mechanism of Na entry across the apical membrane
Proximal tubule	67%	$Na^+ - H^+$ antiporter, Na^+ symporter with amino acid and organic solutes, 1 Na+ $1H^+$ – $2Cl^-$ anion antiporter, paracellular
Loop of Henle	25%	1 Na^+ – $1K^+$ – 2Cl - symporter
Distal tubule	5%	NaCl symporter (early) Na+ channels (late)
Collecting duct	3%	Na^+ channels

In DCT and Collecting Duct

Five percent reabsorption in DCT and three percent reabsorption in collecting duct. In the early part of DCT, entry of NaCl into the cell across the apical membrane is mediated by an Na^+ - Cl^- symporter. Na^+ leaves the cell via the action of Na^+- K^+ ATPase, and Cl^- leaves the cell via diffusion through Cl^- channels.

In the late part of DCT and collecting duct, the reabsorption is via ENaC (epithelial sodium channel) under the influence of aldosterone.

Note

1. *Barter's syndrome:* It is an autosomal recessive genetic disorder characterized by hypokalemia, metabolic alkalosis and hyperaldosteronism. Inactivating mutations in the gene coding for Na^+- K^+ - $2Cl^-$ symporter, the apical K^+ channel, or the basolateral Cl^- channel decrease both NaCl and K^+ reabsorption by thick ascending limb, which in turn causes hypokalemia and a decrease in ECF volume. The fall in ECF volume stimulates renin and aldosterone secretion, which inturn stimulates NaCl reabsorption and H^+ secretion by distal tubule and collecting duct.
2. *Liddle's syndrome:* It is a genetic disorder characterized by an increase in BP secondary to increase in ECF volume. Liddle's syndrome is caused by activating mutations in either the β or γ subunit of ENaC (ENaC is composed of 3 subunits, α, β and γ). These mutations increase the number of Na^+ channels in the apical cell membrane of P cells and thereby the amount of Na^+ reabsorbed by each channel. In Liddle's syndrome, the rate of renal reabsorption is inappropriately high, which leads to an increase in ECF volume and hypertension.

Factors Affecting Sodium Reabsorption

1. *Hydrostatic pressure in peritubular capillaries (P_c)*
   - Increased Pc opposes reabsorption.
   - It is influenced by arterial pressure and the resistances of afferent and efferent arterioles.

$$\uparrow P_c \rightarrow \downarrow \text{Reabsorption}$$
$$\downarrow R_A \rightarrow \uparrow P_c$$
$$\downarrow R_E \rightarrow \uparrow P_c$$
$$\uparrow \text{Arterial Pressure} \rightarrow \uparrow P_c$$

   - Normally it is 10 mm Hg (low) and favors reabsorption.
2. *Colloid osmotic pressure in peritubular capillary (π_c)*
   - Increased favors reabsorption
   - It is influenced by arterial plasma colloidal osmotic pressure (pA) and filtration fraction (FF).

$$\uparrow \pi_c \rightarrow \uparrow \text{Reabsorption}$$
$$\uparrow \pi_A \rightarrow \uparrow \pi_c$$
$$\uparrow FF \rightarrow \uparrow \pi_c$$

3. *Sodium intake:* More the Na intake less the Na^+ reabsorption.
4. *Peritubular capillary filtration coefficient (K_f):* K_f is a measure of the permeability and surface area of capillaries, so increase in K_f raises reabsorption.
5. *GFR:* GFR influences Na^+ reabsorption by two mechanisms
   1. Tubuloglomerular feedback
   2. Glomerulotubular balance

   An increase in GFR, causes an increase in the reabsorption of solutes and consequently water, primarily in the PCT. So that in general, the tubule tends to reabsorb a constant fraction of amount filtered rather than a constant amount.This process is called *glomerulotubular balance.*
6. *Sympathetic stimulation:* Activation of sympathetic nervous system can increase Na reabsorption.
7. *Hormones:*
   a. *Aldosterone:* It increases sodium reabsorption and K secretion by stimulating Na^+-K^+ ATPase pump (on the basolateral side of CT) and promoting the opening of ENaC. Site of action is CT and distal part of DCT.

b. *Angiotensin II:* It increases sodium reabsorption by 3 main effects.
   i. Stimulates aldosterone secretion
   ii. Constricts efferent arteriole (so that Pc decreases)
   iii. Directly stimulates Na reabsorption in PCT, loop of Henle, DCT and collecting duct.
c. Atrial natriuretic peptide (ANP) decreases NaCl and water reabsorption.
d. PGE_2 decreases Na^+ reabsorption.
e. Endothelin and Interleukin I increases the production of PGE_2 and decreases Na^+ reabsorption.
f. Ouabain inhibits Na^+-K^+ ATPase and decrease Na^+ reabsorption.

Reabsorption of Water

Normally 180 L of fliud is filtered /day. But out of this only 1–1.5 L is excreted daily. The rest is reabsorbed from renal tubules. As a result urine osmolality is 1400 mOsm/L. Reabsorption of water occurs from PCT, loop of Henle, DCT and CT.

In PCT

PCT is freely peremeable to water. About 60–70% of water is reabsorbed from PCT. In PCT, passive reabsorption of water occurs along with the active transport of solute. This is called as *obligatory reabsorption.* In PCT water channels called aquaporins are present on the apical surface of epithelial cell. Water channel involved here is aquaporin-1. In PCT fluid is isotonic.

In Loop of Henle

Descending limb is freely permeable to water and not to solutes. Here 15% of water is reabsorbed. Water moves out of tubule and the filtrate becomes hypertonic. At the tip of loop of Henle, filtrate has an osmolarity of 1200 mOsm/L. Ascending limb is impermeable to water, permeable to solutes. So solutes move out, making filtrate hypotonic.

In DCT

It is relatively impermeable to water. Only 5% of filtered water is reabsorbed.

In Collecting Tubule

Here reabsorption is under the control of ADH, so called as *facultative reabsorption.* Collecting tubule has cortical and medullary parts. P cells contain aquaporin-2 through which water is reabsorbed. ADH stimulates the movement of aquaporin-2 to the luminal side of cell membranes. Ten percent of the reabsorption occurs from cortical part where as 5% from medullary part of collecting duct. As a result of reabsorption of water from various segments urine becomes hypertonic (1400 mOsm/L).

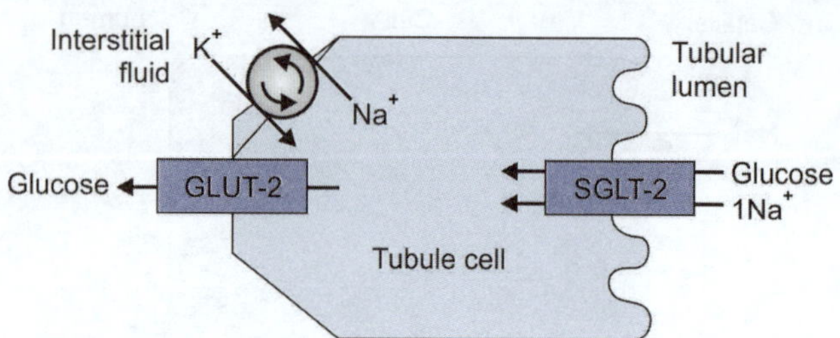

Fig. 6.15: Sodium reabsorption from PCT (SGLT-2: Sodium dependent glucose transporter 2, GLUT-2: Glucose transporter 2)

Note

A part of osmotic flow of water occurs through tight junctions between the epithelial cells. The osmotic water flowing especially in PCT also carries with it some of the solutes, a process referred to as *solvent drag.*

Reabsorption of Glucose

Glucose is completely reabsorbed in the PCT along with Na^+. This reabsorption of glucose occurs along with the reabsorp-tion of Na by symport/cotransport mechanism. Glucose and Na^+ bind to a common carrier SGLT-2 in the luminal membrane. Glucose is carried into the cell as Na^+ moves down its electrical and chemical gradient. The Na^+ is then actively pumped out of the cell into lateral intercellular spaces and interstitium (Fig. 6.15). Glucose combines with another carrier protein GLUT-2 on the basal surface of same cell and moves into the peritubular capillaries by simple diffusion. Thus glucose transport across PCT is an example for secondary active transport.

Note

1. A variety of other substances are transported by secondary active transport via symports with the energy provided by active transport of Na^+ out of the renal tubular cells. These substances include some amino acids, lactate, inorganic phosphate, H^+, and Cl^-.
2. Glucose transport in kidneys is inhibited by phlorhizin, a plant glycoside which competes with glucose for binding to the carrier.
3. Glycosuria is common during pregnancy due to decrease in renal threshold and increase in GFR.

Characteristic of Glucose Transport and Excretion

Rate of filtration of glucose at glomerulus

= Resting plasma level of glucose × GFR

= 80 × (125/100) ml/min

= 100 mg/min

Transport Maximum (T_M)

The substances reabsorbed actively from the renal tubules require some specific transport system. There is a limit to the rate at which solute can be transported. This limit is due to saturation of transport systems involved when maximum solute is delivered to the tubule. The maximum rate at which a substance is reabsorbed from renal tubule is called transport maximum for that substance. For example, the transport maximum for glucose (T_MG) is 375 mg/min in males and 300 mg/min in females.

Renal threshold value for glucose

The renal threshold for glucose is the plasma level at which the glucose first appears in the urine more than the normal minute amounts. This renal threshold is calculated by T_MG / GFR.

Theoretically the renal threshold would be about 300 mg/dl, i.e. 375 mg/min (T_MG) divided by 125 ml/min (GFR). However, the actual renal threshold is about 200 mg/dL of arterial blood or 180 mg/dL of venous blood. This anomaly between predicted value and practical value can be demonstrated by a graph (Fig. 6.16).

The actual curve is rounded and deviates from the 'ideal' curve. This deviation is called ***splay***. It represents the excretion of glucose in urine before the T_MG is reached. It is due to:

a. All the nephrons does not have the same T_MG.
b. Below T_MG levels the interaction between a carrier and glucose is not completely an irreversible process , so some glucose escapes reabsorption.

Reabsorption of Bicarbonate

Reabsorption of HCO_3^- occurs throughout the nephron, except in the descending limb of LH.

In PCT

About 90% of the filtered HCO_3^- is reabsorbed into the PCT. H^+ secretion across the apical membrane of the cell occurs by both Na^+- H^+ antiporter and H^+-ATPase. The Na^+ - H^+ antiporter is the predominant pathway for H^+ secretion and uses the lumen to cell [Na^+] gradient to drive this process. Within the cell, H^+ and HCO_3^- are produced in a reaction catalyzed by CA. The H^+ is secreted into tubular fluid, whereas HCO_3^- exits the cell across the basolateral membrane and returns to the peritubular blood. Movement of HCO_3^- out of the cell across the basolateral membrane is coupled to other ions (Fig. 6.17).

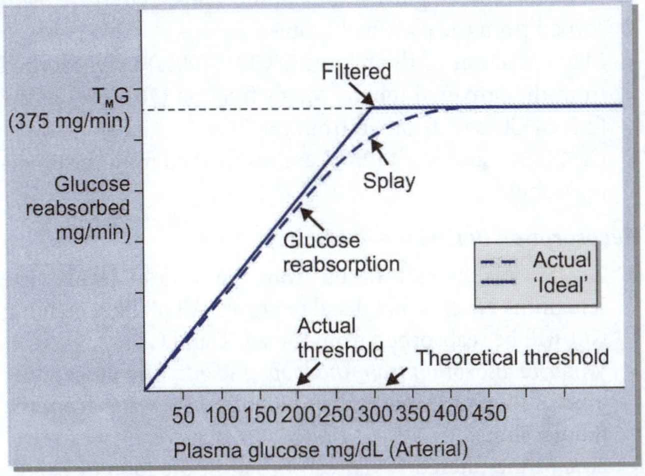

Fig. 6.16: Relationship between the plasma glucose concentration and glucose transport

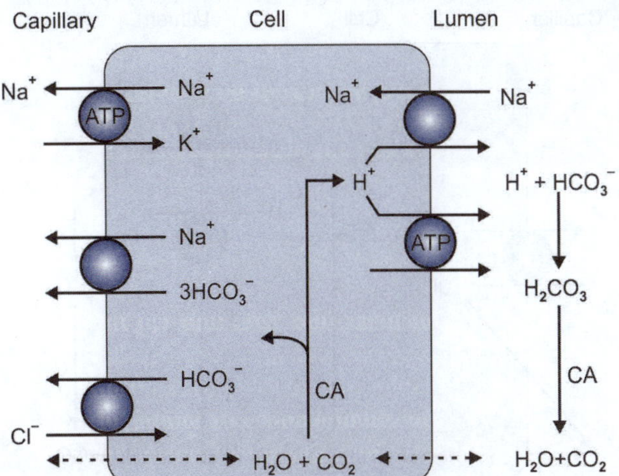

Fig. 6.17: Bicarbonate reabsorption in proximal convoluted tubule

a. The majority of HCO_3^- exits via a symporter that couples with efflux of $1Na^+$ with $3HCO_3^-$ (sodium bicarbonate cotransporter).
b. In addition, some of the HCO_3^- may exit in exchange for Cl^-. CA is also present in the brush border of the proximal tubule cells. This enzyme catalyzes the dehydration of H_2CO_3 in the luminal fluid and thereby facilitates reabsorption of HCO_3^-.

In LH

The cellular mechanism responsible for reabsorption of HCO_3^- in thick segment of LH is very similar to that in PCT. A K^+ - HCO_3^- symporter in the basolateral membrane may also contribute to the exit of HCO_3^- from the cell.

In DCT and CT

Intercalated cells secretes H^+ (reabsorbs HCO_3^-). Within this cell, H^+ and HCO_3^- are produced by the hydration of CO_2, this reaction is catalyzed by CA. The H^+ is secreted into tubular fluid via two mechanisms (Fig. 6.18):

- The first involves an apical membrane H^+-ATPase.
- The second couples the secretion of H^+ with the reabsorption of K^+ via an H^+, K^+-ATPase similar to that found in the stomach. The HCO_3^- exits the cell across the basolateral membrane in exchange for Cl^- (via $Cl^-HCO_3^-$ antiporter) and enters the peritubular capillary blood.

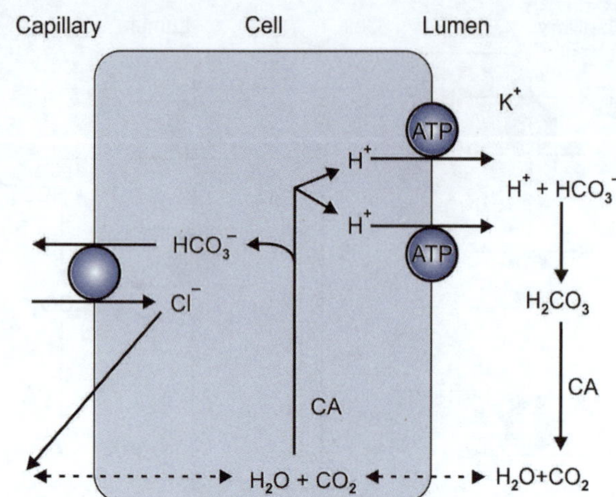

Fig. 6.18: Bicarbonate reabsorption in distal convoluted tubule

Potassium transport

The kidneys play a major role in maintaining K^+ balance. It helps in maintaining a balance between urinary excretion and dietary intake of K^+, thereby ensuring K^+ homeostasis.

Glomerular Filtration

Because K^+ is not bound to plasma proteins, it is freely filtered by glomerulus. The K^+ is the plasma electrolyte that is both reabsorbed and secreted into renal tubules.

Reabsorption of K^+ by Proximal Tubule

About 67% of the filtered K^+ is reabsorbed by active transport in the PCT. In PCT, the amount of K^+ reabsorbed is a constant fraction of the amount filtered.

Reabsorption of K^+ by Loop of Henle

About 20% of the filtered K^+ is reabsorbed through thick ascending limb of loop of Henle along with Na^+ reabsorption.

Reabsorption and Secretion of K^+ by DCT and CT

The distal tubule and CT are able to reabsorb or secrete K^+. The rate of K^+ reabsorption or secretion by DCT and CT depends on variety of hormones and factors. Most of K^+ produced in the urine is due to secretion of the K^+ in the DCT which contributes approximately 75% of excreted K^+. The K^+ secretion from blood into the tubule lumen is a two step process and it involves an active as well as a passive process.

- Uptake of K^+ from blood across the basolateral membrane into the DCT by Na^+-K^+ ATPase. This is the critical step and is associated with active Na^+ efflux via the Na^+-K^+ ATPase.
- The elevated intracelular K^+ so achieved favors the net K^+ diffusion at the apical membrane down a concentration gradient into the tubular lumen.

Factors Affecting K^+ Transport

- Plasma [K^+] is an important determinant of K^+ secretion by the DCT and CT. Hyperkalemia (e.g. resulting from a high K^+ diet or from rhabdomyolysis) stimulates secretion of K^+. Tubular secretion of K^+ is markedly decreased in K^+ and Na^+ depletion.
- In DCT, K^+ and H^+ are both exchanged for Na^+ which is reabsorbed and the two ions compete for the exchange mechanism. Therefore K^+ excretion is decreased when H^+ secretion is increased.
- Flow of tubular fluid: The rate of K^+ secretion is proportionate to the rate of flow of tubular fluid through the distal portion of the nephron, because with rapid flow there is less opportunity for the tubular K^+ concentration to rise to a value that stops further secretion.
- Mineralocorticoids (e.g. aldosterone) increases K^+ secretion by:
  - Increasing the activity of basolateral Na^+- K^+ ATPase, which increases K^+ entry into the DCT.
  - Increasing the permeability of the luminal membrane to K^+.

Summary of Reabsorption Events at Different Parts of a Nephron

180 L of filtrate is formed every day. However, the final urine formation is only about 1–1.5 L/day. It means, the remaining almost 178.5 L of filtrate is reabsorbed by the tubules.

Proximal tubular reabsorption:

- 65–70% of the filtered Na^+ and 60–70% of the filtered water is reabsorbed in the proximal tubule.
- Remaining 30–35% Na^+ and water enter the loop of Henle.
- 65–70% of the filtered K^+ is reabsorbed in the proximal tubule.
- All of the filtered glucose and amino acids (100%) are reabsorbed from the proximal tubule.
- Major fraction of the filtered HCO_3^- (90%) is reabsorbed from the proximal tubule. Major fraction (70–75%) of the filtered Cl^- is reabsorbed from the PCT.
- Ca^{2+} (60%) and Mg^{2+} (25%) are reabsorbed from the proximal tubule.

Reabsorption in the loop of Henle:

- 20–25% Na^+ is reabsorbed from the loop of Henle. The remaining Na^+ reaches distal nephron. All of the remaining Na^+ will be reabsorbed from the DCT and CD.
- *Water reabsorption from the loop of Henle*: The descending limb of loop of Henle reabsorbs some 15% water from the tubular fluids.
- 20% of the filtered K^+ is reabsorbed in the loop of Henle. Some amount (10–15%) of Cl^- is also reabsorbed from the thick ascending limb of loop of Henle.

- Ca^{2+} (20%–25%) and Mg^{2+} (65%) are reabsorbed from the loop of Henle.

Reabsorption from the distal nephron:

- Water reabsorption from the DCT and CD is under the regulation of ADH. Depending on the osmolarity of plasma, ADH will reabsorb water from the tubular fluids. The remaining water will be finally excreted in urine with solutes dissolved in it.
- Collecting duct has two types of cells: (1) Principal cells – They reabsorb Na^+ and secrete K^+; (2) Intercalated cells – They reabsorb K^+ and secrete H^+.
- Ca^{2+} reabsorption in the distal nephron is under the influence of the parathyroid hormone.

Tubular Secretion

Some substances are secreted into the lumen from peritubular capillaries through tubular epithelial cells. It is known as tubular secretion. Secreted substances are H^+, K^+, NH_3, weak acids, steroids, drugs (penicillin).

- H^+ ions are secreted in the PCT. This secretion is to facilitate reabsorption of the filtered HCO_{3^-}.
- Proximal tubule secretes many organic ions. Endogenous substances (e.g. creatinine), toxins, and drugs are secreted by this segment.
- Uric acid can be secreted as well as reabsorbed from the proximal tubule.
- H^+ ions are secreted by the intercalated cells in the collecting duct. This secretion is to achieve acidification of urine (to remove excess acids in the conditions of acidosis of plasma).
- K^+ can be secreted as well as reabsorbed from the distal nephron. Whether net secretion or net reabsorption occurs would depend on the K^+ status of the body. In the conditions of hyperkalemia, net K^+ secretion would occur (via the principal cells).

CONCENTRATION OF URINE

Kidney is able to excrete very concentration urine with osmolarity of 1400 mOsm/L and very dilute urine with osmolarity of 50 mOsm/L. Process of concentration or dilution of urine requires kidney to excrete water and solutes independently. When water intake is decreased, solutes are excreted in excess of water resulting in concentrated urine of maximum osmolarity 1400 mOsm/L. When water intake is increased, water is excreted in excess of solutes resulting in the formation of dilute urine of minimum osmolarity 50 mOsm/L.

Formation of Concentrated Urine

The basic requirement for forming a concentrated urine are:

1. Hyperosmotic renal medulla (Fig. 6.19).
2. Secretion of ADH.

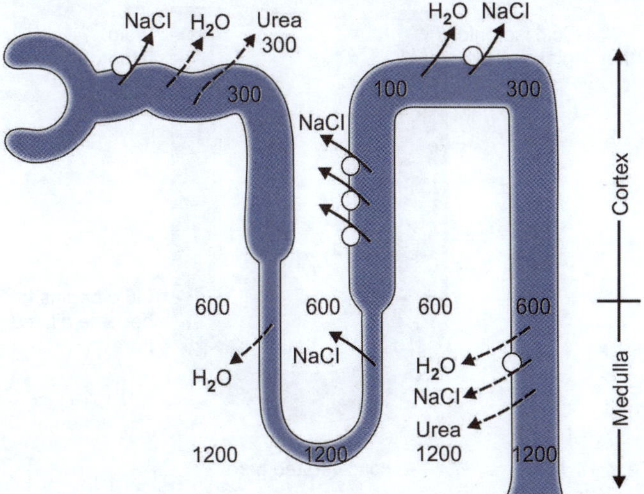

Fig. 6.19: Formation of a concentrated urine when ADH levels are high

Hyperosmotic Renal Medulla

Increasing osmotic gradient that is present along medullary interstitium is produced by combined action of loop of Henle and vasa recta as counter current multiplier and counter current exchanger respectively.

Counter current system is defined as the system in which inflow runs parallel to and in close proximity to outflow in the opposite direction. Thus counter current system has two components:

1. *Countercurrent multiplier system:* Loop of Henle functions as countercurrent multiplier and plays an important role in producing hypertonic medullary interstitium. Ascending limb and descending limb are parallel to each other and in close proximity.
   The descending limb is highly permeable to water. So water moves from the tubular lumen into medullary interstitium (not accompanied by Na^+). The medullary gradient is such that the interstitium becomes more and more hyperosmolar in the deeper parts of the medulla, which is the main reason why water flows from the lumen to interstitium and not in the reverse direction. As a result the tubular fluid becomes more and more concentrated as it descends down the thin descending limb of LH (1200–1400 mOsm/L at the apex of LH) (Fig. 6.20).
   Then, the tubular fluid reaches the ascending limb. The thick segment of ascending limb vigorously reabsorbs Na^+ (along with Cl^- and K^+), but this segment is impermeable to water. Therefore, the tubular fluid loses Na^+, Cl^- and K^+ but no water. This means the tubular fluid begins to become diluted in the ascending limb of LH.
   Because of movement of solutes from ascending limb of LH to interstitium the osmolarity of medullary

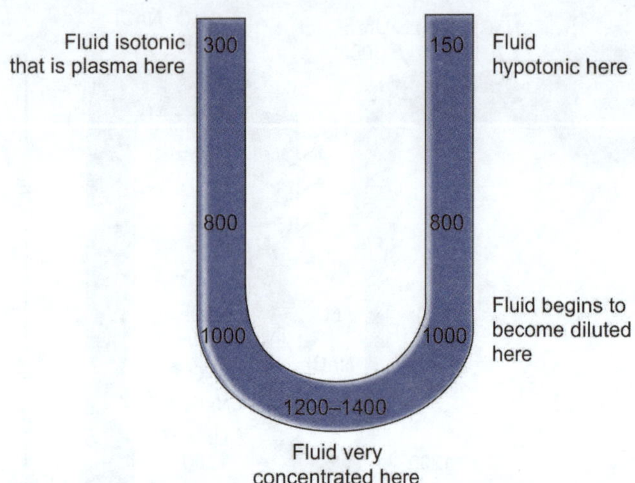

Fig. 6.20: Summary of changes in the osmolality (in mOsm/L) of tubular fluid

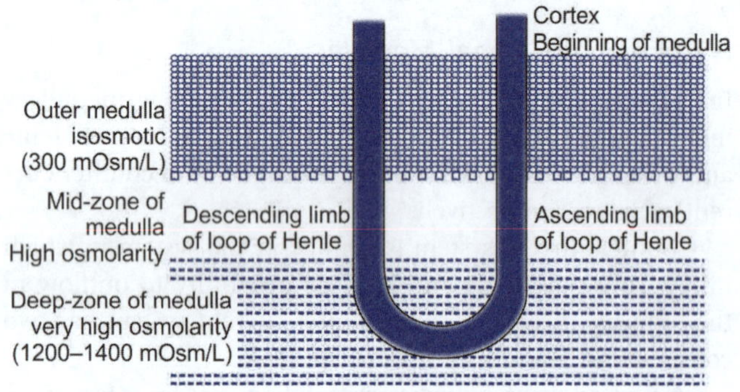

Fig. 6.21: Operation of countercurrent exchange system

interstitium increases and becomes hypertonic (Fig. 6.21). This situation is maximum in JG nephrons because of long LH.

The hypotonic tubular fluid is then delivered to the DCT. In the early DCT, reabsorption of Na^+ continues which causes further dilution of luminal fluid.

Finally the fluid enters the cortical collecting tubule. When ADH acts on cortical collecting tubules, water flows massively from CD to the interstitium through aquaporins. This flow of fluid continues until the osmolality of the CD fluid attains that of interstitium. Thus the urine formed is very concentrated.

Medullary interstitial hypertonicity is also contributed by urea which moves out of inner medullary portion of the collecting tubule. This urea also plays an important role in concentration of urine. This in turn is influenced by a protein diet. So high protein diet produce a high concentration capacity for kidney.

The Figure 6.22 shows the recirculation of urea absorbed from the medullary collecting duct into the interstitial

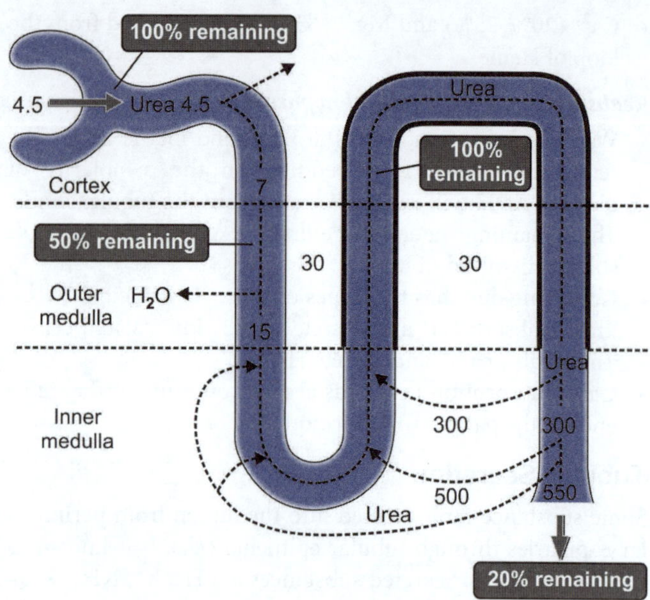

Fig. 6.22: Recirculation of urea absorbed from the medullary collecting duct into the interstitial fluid

fluid, this urea diffuses into the thin loop of Henle,and then passes through the distal tubules, and finally passes back into the collecting duct. The recirculation of urea helps to trap urea in the renal medulla and contributes to the hyperosmolarity of the renal medulla. The heavy dark lines, from the thick ascending loop of Henle to the medullary collecting ducts, indicate that these segments are not permeable to urea. (Numerical values are in milliosmoles per liter of urea during antidiuresis, when large amounts of antidiuretic hormone are present. Percentage of the filtered load of urea that remain in the tubules are indicated in the boxes).

2. *Countercurrent exchanger system:* Vasa recta functions as countercurrent exchanger. It is responsible for maintenance of the hyperosmolarity of medullary gradient developed by countercurrent multiplier system. If blood vessel was straight and the blood flow were high, the solute pumped into renal medulla by countercurrent multiplier system would rapidly dissipate.

   Vasa recta also has a descending and ascending limb. It runs parallel to LH. Both limbs are permeable to water and solutes (except for plasma proteins). Blood entering descending limb has an osmolarity of 300 mOsm/L and osmolarity of blood leaving the AL is 325 mOsm/L. As the blood descends into the medulla it becomes progressively more concentrated, partially by solute (NaCl, urea, etc.) entry from the interstitium and partially by loss of water into the interstitium. By the time the blood reaches the tips of vasa recta, it has a concentration of about 1200 mOsm/L.

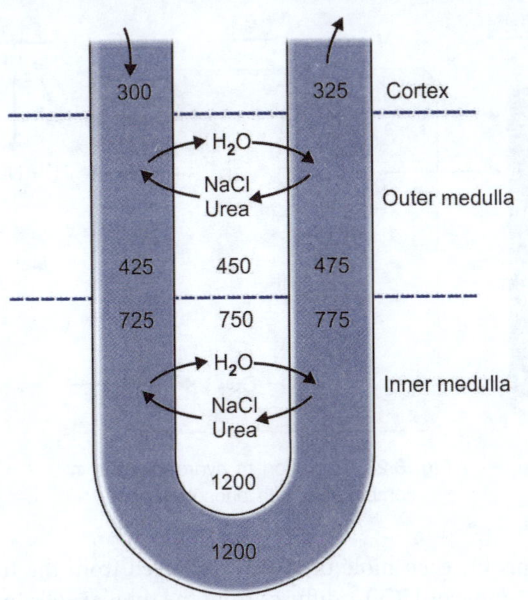

Fig. 6.23: Countercurrent exchange in the vasa recta

As the blood ascends back toward the cortex, it becomes progressively less concentrated as solutes diffuses back out into the medullary interstitium and as water moves into the vasa recta. The blood passing through the AL of vasa recta carry very little amount of NaCl from the medulla. Thus, NaCl and urea are exchanged for water between the AL and DL of vasa recta, hence this system is called countercurrent exchanger (Fig. 6.23).

If vasa recta was straight Na^+ and urea in the interstitium would have been removed by circulation. The sluggishness of blood flow ensures the retention of Na^+ in the medullary interstitium.

Secretion of ADH

In the late distal tubules and cortical collecting tubules, the osmolarity of fluid depends on the level of ADH. With high levels of ADH, these tubules are highly permeable to water.

Formation of Dilute Urine

When water content in the body increases, kidney excrete dilute urine. It is achieved by inhibition of ADH secretion (Fig. 6.24)

ACIDIFICATION OF URINE

Kidneys plays an important role in the maintenance of acid-base balance by excreting H^+ and retaining HCO_3^-. pH of glomerular filtrate: 7.4 (same as plasma). Normally the urine is acidic in nature with a pH of 4.5–6.

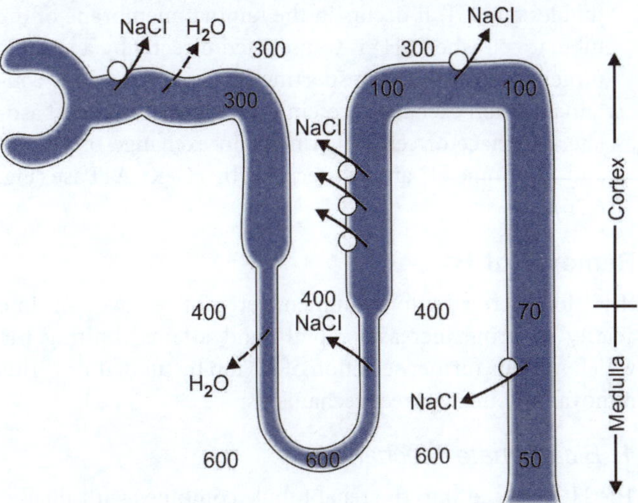

Fig. 6.24: Formation of dilute urine when ADH levels are very low

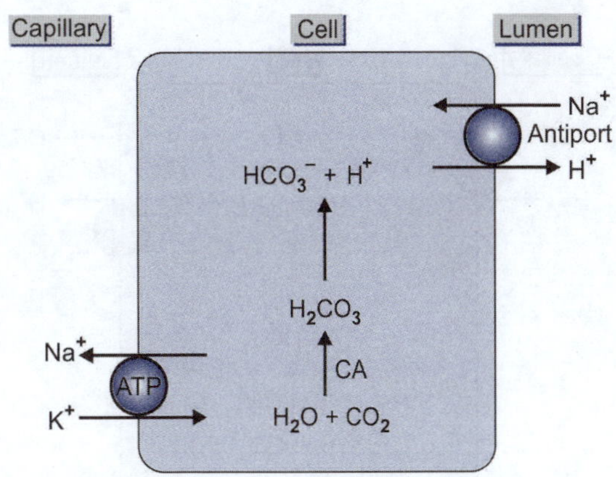

Fig. 6.25: Cellular mechanism for secretion of hydrogen ions into PCT, thick ascending limb of loop of Henle, DT and CT

Secretion of H^+

1. The cells of PCT, thick segment of ascending limb of LH, DT and CT secrete H^+. The reaction that is responsible for H^+ secretion in PCT, thick segment of ascending limb of LH and early distal tubules is Na^+ - H^+ exchange. When Na^+ is reabsorbed from tubular fluid into tubular cell, H^+ is secreted from the cell into the tubular fluid in exchange for Na^+. The H^+ comes from intracellular dissociation of H_2CO_3 and the HCO_3^- formed diffuses into the interstitial fluid. Thus for each H^+ secreted one Na^+ and one HCO_3^- enter the interstitial fluid (Fig. 6.25).
2. In late distal and collecting tubules, H^+ is secreted by an ATP driven proton pump mechanism. Secretion of H^+ occurs in a special type of cell called I cells of late distal

tubules and CT. It occurs in the luminal membrane of the tubular cell where, H^+ is transported directly by a specific protein, a hydrogen-transporting ATPase. The I cells contain an anion exchange protein called band 3 in their basolateral surface of cell which helps in exchange of HCO_3^- and Cl^-. Some H^+ are also secreted by H^+-K^+ ATPase (Fig. 6.26).

Removal of H^+

If H^+ ion secreted into the lumen were not removed in time acidity of urine increases rapidly and attains limiting pH which inhibits further secretion of H^+ ion by tubular cell. This removal is done by three mechanisms:

1. Bicarbonate Mechanism

The H^+ secreted into the renal tubule combines with filtered HCO_3^- forming H_2CO_3. The H_2CO_3 dissociates into CO_2 and H_2O. CO_2 diffuses into cell and it is used to form H_2CO_3 (Fig. 6.27).

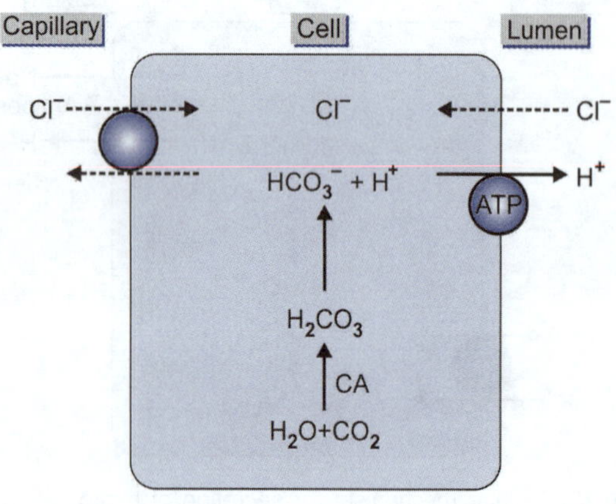

Fig. 6.26: Cellular mechanism for secretion of hydrogen ions into late DT and CT

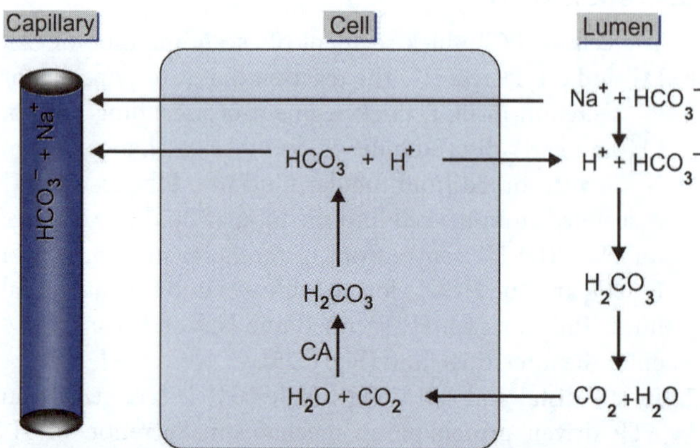

Fig. 6.27: Reabsorption of bicarbonate ions by secretion of hydrogen ions in renal tubule

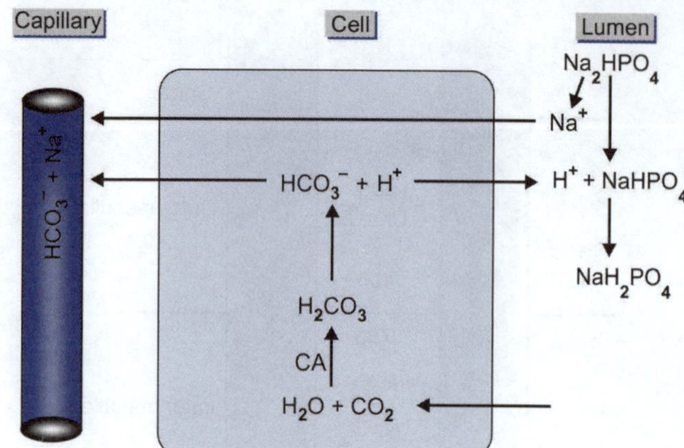

Fig. 6.28: Excretion of hydrogen ions in combination with phosphate ions

Thus for each mole of HCO_3^- removed from the tubular fluid 1 mole of HCO_3^- diffuses from the tubular cells into the blood. This mechanism particularly takes place in proximal tubules since carbonic anhydrase is present in the brush border of the cells.

2. Phosphate Mechanism

In the tubular cell CO_2 combines with H_2O to form H_2CO_3. It immediately dissociates into H^+ and HCO_3^-. HCO_3^- from the tubular cell enters the interstitium, simultaneously Na^+ is reabsorbed. The H^+ is secreted into the tubular lumen it reacts with sodium hydrogen phosphate ($NaHPO_4$) to form sodium dihydrogen phosphate (NaH_2PO_4). NaH_2PO_4 is excreted in urine. This happens mainly in distal tubules and collecting duct (Fig. 6.28).

3. Ammonia Mechanism

In the tubular epithelial cells, NH_3 is formed from glutamine. Glutamine is 1st converted to glutamate by glutaminase. Glutamic dehydrogenase then catalyzes the convertion of glutamate to α ketoglutarate, with the production of NH_3. The NH_3 formed in the tubular cells is secreted tubular lumen in exchange of Na^+ ion. Here it combines with H^+ to form ammonium. (NH_4^+) and is excreted (Fig. 6.29).

Factors affecting H^+ secretion along with HCO_3^- reabsorption

Increase in H^+ secretion

- *Increased pCO_2:* Increase in pCO_2 increases the secretion of H^+ and HCO_3^- absorption. When there is more pCO_2 it results in acidosis.
- *Hypokalemia:* When K^+ concentration is low, no competition with Na^+ for secretion.
- *Increased aldosterone and adrenocortical steroids:* It acts on distal tubule, more Na^+ is reabsorbed and more H^+ is secreted.

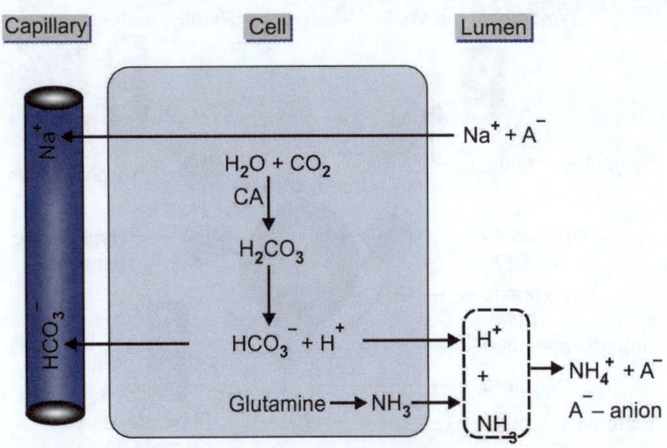

Fig. 6.29: Excretion of hydrogen ions in combination with ammonia

Decrease in H^+ secretion

- Decreased pCO_2
- Hyperkalemia
- Decreased aldosterone
- By carbonic anhydrase inhibitors—this is because H_2CO_3 is not formed.

RENAL CLEARANCE TESTS

These tests are done to assess the functions of different parts of nephrons. Renal clearance of a substance is the volume of plasma that is completely cleared of a substance by the kidneys per unit time. It is calculated from the following formula:

$$C = \frac{U \times V}{P}$$

where,

C = Clearance
U = Concentration of the substance in urine
V = Volume of urine exceted per unit time
P = Concentration of the substance in blood.

Measurement of Glomerular Filtration Rate

A substance that is completely filtered but neither reabsorbed nor secreted should be used to measure GFR. Inulin is an subtance used to measure GFR.

a. Inulin Clearance Test

A large initial dose of inulin is injected intravenously into the body. To maintain a relatively constant arterial plasma level inulin is infused at a constant rate into the body. After sometime concentration of inulin in plasma in venous blood (P_{in}), urinary concentration (U_{in}) and volume of urine excreted per minute (V) are determined. Inulin clearance is the gold standard method. But most widely used marker for GFR is creatinine clearance.

$$\text{Inulin clearance, } C_{in} = \frac{U_{in} \times V}{P_{in}}$$

For example the concentration of inulin in urine is 125 mg%. The plasma concentration is 1 mg%. The volume of urine output is 1 ml/min thus C_{in} gives GFR.

Inulin clearance is used as an indicator of plasma clearance mechanism. A comparison of the clearance of a given substance (C_x) with the clearance of inulin (C_{in}) provides information about the renal mechanisms used to remove the substances from plasma.

- When C_x equals C_{in}, excretion is by filtration alone.
- When $C_x < C_{in}$, excretion is by filtration and reabsorption.
- When $C_x > C_{in}$, excretion is by filtration and secretion.

b. Creatinine Clearance

The most common method to measure GFR in clinical practice is to determine the 24 hour endogenous creatinine clearance. Its determination does not require administration of exogenous creatinine, as creatinine is a product of muscle metabolism.

Normal range for creatinine clearance: 80–110 ml/min. However, some creatinine is reabsorbed by the tubules and some may be secreted. So, when precise measurement of GFR is required, inulin clearance is preferred.

Measurement of Renal Plasma Flow

To measure renal plasma flow, a substance, which is filtered and secreted but not reabsorbed should be used. Such a substance is para-aminohippuric acid (PAH).

a. *PAH Clearance:* A known amount of PAH is injected into the body. After sometime, the concentration of PAH in plasma and urine and the volume of urine excreted are estimated. Since PAH is completely cleared from the plasma, the clearance rate of that substance is equal to the total renal plasma flow.

   PAH clearance,

$$C_{PAH} = U_{PAH} \times \frac{V}{P_{PAH}}$$

   Thus C_{PAH} gives renal plasma flow.

b. *Diodrast clearance* can be also used to measure this.

Measurement of Renal Blood Flow

To determine renal blood flow value of two factors are necessary.

1. Renal plasma flow
2. Percentage of plasma volume in the blood.

Renal blood flow = renal plasma flow/% of plasma in blood

Formula can be also expressed as:

$$\text{Renal blood flow} = \text{RPF} \times \frac{1}{\text{1-Hct}}$$

where Hct = hematocrit.

Renal plasma flow is measured by using PAH clearance. The percentage of plasma volume is calculated indirectly by using PCV. If PCV is 45%, then the plasma volume in blood is 100 – 45 = 55%.

Quantifying Renal Urine Concentration and Dilution

Osmolar Clearance

The total clearance of solutes from blood can be expressed as the osmolar clearance. This is the volume of plasma cleared of solutes each time.

$$C_{OSM} = \frac{U_{OSM} \times V}{P_{OSM}}$$

where,

U_{osm} is the urine osmolarity

V is the urine flow rate

P_{osm} is the plasma osmolarity.

Free Water Clearance

It determines how much water is reabsorbed or lost while concentrating or diluting urine. It is calculated as the difference between urine flow rate and osmolar clearance.

$$C_{H_2O} = V - C_{OSM} = V - \frac{(U_{OSM} \times V)}{(P_{OSM})}$$

Thus rate of free water clearance represents the rate at which solute free water is excreted by the kidneys. When free water clearance is negative, water is conserved. When it is positive excess water is excreted by the kidney.

MICTURITION

Process of voiding the urine is called micturition. It is a reflex process. Although the micturition reflex is a spinal cord reflex, it can also be inhibited or facilitated by centers in the cerebral cortex or brainstem. The main physiological events in the process of micturition are filling of bladder and emptying of bladder.

Innervation of Urinary Bladder

Sympathetic Innervations

Preganglionic fibers of sympathetic nerve arise from 1st and 2nd lumbar segments of spinal cord. They pass through lateral sympathetic chain and terminate in hypogastric ganglion. The postganglionic fibers arising from this ganglion form the ***hypogastric nerve*** and supplies detrusor muscle and internal sphincter (Fig. 6.30). Stimulation of sympathetic nerve results in filling of bladder (by relaxation of detrusor muscle and contraction of internal sphincter). The sympathetic nerves to the bladder have no role in micturition, but they mediate

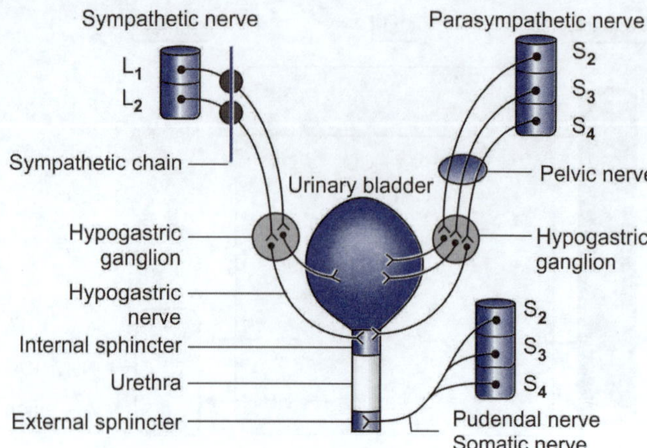

Fig. 6.30: Innervation of urinary bladder

contraction of bladder that prevents semen from entering the bladder during ejaculation.

Parasympathetic Innervation

Preganglionic fibres of parasympathetic nerve form the pelvic nerve ***(nervi ergentis)***. Pelvic nerve arise from 2nd, 3rd, and 4th sacral segments and terminate in hypogastric ganglion. The post ganglionic fibres arise from hypogastric ganglion and innervate detrusor muscle and internal sphincter. Stimulation of parasympathetic nerve results in emptying of bladder (by contraction of detrusor muscle and relaxation of internal sphincter). The pelvic nerve also has the sensory fibers which carry impulses from stretch receptors present on the wall of urinary bladder and urethra to sacral segments of spinal cord.

Somatic Nerve Supply

The external sphincter is innervated by the somatic nerve called the pudendal nerve. It arises 2nd, 3rd, and 4th sacral segments of spinal cord. It maintains tonic contraction of skeletal muscle fibers of external sphincter and keeps external sphincter constricted. During micturition this nerve is inhibited, leading to voiding of urine. Pudendal nerve is responsible for voluntary control of micturition.

Filling of Urinary Bladder

Urine formed in the kidney flows through ureter to urinary bladder. The physiological capacity of the bladder varies with age; 20–50 ml at birth, 200 ml at 1 year and 600 ml in adults. The anatomical capacity of bladder is 1 L.

Volume and Pressure Changes in Bladder During Filling

As bladder is filled up, it adjusts its tone and large volume of urine can be accommodated with minimal alterations in intravesical pressure. Each time urine flows, relaxation

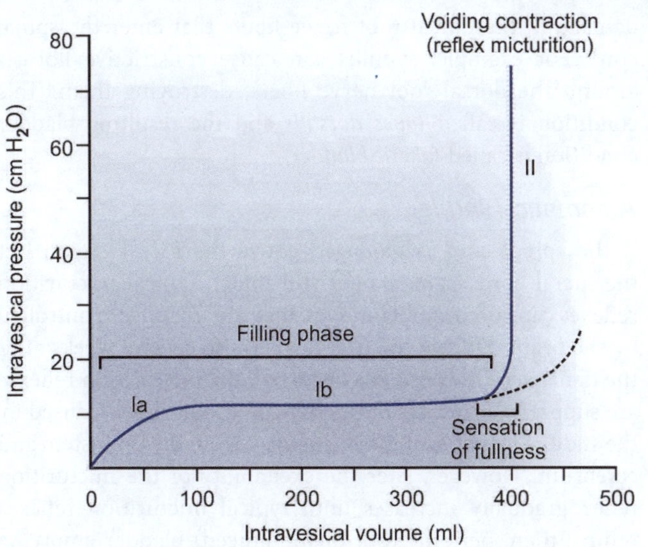

Fig. 6.31: Cystometrogram in a normal human

of detrusor muscle occurs until the physiological limit is exceeded.

Cystometrogram

A plot of intravesicle pressure against volume of fluid in the urinary bladder is called cystometrogram. Normal cystometrogram shows three phases of filling (Fig. 6.31).

Phase Ia

It is the initial phase of filling in which pressure rises to 5–10 cm of H_2O, when about 50 ml of fluid is collected in the bladder.

Phase Ib

- This segment shows plateau, i.e. the intravesical pressure remains more or less at 10 cm of H2O for a volume up to 400 ml of fluid. The flatness of phase Ib is a manifestation of law of laplace.

  Law of Laplace - P= 2T/R .

  where P = pressure in bladder, R = radius of bladder, T = tension on walls.
- In the bladder, tension increases as the urine is filled. At the same time the radius also increases due to relaxation of detrusor muscle. Therefore the pressure increase is slight.

Phase II

- Once the volume reaches 400 ml, pressure suddenly rises. This is shown by phase II of the graph. This is the volume at which micturition reflex occurs.

Note: The 1st urge to void is felt at about 150 ml and a marked sense of fullness at about 400 ml. When it is increased beyond 450 ml, pain and discomfort occurs.

Flowchart 6.2: Micturition reflex

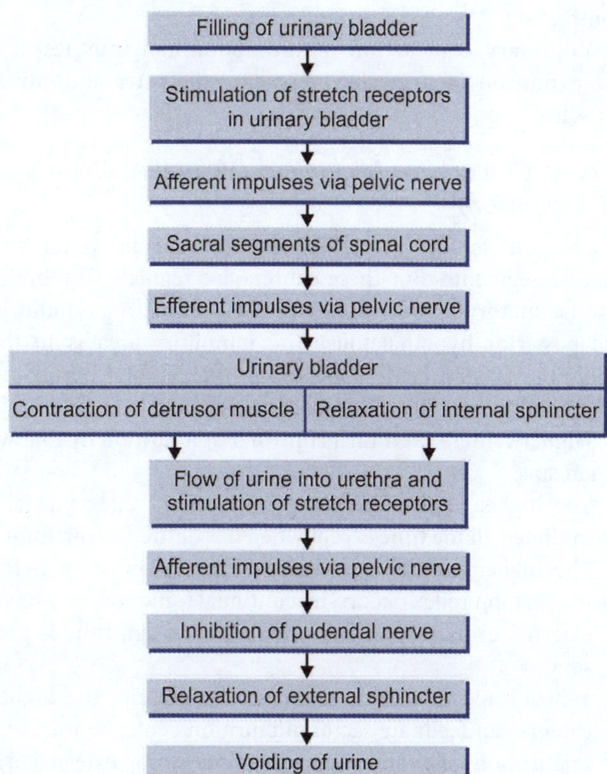

Emptying of Bladder

Micturition Reflex (Flowchart 6.2)

Micturition reflex is initiated by stimulation of stretch receptors located in the wall of urinary bladder. Filling of bladder by 300–400 ml of urine in adults is the normal stimulus for micturition to occur.

The sensory (afferent) impulses from the receptors reach the sacral segments of spinal cord via the sensory fibers of pelvic (parasympathetic) nerve. The motor (efferent) impulses produced in spinal cord, travel through motor fibers of pelvic nerve towards bladder and internal sphincter. The motor impulses cause contraction of detrusor muscle and relaxation of internal sphincter so that urine enters the urethra from the bladder.

Once urine enters urethra, the stretch receptors in the urethra are stimulated and send afferent impulses to spinal cord via pelvic nerve fibers. These impulses inhibit pudendal nerve. So external sphincter relaxes and micturition occurs.

Once a micturition reflex begins it is self regenerative, i.e. initial contraction of bladder further activates the receptors to cause still further increase in sensory impulses from bladder and urethra which cause further increase in reflex contraction of bladder. The cycle thus keeps on repeating itself again and again until the bladder has reached a strong degree of contraction.

Voluntary contraction of the abdominal muscles aids the expulsion of urine by increasing the intra-abdominal muscle.

Higher Centers for Micturition (Voluntary Control of Micturition)

Spinal centers for micturition are present in sacral and lumbar segments. But these centers are regulated by brain. The facilitatory area is located in the pontine region and in the posterior hypothalamus. The inhibitory area is in the midbrain. Several centers located in the cerebral cortex are mainly inhibitory, but can become excitatory.

Higher centers exert final control of micturition by following means:

a. The higher centers keep the micturition reflex partially inhibited all the time except when it is desired to micturate.
b. The higher centers can prevent micturition, even if the micturition reflex occurs, by continual tonic contraction of external urinary sphincter until a convenient time is present.
c. When convenient time to urinate is present, the higher centers can facilitate sacral micturition center to initiate a micturition reflex and at the same time inhibit external urinary sphincter so that urination can occur.

Voluntary Urination

First, a person voluntarily contracts his or her abdominal muscles. This increases the pressure in the bladder and allows extra urine to enter the bladder neck and posterior urethra. This stimulates stretch receptors, which excites the micturition reflex and simultaneously relaxes external urethral sphincter.

Note: In infants and young children micturition is purely a reflex action because the control from higher centers are not well established.

Abnormalities of Micturition

Atonic Bladder

Micturition reflex contraction cannot occur if the sensory nerve fibers from the bladder to the spinal cord are destroyed, thereby preventing transmission of stretch signals from the bladder. When this happens, a person loses bladder control, despite intact efferent fibers from the cord to the bladder and despite intact neurogenic connections within the brain. Instead of emptying periodically, the bladder fills to capacity and overflows a few drops at a time through the urethra. This is called *overflow incontinence.*

A common cause of atonic bladder is crush injury to the sacral region of the spinal cord. Certain diseases can also cause damage to the dorsal root nerve fibers that enter the spinal cord. For example, syphilis can cause constrictive fibrosis around the dorsal root nerve fibers, destroying them. This condition is called *tabes dorsalis* and the resulting bladder condition is called *tabetic bladder*.

Automatic Bladder

If the spinal cord is damaged above the sacral region but the sacral cord segments are still intact, typical micturition reflexes can still occur. However, they are no longer controlled by the brain. During the first few days to several weeks after the damage to the cord has occurred, the micturition reflexes are suppressed because of the state of 'spinal shock' caused by the sudden loss of facilitative impulses from the brainstem and cerebrum. However, later the excitability of the micturition reflex gradually increases until typical micturition reflexes return; then, periodic (but unannounced) bladder emptying occurs. But they are no longer controlled by brain. Voluntary control of micturition is completely lost. Whenever the bladder distention reaches a critical point, micturition reflex is set up and results in urination. Myelination of pyramidal tract will be completed by the age of two years only. So till then, there will be involuntary micturition or automatic bladder which is considered as normal in infants. In adults, automatic bladder may be seen in abnormalities like upper motor neuron lesions.

Uninhibited Neurogenic Bladder

Another abnormality of micturition is also called uninhibited neurogenic bladder, which results in frequent and relatively uncontrolled micturition. This condition derives from partial damage in the spinal cord or the brainstem that interrupts most of the inhibitory signals. Therefore, facilitative impulses passing continually down the cord keep the sacral centers so excitable that even a small quantity of urine elicits an uncontrollable micturition reflex, thereby promoting frequent urination.

DIURESIS

Diuresis is the condition where urine output is increased.

Water Diuresis

Increased water intake leads to decreased plasma osmolarity. This results in decreased secretion of ADH that results in decreased water reabsorption in CD, so dilute urine is excreted which is referred to as water diuresis. Effect of secretion of dilute urine starts 15 minutes after the ingestion of the water load and reaches a maximum at 40 minutes.

Water Intoxication

Maximum urine flow in water diuresis is 16 ml/min. If water is ingested at a rate higher than this for any length of time, swelling of cells because of uptake of water from the hypotonic ECF becomes severe. Swelling of cells in the brain causes convulsions and coma and leads eventually to death. Water intoxication can also occur when water intake is not reduced after administration of exogenous vasopressin or secretion of endogenous vasopressin in response to nonosmotic stimuli such as surgical trauma.

Osmotic Diuresis

Presence of large quantities of unreabsorbed solutes in tubules can cause increased urine output which is referred to as osmotic diuresis. Medullary hypertonicity is decreased when ascending LH cannot reabsorb Na^+ maximally. It causes decreased water reabsorption from descending LH which causes more fluid entry into CD. So there is marked increase in urine volume and increased Na^+ and solute excretion. Osmotic diuresis can be induced by administration of mannitol and infusion of large amount of NaCl and urea.

Difference between osmotic diuresis and water diuresis

In water diuresis, the amount of water reabsorbed in the proximal portions of nephrons is normal and the maximal urine flow that can be produced is about 16 ml/min. In osmotic diuresis, increased urine flow is due to decreased water reabsorption in proximal tubules and loops and very large urine flows can be produced. As the load of excreted solute is increased, the concentration of urine approaches that of plasma in spite of maximal vasopressin secretion because large fraction of excreted urine is isotonic with proximal tubular fluid.

Diuretics

Diuretics are substances which enhance the output of urine. These substances increase the excretion of water, sodium, chloride through urine.

Most diuretics used clinically decreases rate of Na^+ reabsorption in renal tubules. Natriuresis occurs then, in turn increases H_2O output. Tubular reabsorption of many other solutes like K^+, Cl^-, Mg^{2+}, Ca^{2+} are influenced by Na^+ reabsorption secondarily. So, many diuretics increases renal output of these solutes also.

Osmotic diuretics increases osmotic pressure of tubular fluid thereby decreses H_2O reabsorption and increases urine output.

Sites of Action of Various Diuretics (Fig. 6.32)

1. Furosemide and other loop diuretics - thick ascending limb of loop of Henle.
2. Thiazides-early portion of distal convoluted tubule.
3. Aldosterone antagonist (Spironolactone triamterene)-collecting duct.
4. Antagonist to V_2 vasopressin receptors-on collecting duct.

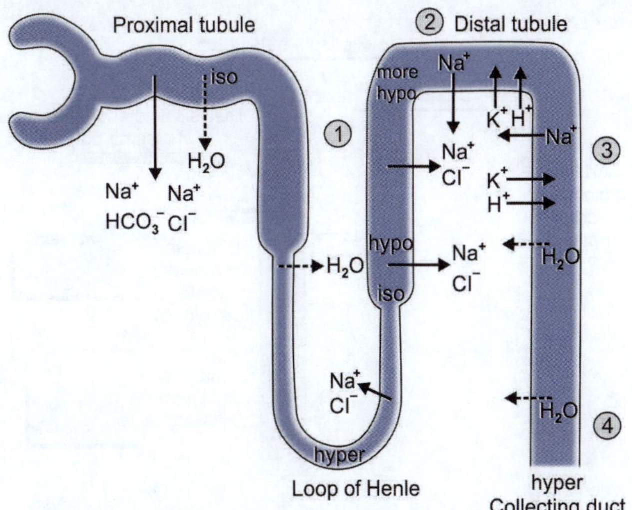

Fig. 6.32: Site of action of various diuretics

Mode of Action

- *Furosemide:* Inhibit Na^+ - K^+ - $2Cl^-$ Cotransport.
- *Thiazides:* Inhibit Na^+ - Cl^- Cotransport.
- *Aldosterone antagonist:* Inhibit action of aldosterone on tubular receptor.
- *Antagonist to V_2 vasopressin receptors:* Inhibits the action of vasopressin.
- *Xanthines like theophylline and caffeine:* Decrease tubular reabsorption of Na^+ and increase GFR.
- *Acetazolamide (carbonic anhydrase inhibitor):* Decrease H^+, with resultant increase in Na^+ and K^+ excretion.
- *Water and ethanol:* Inhibits vasopressin secretion.
- *Glucose and Mannitol:* Produce osmotic diueresis.

DIALYSIS

Severe loss of kidney function, either acutely or chronically is a threat to life and requires removal of toxic waste products and restoration of body fluid volume and composition toward normal. This can be accomplished by kidney transplantation or by dialysis with an artificial kidney.

The basic principle of the artificial kidney is to pass blood through minute blood channels bounded by a thin cellophane membrane. On the other side of the membrane is a dialysing fluid into which unwanted substances in the blood pass by diffusion (Fig. 6.33).

Cellophane is porous enough to allow the constituents of the plasma, except the plasma proteins to diffuse in both directions from plasma into the dialyzing fluid or from the dialyzing fluid back into the plasma.

If the concentration of a substance is greater in the plasma than in the dialyzing fluid, there will be net transfer of the

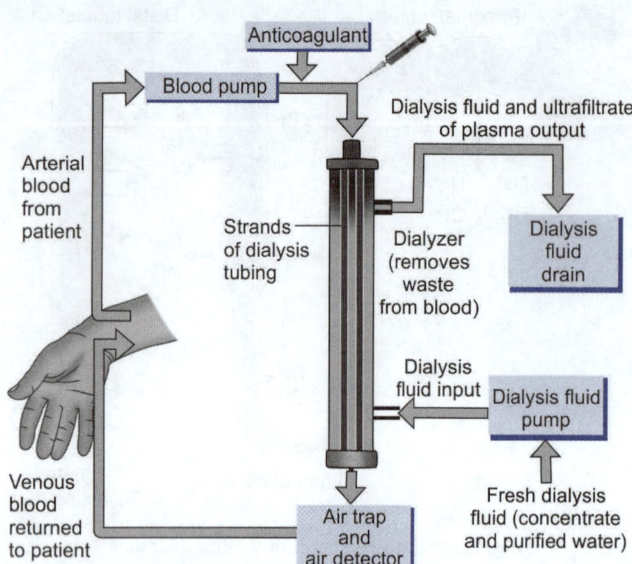

Fig. 6.33: Principles of dialysis

substance from the plasma into the dialyzing fluid. The rate of movement of the solute across the dialyzing membrane depends upon:

1. Concentration gradient of the solute between the two solutions.
2. Permeability of the membrane to the solute.
3. Surface area of the membrane
4. Length of time that the blood and fluid remain in contact with the membrane.

Dialyzing Fluid

The concentration of ions and other substances in the dialyzing fluid are not the same as that in normal plasma or uremic plasma. They are adjusted to levels that are needed to cause appropriate movement of water and solutes through the membrane during dialysis. It contains no creatinine, urea, or other substances to be completely removed from plasma.

Renal Failure

Renal failure refers to the severe deterioration of renal function. It is of two types: acute and chronic.

1. *Acute renal failure:* The onset of this condition is sudden (within days or weeks). It may be due to decreased blood supply to the kidneys, obstruction of the urinary collecting system, etc.
2. *Chronic renal failure:* Refers to a slow (over a period of months), irreversible deterioration of renal functions. It results from diabetes mellitus, glomerulonephritis, pyelonephritis, TB, etc.

Nephrotic Syndrome

It is characterized by loss of large quantities of plasma proteins into the urine. The cause of protein loss in urine is increased permeability of glomerular membrane. So diseases like chronic glomerulonephritis, amyloidosis which increases permeability of membrane can cause nephrotic syndrome. As a consequence of the decreased plasma protein concentration, the plasma colloid osmotic pressure falls to low levels. This causes the capillaries all over the body to filter large amounts of fluid into the various tissues, which in turn causes edema and decreases the plasma volume.

Renal sodium retention in nephrotic syndrome occurs through multiple mechanisms activated by leakage of protein and fluid from the plasma into the interstitial fluid, activation of Na^+ retaining systems such as the renin-angiotensin system, aldosterone, sympathetic nervous system. However, because of the large amount of Na^+ and water retention, the plasma protein concentration becomes further diluted, causing still more fluid to leak into the tissues of the body.

Fanconi Syndrome

It is associated with increased urinary excretion of amino acids, glucose and phosphates. In severe cases other manifestations are also observed such as (a) failure to reabsorb sodium bicarbonate (b) increased excretion of K^+ and Ca^{2+} (c) failure of kidney to respond to ADH. The causes for Fanconi syndrome are hereditary defects in cell transport mechanisms, toxins or drugs that injure the renal tubular epithelial cells, ischemia (causes injury to tubular cell). The proximal tubular cells are especially affected due to tubular injury.

Nocturnal Enuresis

Voiding of urine in the bed during sleep is normal in the infants and young children. Nocturnal enuresis is sometimes seen in older children and adults due to organic leisions. For example, lumbosacral vertebral defect and also due to psychological factors.

Urinary Calculi/Renal Stones

These are mainly composed of calcium stones, i.e. calcium oxalates or calcium phosphates. It may sometimes due to uric acid. They cause obstruction to urine flow. Complications include vomiting, sweating, fever, severe pain and hematuria.

CLINICAL QUESTIONS

1. **A child was brought to the clinic by the parents with complaints of fever, swelling of the face and passing less quantity of urine. On examination there was edema over face and eyelids. Investigations revealed albuminuria.**
   a. Identify the probable condition.
   b. Are plasma proteins normally excreted in the urine?
   c. Explain the features.
2. **A patient with a previous history of Syphilis complains of inability to feel fullness of bladder but voluntary voiding is possible.**
   a. What is this condition?
   b. What is the cause of this condition?
   c. Describe the nerve supply of the bladder.
3. **Calculate effective filtration pressure for GFR from following data.**
   a. Hydrostatic pressure in glomerular capillary = 60 mm Hg
   b. Bowman's capsular fluid pressure = 18 mm Hg
   c. Colloid osmotic pressure in glomerular capillary = 32 mm Hg

Answers for Clinical Questions are given in the Appendix

CHAPTER

7

Temperature Regulation

Normal body temperature depends on balance between heat production and loss.

Body heat is produced by:

- Metabolism of food (basal)
- Food assimilation
- Muscular activities
- Accumulation of brown fat.

Body heat is lost by:

- Radiation
- Conduction
- Vaporization of sweat
- Small amount through urine and feces.

Group of reflex responses that are primarily integrated in hypothalamus, operated to maintain body temperature in a narrow range in spite of wide fluctuation in environment temperature in warm blooded (homeothermic animals) constitute the mechanisms of temperature regulation.

Regulation of body temperature is important because:

- Speed of chemical reaction taking place in the body depends on body temperature.
- Enzymes of body show optimum activity within a narrow range of temperature.

Measurement

Using clinical thermometer,
C = (F–32) × 5/9; Unit is °C.
F = (C × 9/5) +32; Unit is °F.

Normal oral temperature: 36.3–37.1°C/98.3–98.8°F
Scrotal temperature: 32°C to facilitate spermatogenesis.
Oral temperature is 0.5°C less than rectal temperature. Oral temperature is variable but rectal/core temperature is constant.

Hyperthermia is when temperature increases more than 41.6°C (107°F). *Hypothermia* is when temperature decreases less than 25°C (95°F).

Physiological Variation

- Temperature normally increases in the morning and decreases in the evening.
- In females during ovulation body temperature increases
- During exercise body temperature increases to 40°C.

Some adults have chronically above normal temperature known as constitutional hyperthermia. Temperature regulation is less precise in young children, they may normally have a temperature that is 0.5°C or so above the established norm for adults. In females body temperature is normally 0.5°C more than in males (During ovulation and after ovulation, till menstruation, i.e. during luteal/progestational phase).

Pathological Variation

Hyperthyroidism

In hyperthyroidism temperature increases 0.5°C more than normal.

CENTRAL REGULATION OF TEMPERATURE

Hypothalamus is considered as thermostat. Temperature is set at normal level in hypothalamus and when body temperature increases or falls from set point level, various mechanisms gets activated to bring back temperature to set point level.

- Anterior hypothalamus is activated by warmth and is considered to be *heat loss center.*
- Posterior hypothalamus is activated by cold and is known as *heat gain center.*

Various Mechanisms of Temperature Regulation

Afferent impulses reach hypothalamus from receptors in skin, deep tissue, spinal cord, extrahypothalamic region of brain and other parts of brain and activate the following mechanisms (Table 7.1).

Mechanisms Activated by Cold

Increase in Heat Production

- *Shivering:* Shivering is an involuntary response of skeletal muscle to cold which increases skeletal muscle contraction which in turn increases heat production.
- *Increased hunger:* Increased food intake, increases utilization of food which increases body temperature.
- *Increased voluntary activity:* This leads to increase in body temperature.
- Increased production of epinephrine and norepinephrine.

Table 7.1: Mechanisms of temperature regulation

Mechanisms activated by cold (mechanisms of heat gain)	
Increased heat production	**Decreased heat loss**
• Shivering	• Cutaneous vasoconstriction
• Hyperphagia	• Reduced surface area: Curling up
• Increased secretion of catecholamine	• Piloerection: It is important for animals with fur or feathers but not for human
• Increased secretion of thyroxine	
• Exercise (increased voluntary muscle activity)	
• Non-shivering thermogenesis	
Mechanisms activated by heat (mechanisms of heat loss)	
Increased heat loss	**Decreased heat production**
• Cutaneous vasodilation (Earliest response)	• Anorexia
• Sweating	• Lethargy (decreased muscular activity)
• Panting → not important in man	
• The earliest response to heat stress → cutaneous vasodilatation	
• The most important mechanism for the heat loss in response to heat stress → sweating	
• The earliest response to cold stress → cutaneous vasconstriction	
• The major heat production mechanism induced by the cold stress → shivering	

Decrease in Heat Loss

- *Vasoconstriction:* Amount of heat reaching skin from deeper tissues is decreased and will store heat centrally in blood vessels. Cutaneous vessels being cool is more sensitive to catecholamines leads to further constriction of arterioles and venules.
- *Horripilation (Goose wildeness):* Cold intended contraction of piloerector muscles, important in animals. Increased trapping of hair causes increased heat production.
- *Concurrent flow of blood:* In animals at extremities arteries and veins are arranged parallely. Deep veins run along side arteries supplying limbs. Heat transfer between warm arterial blood going to the limbs and cold venous blood coming from extremities cause counter current exchange of heat causing conservation of heat.
- Behavioral changes like curling up.

Mechanisms Activated by Heat

Increase in Heat Loss

Increased heat loss by conduction, convection and radiation

When surrounding temperature is much lower, heat loss takes place mainly through conduction, convection and radiation. When surrounding temperature is close to body tempeature, evaporation becomes major route of heat loss.

Sweating

When body temperature increases, there is increased sweating, thus increased vaporization of water from body surface, which in turn decreases body temperature. Vaporization also occurs through mucous membrane of oral cavity and respiratory packages. Thus, there is certain amount of water loss continuously called insensible loss of water. Vaporization of 1 g of water removes 0.6 kcal of heat.

Cutaneous vasodilatation

Conduction occurs from surface of one object to surface of another object. Temperature of skin determines to a great extent the degree to which heat is gained or lost. Amount of heat reaching the skin, from deeper tissues can be varied by changing the blood flow to the skin. When temperature increases, cutaneous vessels are dilated, warm blood reaches skin and is lost to the surroundings. Rate at which heat is transferred from deep tissues to the skin is called tissue conductance and it increases at high temperature.

Panting

Rapid shallow breathing seen in animals.

Decrease in Heat Production

Generalized lethargy and apathy

Causes decreased muscular activity and thus heat production is decreased.

Loss of appetite

This causes decreased food intake and thus decreased heat production.

Fever

Oldest and most universally known hallmark of diseases. The causes of fever are infection and injuries. During fever, temperature is raised, thermoregulatory mechanism act to regulate body temperature at its new higher levels, i.e. there is apparent reset of thermostat to higher level.

Infection or tissue injury → release endotoxin or pyrogens → Act on RE cells and thereby stimulate monocytes, macrophages, Kupffer cells → produce cytokinins (interleukins, interferons) → cytokinins act on (organum vasculosum of the lamina terminalis (OVLT) → Preoptic area of hypothalamus stimulated (OVLT) → release of local PGs → raise temperature set point → fever resulted.

Advantage of fever is that increased temperature decreases bacterial growth.

CONDITIONS OF HEAT STRESS

Heat stress is the condition of excessive hyperthermia in which impact of heat on the body becomes acute and severe. Such a situation occurs when the heat transport power of the environment overwhelms thermoregulatory competence of the body. The common condition that leads to heat stress is the prolonged exposure to an environment, which is extremely hot and humid. Especially, when physical activity that increases the rate of heat production is increased in such a condition, severe hyperthermia ensues. Evaporation from the skin becomes an important mechanism for heat dissipation in such conditions. But, this is impaired by a higher humidity of the environment that reduces the skin to environment gradient for water vapor pressure, which reduces evaporation. Thus, very hot and humid weather predisposes to progressive hyperthermia and consequent heat stress. The common consequences of heat stress are: heat syncope, heat exhaustion and heat stroke.

- *Heat syncope:* Heat syncope is a state of circulatory failure that occurs due to excessive heat. The major pathophysiologic dysfunction is due to venous pooling of blood that decreases venous return. Venodilation occurs as a compensatory increase in skin blood flow in prolonged exposure to heat. The consequent decrease in end-diastolic volume lowers cardiac output and blood pressure.

  In severe form, it may cause loss of consciousness. As thermoregulatory mechanisms are intact, usually core temperature is not raised. Skin mostly remains wet and cool. In addition to transferring patient from hot environment immediately, treatment aims at improving the diastolic filling of the heart.
- *Heat exhaustion:* Heat exhaustion is a common condition of heat stress. It occurs due to imbalance in cardiovascular homeostasis in a hot environment. This is also called heat collapse.
  - Collapse is usually precipitated during exercise.
  - Decreased diastolic filling of ventricle is the primary pathophysiologic mechanism of heat exhaustion.
  - However, exact mechanism of decreased venous return is not known, though hypovolemia is proposed to be the major contributing factor.
  - Hypotension activates baroreceptors reflex and therefore prevents fainting.

  Features of heat exhaustion include nausea, vomiting, tachycardia, weakness, confusion, headache, ataxia and vertigo. The patient sweats profusely. In severe cases, dilation of pupil may develop and patient may faint.

  Fluid replacement and rest usually improves the condition. Salt intake helps. Though, usually body temperature is normal or slightly elevated in heat exhaustion, hyperthermia and dehydration frequently lead to heat stroke. Hence, it is better to keep the patient in a cool environment.
- *Heat stroke:* Heat stroke is the most perilous disorder of heat stress. It is characterized by high core temperature, neurological deficits and loss of consciousness. Convulsion is the frequent association. There are two forms of heat stroke: classical and exertional.
  1. For classical heat stroke, the major cause is a very high environmental heat that supercedes thermoregulatory mechanisms of the body.
  2. For exertional heat stroke, the major cause is accelerated production of metabolic heat. Usually, exertion in a high ambient temperature predisposes to heat stroke.

The exact pathophysiologic mechanism of heat stroke is not known. Though hyperthermia is the major culprit, state of physical exercise is an important contributor. A triggering factor could be release of endotoxin from bacterial flora which may occur due to intestinal ischemia that allows the toxins to enter circulation and activate inflammatory responses. Treatment should be prompt. Damage to kidney, liver and skeletal muscle are usual complications. In heat stroke, patient rapidly becomes comatose. The skin is dry and body temperature is usually above 106°F. In fact, it is a medical emergency and requires prompt treatment.

- Immediate therapy includes rapid reduction in body temperature, which is effectively accomplished by immersion of the body in cold water.
- Prompt hydration and maintenance of a patent airway prevents complications to develop.

Malignant Hyperthermia

Malignant hyperthermia is a rare condition of very high increase in body temperature that usually occurs on exposure to anesthetics or depolarizing neuromuscular blockers. This is due to mutation of gene coding for ryanodine receptors. This results in increased Ca^{2+} release that severely activates myosin ATPase activity, thereby excessive contraction of muscle occurs, which leads to increased heat production. Halothane anesthesia is known to cause in susceptible individuals. Treatment is by immediate use of dantrolene sodium that decreases the release of calcium from the sarcoplasmic reticulum.

Hypothermia

When body temperature is less than 25°C, ill effects of hypothermia develop. Decreased body metabolism, enzymatic activity, slowing of heart and respiration, and slowing reflex activities are features of hypothermia. If very severe, loss of consciousness occurs, which may further lead to death. The common cause of hypothermia is prolonged exposure to severely cold environment or prolonged immersion in cold water.

Hypothermia occurs earlier and in more severe form in cold water than in cold air. Hypothermia in infants and elderly people is severe than in adults. Peripheral vasoconstriction and shivering do not prevent hypothermia during prolonged exposure in cold water for water's high thermal conductivity. However, a thick layer of insulating fat decreases loss of heat to the water. Therefore, swimmers in cold water apply a thick layer of grease on the skin surface before swimming.

CLINICAL QUESTION

1. **A marathon runner after running the race for 2 hours in hot climate suddenly collapsed. On examination there was tachycardia and BP was low.**
   a. Identify the condition.
   b. What is the cause?
   c. Give physiological basis of the treatment.

Answer for Clinical Question is given in the Appendix

CHAPTER

8

Endocrinology

INTRODUCTION

The biological functions of the multicellular living organism are well-oriented. This coordination is achieved by two main control systems, nervous and the endocrine system. The important endocrine glands include hypothalamus, anterior, pituitary, posterior pituitary, thyroid gland, parathyroid gland, islets of Langerhans, pancreas, adrenal cortex, adrenal medulla, kidney, ovary and testes.

Hormone

Hormones are secretory products of ductless (endocrine) glands released directly into circulation in small amounts in response to a specific stimulus and on delivery in circulation produce response on target cells.

Classification

Depending Upon the Chemical Nature (Flowchart 8.1)

Flowchart 8.1: Classification of hormones based on chemical nature

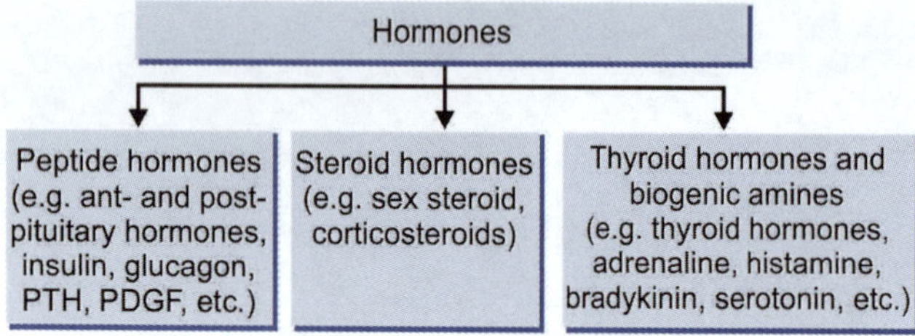

Depending Upon the Mechanisms of Action

1. *Group I hormone:* These act by binding to intracellular receptors and mediate their actions via formation of a hormone receptor complex. These include steroid, thyroid hormones. These hormones have intracellular receptors.
2. *Group II hormone:* These involve second messenger to mediate their effect. These hormones have cell membrane receptors.

Mechanism of Hormone Action

On the target cell, the hormone in combination with the receptor acts by any of the following mechanisms:

- By altering the permeability of the cell membrane.
- By activating the intracellular enzyme.
- Through effect on gene expression.
- Through tyrosine kinase activation.

Action Through Change in Membrane Permeability

Hormone bind with receptors present in the cell membrane (external receptors) leading to its conformational change causing either closing or opening of the ion channels (such as Na^+, K^+ channel), e.g. adrenaline, noradrenaline act by this mechanism.

Action Through Secondary Messengers which Activate the Intracellular Enzyme

The peptides and biogenic amines are two principal classes of hormones which act through second messengers. The hormone, which acts on a target cell is called first messenger. This hormone in combination with the receptor forms hormone-receptor complex. This in turn activates the enzymes of the cell and causes the formation of another substance called the second messenger (cAMP, IP_3, DAG). The release of second messenger is mediated by GTP binding proteins or G proteins (Fig. 8.1).

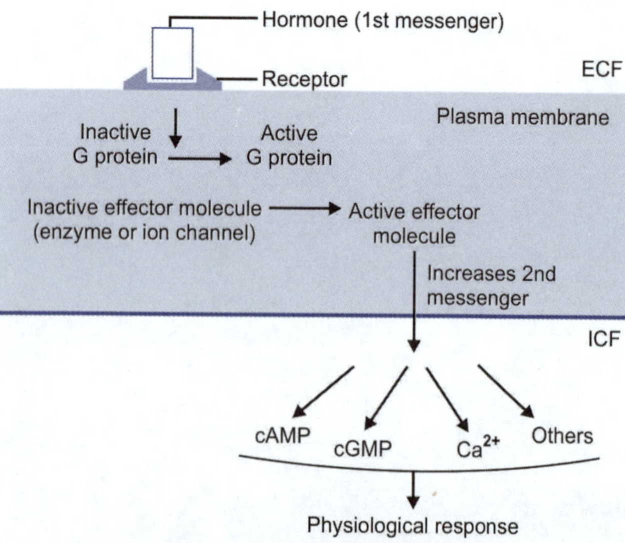

Fig. 8.1: Secondary messenger mediated hormone activity

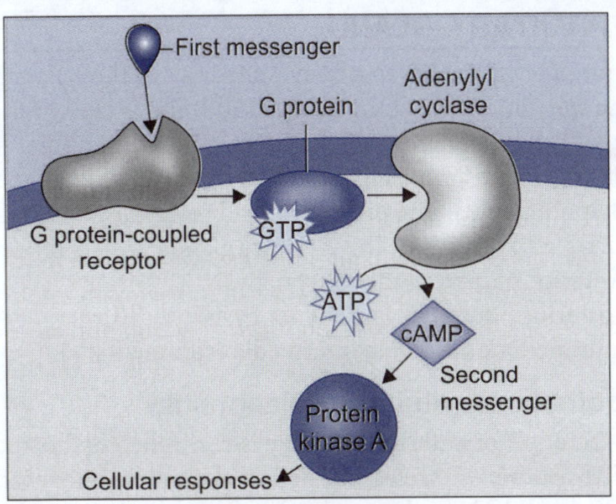

Fig. 8.2: cAMP mediated hormone activity

cAMP as the second messenger (Fig. 8.2)

G protein stimulate the enzyme adenyl cyclase. This increases the formation of intracellular cAMP from ATP. cAMP stimulate protein kinase A. Protein kinase A phosphorylates enzyme protein, thus enzyme is stimulated or inhibited. For examples, epinephrine, norepinephrine, ACTH, LH, GnRH, hCG, TSH.

IP_3 and DAG acts as second messenger (Fig. 8.3)

A signaling molecule binds to a receptor, leading to activation of G protein that stimulates phosholipase C. Phospholipase C cleaves phosphotidyl inositol diphosphate (PIP_2) forming inositol triphosphate (IP_3) and diacylglycerol (DAG). IP_3 and DAG are the second messenger. DAG activates protein kinase C, which phosphorylates its targets. IP_3 quickly diffuses through the cytosol and binds to an IP_3 gated calcium channel in the ER membrane, causing it to open. Calcium ions flowout of the ER, raising the Ca^{2+} level in the cytosol. The calcium ions activate the next protein in one or more signaling pathways. For example, angiotensin-II and vasopressin.

Calcium calmodulin second messenger system

Many hormones act by increasing the calcium ion, which acts as second messenger along with another protein called calmodulin. System operates in response to the entry of Ca into the cells. Ca entry is initiated by:

- Changes in membrane potential that open Ca channels.
- A hormone interacting with membrane receptors that open Ca channels.

On entering a cell, calcium ions bind with the protein calmodulin. Calmodulin has four calcium sites and when three or four of these sites have bound with calcium, the calmodulin changes shape. This initiates multiple effects inside the cell, including activation or inhibition of protein kinases. Activation of calmodulin-dependent protein kinases causes activation or inhibition of proteins involved in the cell's response to the hormone (via phosphorylation).

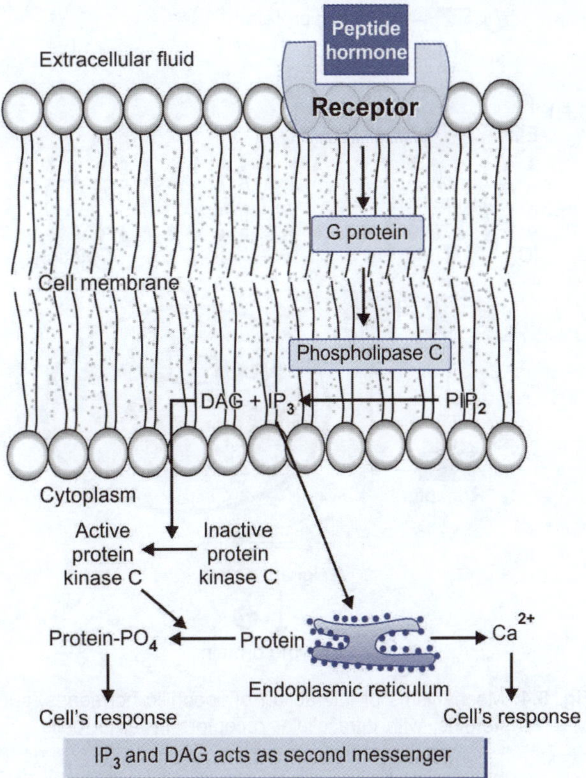

Fig. 8.3: IP_3 and DAG mediated hormone activity

Through Effect on Gene Expression

The mechanism of action of thyroid and hormones is by acting on the genes of the target cells (Fig. 8.4).

Sequence of events are:

1. Transport-after secretion, the hormone is carried to the target tissue on serum binding protein.
2. Internalization-being lipophilic the hormone easily diffuse through the plasma membrane.
3. Receptor hormone complex (RHC) is formed by binding of hormone to the specific receptor inside the cell.
4. Conformational change occurs in receptor protein leading to activation of receptors.
5. The activated RHC then diffuse into the nucleus and binds on specific region on DNA. This initiates transcription.
6. Binding of the RHC to DNA alters the rate of transcription of mRNA.
7. The mRNA moves out of the nucleus and reaches ribosomes. Here it promotes translation process. In this way new proteins are formed which result in specific responses.

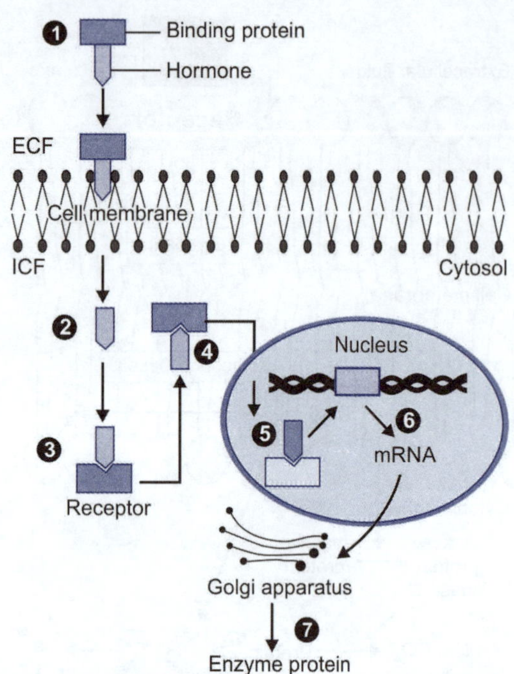

Fig. 8.4: Mechanisms of interaction of lipophilic hormones, such as steroids, with intracellular receptors in target cells

Action Through Tyrosine Kinase Activation

Enzyme-linked hormone receptors

These receptors when activated, functions directly as enzymes or are closely associated with enzymes that they activate. These enzyme linked receptors have their hormone binding site on the outside of the cell membrane and their catabolic or enzyme binding site on the inside. When the hormone binds to the extracellular portion of the receptor, an enzyme immediately inside the cell is activated (or occasionally inactivated). This mechanism of signal generation from plasma membrane receptors does not require G protein intermediaries. For examples, leptin receptor.

The activation of tyrosine kinase occurs by two mechanism:

1. Due to the binding of hormone to the receptor, the receptor itself becomes a tyrosine kinase that phosphorylates tyrosine residue on intracellular protein substrates. This sets into motion a cascade of events leading to enzyme activation and gene expression.
2. Hormone binding to extracellular portion of the receptor can attract intracytoplasmic tyrosine kinases like janus kinase (JAK) and then activates them. This causes phosphorylation of transcription factor proteins and ultimately modulate gene expression, e.g. insulin, IGF, EGF (epidermal growth factor), PDGF, ANF, GABA.

PITUITARY GLAND

The pituitary gland lies in a bony walled cavity, the sella turcica of the sphenoid bone at the base of skull, and is closely associated with hypothalamus of the brain. The infundibular stem (stalk) of the posterior lobe arises in the median eminence of the hypothalamus. The pituitary gland (hypophysis) originate in early embryonic life. The pituitary gland consists of:

1. Anterior pituitary/Adenohypophysis
2. Posterior pituitary/Neurohypophysis
3. Intermediate lobe/Pars intermedia (rudimentary).

Hypothalamo-pituitary Relationship

The secretion of anterior pituitary is controlled by hormones called hypothalamic releasing/hypothalamic inhibitory factors secreted within hypothalamus itself. They are then conducted to anterior pituitary through hypothalamo-hypophyseal portal vessel (Fig. 8.5). In anterior pituitary these releasing and inhibitory hormones act on glandular cells to control their secretion (Flowchart 8.2). Posterior pituitary does not secrete hormones. Posterior pituitary hormones are synthesized by cell bodies located in ***supraoptic and paraventricular nuclei*** of hypothalamus. The hormones are then transported in the axoplasm of nerve fibers to postpituitary. Axons that arise from supraoptic and paraventricular nuclei of hypothalamus pass to posterior pituitary via hypothalamo-hypophyseal tract (Fig. 8.6). The nerve endings contains secretory granules (Herring bodies). They secrete ADH/vasopressin and oxytocin.

Pituitary Hormones

Anterior pituitary has five important cell types that secrete six important hormones. The five cell types are thyrotrope, corticotrope, somatotrope, gonadotrope and lactotrope.

Anterior Lobe

TSH, ACTH, GH, FSH, LH, prolactin and β lipotropin.

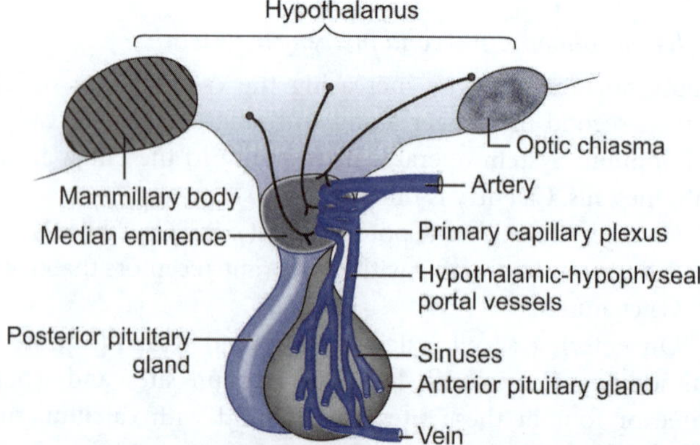

Fig. 8.5: Hypothalamic-hypophyseal portal vessel

Flowchart 8.2: Hypothalamic-pituitary-target organ axis

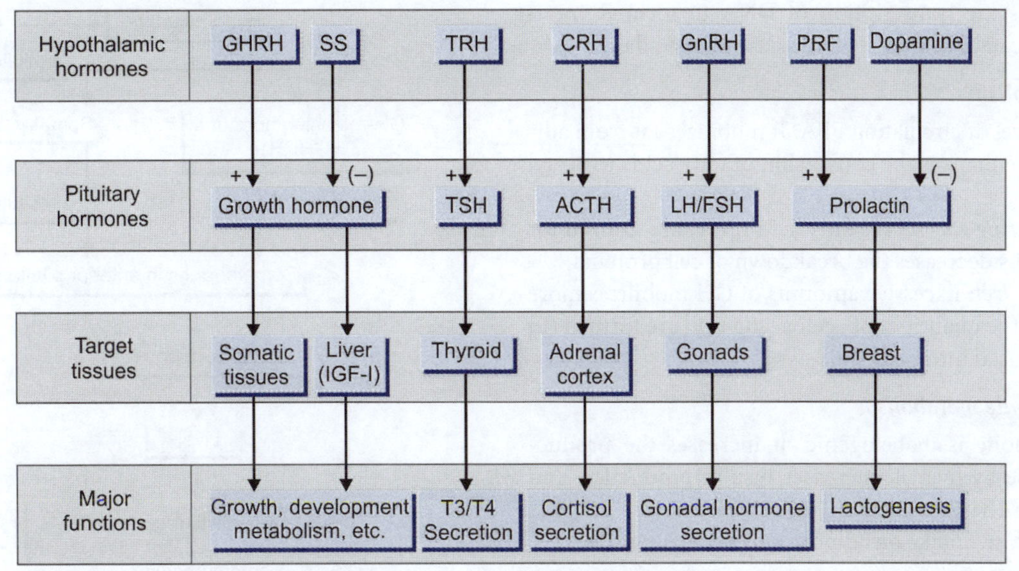

Plus sign (+) indicates stimulation and minus sign (–) indicates inhibition

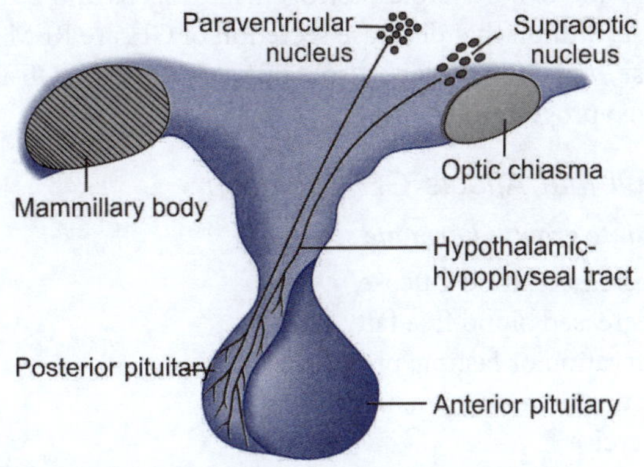

Fig. 8.6: Hypothalamic-hypophyseal tract

Posterior Lobe

ADH and oxytocin.

Intermediate Lobe

α and β melanocyte stimulating hormone.

Growth Hormone

It is also called as somatotropin/somatotropic hormone. It causes growth of almost all tissues of the body that are capable of growing (Fig. 8.7).

Somatomedins: They are polypeptide growth factors secreted by the liver and other tissues. The effects of GH on growth, cartilage and protein metabolism depends on the interaction between GH and somatomedins (Fig. 8.8). They are also called insulin like growth factors (IGFs, their effects on growth are similar to effects of insulin on growth). The principal circulating somatomedins are IGF-I (somatomedin C) and IGF-II.

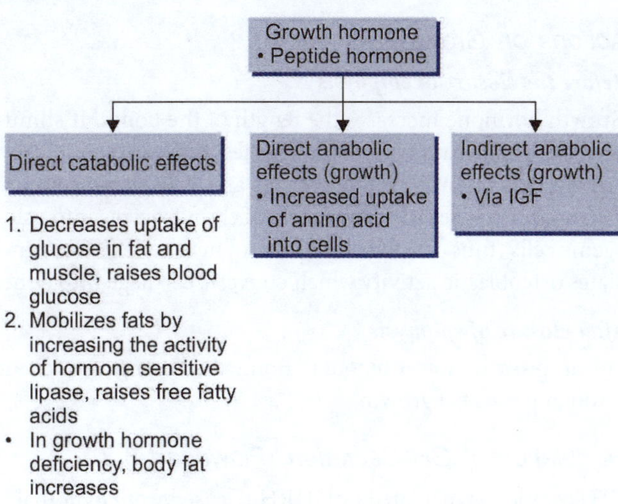

Fig. 8.7: Actions of growth hormone

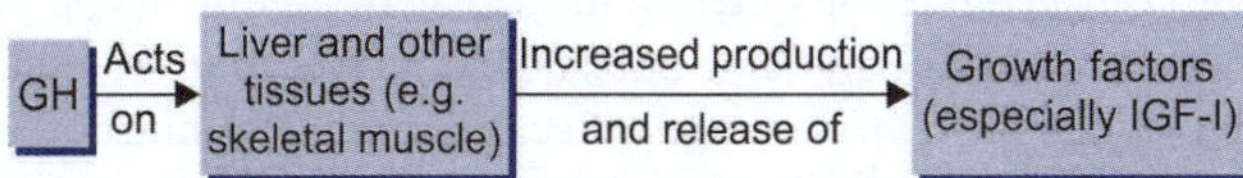

Fig. 8.8: IGF mediated effects of growth hormone

Metabolic Effect of GH

On protein metabolism

Growth hormone has an anabolic effect on protein metabolism. It increases amino acid uptake into the cells. It increases protein synthesis in ribosomes (enhances RNA translation). GH stimulates the transcription of DNA to form RNA. It decreases the catabolism of protein and amino acids.

On fat metabolism

It increases level of circulating FFA. It mobilizes fat from adipose tissue. It enhances the conversion of fatty acids to acetyl CoA.

Protein sparing effect: Free fatty acid (FFA) are utilized for energy and thus decreases the breakdown of cell protein.

Ketogenic effect: Excessive amounts of GH mobilizes more FFA so that large quantities of acetoacetic acid are formed (in liver) and released into body fluids.

On carbohydrate metabolism

Growth hormone is diabetogenic. It increases the production of glucose by liver. It increases insulin production and decreases sensitivity to insulin (insulin resistance) hence it decreases glucose uptake on adipose and skeletal muscle.

On electrolyte metabolism

Intestinal absorption of Ca is promoted. Renal excretion of electrolytes like Na^+, Ca^{2+}, PO_4^{3-} and K^+ is suppressed. Retention of electrolytes and diversion of those electrolyte to growing tissue.

Actions on Growth

Before the closure of epiphysis

Growth hormone increases the length of the bones. It stimulates the proliferation of chondrocytes and osteogenic cells. Protein deposition by chondrocytes and osteogenic cells are increased. It causes the conversion of chondrocytes into osteogenic cells (thus causing deposition of new bones). GH stimulates osteoblastic activity which converts cartilage into bone.

After closure of epiphysis

Linear growth not promoted. Bone thickening can occur through periosteal growth.

Regulation of GH Secretion (Flowchart 8.3)

GH secretion is regulated by GHRH released from hypothalamus. GH is secreted in a pulsatile fashion throughout the life, with elevated rates of secretion immediately after birth and at puberty. Interestingly, large bursts of secretion occur at night during the onset of deep sleep. Secretion of GH requires the presence of normal plasma levels of thyroid hormones. GH secretion is markedly reduced in hypothyroid individuals. The inhibitory effect of IGF-I represents a negative feedback loop to the hypothalamus.

Stimuli that increase secretion of GH are hypoglycemia, exercise, fasting, protein meals, amino acids (like arginine), stress, glucagon, pyrogen, lysine vasopressin, apomorphine, L-dopa and α-adrenergics, estrogen, androgens and 2-deoxyglucose. Stimuli that decrease secretion of GH are REM sleep, glucose, somatostatin, cortisol, FFA, GH itself, IGF-I, and medroxyprogesterone.

Flowchart 8.3: Regulation of growth hormone secretion

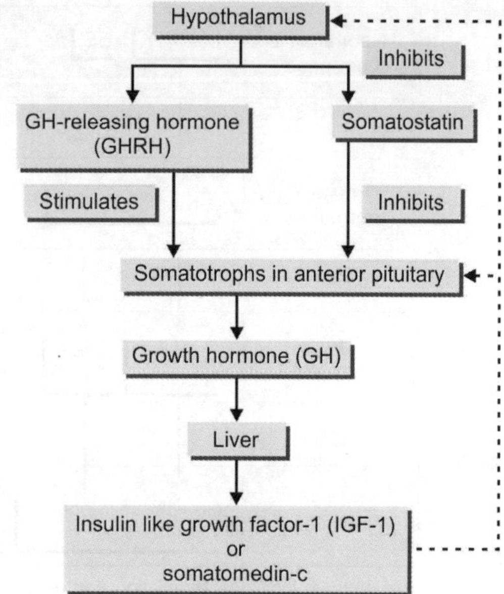

Stimuli that Affects GH Secretion

Stimulate growth hormone secretion

1. Decreased blood glucose
2. Decreased blood free fatty acids
3. Starvation or fasting, protein deficiency
4. Trauma, stress, excitement
5. Exercise
6. Testosterone, estrogen
7. Deep sleep (stages II and IV)
8. Growth hormone-releasing hormone.

Inhibit growth hormone secretion

1. Increased blood glucose
2. Increased blood free fatty acids
3. Aging
4. Obesity
5. Growth hormone-inhibiting hormone (somatostatin)
6. Growth hormone (exogenous)
7. Somatomedins (insulin like growth factors).

Applied Aspects

Gigantism

Due to hypersecretion of GH in growing children before the closure of epiphysis. It is usually caused due to tumor of pituitary gland.

Clinical features
- Abnormal height (6.5–9 feet)
- Large hands and feet
- Bilateral gynecomastia
- Loss of libido/impotence
- Hyperglycemia caused by GH leads to excess insulin secretion
- Over activity of β cells of pancreas ultimately leads to degeneration of these cells and deficiency of insulin resulting in diabetes mellitus.
- The tumor of the pituitary gland itself causes headache and visual disturbances (bitemporal hemianopsia).
- If untreated gigantism ends in hypopituitarism due to destruction of the gland by tumor.

Treatment

Irradiation of tumor.

Acromegaly

Due to hypersecretion of GH in adults after the closure of epiphysis. It can be caused by extrapituitary as well intrapituitary GH secreting tumors and by hypothalamic tumors that secrete GRH. Height will not be increased, but bones become thicker and soft tissues continues to grow. Hypersecretion of growth hormone is accompanied by hypersecretion of prolactin in 20–40% of patients with acromegaly.

Clinical features (Fig. 8.9)
- Hands and feet are enlarged (acral parts)
- Protrussion of lower jaw due to elongation and widening of mandible (Prognathism).
- Overgrowth of the malar, frontal and facial bones combines with prognathism to produce the coarse facial features called acromegalic facies.
- The changes in the vertebra causes a hunched back. (Kyphosis).
- The skeletal changes predisposes to osteoarthritis.
- Excessive growth of internal organs, i.e. cardiomegaly, hepatomegaly, splenomegaly and renomegaly.
- Excessive growth of body hair.
- Bitemporal hemianopsia (optic chiasma is compressed due to pituitary tumor).

In 4% there will be gynecomastia with or without lactation.

Treatment

Surgical resection of the tumor is the preferred treatment. Drugs useful in treatment of acromegaly are somatostatin analogues (somatostatin inhibits growth hormone release), growth hormone receptor antagonist, dopamine agonists.

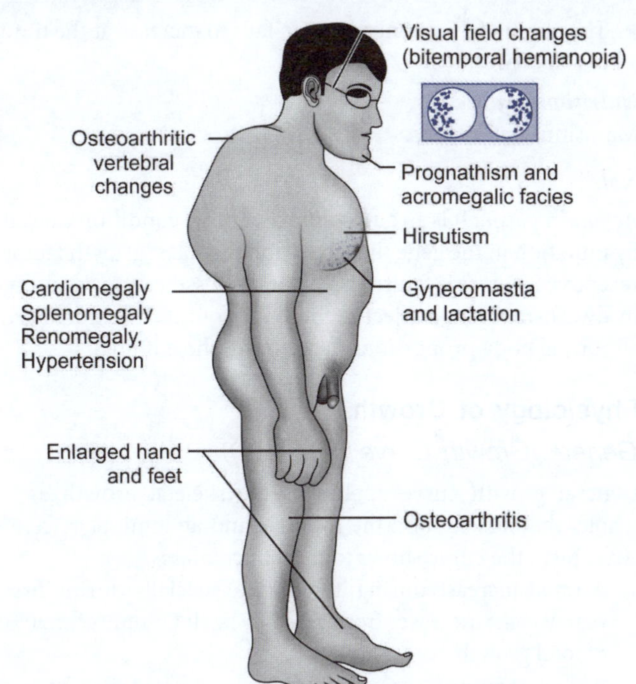

Fig. 8.9: Clinical features of acromegaly

Dwarfism

Endocrinal causes
- *Pituitary dwarf (GH deficiency):* It is due to the GH deficiency secondary to decrease in GHRH. Its characteristic features are plumpness (fatness), immature facies, small genitalia, delicate extremites, delayed skeletal and dental development.
- *Hypothyroid dwarf (cretinism):* It is due to thyroid hormone deficiency. Mental retardation is seen in hypothyroid children. Thyrold hormones are essential for normal mentation. Therefore, mental retardation is an important feature of a thyroid deficiency in infancy and early childhood (thyroid dwarf). This differentiates it from a pituitary dwarf in whom mental activities are apparently normal.

The difference between pituitary and hypothyroid dwarf is given in Table 8.1.

Genetic cause
- *Laron dwarfism (GH insensitivity syndrome):* The plasma GH level is normal or elevated. But the GH receptors are unresponsive (due to mutation in the gene for receptors). Also there is a marked decrease in plasma IGF-I.
- *African pigmies:* They have normal plasma GH levels. Plasma concentration of GH binding protein decreases.

Table 8.1: Difference between pituitary and hypothyroid dwarf

Pituitary dwarf	Hypothyroid dwarf/Cretin
Due to GH deficiency since childhood	Due to thyroid hormone deficiency
Normal mental activity	Mentally retarded
Sexually mature	Sexually immature
Different parts of the body are proportionate	Different parts of the body are disproportionate

The plasma IGF-I concentration fails to increase at the time of puberty.

Nutritional cause

Marasmus and rickets.

Note

Achondroplasia: It is an autosomal dominant condition caused by mutation in the gene that codes for fibroblast growth factor receptor. So there is faulty endochondral ossification resulting in dwarfism. Here subject is mentally sound. It features are abnormal body proportions (large head, short limbs).

Physiology of Growth

General Growth Curve (Fig. 8.10)

General growth curve applies to the skeletal growth as a whole, the muscles and the thoracic and abdominal viscera. After birth the curve shows four distinct phases:

1. A rapid increase during infancy, i.e. specially during first year, weight increases from 3.5–10.5 kg. It accounts for 30% of total growth.
2. A slow progressive growth from 3 to 12 years of age. During this period boys are taller than girls. By the end of 12 years of age, growth reaches 60% of the total growth.
3. A marked increase in growth occurs at the time of puberty also called *growth spurt.* It appears earlier in girls, hence girls mature earlier than boys. Thus, rate of increase of height and weight is the greatest in girls at 12–14 years and in boys at 14–16 years. In girls, the increase in weight is mainly due to increased fat formation and in boys it is due to increased muscular growth.

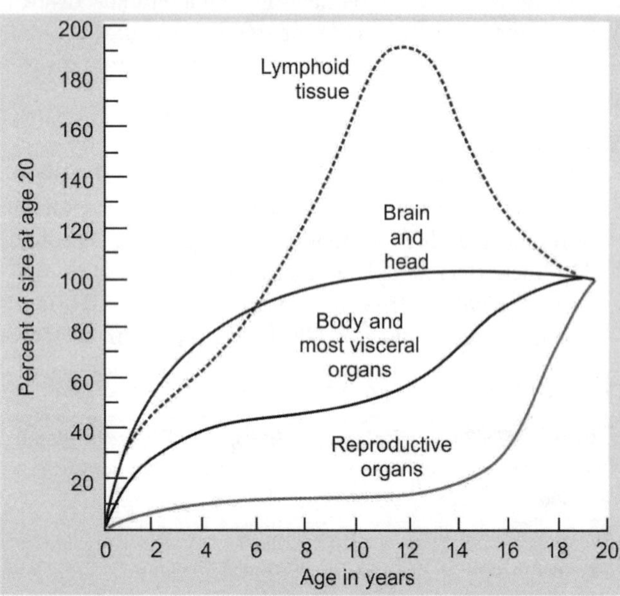

Fig. 8.10: Growth curve

4. Even though pubertal growth has finished at 18 years in girls and 20 years in boys, a small growth occurs until 30 years.

   Thus in humans there are two periods of rapid growth:

1. First in infancy (partly a continuation of fetal growth period).
2. Second at the time of late puberty just before growth stops.

   Certain parts of the body have distinctive growth curves. In both sexes, the rate of growth of individual tissue varies. These are mainly of three types:

   a. *Neural type:* Here there is a rapid initial increase in size of the brain, spinal cord and organs of special senses. They reach 60% and reach 90% of adult size at two and six years of age respectively.
   b. *Lymphoid type:* Lymphoid tissues including thymus, tonsils and lymph nodes throughout the body grow rapidly in early childhood (40% of adult size by the age of two years) and reach their maximum size at puberty, after this lymphoid tissue degenerates.
   c. *Reproductive type:* The gonads and accessory organs of reproduction remain undeveloped until puberty, when very rapid growth begins and continues throughout adolescence. The reproductive system atrophies in women after the menopause.

Note: Certain organs show different type of growth. For example, adrenal glands and uterus. These organs are relatively large at birth, then they lose weight rapidly and then regains just before puberty.

Factors Affecting Growth

Genetic factors

Genetic factors are very important in relation to growth and stature and they are mainly responsible for certain racial differences in the height. For example, achondroplasia. The timing of the adolescent spurt in both males and females appears to be genetically controlled via hypothalamus.

Nutritional factors

The food supply is the most important extrinsic factor affecting growth. The diet must be adequate not only in protein content but also essential in vitamins, minerals and in calories so that ingested protein is not burned for energy. Once the pubertal growth spurt has commenced, considerable linear growth continues even if caloric intake is reduced. Diet deficient in quantity and energy, in proteins, minerals and vitamins, inhibits growth markedly and adversely, therefore:

- If the lack of diet is sufficiently prolonged, the stunting of growth may be irreversible.
- If the lack is less severe or for shorter period, restoration of normal diet leads to a compensatory increase in the rate of growth.

- Undernutrition affects the growth of different organs and tissues unevenly.

Environmental factors

- *Diseases:* Ill health causes temporary depression of growth, but during recovery the lost ground is regained. Thus, following illness and starvation in children, there is a period of catch-up growth which takes place when the growth rate is greater than the normal. The accelerated growth usually continues until the previous growth curve is reached at which point growth slows to normal.
- *Exercise:* Repeated exercise of skeletal can increase in their mass by producing enlargement of individual fibers.
- *Emotional disturbances:* Emotional disturbances can cause decrease in rate of growth in children taking an adequate diet.
- *Old age:* Aging is characterized by:
  - Cellular degeneration due to degradative changes in the properties of multiplying cells
  - Impairment of various functions due to loss of non-multiplying cells.

Hormonal factors

Contribution of hormones to growth after birth:

- Rapid growth during infancy—GH and TH
- Spurt of growth at puberty—GH and androgens
- In between continuous growth—TH and GH
- After attainment of puberty and rest of life—TH, GH, androgens.

Growth hormone: Growth *in utero* and neonatal growth are independent of growth hormones (GHs).

- *Clinical features due to GH deficiency:* Normal birth weight, subsequent severe retardation of growth and tendency to obesity, low fasting blood sugar and delayed recovery from insulin hypoglycemia.

Thyroid hormone: It is necessary for a completely normal rate of GH secretion. Hypothyroidism decreases the synthesis, storage, and release of growth hormone and retards growth.

Thyroid hormone (TH) has widespread effects on ossification of cartilage, growth of teeth, contours of face and proportions of body. Cretins are therefore dwarfed and have infantile features.

Patients who are dwarfed due to panhypopituitarism have features consistent with their chronological age until puberty, but since they do not mature sexually, they have juvenile features in the adulthood.

Note: GH and TH show *permissive action,* i.e. either of the two cannot produce normal growth, but when administered together they will stimulate growth (possibly *via* potentiation of the actions of somatomedins).

Androgens

In males, testes (mainly) and adrenal cortex whereas in females the main androgen sources are adrenal cortex (mainly) and ovaries.

- It is a protein anabolic hormone and is responsible for growth spurt
- It produces an increase in GH secretion that in turn increase IGF-I secretion
- Although androgen stimulates growth but, ultimately it terminates growth by causing epiphysial closure thereby decreases linear growth
- Estrogen have similar effects due to stimulation of androgen secretion by the adrenals. Sex steroids (estrogen and androgen) stimulate both synthesis and release of GH which in turn increases IGF-I secretion to cause growth.

Others

- Adrenocortical hormones exert permissive action on growth.
- Insulin: Diabetic children fail to grow because of increased breakdown of proteins and fats.

Prolactin

Prolactin is structurally similar to GH. Prolactin is physiologically involved in lactation. In a breast which has been primed by female hormones (estrogen and progesterone), prolactin induces and maintains lactation by stimulating synthesis of milk. Prolactin is the only pituitary hormone which is primarily under inhibitory control of hypothalamus. Its secretion is suppressed by dopamine (prolactin inhibitory substance) secreted by hypothalamus. The normal prolactin level is < 20 ng/ml. Moderate elevation (30–200 ng/ml) of prolactin can occur in postpartum period, renal failure, liver failure, hypothyroidism, stress, drugs (dopamine antagonists) and prolactinoma. It is called lactogenic/mammotrophic/galactopoietic hormone.

Actions (Fig. 8.11)

Breast growth

During pregnancy under the influence of prolactin, mammary duct gives rise to lobules of alveoli.

Lactogenic effect

Prolactin acts on alveolar epithelium and stimulates the secretory activity. It stimulates galactosyltransferase activity, leading to the synthesis of lactose.

Suppression of ovarian cycle in nursing mothers

It inhibits the secretion of GnRH from hypothalamus. Therefore, FSH and LH secretion from anterior pituitary decreases and account for the antireproductive and antigonadal effects of prolactin, which account for amenorrhea (stoppage of periods) during postpartum lactation.

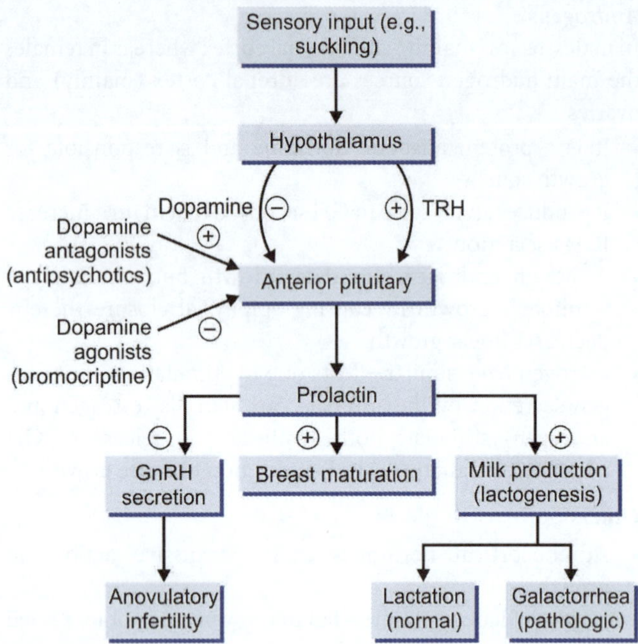

Fig. 8.11: Physiological action and regulation of prolactin secretion

Table 8.2: Factors influencing prolactin secretion

Stimuli that increases secretion	Stimuli that decreases secretion
Exercise and stress	Prolactin inhibitory factor
Dopamine antagonists (phenothiazine, tranquilizers), adrenergic blockers, serotonin agonist	Dopamine agonist (bromocriptine, apomorphine)
Pregnancy	Serotonin antagonist
TRH	

Regulation of Prolactin Secretion (Table 8.2)

- *By hypothalamus:* Prolactin releasing hormone (PRH) and prolactin inhibiting hormone (PIH) regulate prolactin secretion. PIH is a dopamine and is more important than PRH. Prolactin stimulates the secretion of PIH from hypothalamus and brings about its inhibition.
- *Estrogen and progesterone:* High levels of these hormones inhibit and low levels facilitate prolactin secretion.
- *Suckling of breast* and stimulation of the vagina during coitus stimulate prolactin secretion.
- *Bromocriptine* is a dopamine agonist and so it decreases prolactin secretion. This is used in the treatment of prolactin dependant breast tumors.

Oxytocin

Synthesized by paraventricular nucleus of hypothalamus. It acts on the myoepithelial cells of mammary gland and the uterus.

Oxytocin secretion is inhibited by sympathetic discharge and circulating catecholamines, by pain and enkephalins, by emotional stress, especially fear and by alchohol.

Actions

On mammary glands

It causes the ejection of milk from the mammary gland. Oxytocin causes the contraction of myoepithelial cells. It squeezes milk from alveoli to the exterior through the duct system and nipple. The process by which the milk is ejected from the alveoli of lactating breastmilk ejection reflex (details given in reproductive system).

On uterus

On pregnant uterus: It causes contraction of smooth muscles of uterus and helps in the expulsion of fetus. Sensitivity of the uterine musculature to oxytocin is enhanced by estrogen and inhibited by progesterone. In late pregnancy, the uterus becomes very sensitive to oxytocin (due to increase in oxytocin receptors). Oxytocin secretion is increased during labor. At the onset of labor, cervix dilates and the fetus descends through the birth canal. Expansion of birth canal stimulate stretch receptors.

From them impulses goes to pituitary through afferent fibers which in turn increases oxytocin in blood. This will reach uterus through general circulation. This enhances further strong contraction of uterus and favors delivery of the baby.

On nonpregnant uterus: Oxytocin acts on the nonpregnant uterus to facilitate sperm transport. Oxytocin released causes uterine contraction and facilitate sperm transport.

Other actions

In males at the time of ejaculation it causes increased contraction of smooth muscle of vas deferens, propelling sperm towards the urethra.

Vasopressin

Antidiuretic hormone (ADH) is secreted mainly by supraoptic nucleus of hypothalamus. It is an antidiuretic hormone. The most important stimulus for secretion of ADH is an increase in osmolarity of plasma. The increased osmolarity is sensed by osmoreceptors located in the hypothalamus. The response to stimulation of osmoreceptors is an increase in the synthesis and release of ADH.

Vasopressin Receptors

V_{1A}: Located in blood vessels, liver brain.
V_{1B} (also called V3 receptors): Located in anterior pituitary.
V_{2-}: Located in kidney.

Actions

Water retention

The major function of ADH is retention of water by acting on kidney (activated by V_2). Main site of action is at distal nephron. It increases the permeability of collecting ducts of kidney. Due to increased permeability water enters hypertonic medullary interstitium. Thus diuresis is prevented. Water is retained in the kidney and urine becomes concentrated. Water is reabsorbed through aquaporin II (ADH responsive water channel).

Vascular effect

In large amounts ADH causes constriction of vascular smooth muscles (mediated by V_{1A}). Due to vasoconstriction BP increases.

Other actions

Acts on anterior pituitary and cause ACTH release (mediated by V_{1B}). It is a neurotransmitter in brain and spinal cord. Vasopressin causes glycogenolysis in the liver (mediated by V_{1A}).

Regulation of ADH Secretion

Vasopressin secretion is regulated by osmoreceptors located near the anterior hypothalamus. They are located outside the blood brain barrier. Two important factors that regulate ADH secretion are osmolality and ECF volume. Vasopressin secretion is increased by: 1. Increased osmolarity (osmotic pressure) of plasma, 2. Decreased ECF volume, 3. Pain, emotion, stress, exercise, 4. Nausea and vomiting, 5. Standing, 6. Clofibrate, Carbamazapine, 7. Angiotensin.

Vasopressin secretion is decreased by: 1. Decreased osmolarity of plasma, 2. Increase ECF volume, 3. Alcohol.

Effect of Osmolality (Flowchart 8.4)

Flowchart 8.4: Effect of osmolality on ADH secretion

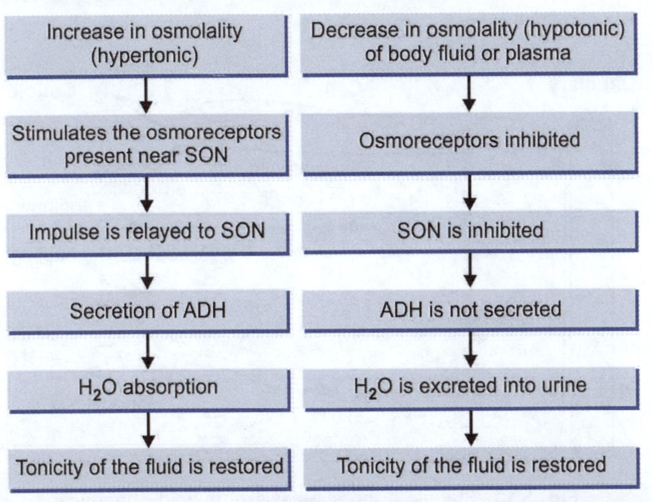

Effect of ECF Volume (Flowchart 8.5)

Flowchart 8.5: Effect of ECF volume on ADH secretion

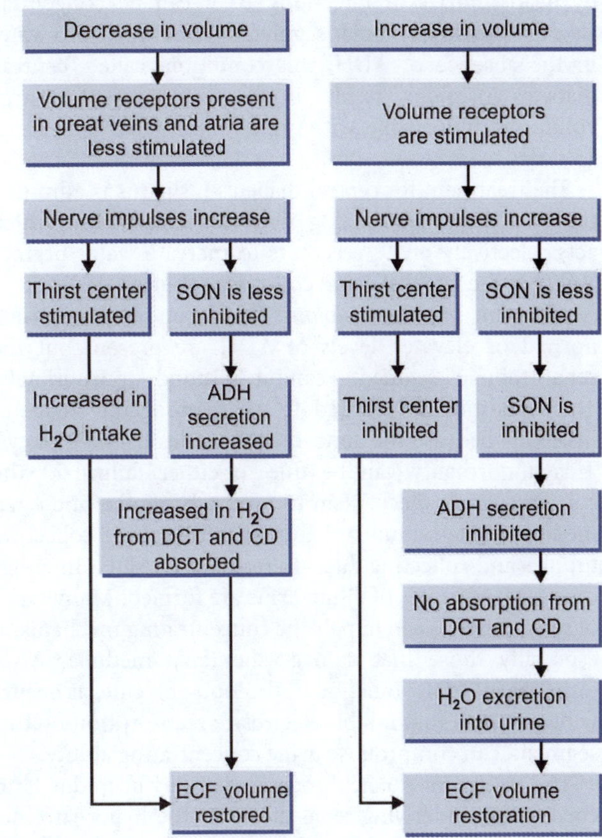

Other Stimulants

Pain, emotion, stress, exercise, vomiting, angiotensin II.

Other Inhibitors

Alcohol

Clinical

1. Patients highly sensitive to vasopressin are prone to develop hypertension.
2. In massive hemorrhage and shock, vasopressin is secreted in high amounts. The pressor action of vasopressin raises the BP.
3. *Diabetes insipidus:* The deficiency of ADH causes diabetes insipidus. This disease is characterized by excessive excretion of water through urine (polyuria), increased water intake (polydypsia).

Causes

It can be due to failure of production of ADH (cental diabetes insipidus) or due to inability of the kidneys to respond to ADH (nephrogenic diabetes insipidus).

- *Central diabetes insipidus:* It is due to inability to produce or release ADH from the posterior pituitary. It can be caused by head injuries or infections, or it can be congenital. Because the distal tubular segments cannot reabsorb water in the absence of ADH, this condition, called 'central' diabetes insipidus, results in the formation of a large volume of dilute urine, with urine volumes that can exceed 15 L/day.

  The treatment for central diabetes insipidus is administration of a synthetic analog of ADH, desmopressin, which acts selectively on V_2 receptors to increase water permeability in the late distal and collecting tubules.
- *Nephrogenic diabetes insipidus:* It is a condition in which normal or elevated levels of ADH are present but the renal tubular segments cannot respond appropriately. This condition is referred to as 'nephrogenic' diabetes insipidus because the abnormality resides in the kidneys. This abnormality can be due to either failure of the countercurrent mechanism to form a hyperosmotic renal medullary interstitium or failure of the distal and collecting tubules and collecting ducts to respond to ADH. In either case, large volumes of dilute urine are formed. Many types of renal diseases can impair the concentrating mechanism, especially those that damage the renal medulla. Also, impairment of the function of the loop of Henle, as occurs with diuretics that inhibit electrolyte reabsorption by this segment, can compromise urine concentrating ability.

  The treatment for nephrogenic diabetes insipidus is to correct the underlying renal disorder. The hypernatremia can also be attenuated by a low-sodium diet and administration of a diuretic that enhances renal sodium excretion, such as a thiazide diuretic.

THYROID GLAND

The two principal hormone secreted by thyroid gland are thyroxine (T_4) and triiodothyronine (T_3). Small amount of reverse T_3 are also found (inactive form). T_3 is more active than T_4.

Parafollicular cells of thyroid gland secretes calcitonin, a calcium-lowering hormone. The thyroid gland is composed of large number follicles. Each follicle is lined with cuboidal epithelial cells (thyroid cells) and filled with a secretory substance called colloid.

Note: When the gland is inactive, the colloid is abundant, follicles are large and the cells lining them are flat. When the gland is active, the follicles are small, the cells are cuboid or columnar and the edge of the colloid is scalloped forming many small reabsorption lacunae (Fig. 8.12).

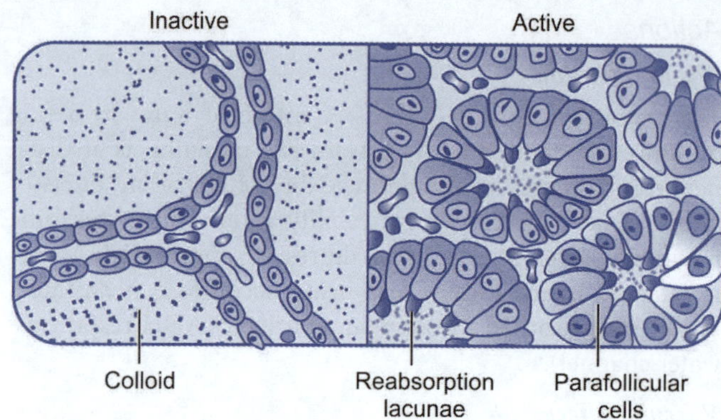

Fig. 8.12: Histology of thyroid gland during inactive and active state

Synthesis of Thyroid Hormones

Iodine and tyrosine are essential for the formation of thyroid hormones. Iodine consumed through diet is converted into iodide and is absorbed from GIT. Tyrosine is also consumed through diet.

Stages in the Synthesis of Thyroid Hormones

Thyroglobulin synthesis

The ER and golgi apparatus in the thyroid cells synthesize and secrete a glycoprotein molecule called thyroglobulin into the colloid. It contains 123 tyrosine residues that combines with iodine to form thyroid hormones. The hormone remain bound to thyroglobulin until secreted (Fig. 8.13).

Iodide trapping

Iodide trapping is the picking up of iodide by thyroid gland. Na^+ and I^- are co-transported into the thyroid gland and the Na^+ is pumped into the interstitium by Na^+- K^+ ATPase (secondary active transport).

Oxidation of iodide

Iodide has to be oxidized to iodine because only iodine is capable of combining with tyrosine. The process of oxidation is promoted by an enzyme thyroid peroxidase (H_2O_2 accepts the electron).

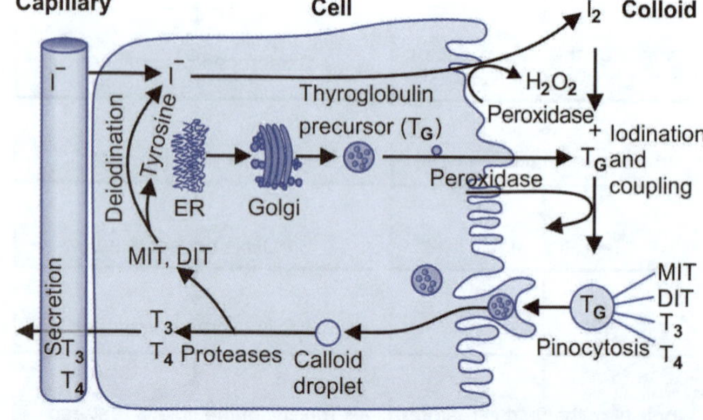

Fig. 8.13: Stages in the synthesis of thyroid hormones

Iodination of tyrosine

The binding of iodine with thyroglobulin molecule is called organification of thyroglobulin. Tyrosine (of thyroglobulin) is 1st iodinated (at 3rd position) to form monoiodotyrosine. (MIT). MIT is next iodinated (at 5th position) to diiodotyrosine (DIT).

Coupling

DIT+MIT = T_3 (Triiodothyronine)
DIT+DIT = T_4 (Tetraidothyronine/thyroxine)
The enzyme peroxidase is required for coupling.

Note: MIT + DIT = Reverse T_3.

Storage

In combination with thyroglobulins, thyroid hormone can be stored in the follicles for several months. Therefore, when synthesis of thyroid hormones ceases, the physiological effects of deficiency are not observed for several months.

Release of thyroid hormones

Thyoglobulin itself is not released into the bloodstream. The hormones are 1st cleaved from thyroglobulin. The process occurs as follows:

The apical surface of thyroid cells sends out pseudopod like extensions, that close around small portions of colloid to form pinocytic vesicles. These vesicles then enter the thyroid cell. Then the lysosomes of the cell fuses with the vesicles. The digestive enzymes present in the lysosomes digest the thyroglobulin and release T_3 and T_4 in free form. These then diffuses through the base of thyroid cell into the surrounding capillaries. The T_4-T_3 secretion ratio is 10 : 1.

Transport of T_3 and T_4

Over 99% of T_3 and T_4 combines immediately with plasma proteins like thyroxine binding globulin (mainly) and thyroxine binding prealbumin and albumin (to lesser extent). The rest circulate unbound in the plasma.

Table 8.3: Comparison of T_4 and T_3

T_4	T_3
Considered as a precursor of T_3 and is solely secreted by the gland	Considered as a physiologically active form and plasma T_3 comes from • Deiodination of T_4 in the tissue • Secretion by the gland
T_4 combines less freely with DNA receptor	It has more affinity to the receptor on the DNA
Amount secreted is ten to twenty times more	Amout secreted is less
More bound to protein, less free form	Less bound to protein, more free form
Slow and sustained	Fast action
Gets metabolized slowly	Gets metabolize faster

Differences between T_4 and T_3 (Table 8.3)

Actions

Metabolic

Calorigenic action: Thyroid hormone in general stimulates the metabolic activities and increases O_2 consumption and heat production in most tissues of the body except adult brain, testis uterus, lymph nodes, spleen and anterior pituitary. Thus, it increases the BMR. They increases activity of Na^+- K^+ ATPase (Table 8.4).

Effects on carbohydrate metabolism

- Increased uptake of glucose by the cells
- Enhanced gluconeogenesis
- Increased rate of absorption from GIT
- Increased insulin secretion.

Effects on fat metabolism

- Mobilization of fat from adipose tissue
- Increase the level of free fatty acids

Table 8.4: Summary of effects of thyroid hormones

Target tissue	Effect	Mechanism
Heart	Chronotropic and inotropic	• Increased number of β-adrenergic receptors • Enhanced responses to circulating catecholamines • Increased proportion of α-myosin heavy chain (with higher ATPase activity)
Adipose tissue	Catabolic	Stimulates lipolysis
Muscle	Catabolic	Increase in protein breakdown
Bone	Developmental	Promote normal growth and skeletal development
CNS	Developmental	Promote normal brain development
GI tract	Metabolic	Increased rate of glucose absorption
Cholesterol	Metabolic	Increased clearance by formation of LDL receptors
Throughout the body	Calorigenic	• Stimulates O_2 consumption • Increase in basal metabolic rate • Exceptions are testes, uterus, lymph nodes, spleen, anterior pituitary

- Enhances the oxidation of free fatty acids by cells
- Lowers circulating cholesterol levels (due to increased secretion of cholesterol in bile; cholesterol secretion is increased by inducing the formation of LDL receptors in the liver, resulting in increased hepatic removal of cholesterol)
- Plasma levels of triglycerides and phospholipids are also decreased.

Effects on protein metabolism

In physiological amounts thyroid hormones function as anabolic hormone. They cause increase in RNA and protein synthesis. In high concentration they have catabolic effect.

Effect on vitamin metabolism

Thyroid hormones increase the quantity of enzymes. Vitamins are essential parts of some enzymes and coenzymes. Therefore, thyroid hormones cause increased need for vitamins leading to relative vitamin deficiency in hyperthyroidism.

Growth and Development

Effects on growth

Thyroid hormones are essential for normal growth and skeletal maturation. They exert their effect directly by increasing protein synthesis and enzymes and indirectly by increasing the production of GH and potentiating their effect on the tissues. They also promote growth and development of brain during fetal life and for 1st few years of postnatal life.

Effect on other endocrine glands

They increases the rate of secretion of other endocrine glands. They also increases the need of tissues for hormones (insulin, parathyroid, catacholamines, etc.).

Effect on body weight

Greatly increased thyroid hormone always decreases the body weight, and greatly decreased hormone almost increases the body weight.

Systemic

Cardiovascular effects

Effect on heart

- Increased heart rate
- Increased stroke volume
- Increased cardiac output.

Cardiac output is increased due to increase in metabolism, increase in β-adrenergic receptors (both number and affinity) and increase in level of α- MHC (Myosin heavy chain).

Effect on blood vessels

Systolic BP is increased due to increase in cardiac output. Diastolic BP is decreased due to the peripheral vasodilatation. Vasodilatation is due to increase in heat production and increased metabolites. This results into the increased pulse pressure and increased velocity of blood flow causing increase in circulation (hyperdynamic circulation).

Respiratory effects

The increased rate of metabolism increases the utilization of O_2 and formation of CO_2. These effects activate all the mechanisms that increases rate and depth of respiration.

Effect on GIT

They increase appetite and food intake. Thyroid hormones also increases secretions and motility of GI tract.

Effect on CNS

They are essential for brain development (especially cortex, basal ganglia and cochlea) during fetal life and for 1st few years of postnatal life. Normal functioning of brain need thyroid hormone. The hyperthyroid individuals may develop psychoneurotic problems like anxiety, complexes, extreme worry, etc. Reaction time of stretch reflex is shortened in hyperthyroidism and it is prolonged in hypothyroidism.

Thyroid hormones are essential for normal formation of synapses and myelination in the developing brain. In hypothyroidism there will be abnormal development of synapses, decreased myelination and decreased growth and branching of dendrites. This decrease in number of neurons is responsible for mental retardation.

Effect on skeletal muscle

Slight increase in thyroid hormone can make the muscle to work with more vigor. But excessive secretion causes weakness in muscles due to catabolism of proteins. Fine muscle tremor is a characteristic sign of hyperthyroidism.

Effect on sleep (due to activity on RAS)

Hypersecretion of thyroid hormone causes excessive stimulation of muscles and CNS. So the person feels tired but because of excitable effects of thyroid hormone on synapses it is difficult to sleep. On the other hand hyposecretion causes excessive sleep (somnolence).

Effect on reproductive system

For normal function thyroid hormones are essential. In males, lack causes loss of libido and excess causes impotence. In females lack causes menorrhagia (excessive bleeding) and polymenorrhagia (frequent menstruation). Hypersecretion in women causes oligomenorrhea (reduced bleeding).

Regulation of Secretion

Thyroid activity is controlled by TSH secreted by basophils in the anterior pituitary. TSH stimulates almost all steps in thyroid hormone synthesis. TRH provides a constant and

Flowchart 8.6: Negative feedback control of thyroid hormone release

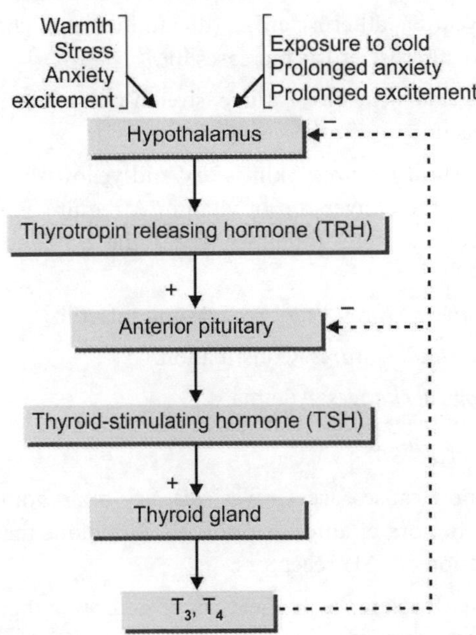

necessary stimulus for TSH secretion. In the absence of TRH, the secretion of TSH (and T_4) decreases to very low-levels. The target tissue for TSH is the thyroid, where it increases the secretion mainly of T_4.

Thyroid secretion is regulated in a classical negative feedback mechanism (Flowchart 8.6).

Because the main circulating form is T_4, it is T_4 that is responsible for most of the negative feedback. An increase in thyroid hormone level suppress TSH and TRH secretion. On the other hand, a decrease in thyroid hormone level stimulates TSH and TRH secretions. Besides TSH, TRH also stimulates the secretion of growth hormone (GH) and prolactin. Therefore, TRH stimulation test is useful in disorders of GH.

Autoregulation of Thyroid Gland

The secretions of thyroid gland is regulated by food iodine contents. If there is deficiency of iodine content in the diet then the iodine trapping mechanism of the thyroid cells become super efficient and vice-versa if there is excess of iodine content in the diet. In this way iodine availability for thyroid hormone synthesis remains constant and this phenomenon is called autoregulation.

Note: In normal individuals, large doses of iodines act directly on thyroid to produce a mild and transient inhibition of organic binding of iodide and hence of hormone synthesis. This inhibition is known as the ***Wolff-Chaikoff effect.***

Antithyroid Drugs

Drugs that depresses thyroid secretion are called antithyroid drugs.

Mechanism

- Interfering iodide trapping
- Blocking the organic binding of iodine.

For example: (1) Thiocyanate, (2) Propylthiouracil, (3) High concentrations of inorganic iodides.

Thiocyanate ions decrease iodide trapping: Administration of thiocyanate in high concentration causes competitive inhibition of iodide transport into the cell (thiocyanate and iodide ions have the same active pump).

Propylthiouracil decreases thyroid hormone formation: Prevents formation of thyroid hormone from iodides and tyrosine. Mechanism-block the peroxidase enzyme required for iodination of tyrosine and partly to block the coupling of two iodinated tyrosines to form thyroxine and triiodothyronine.

Iodides of high concentration decrease thyroid activity and thyroid gland size. When iodides are present in high concentration most activities of thyroid gland are decreased to reduce rate of iodide trapping. So the rate of iodination of tyrosine to form thyroid hormones are decreased.

Thyroid Function Test

- Sleeping pulse rate >100 in hyperthyroidism.
- BMR: Normal value is 37–40 kcal/m^2 of body surface/hours. BMR is increased in hyperthyroidism (50), decreased in hypothyroidism (20).
- Serum cholesterol: Increases in hypothyroidism, decreases in hyperthyroidism.
- Serum T_3 and T_4: Estimated by radioimmunoassay. Normal T_3 = 0.15μg/dl, T_4 = 8 μg/dl.
- Ankle jerk (Achilles reaction time): Normally 2–3 msec. In hypothyroidism it is prolonged, and in hyperthyroidism it is shortened.
- Radioactive iodine uptake studies: I_{131} is given orally in 100 ml water and thyroid uptake is determined by placing a X-ray counter over the neck. Normally 20–40% is taken up.
- Scanning technique.
- Thyroid biopsy: To detect any malignant process.
- TRH/TSH stimulation test: To know whether pituitary/thyroid disorder.

Applied Aspects

Hypothyroidism

Caused by low levels of circulating thyroid hormones. Depending upon the cause it can be:

- Primary hypothyroidism: Disorder of thyroid gland.
- Secondary hypothyroidism: Diseases of anterior pituitary or hypothalamus.

It leads to myxedema in adults and cretinism in children.

Cretinism

Cause

- Congenital absence of thyroid gland
- Genetic disorder
- Lack of I_2.

Symptoms

- Appear 1–3 weeks after birth
- Appearance-idiotic, ugly, obese, short child
- Mental retardation in children
- All milestones of development are delayed
- Skeletal growth is more affected than soft tissues (so stunted body with pot belly)
- Tongue larger (macroglossia) and protrude out of the mouth
- Big tongue obstructs swallowing and breathing
- Sexual development is affected
- Skin is dry, coarse and wrinkled
- Hair is sparse and scanty
- Temperature is subnormal.

Treatment

Treatment of neonate with cretinism at any time with adequate iodine or thyroxine returns normal physical growth, but unless the cretinism is treated within few weeks after birth, mental growth remains permanently retarded.

Myxedema

General features: Tiredness, weight gain, intolerance to cold, mental sluggishness, poor memory, decreased BMR, lower body temperature, husky and slow voice (frog like voice), hair coarse and sparse, extreme sleep (Fig. 8.14).

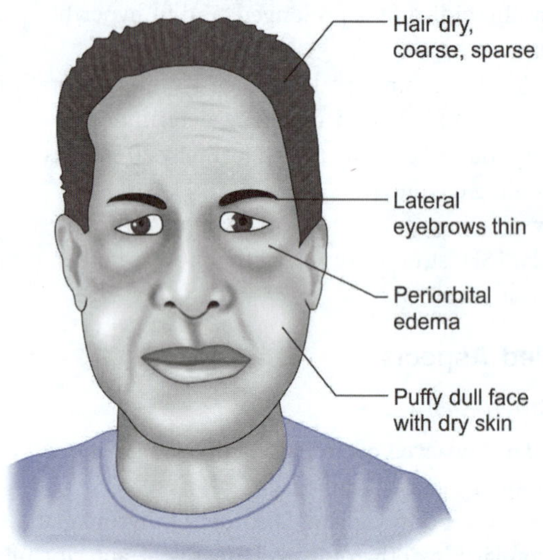

Fig. 8.14: Patient with myxedema

Cardiovascular features: Adrenergic activity is decreased causing bradycardia, atherosclerosis (due to increased cholesterol level) and atherosclerosis increases BP.

Neuromuscular features: Fatigue, stretch reflex reaction time is prolonged.

Dermatological features: Skin is dry and yellowish (carotenemia, since the conversion of vitamin A require T_3 and T_4), swelling of the face, puffiness under the eyes, nonpitting edema.

Reproductive features: Menorrhagia and infertility.

Gastrointestinal features: Constipation.

Hematological changes: Anemia.

Hyperthyroidism

Its common causes are Graves' disease, toxic goiter, TSH secreting tumors of anterior pituitary, mutations that causes the activation of TSH receptors.

Symptoms: Intolerance to heat, increased sweating, weight loss, nervousness, muscle weakness, extreme fatigue but inability to sleep, diarrhea, tremor of hands, goiter, atrial fibrillation, tachycardia, exophthalmos.

Treatment: Surgical removal of thyroid gland.

Clinical Note

Iodine preparation is given before thyroidectomy. Iodides in high concentration decrease all phases of thyroid activity, they slightly decrease the size of the thyroid gland and decrease its blood supply. This decreases the necessary amount of surgery, the amount of bleeding.

Graves' disease

It is an autoimmune disease. It is characterized by development of TSH receptor stimulating antibodies. These antibodies bind to TSH receptors and mimic TSH action, making the gland hyperactive. In Graves' disease there is marked stimulation of secretion of thyroid hormones and high circulating T_4 and T_3 levels. This will inhibit TSH secretion. Increased levels of thyroid hormones tend to cause increased formation of antibodies. Exophthalmos is often seen.

Exophthalmos: Exophthalmos means protrusion of eyeballs. The cause of protruding eyes is edematous swelling of retro-orbital tissues and degenerative changes in the extraocular muscles (Fig. 8.15). Sometimes eyeball protrusion stretches the optic nerve enough to damage the vision. Due to the protrusion of eyeballs, the eyelids cannot be closed completely while blinking or sleep. So the constant exposure of eyeball to atmosphere causes dryness of the cornea leading to irritation and infection, finally resulting in ulceration of cornea.

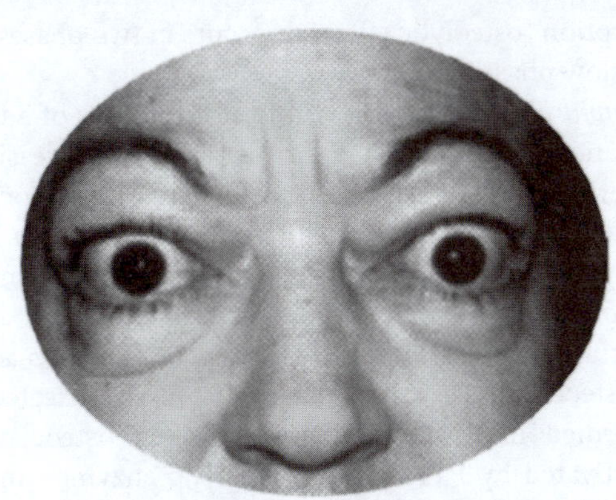

Fig. 8.15: Exophthalmos

Goiter

Goiter refers to any abnormal increase in size of thyroid gland. Goiter does not denote functional state of the thyroid gland. It may be associated with euthyroid, hypothyroidism or hyperthyroidism. Antithyroid substances that cause enlargement are called goitrogens. Goitrogens decreases thyroid hormone synthesis leading to feedback increase in TSH secretion. TSH is responsible for the formation of hypertrophic thyroid gland (goiter). Goiter in hyperthyroidism-toxic goiter. Goiter in hypothyroidism are of two types

1. *Endemic colloid goiter:* Also called iodine deficiency goiter (intake below 10 µg/day). TSH (produced due to feedback mechanism) stimulates thyroid cells to secrete tremendous amounts of thyroglobulin. Due to iodine deficiency T_3 and T_4 production does not occur and the thyroglobulin remains as such and gets accumulated in the follicles of the gland. This increases size of gland.
2. *Idiopathic nontoxic colloid goiter:* Enlargement of thyroid gland occurs even without iodine deficiency.

Causes: Thyroiditis, abnormal enzyme system, goitrogenic substances like propylthiouracil present in turnips and cabbages.

PARATHYROID GLANDS

Parathormone secreted by parathyroid gland is essential for maintenance of blood calcium level.

Calcium Metabolism

Calcium is essential for bone formation, neuromuscular activity, normal cardiac rhythmicity, coagulation of blood, formation of milk, mediation of intercellular action of hormones, fetal development during pregnancy, membrane integrity and permeability. Normal Ca level in blood is 9–11 mg/dl. The percentage of dietary calcium absorbed from the gut is inversely related to intake. The dietary intake of and the percentage of calcium absorbed is diminished in the elderly. Ingested phosphate is also absorbed by the gut. Both calcium and phosphate absorption in the GI tract are stimulated by the active form of vitamin D (calcitriol).

Types of Calcium

1. *Calcium in plasma exists in diffusible and non-diffusible forms.*
   - Diffusible Ca is in the form of ionic Ca (about 50%) or complexed to HCO_3^-, citrate, etc. (about 10%). Ionized Ca^{2+} is required for—(a) muscle contraction, (b) cardiac activity, (c) blood coagulation.
   - Non-diffusible is bound with albumin or globulin (about 40%).
2. *Calcium in bones is of two types:*
   - Readily exchangeable form (1%)
   - Stable calcium (99%) can be mobilized only through the action of PTH.

Regulation of Blood Calcium Level

Calcium that is taken through dietary sources are absorbed from GI tract. Through blood it is distributed to various parts of the body. Depending upon the blood level, the calcium is either deposited or removed from the bone. All these process are finely regulated by three hormones (Flowchart 8.7).

1. Parathormone.
2. 1, 25–dihydroxycholecalciferol.
3. Calcitonin.

In addition to the above mentioned three hormones, growth hormone and glucocorticoids also regulates blood calcium level. Growth hormone increases the blood calcium level by increasing intestinal calcium absorption. Glucocorticoids

Flowchart 8.7: Regulation of blood calcium level

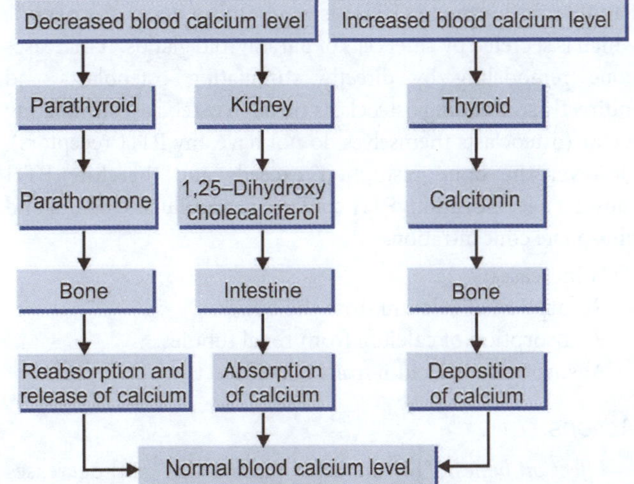

PHYSICON—The Reliable Icon in Physiology

decreases blood calcium level by inhibiting intestinal absorption and increasing the renal excretion of calcium.

Relationship between calcium and phosphate

Bone is a complex precipitate of calcium and phosphate to which hydroxide and bicarbonate ions are added to make up the mature hydroxyapatite crystals, which are laid down in a protein (osteoid) matrix. Whether calcium and phosphate are laid down in bone (precipitate from solution) or are resorbed from bone (go into solution) depends on the product of their concentrations rather than on their individual concentrations. When the product exceeds a certain number (solubility product or ion product), bone is laid down:

$[Ca^{2+}] \times [PO_{-4}] >$ solubility product = bone deposition

Under normal conditions, the ECF product of calcium times phosphate is close to the solubility product. Thus, an increase in the interstitial fluid concentration of either Ca^{2+} or phosphate increases bone mineralization. For example, an increase in plasma phosphate would increase the product of their concentrations, promote precipitation, and lower free calcium in the interstitial fluid. When the product is below the solubility product, bone is resorbed:

$[Ca^{2+}] \times [PO_{-4}] <$ solubility product = bone resorption

Thus, a decrease in the interstitial concentration of either Ca^{2+} or phosphate promotes the resorption of these salts from bone (demineralization). For example, a decrease in plasma phosphate alone would promote bone demineralization. Increasing renal excretion of phosphate would promote bone demineralization and a rise in interstitial free calcium.

It is the free Ca^{2+}, not the phosphate, that is regulated so precisely. Hormonal control of free Ca^{2+} levels is via a dual hormonal system, parathyroid hormone and vitamin D.

Parathormone

Parathyroid hormone (PTH) is a 84 amino acids polypeptide which is secreted by chief cells of parathyroid glands. It increases bone remodeling by directly stimulating osteoblasts and indirectly stimulating osteoclasts through osteoclast stimulating factor (osteoclasts themselves do not have any PTH receptors). However the bone resorption exceeds and therefore PTH causes a net resorption. PTH controls extracellular calcium and phosphate concentration.

PTH increases:
- Resorption of calcium from the bones.
- Reabsorption of calcium from renal tubules.
- Absorption of calcium from the GI tract.

Actions

- *Effect on bones:* PTH increases plasma Ca^{2+} and decreases plasma phosphate concentration by promoting bone resorption (osteolytic effect). It occurs in two phases: rapid and slow phase.
  - *Rapid phase:* It is seen within few minutes of administration of PTH. Plasma Ca^{2+} is raised by increasing the permeability of osteoclasts, osteoblast and osteocytes to calcium. It increases calcium pump mechanism, allowing Ca^{2+} ions to move from these cells to plasma.
  - *Slow phase:* It occurs hours or days after PTH administration. There occurs increased osteoclastic activity. Osteoclasts are large phagocytic multinucleated cells formed in the bone marrow. When osteoclasts are activated by PTH some proteolytic enzymes and several acids like citric acid and lactic acid are released. The enzymes digest or dissolve the organic matrix of the bone and acids dissolves the bone salts. Eventually Ca^{2+} ions are released into plasma. Along with Ca^{2+} resorption, PTH also increases phosphate absorption from the bones.
- *Effect on kidney:* PTH increases the resorption of calcium mainly from distal tubules, collecting tubules and to a lesser extent from ascending limb of loop of Henle. It decreases phosphate reabsorption.

  Reabsorption of Mg^{2+} and H^+ are increased while the reabsorption of Na^+, K^+ ions and amino acids are decreased.
- *Effect on intestine:* Increases intestinal absorption of Ca and phosphates.

Role of PTH in activation of vitamin D

Vitamin D is essential for calcium absorption from intestine. But vitamin D has to be converted to 1,25–dihydroxycholecalciferol (active form).

Steps (Fig. 8.16)

- Cholecalciferol (vitamin D_3) is formed in the skin.
- Cholecalciferol is converted to 25–hydroxycholecalciferol in liver.
- 1,25–dihydroxycholecalciferol is formed in the kidney. This step is under the control of PTH.

When blood Ca level increases it inhibits the formation of 1, 25-dihydroxycholecalciferol. The mechanism involved in the inhibition of formation of 1,25-dihydroxycholecalciferol is:
- Ca ion itself has a slight effect in preventing the conversion of 25 hydroxycholecalciferol to 1,25-dihydroxycholecalciferol.
- Increase in Ca ion concentration decreases the PTH secretion which in turn suppresses the conversion of 25 hydroxycholecalciferol to 1,25 dihydroxycholecalciferol.

Actions of 1,25-dihydroxycholecalciferol

- Promotes intestinal Ca absorption
- Promotes intestinal phosphate absorption
- Decreases excretion of Ca and phosphate from kidney

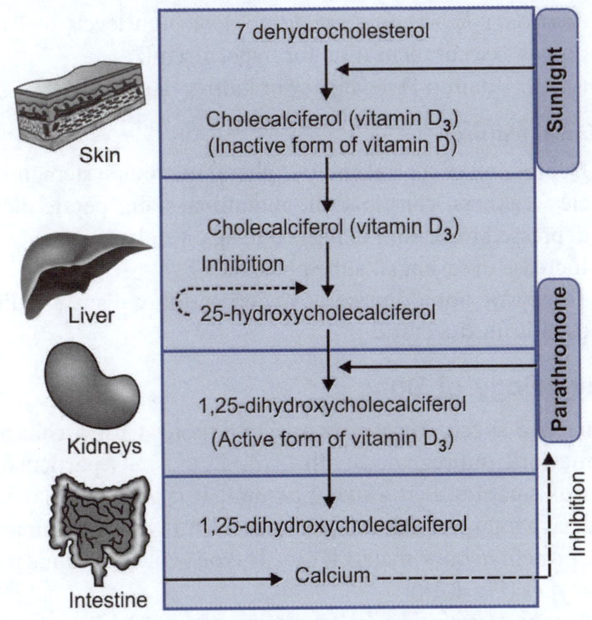

Fig. 8.16: Activation of vitamin D

- Extreme quantities of vitamin D causes absorption of bone. In the absence of vitamin D the effect of PTH in causing bone absorption is greatly reduced
- Vitamin D in smaller quantities promotes bone calcification.

Regulation of Parathyroid Secretion

- Ca concentration in the blood is the main factor.
- Increased phosphate stimulates PTH secretion (by lowering plasma Ca and 1,25-dihydroxycholecalciferol).
- 1,25-dihydroxycholecalciferol acts directly to decrease prepro PTH mRNA and decreases PTH secretion.
- Mg deficiency cause impaired PTH release along with diminished target organ responses to PTH.

Calcitonin

Calcitonin is a polypeptide hormone which is produced by parafollicular 'C' cell of thyroid (major source). Parathyroids, thymus and cells of medullary carcinoma of thyroid also contain calcitonin. Synthesis and secretion of calcitonin is regulated by plasma Ca^{2+} concentration itself: rise in plasma Ca^{2+} increases, while fall in plasma Ca^{2+} decreases calcitonin release. Calcitonin decreases calcium levels in general counteracts PTH.

Summary of major hormones that affect calcium and phosphate levels are given in Table 8.5.

Actions

On bones

- Facilitates the deposition of Ca on bones
- Suppresses the activity of osteoclast
- Inhibits development of new osteoclast in bones.

On kidney (minor effect): Increases the excretion of Ca through urine.

On intestine (minor effect): Prevents the absorption of Ca from intestine into blood.

Applied Aspects

Hypoparathyroidism

Decreased secretion of PTH.

Causes

- Surgical removal of parathyroid gland
- Removal of parathyroid glands during surgical removal of thyroid gland
- Deficiency of receptors for PTH in target cells.

When total serum Ca level is decreased below six mg%, it results in hypocalcemic tetany. Simultaneously serum phosphate is also decreased.

Table 8.5: Summary of major hormones that affect calcium and phosphate

	PTH	Vitamin D	Calcitonin
Major stimulus for secretion	Decrease in serum calcium	• Decrease in serum calcium • Decrease in serium phosphate • Increase in PTH	Increase in serum calcium
Action on bone	Increases bone resorption	Capable of both bone mineralization and resorption	Inhibits bone resorption
Action on intestine	Indirectly acts by increasing vitamin D	Increases calcium and phosphate absorption	
Action on kidney	• Increases calcium resorption • Increases phosphate excretion (phosphaturic)	Increases calcium and phosphate resorption	Increases calcium excretion
Overall effect	• Increases serum calcium • Decreases serum phosphate	Increases serum calcium and phosphate	Decreases serum calcium

PHYSICON—The Reliable Icon in Physiology

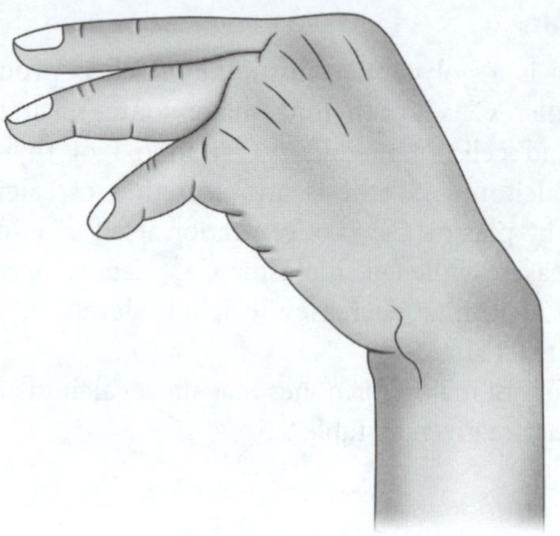

Fig. 8.17: Carpopedal spasm (obstetric hand)

Treatment

- Administration of 1,25-dihydrocholecalciferol.
- Administration of PTH (usually not treated).

Tetany

Refers to a clinical condition resulting from increased neuromuscular excitability. When ECF concentration of Ca ions falls below normal, neuronal membrane permeability to Na increases, allowing easy initiation of action potentials.

Clinical features

Carpopedal spasm (obstetric hand) (Fig. 8.17): It is a peculiar attitude of hand in tetany.

There is flexion at the wrist and thumb with hyperextension of remaining fingers.

Laryngeal stridor: Due to the spasm of laryngeal muscles.

Visceral manifestations: It includes intestinal colic, biliary colic, bronchospasm, profuse sweating.

ECG changes: QT segment is prolonged with abnormal T wave.

Trousseau's sign: Occluding the blood supply to a limb by inflation of sphygmomanometer cuff produces characteristic carpopedal spasm.

Chvostek's sign: Tapping the facial nerve at the angle of jaw produces ipsilateral contraction of the facial muscles (due to increased excitability of nerves to mechanical stimuli).

Hyperparathyroidism

Increased secretion of PTH. Based on cause, it is divided into primary and secondary hyperparathyroidism.

- *Primary hyperparathyroidism:* Abnormality of parathyroid causes excess PTH secretion.
  Cause: Tumor of parathyroid gland.
  Here Ca ion concentration is elevated (due to extreme osteoclastic activity). Phosphate ion concentration is decreased (due to increased renal excretion of phosphate).
- *Secondary hyperparathyroidism:* Here high levels of PTH occurs as a compensation for hypocalcemia.
  Cause: Vitamin D deficiency or kidney damage.

Clinical features

- Depression of central and peripheral nervous system, muscle weakness, constipation, abdominal pain, peptic ulcer, depressed relaxation of heart during diastole.
- Increase in serum alkaline phosphatase.
- The cystic bone disease of hyperparathyroidism is called osteitis fibrosa cystic.

Physiology of Bone

Bone is a special type of connective tissue with a collagen framework impregnated with Ca^{2+}, PO_4^{3-} salts particularly hydroxyapatites. It is a living tissue that is well vascularized and has a total blood flow of 200–400 ml/min in adult humans. The protein in bone matrix is mostly type I collagen. Bone is of two types (Fig. 8.18):

1. *Compact/cortical bone:* It makes up the outer layer of most bones. It accounts for 80% of the bone in the body. Surface-to-volume ratio is low. Bone cells (osteocytes) lie in lacunae and they receive nutrients via Haversian canals.
2. *Trabecular/spongy bone:* It lies inside the cortical bone. They are made up of spicules or plates makes up remaining 20% of bone in the body. Surface to volume ratio is high. Bone cells lie on the surface of plates. In spongy bone, nutrients diffuse from bone ECF into the trabeculae.

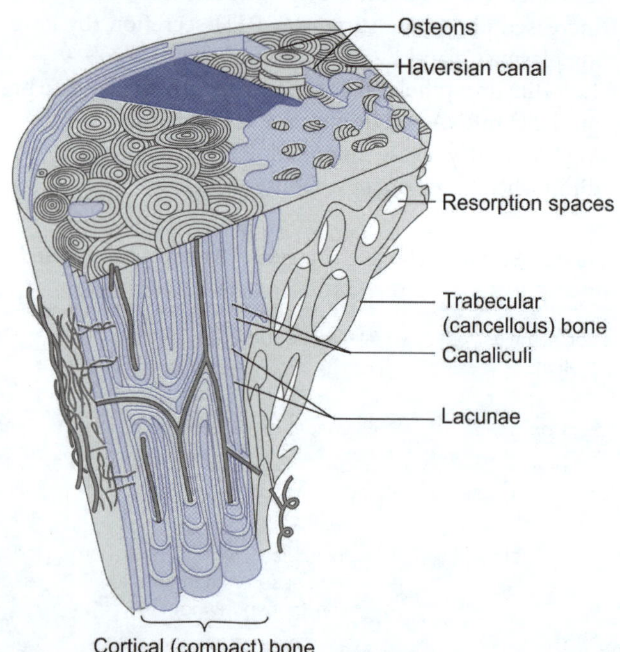

Fig. 8.18: Composition of bone

Bone Growth

During fetal development, most of the bone are modelled in cartilage and then transformed into bone by ossification-endochondral bone formation.

Certain bones (bones of skull) are formed directly from mesenchymal cells-intramembranous bone formation.

During growth, specialized areas at the ends of each long bone (epiphysis) are separated from the shaft of bone by a plate of actively proliferating cartilage, the epiphysial plate. The width of the epiphysial plate is proportionate to the rate of growth and is affected by a number of hormones like growth hormone and IGF-1. Linear bone growth ceases after the epiphyses unit with the shaft (epiphysial closure).

Bone Formation and Resorption

Bone is constantly being reabsorbed and reformed, which is under the cellular control of osteoblasts, osteocytes and osteoclasts. The cells responsible for bone formation are osteoblasts and the cells responsible for bone resorption are osteoclasts.

- *Osteoblasts:* They are bone forming cells. They are found on the outer surfaces of the bones and in bone cavities. They synthesize and secrete collagen, forming a matrix around themselves which then calcify and form new bone. They have abundant alkaline phosphatase activity.
- *Osteoclasts:* They are phagocytic multinuclear giant cells containing numerous lysosomes. They erode and resorb previously formed bone. They contain several acids and appear to phagocytose bone, digesting it in their cytoplasm.
- *Osteocytes:* They are bone cells surrounded by calcified matrix. Osteocytes remain in contact with one another and with osteoblasts via long protoplasmic processes that run through channels in the bone forming functional syncytium. Osteocytes provide rapid and transient movement of Ca from bone into the ECF space.

Mechanism of Bone Formation

- The initial stage in bone production is secretion of collagen molecules (called collagen monomers) and ground substances (proteoglycans) by osteoblasts. The collagen monomers polymerize rapidly to form collagen fibers; the resultant tissue becomes osteoid. As the osteoid is formed, some of the osteoblasts become entrapped in the osteoid. At this stage they are called osteocytes.
- During the normal process of mineralization, minerals accumulate within membrane bound vesicles. Within a few days after osteoid is formed, calcium salts begin to precipitate on the surfaces of collagen fibers. This process is controlled by PTH, calcitonin, 1-25 DHCC (Fig. 8.19).
- PTH increase and CT decreases the permeability of the bone cells to Ca^{2+} while 1-25 DHCC facilitates the active transport of Ca^{2+} from osteoblasts into ECF. In this way calcium and phosphate concentrations in bone fluid is regulated.

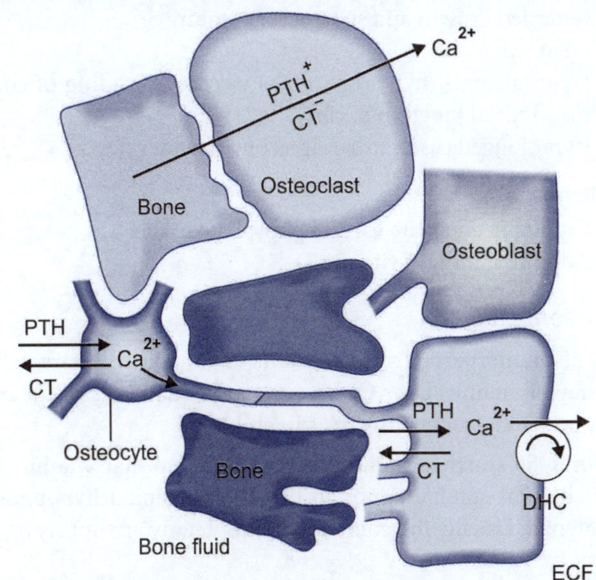

Fig. 8.19: Organization of bone cells and mechanism of bone formation

- Osteoblast secrete an alkaline phosphatase that hydrolysis phosphate esters and the phosphate is released. Thus whenever $[Ca^{2+}] \times [PO_4^{3-}]$ exceeds solubility product, calcium phosphate precipitates.

Reabsorption of Bone

It is a process that involves the destruction of entire matrix followed by the removal of calcium. It is brought about by osteoclasts. Osteoclasts are large phagocytic multinucleated cells formed in the bone marrow. When osteoclasts are activated by PTH some proteolytic enzymes and several acids like citric acid and lactic acid are released. The enzymes digest or dissolve the organic matrix of the bone and the acids cause solution of the bone salts. All the dissolved materials are then released into the blood.

Metabolic Bone Diseases

Rickets

Defective calcification of bone matrix in children due to Ca or phosphate deficiency caused by the lack of vitamin D.

Causes: Inadequate intake of provitamins, inadequate exposure to sun, kidney failure, liver failure, congenital hypophosphatemia (congenital reduced uptake of phosphate by renal tubules).

Clinical features

- Weakness and bowing of weight-bearing bones
- Thickening of wrist and ankles

- Retarded growth and shortness of stature
- Dental defects
- Hypocalcemia, hypotonia, rickety rosary (beading of costochondrial junction of ribs)
- In prolonged cases, usual signs of tetany develop.

Treatment

- Supplying adequate Ca and phosphate in diet.
- Administration of vitamin D.

Osteomalacia

Adult counterpart of rickets. Adults seldom have dietary deficiency of vitamin D or Ca because large quantities of Ca are not needed for bone growth as in children.

Causes: Steatorrhea (failure to absorb fat, so that vitamin D which is fat soluble is not absorbed), congenital hypophosphatemia. Usually the complications of tetany are not seen.

Note

- *Vitamin D resistant rickets:* Rickets due to congenital hypophosphatemia (congenital reduced reabsorption of phosphates by renal tubules) must be treated with phosphate compounds instead of Ca and vitamin D.
- *Renal rickets:* It is a type of osteomalacia that results from prolonged kidney damage. The cause of this condition is mainly failure of the damaged kidneys to form 1,25-dihydrocholecalciferol.

Osteoporosis

Osteoporosis is a loss of bone mass (both mineralization and matrix) with fractures, due to normal age-related changes in bone remodeling as well as additional factors that exaggerate this process. Usually occurs in old age.

Causes: Lack of physical stress on bones, malnutrition, lack of vitamin C (essential for secretion of intercellular substances), lack of estrogen secretion (estrogen decrease the number and activity of osteoclast), old age, Cushing's syndrome (here osteoblastic activity as well as deposition of protein in bone is decreased).

PANCREAS

Secretes enzymes and hormone. Exocrine-secrete enzymes that promote the digestion of carbohydrates, proteins and fats. Cells in endocrine part secrete hormones (Fig. 8.20).

- *A cells or α cells (15–20%):* Glucagon (hyperglycemic hormone).
- *B or β cells (70–80%):* Insulin-hypoglycemic hormone.
- *D cells (1–8%):* Somatostatin (GHIH) and gastrin (in small amounts).

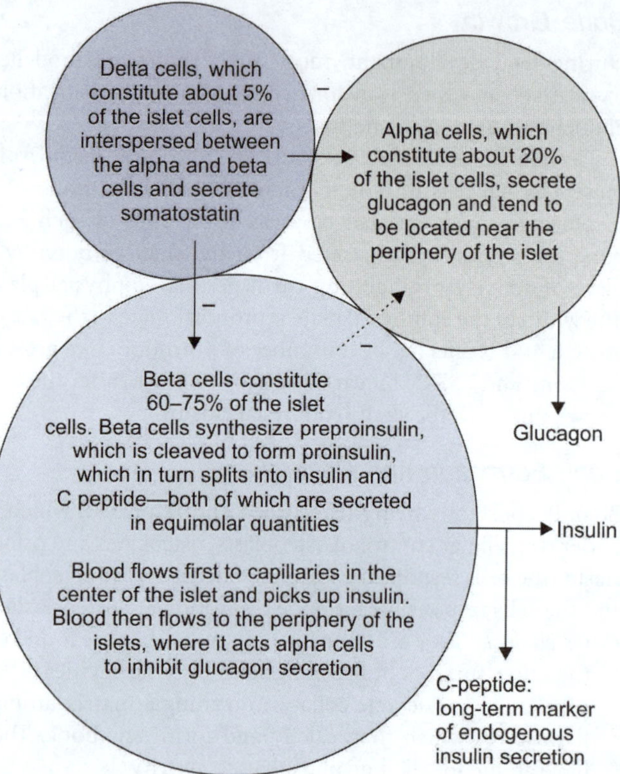

Fig. 8.20: Hormones of the pancreatic islets

- *F Cell:* Pancreatic polypeptide (decreases the absorption of food from GIT).

Nerve supply: ANS

Blood supply: Portal vein

Insulin (Fig. 8.21)

Structure of Insulin

Proinsulin is made up of A and B chain connected by a connecting peptide (C-peptide or C-chain). C peptide is detached in the granules before secretion. Normally, 90–97% of the product released from B cells is insulin along with equimolar amounts of C-peptide. Insulin is a two chain polypeptide having 51 aminoacids. The A chain has 21 while B chain has 30 amino acids.

Synthesis and Excretion

Insulin is synthesized by ribosomes on ER (proinsulin). It is then transported to the Golgi apparatus to form insulin. Here the formation of insulin continues within the storage granules which, therefore contain proinsulin, insulin and C peptide. These granules move to the cell wall and their membranes fuse with the membrane of the cell, expelling the insulin to the

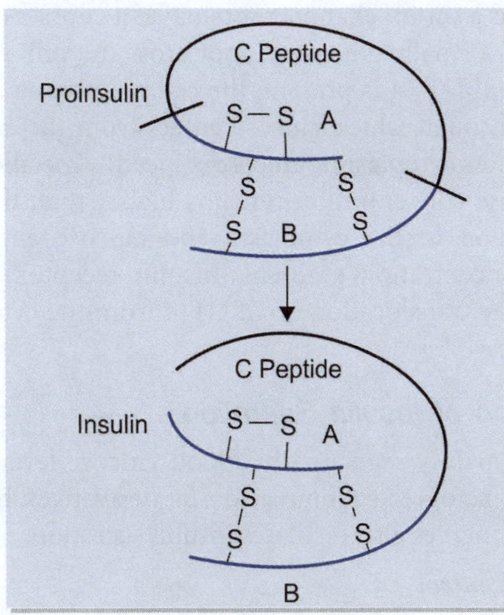

Fig. 8.21: Insulin

exterior by exocytosis. Insulin is formed after detaching connecting (C) peptide before secretion. The process of release of insulin requires ATP, cAMP and presence of Ca^{2+} and K^{+}. Normal fasting insulin concentration is 10–50 U/ml. Insulin is 10–20 times more active than proinsulin.

Transport and Distribution

Binds with circulating plasma protein of *anti-insulin* activity called synalbumin. Insulin fixes to insulin receptors (glycoprotein) on the cell membrane of may tissues. Insulin exerts its effect without entering the cell on which it acts.

Metabolism

Half life is about 5 minutes. 80% gets metabolized by the liver and kidneys by hepatic glutathione insulin dehydrogenase (HGIT) which breaks disulfide bridge to SH groups with separation of α and β chains. 20% in rest of body tissues and is destroyed by insulin protease.

Actions (Fig. 8.22)

On cell membrane permeability

Promotes glucose entry into cell (except RBC liver and brain cell).

On metabolism

- *Carbohydrate metabolism*
  - Peripheral utilization of glucose is increased.
  - Increased uptake of carbohydrates (by liver cells)
  - Insulin responsible for stimulation of GLUT
  - Stimulates phosphorylation of glucose by stimulating glucokinase

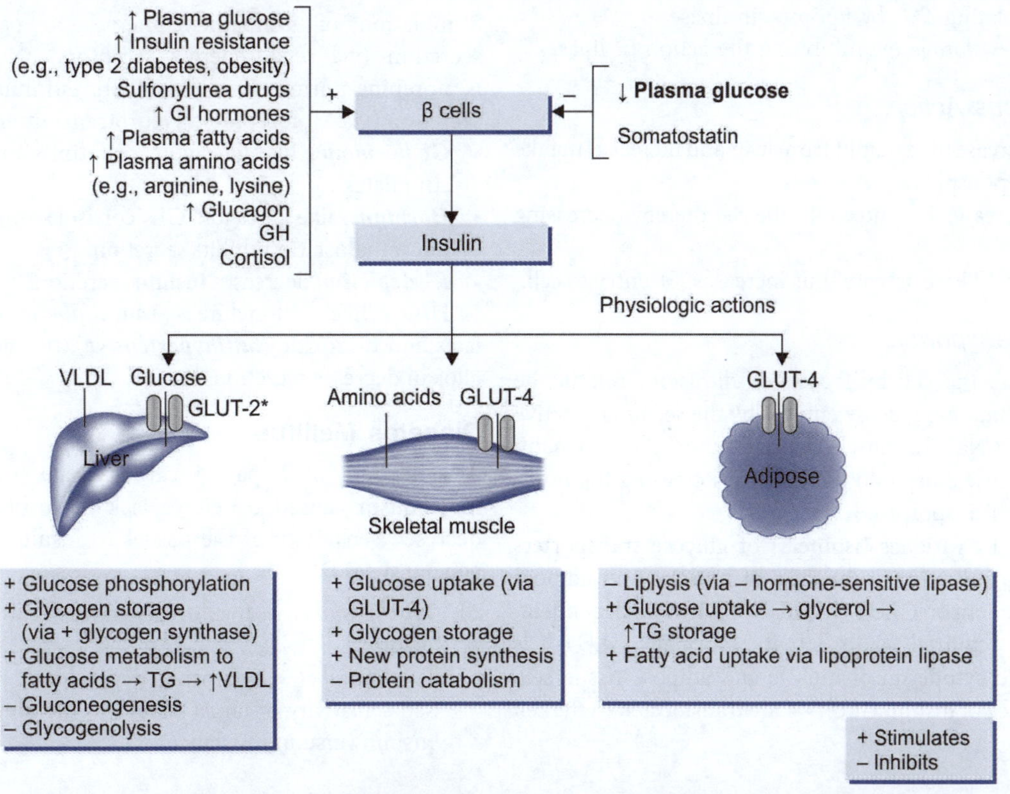

Fig. 8.22: Regulation of insulin secretion and physiological actions of insulin

- Activates glycogen synthetase. Helps glycogen synthesis in liver and muscle
- Inhibits glycogenolysis and gluconeogenesis
- Inhibits secretion of glucagons.

In hyperinsulinemia, patients suffer from hypoglycemia (decrease in blood sugar), brain cells are affected and produce convulsions.

Insulin dysfunction-glucose utilization severely affected.

- *Protein metabolism:*
  - Its action is anabolic.
  - Facilitates the transport of amino acids into the cell from blood (by increasing the permeability of cell membrane)
  - Accelerates protein synthesis by influencing translation of mRNA.
  - Inhibits gluconeogenesis, thus decrease protein breakdown.
  - Promotes growth-acts synergistically with GH.
- *Fat metabolism.*
  - **Promotes fat synthesis by**:
    - Increasing the transport of glucose into liver cells and this glucose is utilized for synthesis of fatty acids and triglycerides
    - Acetyl CoA carboxylase is activated (enzyme for fatty acid synthesis)
    - Increases the deposition of TGs by breaking down circulating TGs by lipoprotein lipase.
  - *Promotes storage by:* Inhibiting the action of lipases.

Miscellaneous Action

- Insulin increase urea output from liver and increases uptake of K+ and phosphate
- Insulin increases K+ entry into the cell thereby decreasing ECF [K+]
- It activates ATPase activity thus increases K+ entry to cell.

Glucose Transporters

Glucose enters the cell by facilitated diffusion. But in the intestine and kidneys glucose entry is by the secondary active transport with Na^+. In muscle, fat and other tissues, insulin facilitates glucose entry into the cells by increasing the number of glucose transporters.

There are 14 varieties (isomers) of glucose transporters (GLUT). Glucose entry in the cells of muscles and adipose tissue is dependent on GLUT-4. GLUT- 4 is insulin dependent, i.e. insulin is required for its activity. Normally GLUT-4 is present in the cytoplasm of muscle and adipose tissue cell. But in presence of insulin GLUT- 4 are translocated in the cell membrane.

GLUT is a sort of channel protein, i.e. it contains a channel within it. Normally glucose cannot cross the cell membrane, but when GLUT- 4 is present, the cell membrane contains a channel, through which glucose enters from the ECF to the cytoplasm. As cytoplasmic glucose is speedily metabolized, the ECF glucose concentration remains higher than the glucose concentration in the cytoplasm and glucose entry occurs due to concentration gradient. Insulin receptor substrates facilitate the translocation of GLUT-4 from the cytoplasm to membrane.

Regulation of Insulin Secretion

Insulin is mainly regulated by blood glucose level. In addition other factors like amino acids, fat derivatives, hormones, autonomic nerves also regulates insulin secretion.

Substrate control

- *Blood glucose:* Stimulates insulin secretion. Note that sugars like 2-deoxyglucose, mannoheptulose decreases secretion.
- *Amino acids:* Arginine and lysine (most potent) and certain other amino acids stimulates.
- *Fat derivatives:* β ketoacids stimulates.

cAMP and various cAMP generating substances

Stimuli that increase cAMP levels in β cells increase insulin secretion (increasing intracellular Ca^{2+}).

Autonomic nerves

Stimulation of sympathetic nerves to pancreas inhibit secretion (via α adrenergic receptors). Neurotransmitter is norepine-phrine. Parasympathetic stimulation increases secretion (via M_4 receptors). Neurotransmitter is ACh.

- ***GI hormones*** like glucagon, secretin, gastrin, CCK, GIP stimulates.
- ***Hormones*** like glucagon, GH, cortisol stimulates and insulin, somatostatin inhibits secretion.
- ***K^+ depletion*** decreases insulin secretion.

Drugs like sulfonylureas ***(antidiabetic agents)*** stimulates and diazoxide ***(antihypertensive)***, thiazides, phenytoin, alloxan decreses secretion.

Diabetes Mellitus

A syndrome of impaired carbohydrate, fat and protein metabolism caused by either lack of insulin secretion or decresed sensitivity of the tissues to insulin. There are two general types DM.

1. *Type I diabetes:* Insulin dependent; caused by lack of insulin.
2. *Type II diabetes:* Noninsulin dependent; caused by decreased sensitivity of target tissues to the metabolic effect of insulin (insulin resistance).

Clinical Characteristics (Table 8.6)

Table 8.6: Differentiating features of type I and type II diabetes mellitus

Feature	Type I	Type II
Age of onset	Usually < 20 years	Usually > 30 years
Body mass	Low (wasted) to normal	Obese
Plasma insulin	Low or absent	Normal to high initially
Plasma glucagon	High, can be suppressed	High, resistant to suppression
Plasma glucose	Increased	Increased
Insulin sensitivity	Normal	Reduced
Therapy	Insulin	Weight loss, thiazolidinediones Metformin Sulfonylureas, insulin

Signs and Symptoms

Various manifestations develop because of three major setbacks of insulin deficiency:

1. Increased blood sugar level due to reduced utilization by tissues.
2. Mobilization of fat from adipose tissue (for energy purpose) elevates fatty acid content in the blood; atherosclerosis.
3. Depletion of proteins from tissue.

Features

Polyuria (due to osmotic effect, more water accompanies the glucose), polydypsia (to compensate for the loss of water, thirst center is activated and more water is taken), polyphagia (to compensate the loss of glucose and protein), glucosuria, osmotic diuresis, asthenia (lack of energy), ketoacidosis, acetone breathing, Kussmaul breathing, coma. Difference between diabetes mellitus and diabetes insipidus is given in Table 8.7.

Complications of DM (Flowchart 8.8)

- Predisposition to infection (intracellular glucose are converted to advanced glycosylation end products (AGEs) and these AGEs interfere with leukocyte response to infection).
- Atherosclerosis.
- Diabetic neuropathy-degeneration of autonomic and peripheral nerve.
- Diabetic retinopathy-degenerative changes in retina.
- Diabetic nephropathy-degenerative changes in kidney.
- Stroke and MI.

Table 8.7: Comparison between diabetes mellitus and diabetes insipidus

Features	Diabetes mellitus	Diabetes insipidus
Etiology	• Deficient insulin secretion from pancreas • Lesions of pancreas	• Deficient ADH secretion from posterior pituitary • Lesions of pancreas supraoptic nucleus of hypothalamus
Major metabolic changes	• Storage of glucose as glycogen in muscles is impaired • Liver glycogen breakdown is increased • Fat breakdown increased • Ketone bodies formation increased	• No such effects
Urine output	• Large volume of urine is voided-polyuria	• Large volume of urine is voided-polyuria
Cause of polyuria	• Water reabsorption is prevented by the osmotic pressure effect of glucose in the lumen of renal tubule. So more water is lost through urine.	• ADH deficiency decreases water reabsorbtion at DCT and collecting duct. So more water is lost
Presence of glucose in urine	• Present-glycosuria	• Absent
Taste of urine	• Sweet	• No sweet taste
Specific gravity	• High-as glucose is present in urine	• Low-dilute hypotonic urine. • Specific gravity-1.002–1.006
Blood glucose level	• High-hyperglycemia	• Normal
Ketone body concentration in blood	• High-ketosis	• Not seen
Symptoms	• Increased thirst, hunger, ketonuria, poor wound healing	• Increased thirst. Other effects are absent.
Treatment	• Oral hypoglycemic agents • Insulin injection	• ADH injection

Flowchart 8.8: Complications of DM

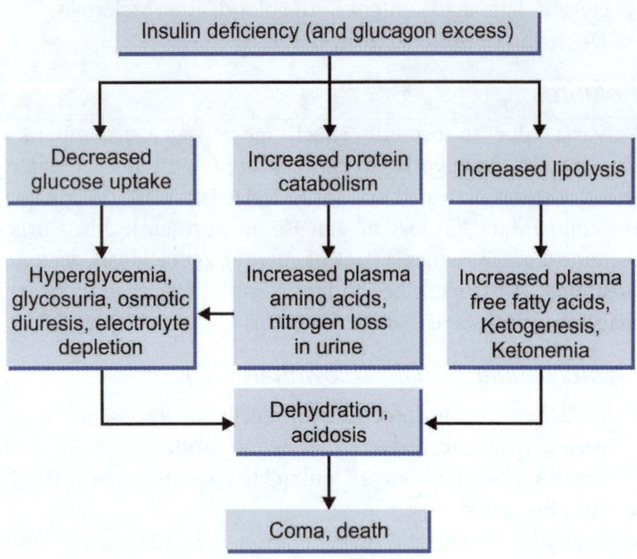

Treatment

Type I: Administration of insulin.

Type II: Diet controlling, exercise (to induce weight loss and reverse insulin resistance). If this fails drugs are administrated to stimulate increased production of insulin/decreased hepatic glucose production.

Glucagon

Secreted from α cells in islets of Langerhans. It has several functions that are opposite to that of insulin. Normal fasting glucagons concentration is 100–150 pg/ml. Metabolism same as that of insulin.

Actions

Glucagons is glycogenolytic, gluconeogenic, lipolytic and ketogenic. It favors breakdown of stored nutrients.

On carbohydrate metabolism

Glucagon increases the blood glucose level by:

Stimulates glycogenolysis

It increases breakdown of liver glycogen to glucose, which in turn increases blood glucose by:

- Inhibiting glycogen synthetase.
- By activating cAMP formation (via its action on Gs) → activates protein kinase → activates phosphorylase enzyme which converts glycogen to glucose-6-phosphate.

$$\text{Glucose-6-phosphate} \xrightarrow{\text{Liver phosphatase}} \text{glucose}$$

- Act on liver cells to activate phospholipase C and results in intracellular Ca^{2+}, thus stimulating glycogenolysis.

Promotes gluconeogenesis

Promotes formation of glucose from lactate, pyruvate, glycerol and amino acids by:

- Increases rate of amino acid uptake by liver cells.
- Activates the enzymes, which convert pyruvate to phosphoenol pyruvate (rate limiting step).
- Increasing deamination of amino acids in the liver.

On protein metabolism

Increases transport of amino acids into liver cell.

On lipid metabolism

Shows lipolytic and ketogenic actions. It increases the release of free fatty acids from adipose tissue and makes free fatty acids available for peripheral utilization. The lipolytic activity of glucagon in turn promotes ketogenesis.

Other Actions

- Inhibits secretion of gastric juice
- Stimulates secretion of GH, insulin and pancreatic somatostatin
- Increases force of contraction of heart by increasing cAMP
- Increases blood flow in some tissues like kidney
- Enhances bile secretion.

Regulation of Glucagon Secretion

Controlled mainly by blood glucose amino acid level in blood.

Blood glucose level (most potent factor)

Increased blood inhibits glucagon secretion.

Amino acid level in blood

Increased amino acids stimulates the secretion of glucagon. Thus in this instance glucagon and insulin responses are not opposite.

Other Factors

- *Stimulators:* Exercise, stress, gastrin, CCK, cortisol, β adrenergic stimulations.
- *Inhibitors:* Somatostatin, secretin, FFA, insulin, ketones, GABA, α adrenergic stimulations.

Somatostatin

Somatostatin is secreted by δ cells of the islets. It inhibits glucagon, insulin and pancreatic polypeptide. Somatostatin secretion is stimulated by glucose-amino acid meals. It is also increased by CCK. Apart from islet cells, somatostatin is secreted from various sites of our body, like: (i) Brain and CNS (ii) GI tract. Hypothalamic somatostatin inhibits GH hormone. That is why, it is also called growth hormone inhibiting hormone (GHIH). Somatostatin inhibits gastric secretion and gastric motility.

Pancreatic Polypeptide

F-cells of the islets produce pancreatic polypeptide which is a polypeptide hormone containing 36 amino acids and is structurally related to the neurotransmitter neuropeptide Y in the CNS and polypeptide YY found in the intestine. Fasting and hypoglycemia increase the secretion of pancreatic polypeptide. Physiological significance of this hormone is uncertain.

ADRENAL CORTEX

The adrenal glands are paired structures situated above the kidney. Hence, the name adrenal, i.e. adjacent to renal or suprarenal gland, i.e. superior to renal (kidney). The adrenal gland consists of an outer cortex and inner medulla. The hormones secreted by the adrenal cortex are called corticosteroids, which are classified into glucocorticoids, mineralocorticoids and androgen. The hormones secreted by the adrenal medulla are epinephrine and norepinephrine. The adrenal cortex is essential for life, the adrenal medulla is not. Adrenal cortex has three layers: zona glomerulosa, zona fasciculata and zone reticularis. The zone glomerulosa is the outermost layer and is the site of mineralocorticoid synthesis. The middle layer (zona fasciculata) synthesize and secrete glucocorticoids and inner layer (zona reticularis) secretes androgens (Fig. 8.23).

Mineralocorticoids

Aldosterone

The chief mineralocorticoid (90%). Other mineralocorticoids are deoxycorticosterone, 9 α-fluorocortisol (synthetic). They are life saving hormones.

- *Effects on renal tubules:*
  - Na^+ reabsorbtion from the tubular fluid into tubular epithelial cell.
  - Potassium excretion (active reabsorption of Na occurs in exchange of K and H).
  - H^+ excretion.
- *Effect on ECF volume:* When Na^+ are reabsorbed from renal tubules, simultaneously water is also reabsorbed which causes increase in volume of ECF.
- *Effect on blood pressure:* Blood pressure (BP) is increased due to increase in ECF volume or blood volume.

Aldosterone escape

When aldosterone secretion increases, ECF volume and blood volume, is increased leading to rise in BP elevated BP stimulates the secretion of ANP from atrial muscles. It causes excretion of excess salt and water through urine *(pressure natriuresis and pressure diuresis).* Content of salt and water in ECF comes to normal in spite of increase in secretion of aldosterone.

- *Effect on salivary gland and sweat gland:* Na^+ reabsorption from sweat gland and loss of Na^+ is prevented.
- *Effect on intestine:* Enhance Na^+ absorption from intestine especially in the colon and prevents loss of Na^+ through feces.

Mechanism of Action

Aldosterone binds to a cytoplasm receptor, and the receptor-hormone complex moves to the nucleus where it alters the transcription of mRNAs. This in turn increases the production of proteins that alter cell function. The aldosterone-stimulated proteins have two effects-a rapid effect, to increase the activity of epithelial sodium channels (ENaCs); and a slower effect to increase the synthesis of ENaCs. Aldosterone activates the gene for ***serum and glucocorticoid regulated kinase (sgk)*** and sgk increases ENaC activity. Aldosterone also increases the mRN. As for the three subunits that make up ENaCs. Aldosterone increases the activity of membrane Na^+-K^+ exchangers. This produces an increase in intracellular Na^+.

Regulation of Aldosterone Secretion (Flowchart 8.9)

Mineralocorticoid secretion is stimulated by hyperkalemia, angiotensin II, ACTH and hyponatremia.

- Aldosterone secretion in response to hyperkalemia is the most important and forms the basis for renal regulation of body potassium balance.

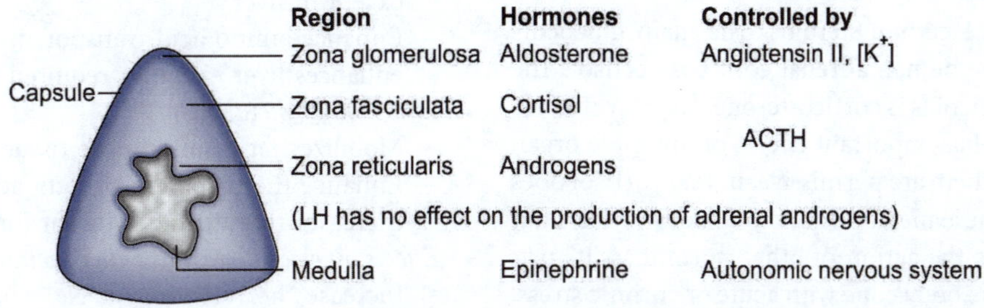

Fig. 8.23: Adrenal gland

Flowchart 8.9: Regulation of aldosterone secretion

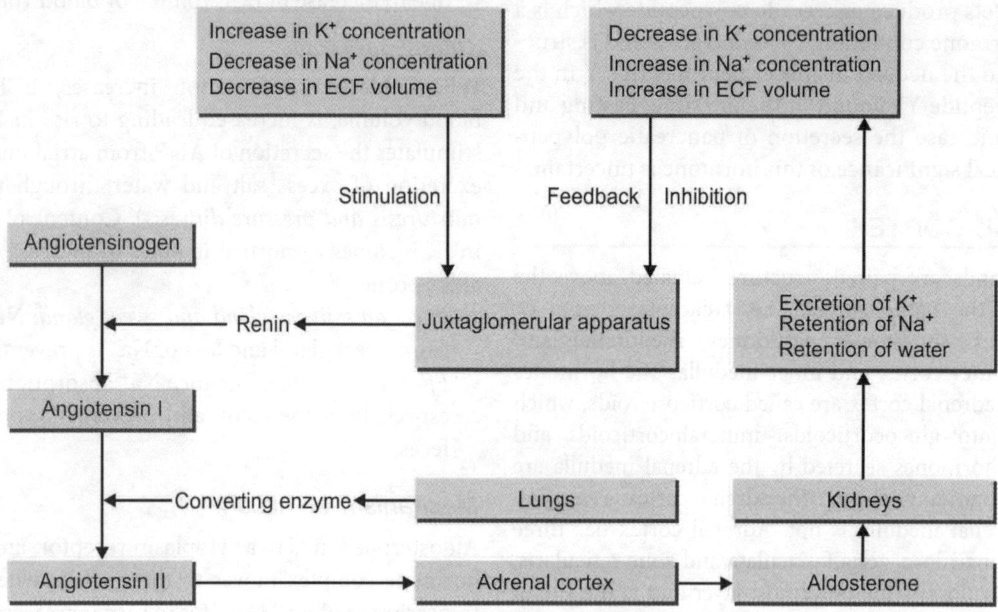

- Stimulation of aldosterone by angiotensin II (through renin-angiotensin system) is important for the correction of hypovolemia and hypotension in conditions like salt depletion or renal ischemia.
- Stimulation of aldosterone secretion by ACTH results in diurnal variation of aldosterone secretion. However, ACTH is not an important physiological regulator for aldosterone secretion.
- Hyponatremia is a weak stimulator of aldosterone secretion.

The stimulatory agents for aldosterone secretion are given below in the order of importance:

- Increase in K^+ ion concentration in the ECF
- Increased activity of renin-angiotensin system
- Decrease in Na ion concentration
- ACTH.

Glucocorticoids

Glucocorticoids are 21 carbon steroids. The main glucocorticoids secreted by the human adrenal cortex is cortisol. The other major glucocorticoids is corticosterone. Glucocorticoids is essential for life. It has important effects on multiple organ systems, but most of them are permissive, in that cortisol does not directly initiate these metabolic or circulatory process but its presence facilitates the action of other hormones. Its primary role is to help the body cope with acute or chronic stress, to execute the 'fight-or-flight' response.

Actions

Metabolic effects

- *Effects on carbohydrate metabolism:* Exerts anti-insulin effect by
  - Increases gluconeogenesis by:
    - Enhancing breakdown of protein in extrahepatic cells.
    - Increasing synthesis of enzymes required for gluconeogenesis.
  - Inhibiting glucose uptake and utilization by peripheral cells.
- *Effects on protein metabolism:* Decrease cellular protein and increase liver and plasma proteins by:
  - Decreasing the protein synthesis by inhibiting amino acid transport into extrahepatic cells and inhibiting the formation of RNA
  - Stimulates catabolism of proteins in all body cells except in liver
  - Enhance amino acid transport into liver cells and also enhances liver enzymes required for protein synthesis.
- *Effect on fat metabolism*
  - Mobilizes fat from adipose tissue
  - Enhance the oxidation of fatty acids in cells
  - Increases the utilization of fat for energy.
- *Effects on electrolyte and water metabolism*
  - Increase the retention of Na^+ and excretion of K^+ by the kidney

– Accelerates the excretion of water; adrenal insufficiency causes water retention.

Physiological Actions on Various Organs and Systems

- *Effects on muscle:* Hypersecretion causes muscular weakness (due to protein catabolism).
- *Effects on bone*
  - Increased bone resorption.
  - Inhibition of bone formation.
- *Effects on vascular system:* Essential for constrictor action of adrenaline and noradrenaline. In adrenal insufficiency, blood vessels fail to respond to adrenaline and noradrenaline leading to vascular collapse.
- *Effects on CNS:* Insufficiency causes personality changes like irritability and lack of concentration.
- *Effects on blood cells and lymphatic organs:*
  - Decrease circulating eosinophils and basophils
  - Increase number of neutrophils, platelets and RBCs
  - Decrease circulating lymphocyte count and size of lymph nodes and thymus.

Permissive Action

Actions of some hormones are executed only in presence of glucocorticoids. For example:

- Calorigenic action of glucagon
- Pressor activity of catecholamine
- Bronchodilation of catecholamine
- Lipolytic effect of catecholamine.

Effects in resistance to stress

Exposure to any type of stress increases secretion of ACTH, which in turn increases the secretion of glucocorticoids. It enhance resistance by:

- Immediate release of amino acids → synthesis of new protein.
- FA released from cell → energy supply.
- Enhances vascular reactivity to catecholamine.
- Prevent the severity of other changes in body caused by stress.

Anti-inflammatory effects

Blocks the early stages of inflammation process before inflammation begins. If inflammation has already begun, it causes rapid resolution of inflammation and increased rapidity of healing. These effects are by:

- Stabilizing lysosomal membranes so that proteolytic enzymes are not released
- Decreasing permeability of capillaries so that loss of plasma is prevented
- Decreasing both migration of WBCs into inflamed area and phagocytosis of damaged cell (by decreasing the release of PG and leukotrienes)
- Suppression of T-cells and other leukocytes so that there is decrease in reaction of tissue
- Reducing the release of IL-1 (so temperature is reduced, which in turn reduces vasodilation)
- Inhibit phospholipase A2 → less arachidonic acid is formed.

Anti-allergic effects

Prevents various reactions in allergic condition.

Regulation of Cortisol Secretion (Flowchart 8.10)

The adrenal cortex is under the control of hypothalamo-hypophysial axis. The secretion of glucocorticoids by adrenal cortex is regulated by anterior pituitary gland through ACTH (corticotropin). ACTH secretion itself is regulated by hypothalamus through corticotropin releasing hormone (CRH). The chain is called hypothalamus-pituitary-adrenal-axis. The secretion of ACTH and consequently that of cortisol follows a circadian rhythm due to hypothalamic control. ACTH secretion is minimum during night and maximum early in the morning (6–8 am). The hypothalamo-hypophyseal axis

Flowchart 8.10: Regulation of cortisol secretion

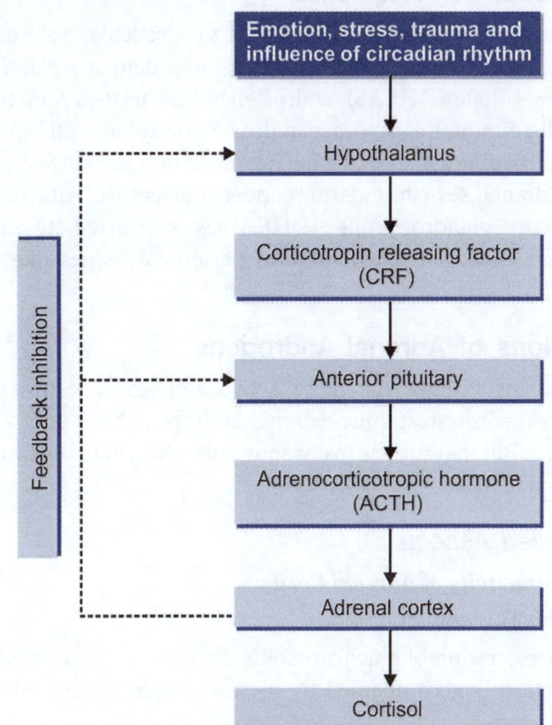

PHYSICON—The Reliable Icon in Physiology

is susceptible to feedback control by cortisol. The secretion of ACTH and CRH is subjected to negative feedback (inhibition) by glucocorticoids which keeps glucocorticoids secretion within normal limits. Stress can stimulate the hypothalamus to release more CRH that in turn increases ACTH secretion. Consequently, glucocorticoid secretion is elevated in stress.

Circadian Rhythm of Glucocorticoid Secretion

The secretory rates of CRF, ACTH and cortisol are high in the early morning but low in the late evening. This effect results from 24 hours cyclical alteration in the signals from the hypothalamus that cause cortisol secretion.

Note

Stages of inflammation:

- Substances that activate inflammation process such as histamine, bradykinin, proteolytic enzymes, PG and leukotrienes are released from damaged cells.
- Increase in blood flow in the inflamed area.
- Leakage of plasma out of the capillaries into the damaged areas (due to increased capillary permeability) followed by clotting of tissue fluid causing nonpitting type of edema.
- Infiltration of the area by leukocytes.
- After days or weeks, ingrowth of fibros tissue that often help in healing process.

Adrenal Sex Hormones

Adrenal sex steroids produced from zona reticularis are dehydroepiandrosterone (DHEA, major one), dehydroepiandrosterone sulfate (DHEAS), androstenedione, testosterone (only small amounts). Dehydroepiandrosterone sulfate (DHEAS) is the most abundant circulating hormone in humans. Secretion of adrenal sex steroids are under the control of ACTH. Dehydroepiandrosterone (DHEA) is converted to more potent androgen testosterone in peripheral tissues like hair folicles, breast.

Actions of Adrenal Androgens

Since males have the more active androgens testosterone and dihydrotestosterone, adrenal androgens have only weak effects. But they are the major source of estrogen in postmenopausal females.

Applied Aspects

Hyperactivity of Adrenal Cortex

Cushing's syndrome

Hypersecretion of glucocorticoids. Increase in glucocorticoid secretion is accompanied by increased secretion of adrenal androgens.

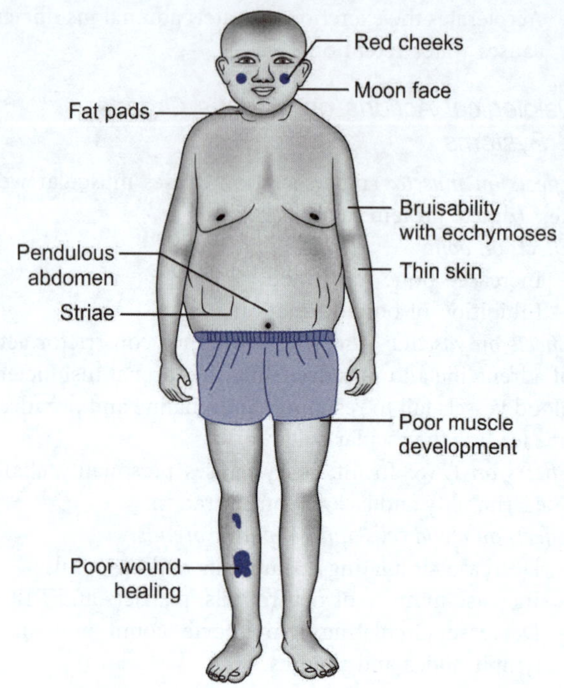

Fig. 8.24: Clinical features of Cushing's syndrome

Causes

- Adenomas of anterior pituitary that secrete ACTH.
- Abnormal functions of hypothalamus that causes high levels of CRH.
- Ectopic secretion of ACTH by a tumor elsewhere in the body.
- Adenomas of adrenal cortex.

Cushing's syndrome due to anterior pituitary tumors are called ***Cushing's disease.***

Signs and symptoms (Fig. 8.24)

1. Disproportionate distribution of body fat producing following features:
   a. Moon face-due to fat accumulation on face.
   b. Buffalo hump-due to fat accumulation in upper back.
   c. Pot belly-due to fat accumulation in upper abdomen.
   d. Purple striae-reddish purple stripes on abdomen due to:
      - Stretching of abdominal wall by increased subcutaneous fat
      - Deficiency of collagen fibers due to protein depletion (cause thinning of skin)
      - Rupture of subdermal tissues due to stretching.
2. Thinning of extremities.
3. Muscle are poorly developed due to protein catabolism.
4. Facial hair growth and acne (effect of androgens).

5. Wounds heal poorly and minor injuries cause bruises and ecchymoses.
6. Hyperglycemia due to gluconeogenesis.
7. Bone resorption and osteoporosis.
8. Mental abnormalities.
9. Blackening of skin due to pigmentation of skin by MSH like activity of ACTH.
10. Hypertension due to increased retention of sodium and water.

Treatment

1. Removal of adrenal tumor.
2. Tumors in the pituitary gland that over secrete ACTH can be surgically removed or destroyed by radiation.
3. Serotonin antagonist and GABA transaminase inhibitors (inhibit ACTH secretion).
4. Bilateral adrenalectomy if ACTH secretion cannot be decreased.

Hyperaldosteronism

Depending upon the causes, it is classified as:

- *Primary hyperaldosteronism:* It is called *Conn's syndrome.* Renin secretion is depressed (due to feedback suppression). The most important effects are hypokalemia, slight increase in ECF and blood volume, hypertension. Due to hypokalemia muscles are paralyzed.
  Causes: Adenoma of zona glomerulosa, adrenal hyperplasia, adrenal carcinoma.
  Treatment: Surgical removal of tumor or adrenal tissue when hyperplasia is the cause.
- *Secondary hyperaldosteronism:* Occurs due to extraadrenal causes.
  Causes: Cirrhosis, heart failure and nephrosis.

Adrenogenital Syndrome (Virilism)

Tumor of zona reticularies of adrenal cortex cause intense musculinizing effects through out the body. In females they cause development of male secondary sexual characteristics such as beard, deeper voice, muscular body, enlargement of clitoris, baldness, etc. In prepubertal males it produces same characteristics as in females along with rapid development of male sex organs. In males the effects are usually masked due to effects produced by testosterone.

Hypoactivity of Adrenal Cortex

Addison's disease

Due to insufficiency of mineralocorticoids as well as glucocorticoids.

Cause: Complication of TB, autoimmune inflammation of adrenal.

Signs and symptoms: Glucocorticoid deficiency produces weight loss, nausea, vomiting, weakness, tiredness, etc. Since glucocorticoids are essential for adaptation to stress, therefore in Addison's disease, exposure to any type of stress may be fatal. Mineralocorticoid deficiency produces hyponatremia, hyperkalemia, acidosis, decreased ECF volume with hypotension. They have small heart (hypotension decreases work of heart). Increased ACTH secretion occurs due to feedback mechanism and causes pigmentation of skin and mucous membrane (because of its MSH like activity).

Treatment: Administration of mineralocorticoids and glucocorticoids daily.

Clinical Note

Addisonian crisis

Great quantities of glucocorticoids are occasionally secreted in response to different types of physical or mental stress. In a person with Addison's disease, the output of glucocorticoids does not increase during stress. Yet whenever different types of trauma, disease, or other stresses, a person is likely to have an acute need for excessive amounts of glucocorticoids (often must be given 10 or more times the normal quantities of glucocorticoids to prevent death). This critical need for extra glucocorticoids and the associated severe debility in times of stress is called an addisonian crisis.

ADRENAL MEDULLA

Adrenal medulla constitutes central 20% of the gland. Epinephrine (adrenaline), norepinephrine (noradrenaline) and dopamine are secreted by adrenal medulla. These hormones are called catecholamines. It secretes epinephrine and norepinephrine in response to sympathetic stimulation. Adrenal medulla is referred as a modified sympathetic ganglion.

Mechanism of Release of Catecholamines

Stimulation of preganglionic splanchnic fibers → release of ACh → stimulate medullary chromaffin cells, by promoting inward movement of Ca^{2+} → secretion of epinephrine and NE into blood by exocytosis (Fig. 8.25).

- *Adrenergic receptors:* Adrenergic receptors are divided into α and β types: Epinephrine and norepinephrine both act on α and β receptors, with norepinephrine having greater affinity for α adrenergic receptors and epinephrine for β adrenergic receptors.

Alpha adrenergic receptors

They are sensitive to both epinephrine and NE. They are mainly excitatory, except inhibition of intestinal motility. They are of two kinds α_1 and α_2.

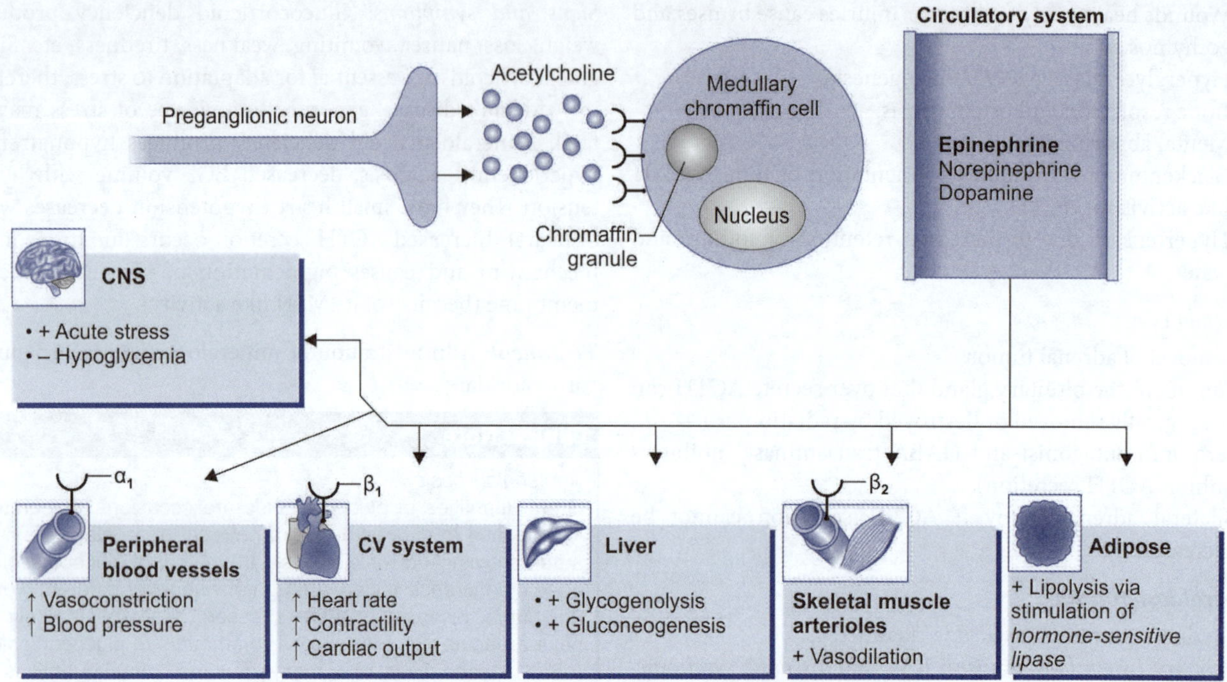

Fig. 8.25: Synthesis and physiological actions of catecholamines

1. α_1 Mainly excitatory (receptor located on postsynaptic membranes).
2. α_2 They are inhibitory (located on presynaptic nerve terminals of cholinergic and adrenergic nerves).

Beta adrenergic receptors

They respond to epinephrine and in general are relatively insensitive to NE. They are mainly inhibitory except excitation of myocardium. They are of three types: β_1 β_2 and β_3.

β_1: Its activation produce tachycardia and increased myocardial contractility (receptors located on cardiac muscle).

β_2: Associated with relaxation of smooth muscle.

In humans β_1-adrenergic mechanism predominates.

Actions of Epinephrine and Norepinephrine

On CVS

Heart

Epinephrine and norepinephrine are powerful cardiac stimulants. They act mainly by interacting with β_1 receptors and produces various effects as follows:

- Increase in heart rate (positive chronotropic)
- Increased myocardial contractility (positive inotropic)
- Increase in conduction velocity (positive dromotropic)
- Increase in cardiac output
- Increase in automaticity
- Increase in cardiac work and its oxygen requirement
- Increase in excitability and tendency to cause cardiac arrhythmias.

Blood vessels and blood pressure

Blood vessels of the skin and mucous membranes predominantly contain α_1 receptors, hence are constricted by epinephrine and norepinephrine. Both epinephrine and norepinephrine also constricts renal, mesenteric, pulmonary and splanchnic vessels. But epinephrine dilates the blood vessels of skeletal muscle and coronary vessels; via β_2 (norepinephrine does not produce this action as it has no β_2 action).

Normally adrenaline acts through α and β receptors. α receptors are vasocontrictors and β are dilators. α receptors are not as sensitive as β to levels of adrenaline. Intravenous administration of adrenaline in moderate doses produces typical biphasic effect.

There is an initial rise in BP due to α_1 (blood vessels) and β_1 (heart) actions, followed by a fall in BP due to β_2 mediated vasodilatation in skeletal muscle. Administration of adrenaline after α_1 blocker produces only a fall in BP (β_2, vasodilatation). This is referred to as ***Dales vasomotor reversal.***

Carbohydrate Metabolism

Catecholamines increase blood sugar (via β receptors increases glycogenolysis by increasing phosphorylase activity and via α receptors increases glycogenolysis by increasing intracellular Ca^{2+}).

Catecholamines via β receptors increases the secretion of insulin and glucagon, but inhibit the secretion of these hormones via α receptors.

Lipid metabolism

Catecholamines by β receptors stimulates hormone sensitive lipase, breaks down stored triglycerides to free FFA and glycerol. In liver, excess fatty acids are converted in to ketone bodies.

- *On BMR:* Catecholamines increase BMR (calorigenic action) in the presence of T_4 and adrenal cortex. Epinephrine shows more calorigenic action than norepinephrine.
- *On CNS:* Catecholamines show stimulatory effect on CNS and produce anxiety, hyperventilation and coarse tremors of extremities. It inhibits the release of ADH.
- *On eyes:* Receptors cause contraction of radial muscles producing mydriasis. β receptors cause relaxation on ciliary muscles and increases tone of eye muscles.
- *On GIT:* Epinephrine decreases tone and mobility (via β receptors).It causes sphincteric constriction (via β receptors), thus produces constipation.
- *On urinary bladder:* Epinephrine via β receptors causes relaxation of detruser muscle and via α receptors cause contraction of trigone and shinctors; thus produces retention of urine.
- *On skin:* Catecholamines (via α receptors) produce piloerection of hair.
- *On sweat glands:* Produce localized sweating on palm and sole called adrenergic sweating.
- *On skeletal muscles:* Improves skeletal muscle blood supply (via $β_2$) and increases force of contraction.
- *On bronchial muscles:* Epinephrine relaxes bronchial musculature producing bronchodilatation (via $β_2$ receptors).
- *On blood:*
  - *Epinephrine:*
    - Decreases clotting time due to increase in activity of factor five.
    - Increases RBC count, PCV, Hb concentration.
    - Increases plasma protein concentration.
    - Cause increase in neutrophils.

Miscellaneous

Initially cause hyperkalemia followed by hypokalemia due to increased K^+ influx into skeletal muscle.

Actions of dopamine

- It produces generalized vasoconstriction by releasing NE.
- It increases contractility of heart (via β receptors).
- Increases in SBP and does not affect DBP.
- On kidneys it produces natriuresis (by inhibiting Na^+- K^+ ATPase) and vasodilation.

Because of these actions, dopamine is usefuel in the treatment of traumatic and cardiogenic shock.

Regulation of Catecholamine Secretion

- Secretion is entirely controlled by splanchnic nerves. These fibers are preganglionic sympathetic fibers and release ACh as their transmitter. Splanchnic nerve activities are controlled by centers in the reticular formation in the medulla and hypothalamus. Adrenal medullary activation occurs as a part of sympathetic response to any emergency situation like fear, anxiety, pain, trauma, hemorrhage, hypoxia.
- Secretion of glucocorticoids promotes conversion of NE to epinephrine.
- Hypoglycemia is a potent stimulus to catecholamine secretion.

Applied Aspect

- *Hyposecretion of catecholamines:* It usully produces no clinical signs and symptoms because catecholamine production from sympathetic nerve endings appears to satisfy the normal biological requirements.
- *Hypersecretion of catecholamines:* Seen in tumors of chromaffin tissue called pheochromocytoma.

Features

- Sustained hypertension, headaches
- Sweating, anxiety
- Palpitations and chest pain
- Increased body temperature, hyperglycemia, glycosurea and increase in BMR
- Increased in urinary excretion of catecholamines, metanephrines and VMA.

Summary of the different hormones in human body (Table 8.8).

Table 8.8: Hormones showing type, excess, deficiency and effects

Hormone	Source	Type	Excess	Deficiency	Effects
Insulin	Beta cells of pancreas	Small protein or polypeptide	Hypoglycemia	Diabetes mellitus	Glycogen synthesis in liver and muscle Lipogenesis in adipose tissue
Glucagon	Alpha cells of pancreas	Polypeptide	Hyperglycemia	Hypoglycemia	Glycogen breakdown, glyconeogenesis
Parathormone (PTH)	Chief cells, parathyroid	Polypeptide	Hypercalcemia, Hypercalcuria, Phosphate bone	Tetany, abnormal conduction, calcification	Increased vitamin D activity, increase bone reabsorption
Calcitonin	Parafollicular cells of thyroid	Polypeptide	No known effects	No known effects	Decreased serum calcium and decreased bone reabsorption
ADH	Posterior pituitary	Peptide	Hypertension, Hyponatremia, SIADH	Diabetes insipidus	Increased reabsorption of water, increased permeability of the collecting ducts

Contd...

Contd...

Hormone	Source	Type	Excess	Deficiency	Effects
Oxytocin	Posterior pituitary	Peptide	—	—	Uterine contraction and milk ejection reflex
GH	Acidophils of anterior pituitary	Polypeptide	Acromegaly (adults)	Dwarfism	Increased protein synthesis, somatomedins, lipolysis, and calcium absorption
ACTH	Basophils of anterior pituitary	Protein	Cushing's syndrome	Secondary Addison's disease	Increase cortisol and androgen
Cortisol	Adrenal zona fasciculata	Steroid	Cushing's syndrome	Stress intolerance, Addison's disease	Increased protein and fat catabolism and increased glycogenesis and increased gluconeogenesis
Aldosterone	Adrenal zona glomerulosa	Steroid	Conn's syndrome	Hypotension	Na^+ retention in the kidneys
Adrenal androgens	Adrenal zona reticularis	Steroid	Virilism	Poor secondary sexual character development, hypogonadism	Contribute to the secondary sexual characters

CLINICAL QUESTIONS

1. **A patient came to the clinic with the complaints of severe thirst and polyuria. On urine examination showed.**
   - **Total volume—20 l/day**
   - **Specific gravity of urine—1.002**
   - **Benedict's test was negative**

   a. What is the condition?
   b. Explain the features.
   c. What is the physiological basis of treatment?

2. **As a 35-year-old patient was entering the clinic, the doctor observed that he had prognathism, kyphosis and enlarged hands and feet.**
   a. What is the condition?
   b. What is the cause?
   c. Explain the observations.

3. **A two-year-old boy was having delayed milestones, potbelly and moon face.**
   a. What is the condition?
   b. What is the cause?
   c. What is the physiological basis of treatment?

4. **During postoperative period following thyroidectomy, patient developed laryngeal stridor, facial muscle irritability and carpopedal spasms.**
   a. What is the probable condition?
   b. Explain the signs.
   c. Give physiological basis of treatment.

5. **An elderly lady came to the doctor with complaints of swelling in the neck and protrusion of the eyeballs. Examination revealed fine tremors at rest and sleeping pulse rate was 110 /minute.**
   a. What is the probable diagnosis?
   b. How will you confirm the diagnosis?
   c. Outline the physiological basis of treatment.

6. **A 45-year-old lady came with complaints of intolerance to warmth, weight loss and palpitations. On examination she was found to have sleeping pulse rate 100/min and protruding eyeballs.**
   a. Identify the condition.
   b. Explain the findings.
   c. How will you confirm the diagnosis?

7. **A 45-year-old lady came with complaints of weight gain in spite of loss of appetite and tiredness. On examination resting pulse rate was 50/min. There was generalized non-pitting edema and tendon jerks were found sluggish.**
   a. Identify the condition.
   b. Explain the findings.
   c. How will you confirm the diagnosis?

8. **In a routine checkup, a 46-year-old patient was found to have: Blood sugar–fasting 200 mg%, Postprandial 260 mg%. Urine–sugar present.**
   a. Identify the condition.
   b. Outline the principles of treatment.

9. **A 50-year-old patient came with non-healing wound on left foot. His investigation showed: Blood sugar-Fasting 250 mg%, Postprandial—320 mg%. Urine sugar present.**
   a. What is the diagnosis?
   b. How is blood sugar level regulated?

Answers for Clinical Questions are given in the Appendix

CHAPTER

9

Reproductive System

INTRODUCTION

Reproductive system is unique because it ensures the continuation of the species. The main difference from other system like cardiovascular system, respiratory system is that other system function for the survival of the individual but function of reproductive system is not necessary for the survival of the individual.

In both sexes, the gonads have a dual function: The production of germ cells (gametogenesis) and the secretion of sex hormones. The androgens (e.g. testosterone) are male sex hormone and estrogens are female sex hormone. Both types of hormones are secreted by both sexes. The testes (male gonads) secrete large amounts of androgens, principally testosterone, but they also secrete small amount of estrogens. The ovaries (female gonads) secrete large amount of estrogens and small amounts of androgens (testosterone). Ovaries also secrete progesterone, inhibin and relaxin.

The organs of reproductive system can be divided into two portions:

1. Internal reproductive organs
2. External genital organs.

ABNORMAL SEXUAL DIFFERENTIATION

Chromosomal Abnormalities

Turner's syndrome (44-XO) (gonadal dysgenesis or ovarian agenesis)

- Here gonads are rudimentary and absent.
- Female external and internal genitalia.
- Stature is short and puberty changes do not occur.

Klinefelter's syndrome (44-XXY)

- Genitalia of a normal male.
- Testosterone secretion at puberty is normal but the seminiferous tubule are absent.
- Mental retardation.

Down's syndrome

Autosomal dysjunction of chromosome 21 produce trisomy 21 (mongolism). Symptoms are broad face, epicanthus, hand with single transverse crease and consistent infections that leads to death.

Hormonal Abnormalities

- *Female pseudohermaphroditism:* Male genetic development occur in genetic female exposed to androgens from other source during the 8th to 13th week of gestation.
- *Male pseudohermaphroditism:* Development of female external genitalia in genetic males.

Causes

1. Embryonic testes are defective.
2. Androgen resistance.

Note

Barr bodies/sex chromatin: A Barr body is highly coiled, genetically inactive X chromosome seen in the female (where other X chromosome is active). It can be detected in sex chromosome from buccal cells, vaginal mucous cells and spinous epidermal cells.

No. of barr bodies = No. of X Chromosome–1

MALE REPRODUCTIVE SYSTEM

The reproductive functions of male can be divided into three major subdivisions which includes:

1. Spermatogenesis: Formation of sperm.
2. Performance of male sexual act.
3. Regulation of male reproductive functions by various hormones.

Blood-Testis Barrier

Tight junctions between adjacent Sertoli cells near the basal lamina form a blood-testis barrier (Fig. 9.1). These creates a specialized, immunological safe microenvironment for developing sperm. Steroids can penetrate this barrier with ease. Mature germ cell pass through this barrier as they move to lumen through the formation and breakdown of these junctions.

Functions

1. Prevents large molecules from passing from the interstitial tissue and the part of tubule near the basal lamina.
2. Maintenance of composition of fluid in the lumen of seminiferous tubule (little protein, glucose but rich in

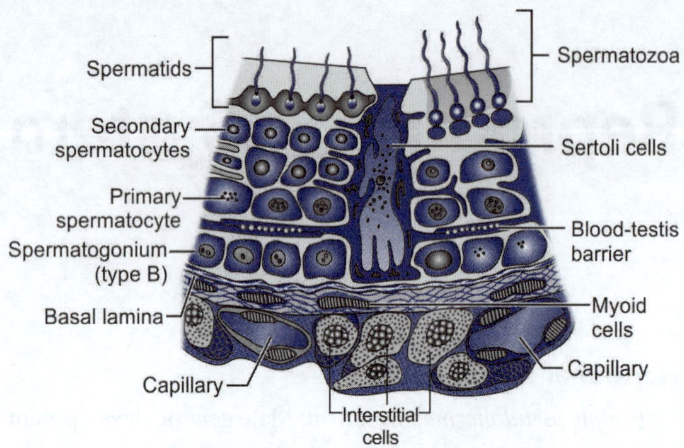

Fig. 9.1: Stages in the development of sperm from spermatogonia

androgens, estrogens, K^+, inositol and glutamic and aspartic acids) depends on blood-testis barrier (BTB).

3. Protect the germ cell from blood borne noxious agent.
4. Establish an osmotic gradient that facilitates movement of fluid into the tubular lumen.

Spermatogenesis

The process by which new spermatozoa are created from spermatogonia is called spermatogenesis (Fig. 9.2). In human it takes an average of 74 days. The estimated number of spermatids formed from single spermatogonia is 512.

Phases of Spermatogenesis

1. *Phase of mitotic division of spermatogonia:* Spermatogonia divides mitotically 7 times to form 128 spermatogonia
2. *Phase of formation of primary spermatocyte by maturation:* 128 spermatogonia undergoes maturation to form 128 primary spermatocytes. They are large cell with diploid number of chromosome.
3. *Phase of formation of secondary spermatocyte by 1st meiotic division:* During 1st meiotic (reductional division), 128 primary spermatocyte is converted into 256 secondary spermatocytes with haploid number of chromosomes.
4. *Phase of formation of spermatid:* Each secondary spermatocyte undergoes 2nd meiotic division(similar to mitotis) to give rise to 2 spermatids. Thus a total of 512 spermatids is formed having haploid number of chromosomes.
5. *Phase of formation of spermatozoan:* Spermatids do not divide further but undergoes morphological changes to form sperms or spermatozoa.

Spermiogenesis

Conversion of spermatids to sperms. This process takes place within the cytoplasm of the Sertoli cells and depends on the presence of androgen.

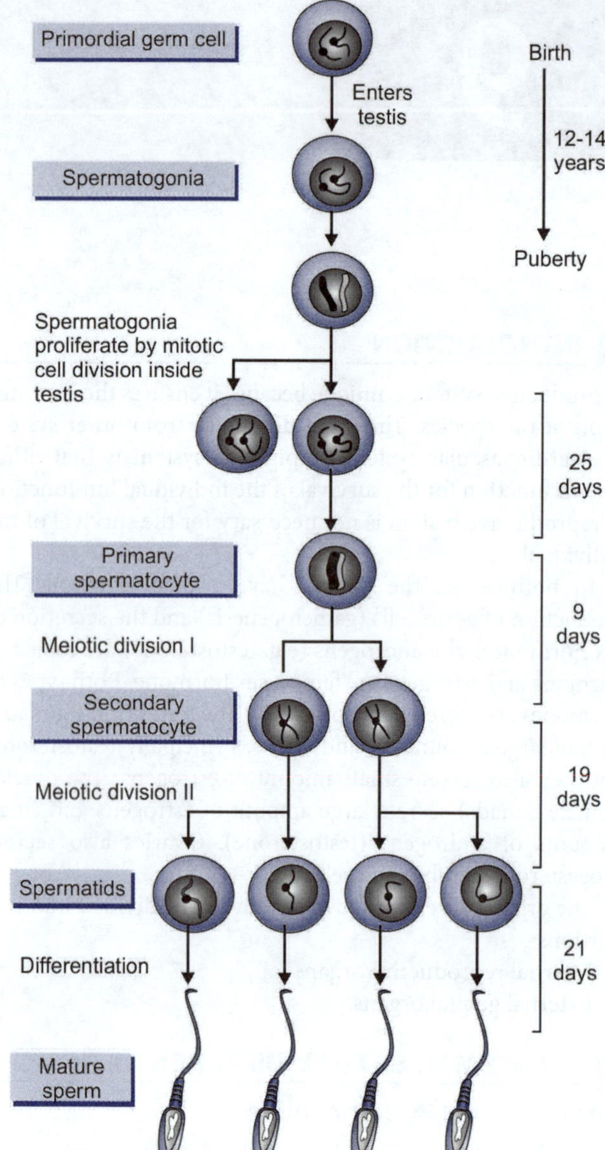

Fig. 9.2: Cell division during spermatogenesis

Factors Influencing Spermatogenesis (Table 9.1)

1. Testosterone in high concentration is essential for growth and division of testicular germinal cells, which is the first stage in forming sperm.
2. *LH:* It is secreted by anterior pituitary gland helps by stimulating the Leydig cells to produce testosterone which is essential for spermatogenesis.
3. *FSH:* It is the key gonadotropin for spermatogenesis. It is secreted by anterior pituitary. It help in the conversion of spermatid to sperm by stimulating the Sertoli cells to produce some local factors. FSH, along with a very

Table 9.1: Factors influencing spermatogenesis

Stage of spermatogenesis	Hormone necessary
Stage of proliferation	• FSH • Growth hormone
Stage of growth	• Testosterone • Growth hormone
Stage of maturation	• Testosterone • Growth hormone
Stage of transformation	• Testosterone • Estrogen

high level of testosterone from the neighboring Leydig cells, produces growth factors necessary for growth and maturation of the sperm. FSH and testosterone induce the synthesis of androgen binding protein which helps maintain high local levels of testosterone. FSH stimulates aromatase, which aromatizes testosterone into estradiol, an important hormone for growth and maturation of the sperm.

4. *Growth hormone:* It is necessary for controlling the background metabolic functions of the testis. It specially promotes early division of spermatogonia themselves.
5. *Estrogen:* It is formed from testosterone by the Sertoli cells when they are stimulated by FSH. They are also essential for spermiogenesis.
6. Sertoli cells secrete androgen binding factors (ABP), inhibin and MIS (mullerian inhibiting substance). They do not synthesize androgens, but contain aromatase, the enzyme responsible for conversion of androgens to estrogens (promotes spermatogenesis)
   - ABP helps to maintain a high stable supply of androgens in the tubular fluid.
   - Inhibin inhibits FSH secretion.
   - MIS causes regression of the mullerian ducts in males during fetal life.
7. Seminal fluid with fructose content help in maturation of sperms.
8. Vitamin E, C and several members of B complex are required for normal spermatogenesis.
9. *General factors:*
   a. Temperature—optimum 32°C
   b. Radiation—degenerates seminiferous tubule
   c. Vasectomy
   d. Age.

Figure 9.3 illustrates the source and nature of the hormones controlling testicular function.

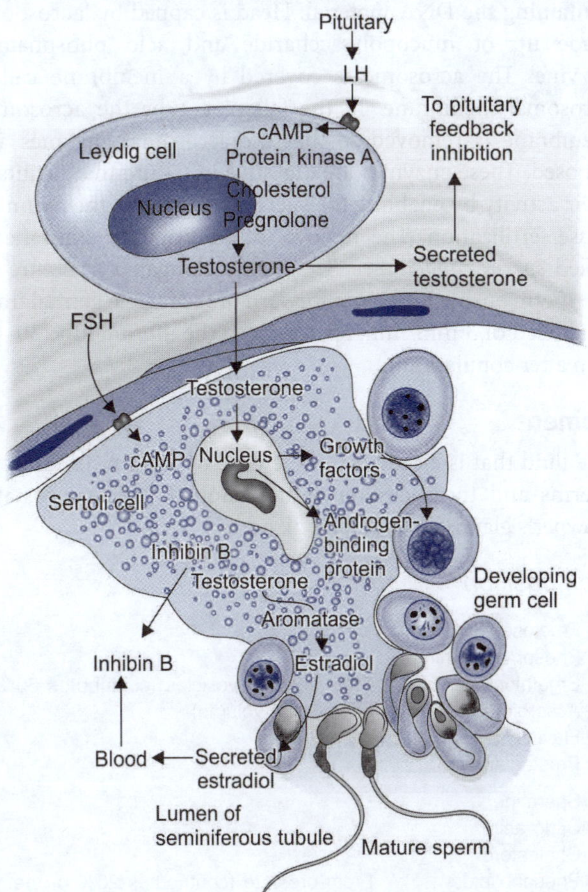

Fig. 9.3: Testicular hormones and spermatogenesis

Spermatozoan (The sperm)

The sperm (Fig. 9.4) about 60 μm long is a long single cell which has a 'head' and a 'tail'. The head is the nucleus of the cell

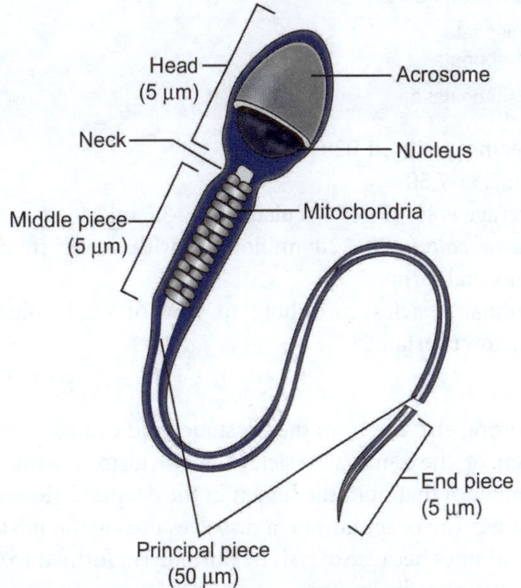

Fig. 9.4: Structure of human spermatozoan

PHYSICON—The Reliable Icon in Physiology

containing the DNA material. Head is capped by 'acrosome' made up of mucopolysaccharide and acid phosphatase enzyme. The acrosome is covered by a membrane called acrosomal membrane. In the fallopian tube the acrosomal membrane is removed so that the acrosomal enzymes are exposed. These enzymes are digestive in nature that facilitate their activity by enabling the sperm to penetrate the ovum to cause fertilization. The removal of acrosomal membrane is called *sperm capacitance.* The highly elongated structure of the sperm enable it to swim forward in the female genital tract at a speed of 3 mm/min. Sperm reach the uterine tube 30–60 min after copulation.

Semen

The fluid that is ejaculated at the time of orgasm. It contains sperms and the secretion of the seminal vesicle, prostate, Cowper's glands and urethral gland.

Composition

• Fructose • Phosphorylcholine • Ergothioneine • Ascorbic acid • Flavins • Prostaglandins	From seminal vesicles (contributes 60% of the total volume)
• Spermine • Citric acid • Cholesterol • Phospholipids • Fibrolysin • Fibrinogenase • Zinc • Acid phosphatase	From prostate (contributes 20% of the total volume)
• Phosphate • Bicarbonate	Buffers
• Hyaluronidase	

- Specific gravity: 1.028
- pH: 7.35-7.50
- Average volume per ejaculate is 2.5–3.5 ml.
- *Sperm count:* 80–120 million/ml with fewer than 20% abnormal forms.

Seminal vesicles contribute to 60% of total volume of semen and prostate 20%.

Note:

a. Clotting enzyme from the prostatic fluid causes the fibrinogen of the seminal vesicle fluid to form a weak fibrin coagulum that hold the semen in the deeper regions of the vagina. The coagulum then dissolves during the next 15 to 30 minutes because of lysis by fibrinolysin formed from the prostatic profibrinolysin.
b. Nutrition to sperms is mainly provided by fructose.
c. Fertilization is enhanced by the prostaglandin present in seminal vesicle.

Sertoli Cells

Sertoli cells are large, complex glycogen containing cells that stretch from the basal lamina of the tubule to the lumen.

Functions

1. Sertoli cell secrete androgen binding factors (ABP), inhibin, activin, MIS (mullerian inhibiting substance).
2. They have receptors for FSH and testosterone. After combining with FSH, Sertoli cells stimulates the first half of spermatogenesis. Subsequently testosterone-sertoli cells binding causes development of last half of spermatogenesis
3. Sertoli cells are components of blood-testis barrier.
4. They produce estradiol from testosterone.
5. They provide nutrition to the germ cells.
6. Converts testosterone into 5 alpha dihydrotestosterone.
7. Sertoli cells and epithelium of the epididymis secrete a special nutrient fluid that is ejaculated along with the sperm.

Testosterone

Testosterone, the principal hormone of the testis is a C19 steroid with an OH group in the 17th position.

- *Synthesis:* It is produced from cholesterol in the Leydig cells and is also formed from androstenedione secreted by the adrenal cortex.
- *Secretion:* The testosterone secretion rate is 4-9 mg/day in normal adult males. Small amount of testosterone are also secreted in females. The secretion is under the control of LH.
- *Transport:* Ninety-eight percent of testosterone in plasma is bound to plasma protein. Sixty-five percent is bound to β globulin called gonadal steroid binding globulin or sex-binding globulin and thirty-three percent bound to albumin.

Mechanism of Action of Testosterone

Testosterone has several target cells.

In the target cell of prostate, seminal vesicles, epididymis, penis and skin testosterone crosses the cell membrane and is converted to dihydrotestosterone (DHT) by an enzyme 5 alpha reductase. In these cells DHT is the final hormone (testosterone in these cells is merely a prohormone).

In the hypothalamus, muscle mass and anterior pituitary, testosterone is the final active agent as no DHT is formed.

The androgen (either DHT or testosterone itself, depending upon the tissue) combines with its receptor and the receptor losses its heat shock protein. Now the androgen receptor complex moves to the target chromosome and various proteins are synthesized and acts on target cells.

Actions

On the sex organs, secondary sex characteristics and sex behavior

In the fetus

i. Testosterone is formed in the 7th week of intrauterine life. It is responsible for the sex differentiation of male fetus.
ii. Exposure of some part of brain to testosterone in fetal life, determines the sexual behavior in adult life.

In the puberty

i. Testosterone causes growth of the external genitalia and accessory sex organs in pubertal stage.
ii. It also causes the appearance of secondary sexual characters in boys, i.e. beard, moustache, hairs (on chest and abdomen, as well as axillary and pubic hairs), linear growth, muscular growth, deepening of voice and male psyche.

In adults

i. Maintenance of the accessory sex organs.
ii. Development of sebaceous glands and acne vulgaris.
iii. Necessary for spermatogenesis and sperm motility.

On metabolism

Anabolic effects

Proteins

Increase the synthesis and decrease the breakdown of protein, leading to an increase in the rate of growth.

Bone

- Cause epiphysis to fuse with the long bone.
- Increase growth.
- Favors calcium deposition.

Muscle

Promotes growth of muscle and muscle mass get doubled.

On electrolytes

Retention of Na, K, Ca, H_2O, PO_4, SO_4.

Note

Androgenic drugs like nandrolone are used as anabolic steroids. These agents are not easily converted into DHT. So they have minimal action on sex organs, but they act on muscles to increase muscle bulk and strength. Unscrupulous sports persons misuse this drug to increase their muscular efficiency, this is called **doping.**

Regulation of Secretion

Secretion of testosterone from Leydig cells during fetal stage is caused by hCG from placenta. After birth, its secretion is absent till adolescence. During adolescence it starts again under the influence of GnRH. The factors involved in the overall control of adult male hormone secretion are summarized in Flowchart 9.1 and Figure 9.5.

Flowchart 9.1: Regulation of male reproductive functions

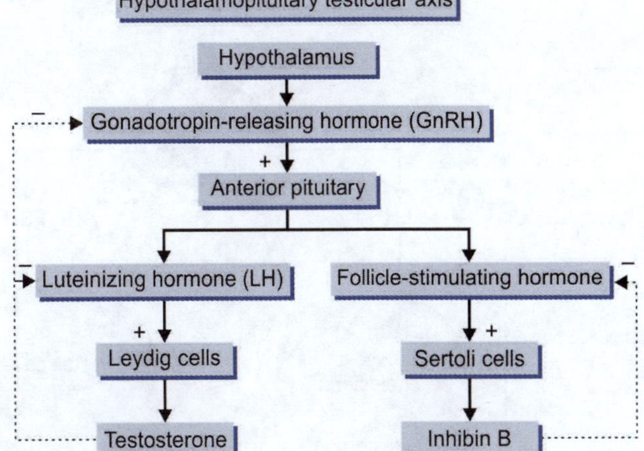

Applied Aspects

1. *Cryptorchidism:* The testis develops in the abdominal cavity and migrate to scrotum during the fetal development in the 7th week. The failure of descent of testis cause the testis to remain in abdominal cavity or inguinal canal leading to sterility called cryptorchidism.
2. *Testicular feminizing syndrome:* Due to congenital lack of androgen receptors. Testis and testosterone secretion is normal but testosterone cannot act due to lack of receptors. So, there is development of female genitalia and there is also enlargement of breast.

Test for Male Infertility

1. *Semen analysis:* Here the masturbation sample of semen is obtained and examined for sperm morphology, motility and count. Normally, the volume of an ejaculate is 2-6 ml. If analyzed within an hour of ejaculation, more than 60% of the sperm should be normal in morphology, more than 60% of the sperm should be motile, and the sperm number in the ejaculate should be more than 60 million.
2. At testicular level, function may be assessed by measuring testosterone levels—free and protein bound.
3. *Sex hormone binding globulin (SHBG)* may be measured in abnormal testosterone levels.

FEMALE REPRODUCTIVE SYSTEM

During the reproductive years of female, between 13–46 years of age, 400–500 primordial follicles develop enough to expel their ova. One ova is expelled each month and the remaining degenerate at the end of reproductive life. At menopause only few

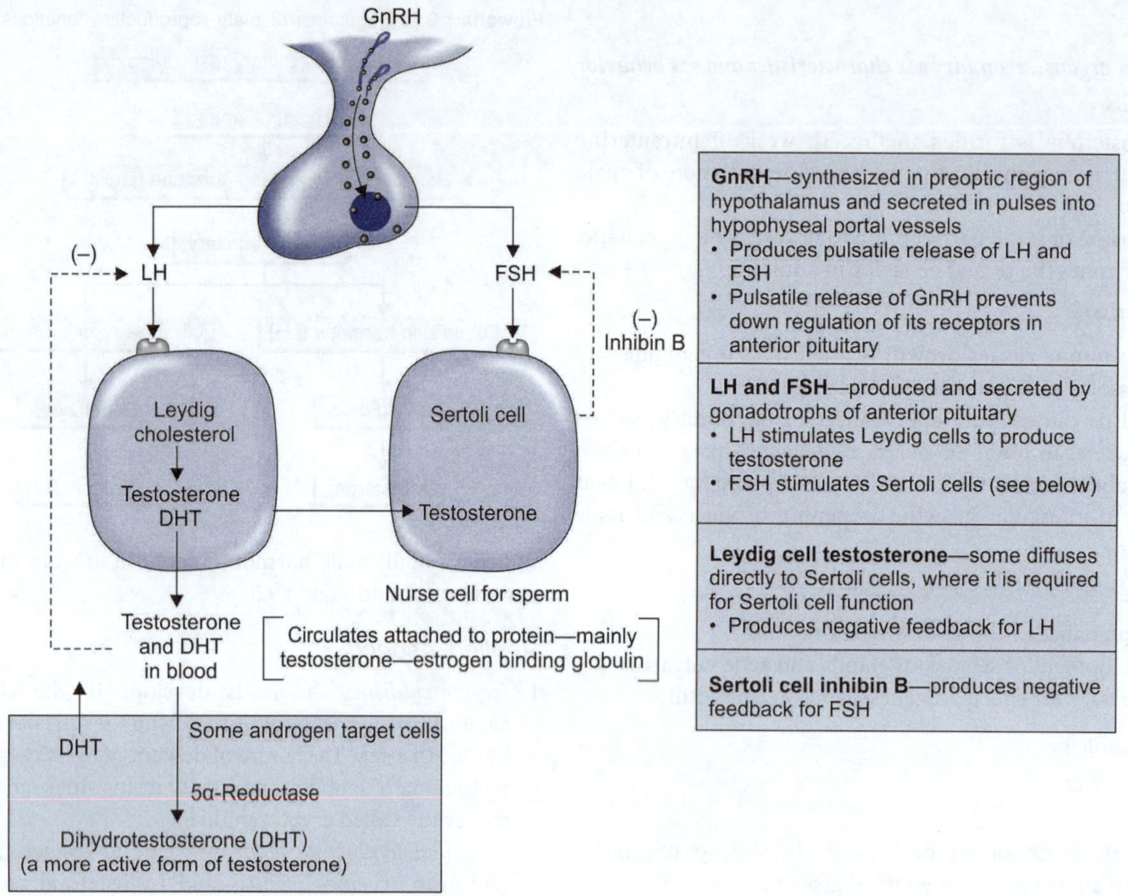

Fig. 9.5: Factors involve in the regulation of testosterone secretion

primordial follicle remains and even this degenerate. The most prominent part of this reproductive cycle is menstrual cycle.

Menstrual Cycle

Menstrual cycle is defined as periodic regular rhythmic changes that occur in female reproductive organs characterized by periodic vaginal bleeding associated with endometrial shedding. The average duration of the cycle is 28 days but the normal range is quite wide (20–45 days). The days are numbered in terms of menstrual bleeding, day one of the cycle being the 1st day of menstrual bleeding. Ovulation takes place at about 14th day of the cycle. If the cycle length is shorter or longer than 28 days, the variation is generally in the period before ovulation. That is, the interval between ovulation and end of the cycle is essentially constant at 14 days irrespective of the cycle length. It consists of four cycles:

1. Ovarian cycle
2. Uterine cycle
3. Cervical cycle
4. Vaginal cycle.

Ovarian Cycle

Depends on gonadotropin secretion which begins at puberty (8–13 years). During 8th year, large quantity of GnRH is secreted which initiates the monthly sexual cycle. GnRH shows increase or decrease in secretion which is responsible for the cyclical changes in the ovary. There are three phases in ovarian cycle:

1. Follicular phase/estrogenic
2. Ovulation
3. Luteal phase/progestational phase.

Follicular phase

During fetal development, ovaries contain seven million primordial follicles. However, many undergo atresia (involution) before birth and others are lost after birth. At the time of birth, there are two million ova, 50% of these are atretic. The normal ova undergo the 1st part of the first meiotic division and enter a stage of arrest in the prophase which persists until adulthood. Atresia continues during development, and the number of ova in the both of the ovaries at puberty is less than 300,000. Only one of those ova per cycle (500 in a normal reproductive life) normally reaches maturity; the remaining degenerates. Just before ovulation the first meiotic division is completed. One of the daughter cells, the secondary oocyte immediately begins the 2nd meiotic division, but this division stops at metaphase and is completed only when a sperm penetrates the oocyte.

At the start of each cycle, several of these follicles enlarges, one of follicle in one ovary start to grow at 6th day and become dominant follicle and other regress forming atretic follicle (Fig. 9.6). Follicle secretes estrogen for final maturation. The cells of the theca interna of follicle are the primary source of circulating estrogen.

Ovulation

The rupture of graafian follicle releases 2° oocyte occurs on 14th day by LH hormone. This process is called ovulation. The 2° oocyte moves towards surface of ovary and protrudes through the outer layer. The protruding outer wall of follicle swells rapidly and a small area in the center of the follicular capsule, called the stigma protrudes like a nipple. In another 30 minutes the fluid begins to ooze from the follicle through the stigma. And about 2 minutes later the stigma ruptures widely allowing more viscous fluid, which has occupied the central portion of the follicle to evaginate outward. This viscous fluid contain ovum surrounded by a mass of several thousand small granulosa cells called corona radiata.

The follicle that ruptures at the time of ovulation is promptly filled with blood and is called as corpus hemorrhagicum. The granulosa and theca cells of the follicle lining promptly begins to proliferate, and the clotted blood is rapidly replaced by yellowish, lipid-rich luteal cells, forming the corpus luteum. This initiates the luteal phase of the menstrual cycle.

Mechanism of ovulation

Follicle secrete estrogen which stimulate hypothalamus and pituitary to release LH (6-10 times called LH surge) and FSH (2 folds). LH and FSH are required for the final maturation of follicle. Estrogen in high dose results in positive feedback effect where as in moderate dose negative feedback effect is produced.

Luteal phase

Granulosa and theca cells of follicle begin to proliferate, and the clotted blood is replaced by yellowish, lipid rich luteal cells, forming corpus luteum. Luteal cells secrete estrogens and progesterone.

- If fertilization persists LH maintains pregnancy.
- No pregnancy corpus luteum degenerates to form corpus albicans.

Uterine Cycle

Changes occurring in endometrium to prepare it to receive the fertilized ovum, then for implantation constitute the uterine cycle (Fig. 9.7).

Phases

1. Proliferative phase (5–14 days)-Estrogen.
2. Secretory phase (15–28 days)-Progesterone and estrogen
3. Menstrual phase (1–4 days) can prolong up to 8 days.

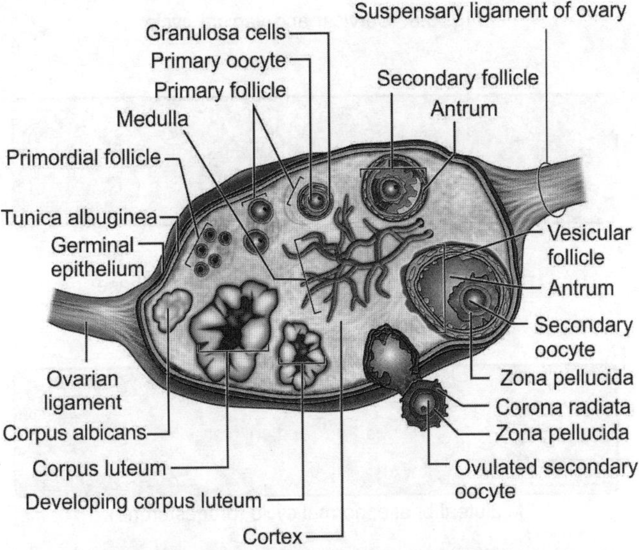

Fig. 9.6: Stages of follicular growth in ovary

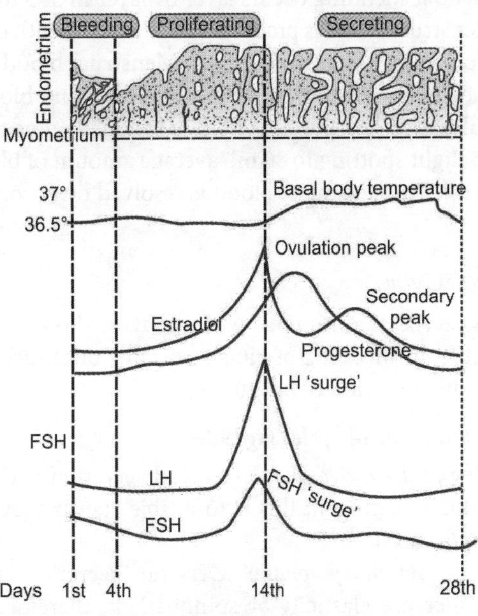

Fig. 9.7: Uterine cycle

1. *Proliferative phase/Estrogenic phase:* It is the period between menstruation and ovulation and it represents the restoration of the epithelium from the preceding menstruation. It corresponds to follicular phase of ovarian cycle. The estrogen secreted from the developing ovarian follicles under the influence of FSH is responsible for this phase.
   Changes occurring during proliferation phase:
   - Proliferation of endometrial tissue from 2-4.5 mm in 5 to 14 days of menstrual cycle. As the thickness increases, the uterine gland is drawn out so that they lengthen.
   - Proliferation of glands and blood vessels.
   - Restoration of epithelium of the endometrium within 7 days.
2. *Secretory/Progestational phase:* It is the period between ovulation and next menstruation. It corresponds to luteal phase of ovarian cycle and so the hormone responsible is progesterone and estrogen. Here endometrial thickness increase from 6 to 8 mm. Endometrial gland become tortuous and begins to secrete.

   Proliferation of cytoplasm, deposition of lipids and glycogen is seen. There is increased vascularity of endometrium which is proportional to activity of gland. The spiral arteries become more tortuous. Arteriovenous anastomosis and anastomosis between veins occur.
3. *Menstrual phase:* Corpus luteum regresses, so that the hormone support is withdrawn and thus endometrium becomes thin. The spiral arteries become more tortuous and they undergo vasospasm by PGF2α. This leads to ischemia and necrosis of tissue and the walls rupture. Sequential shedding occurs layer by layer in 3–5 days.

   Menstrual blood is predominantly arterial with only 25% of blood being venous in origin. Menstrual blood consists of shed endometrium, secretion of glands and blood from spinal artery. The amount of blood lost may range normally from slight spotting to 80 ml, average amount of blood lose is 30 ml. The clotting of blood is resolved by fibrolysin system.

Cervical Cycle

Though cervix is continuous with uterus it shows a separate cycle. Here no shedding of mucosa occurs, but mucous show changes due to action of hormone.

Changes in cervical cycle (Fig. 9.8)

a. *During proliferative phase:* Cervical secretion is thin alkaline due to estrogen; this is to enable sperm survival and transportation.
b. *During ovulatory phase:* Cervical secretion is thinnest, increase elasticity or spinnbarkeit, therefore can be stretched to 8–12 cm. More ever it dries in an arborizing fern-like pattern when a thin layer is spread on a slide (Fig. 9.9).
c. *Secretory phase:* Cervical secretion is thick, tenacious and cellular (Fig. 9.10).

Vaginal Cycle

During proliferative phase under the influence of estrogen, vaginal epithelium becomes cornified and can be identified as vaginal smear. During secretory phase under influence of progesterone, a thick mucus is secreted and the epithelium proliferates and become infiltrated with leukocytes.

Hormonal Control of the Menstrual Cycle (Fig. 9.11)

The regulation is based on the hypothalamo-pituitary-gonadal axis and feedback actions of estrogen and progesterone(1). GnRH is secreted in episodic bursts to stimulate secretion of FSH and LH from anterior pituitary which then act on ovary(2).

At the start of cycle there are very low levels of estrogen and progesterone, therefore minimum feedback inhibition. So GnRH secretion increases and there is increased FSH and LH.

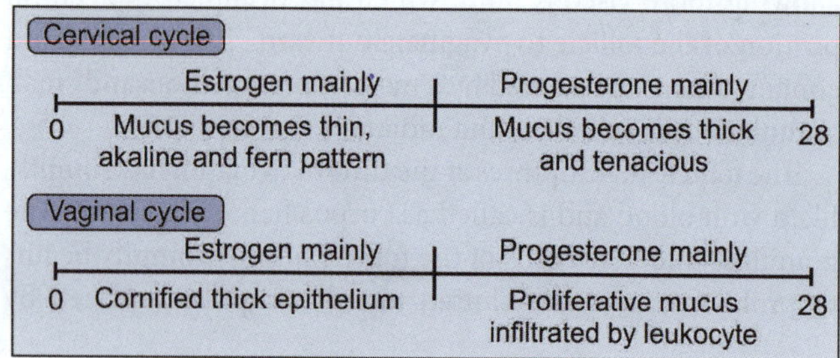

Fig. 9.8: Cervical and vaginal cycle

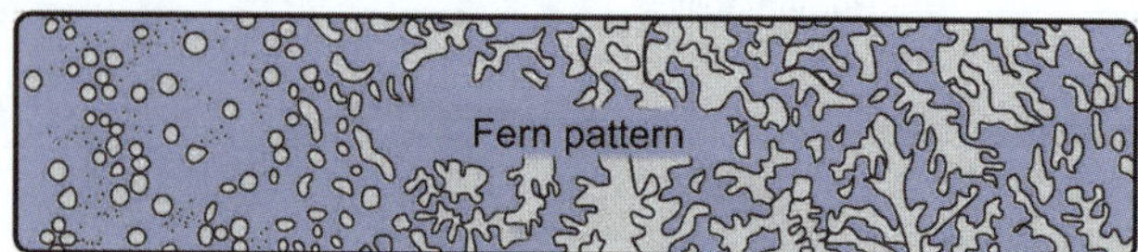

Normal cycle, 14th day estrogen

Fig. 9.9: Ferning pattern in proliferative phase

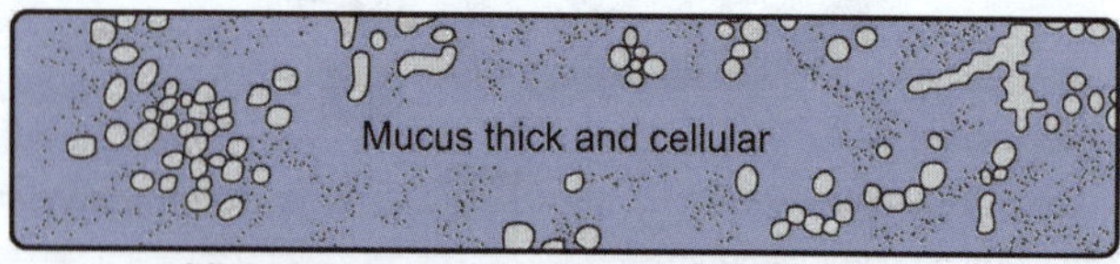

Midluteal phase, normal cycle (progesterone)

Fig. 9.10: Cervical mucus thick and cellular in secretory phase

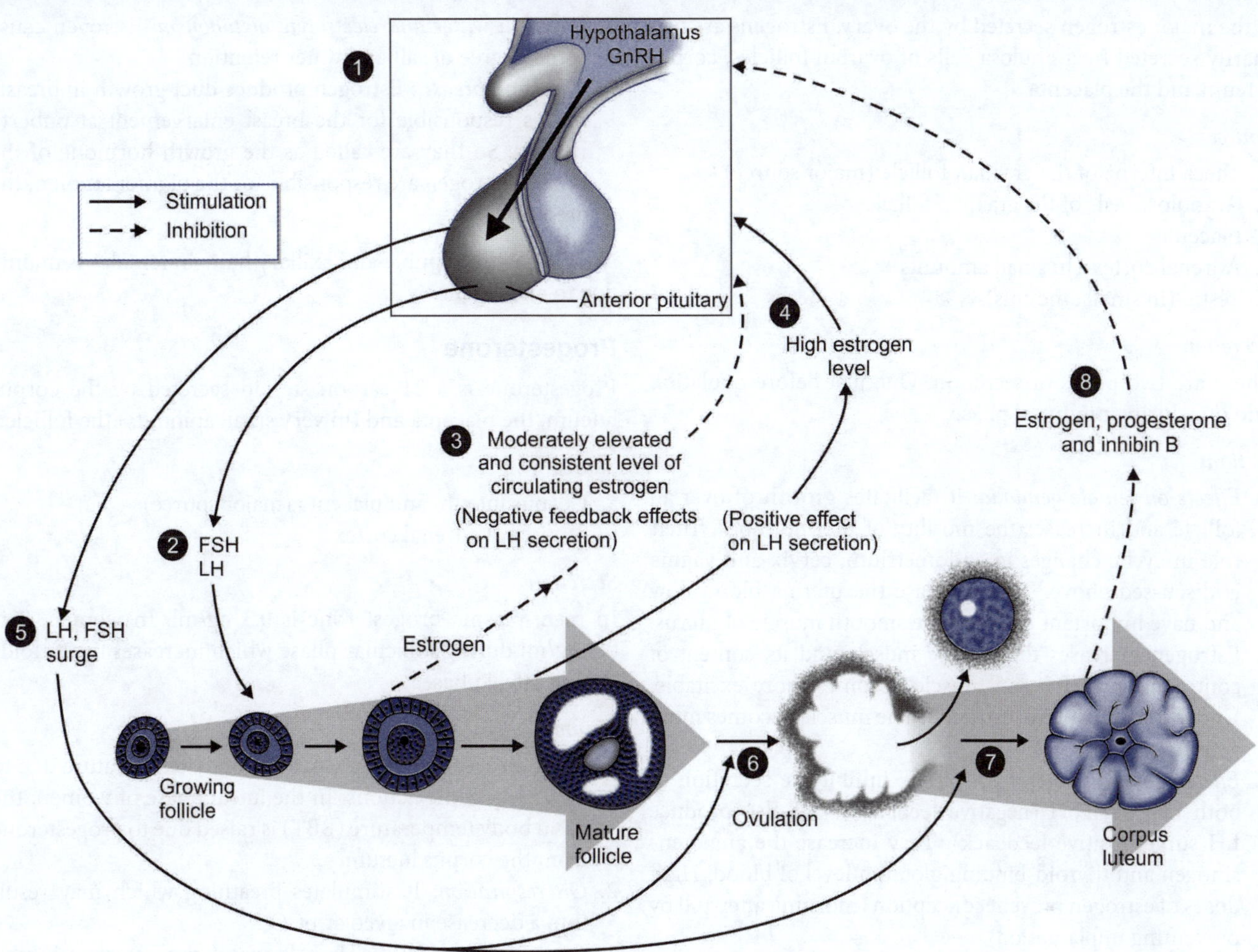

Fig. 9.11: Feedback interaction involved in the control of ovarian activity

Follicle stimulating hormone now causes development of the follicle and LH receptors (LH does not act on follicle). The LH acts on the theca cells which produces androgens. These androgens are subsequentially converted into estrogen in granulosa cell. Estrogen at this stage causes feedback inhibition of LH, FSH, and GnRH(3), but more on FSH, which is further helped by inhibin acting at the level of pituitary. Towards the middle of the cycle, due to further development of the follicle, estrogen secretion increases further(4). This persistent high level of estrogen increases responsiveness of the pituitary gonadotropins to GnRH. There is also increased secretion of GnRH. All these result in positive feedback action and there is rapid rise of LH secretion(5), called LH surge which is thought to cause ovulation(6). The estrogen level increases 25 hours before and the LH surge occurs about 9 hours before the ovulation, i.e. after estrogen peak. At this time there is also FSH peak due to both estrogen and progesterone.

After ovulation corpus luteum(7) is formed which secretes both estrogen and progesterone(8), so there is feedback inhibition on both LH and FSH. At this stage positive feedback action by estrogen cannot occur due to inhibitory effects of high levels of progesterone.

Towards the end of cycle, estrogen progesterone level become very much low again. This removes the feedback inhibition, so there is rise of GnRH pulses as well as increased output of FSH and LH to start the cycle again.

Ovarian Hormones

Two important ovarian hormones are estrogen and progesterone.

Estrogen

All estrogens are steroid hormones with cholesterol as the main precursor. Naturally occurring estrogens are estradiol, estrone and estriol. Estrogens are 18 carbon steroids. Estradiol is the major estrogen secreted by the ovary. Estrogens are primarily secreted by granulosa cells of ovarian follicles, corpus luteum and the placenta.

Source

a. Theca interna of the graafian follicle (major source)
b. Granulosa cells of the graafian follicle
c. Placenta
d. Adrenal cortex-(in small amounts)
e. Testis-(in small amounts).

Secretion

There are two peaks of secretion. One just before ovulation and one during midluteal phase.

Actions

1. *Effects on female genitalia:* It facilitates growth of ovarian follicle and increases the motility of uterine tubes. Their role in cyclic changes in endometrium, cervix and vagina is discussed above. They increase the uterine blood flow and have important effect on the smooth muscle of uterus. Estrogen increases the uterine muscle and its content of contractile proteins and muscle becomes more excitable. Under the influence of estrogens, the muscle becomes more active and excitable.
2. *Effects on endocrine organs:* They inhibit the secretion of both LH and FSH (negative feedback), but also produce LH surge(positive feedback). They increase the angiotensinogen and thyroid-binding globulin level of blood. High doses of estrogen prevent conception (morning after-pill by preventing implantation).
3. *Effects on CNS:* Estrogen is responsible for the female type of behavior and also it increases the libido in females. It also increases the proliferation of dendrites on neurons and the number of synaptic knobs.
4. *Effects on CVS:* Estrogens have a significant plasma cholesterol lowering action and they rapidly produce vasodilatation by increasing the local production of nitric oxide (NO). These action inhibit atherogenesis and contribute to low incidence of myocardial infarction (MI). However large doses of orally active estrogen promotes thrombosis, because they reach the liver in high concentration and alter hepatic production of clotting factors.
5. *Effect on female secondary sex characteristics:* The body changes that develop in girls at puberty in addition to enlargement of breast, uterus and vagina are due to estrogen, which is called the 'feminizing hormones'. Women have narrow shoulders and broad hips, thighs that converge and arms that diverge (carrying angle). This body configuration, plus the female distribution of fat in breast and buttocks is due to estrogen.
6. *Effect on water and electrolyte metabolism:* Estrogen cause some degree of salt and water retention.
7. *Effects on breasts:* Estrogen produce duct growth in breasts and is responsible for the breast enlargement at puberty in girls. So they are called as the growth hormone of the breast. Estrogen are responsible for the pigmentation of the areolas.

Note: Growth of pubic and axillary hairs in females is mainly due to androgens.

Progesterone

Progesterone is a 21 carbon steroid secreted by the corpus luteum, the placenta and (in very small amounts) the follicle.

Source

a. Corpus luteum and placenta (major source)
b. Testis and adrenal cortex.

Secretion

In men, plasma progesterone is 0.3 ng/ml. In women, it is 0.9 ng/ml during follicular phase which increases by 20-folds during luteal phase.

Actions

1. *BMR:* Progesterone increases the body temperature due to its thermogenic actions. In the luteal phase of women, the basal body temperature (BBT) is raised due to progesterone from the corpus luetum.
2. *On respiration:* It stimulates breathing which may result into a decrease in alveolar pCO_2.
3. *On endocrine glands:* High levels of progesterone inhibit the LH secretion.
4. *On reproductive system:* Progesterone is responsible for the progestational changes in the endometrium and the cyclical changes in the cervix and vagina. It has an antiestrogenic effect on the myometrial cells, decreasing their excitability. It also decreases the number of estrogen receptors on the endometrium.
5. *On mammary gland:* It causes the development of alveoli of the mammary glands. Along with estrogen it prepares the gland for lactation.
6. *On renal system:* Large doses of progesterone produces natriuresis, probably by blocking the action of aldosterone on the kidney.

Clinical Note

During the first three months of pregnancy, corpus luteum in the ovaries secrete estrogen and progesterone, the hormone maintaining pregnancy and later only the placenta takes over. So removal of ovaries in early stages of pregnancy results in termination of pregnancy.

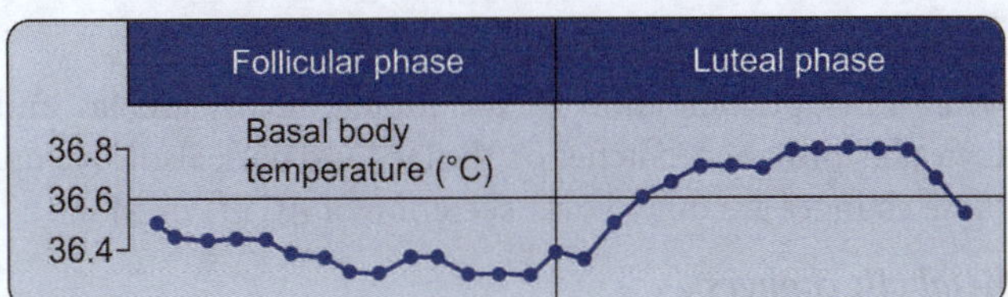

Fig. 9.12: Changes in basal body temperature in follicular and luteal phase

Relaxin

Relaxin is a polypeptide hormone that is produced in the corpus luteum, uterus, placenta and mammary gland in women and in the prostate gland in men.

Actions

During pregnancy, it relaxes the pubic symphysis and other pelvic joints, softens and dilates the uterine cervix. Thus it facilitates delivery. It also inhibits uterine contractions and may play an important role in the development of mammary glands.

Indicators of Ovulation

1. *Basal body temperature:* It shows a rise by 0.3–0.5°C after ovulation due to increase in progesterone secretion, since progesterone is thermogenic (Fig. 9.12). The temperature (oral or rectal) should be recorded in the morning before leaving the bed.
2. *Cervical mucus pattern:* Cervical mucus when spread on a slide and dried, shows a fern-like pattern under microscope this pattern are lost after ovulation.
3. Vaginal cornification disappear after ovulation.
4. Pregnandiol, a metabolite of progesterone appears in urine after ovulation.
5. Estimation of plasma progesterone level shows a gradual rise after ovulation.
6. Estrogen, FSH, LH estimation—peaks just before ovulation.
7. *Mittelschmerz sign:* Pain in lower abdomen due to minor bleeding from the follicle into peritoneum.

Mammary Gland

It is a modified apocrine gland for the supply of nutrition to the young ones.

- Estrogen stimulates the proliferation of mammary duct and deposition of fat to give the breast mass. Far greater growth occurs during high estrogen state of pregnancy (Fig. 9.13).
- Progesterone is essential for the development of lobules.
- Glucocorticoids, insulin and growth hormone are necessary for mammary development in response to other hormones, but they do not themselves cause growth of breasts.

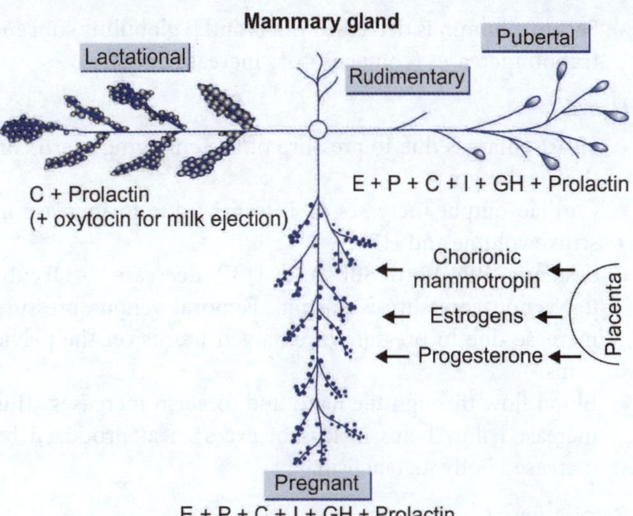

Fig. 9.13: Hormonal actions on mammary gland

- Prolactin is not very high in nonpregnant state, hence not important for the mammary gland. During pregnancy its level increases to make alveolar cells ready for milk production. Prolactin needs prior activity of estrogen and progesterone and also presence of other hormones.

PREGNANCY

Physiological Changes in Pregnancy

Changes in uterus

Uterus increase in weight from 30–60 gm in the nonparous women to 800-1000 gm at full term. This is due to:

- Hypertrophy of pre-existing muscle cells (mainly) both in width and length by approximately 5–9 times.
- Increase in amount of connective tissue and elastic tissue between the muscle fibers.

All these effect are seen during the first 2–3 months of pregnancy due to estrogen. Subsequent enlargement of uterus is due to growing fetus which causes uterine wall to become thinner.

Changes in the body system and organs

Blood

- *Blood volume:* It increases by 30% (4 L to 5.4 L) mainly due to increase in plasma volume. Therefore RBC count, PCV, Hb concentration decreases producing anemia called physiological anemia of pregnancy. Its characteristic features are of iron deficiency anemia as iron demand increases during pregnancy.
- *Plasma proteins:* Total plasma concentration decreases. Serum fibrinogen increases which increases the ESR.

Serum albumin is decreased but α and β globulins concentration increases (compensatory increase).

Heart

- Heart enlarges due to pressure of the enlarging uterus on the diaphragm.
- Cardiac output increases (5 L to 6 L) due to increase in stroke volume and HR.
- Systemic BP: Both SBP and DBP decrease. Antecubital venous pressure is normal. Femoral venous pressure increase due to pressure of enlarged uterus on the pelvic veins.
- Blood flow through the hand and forearm increases. This increased flow helps in loss of excess heat produced by increased body metabolism.

Respiration

- *Vital capacity (VC):* No change as any change in VC due to upward displacement of the diaphragm gets compensated by increase in width of pleural cavity.
- Pulmonary ventilation increases due to increase in tidal volume (TV) and frequency of breathing. This may be due to increase in progesterone level which increase the sensitivity of respiratory center to CO_2 and causes fall in arterial pCO_2.
- Body O_2 consumption increases by 15%.

GIT

- There is morning sickness feeling of nausea and vomiting in early months of pregnancy.
- Hypochlorhydria.
- Decrease in motility of stomach and colon.

Urinary system:

- RBF and GFR increases in parallel with increase in cardiac output.
- Increased GFR increases the load of solutes presented for reabsorbtion. This may account for the glycosuria of pregnancy.

Endocrine glands:

- Thyroid gland shows mild enlargement with hyperplasia and increased thyroxine output. But here there is no signs of hyperthyroidism.
- Adrenal cortex shows enlargement of zona fasciculata layer in particular, therefore cortisol secretion increases but no signs of Cushing's syndrome.
- Placental hormones are secreted.

Nervous system

Nervous system shows mild mental changes which vary from craving from unusual articles of diet to alteration in mood and behavior. In some, a true psychosis may also develop.

Skin

Skin shows pigmentation of the nipple, breast areolas and linea alba, brownish patches on the face and neck also develop. These changes are due to over secretion of ACTH or MSH.

Metabolic changes

- During pregnancy there is marked *increase in body weight*, on an average of 12.5 kg.
- *Water metabolism:* During the early months of pregnancy there is marked diuresis, sweating and a weight loss of approximately 2.5 kg. During later months (5–6 month onwards) of pregnancy excess of water is retained in the fetus, placenta, amniotic fluid, breast, uterus and other tissues. The retention of water is due to fall in plasma protein concentration, especially albumin (thus colloidal osmotic pressure decreases). Retention of sodium due to the steroidal sex hormones.
- *Protein metabolism:* There is a positive nitrogen balance during pregnancy and lactation period.
- *Carbohydrate metabolism:* Renal threshold of glucose decreases during pregnancy producing glycosuria.
- *Fat metabolism:*
  - There occurs increase in blood concentration of cholesterol, phospholipids and neutral fats.
  - Adipose tissue fat increases to supply energy in the later stages of pregnancy and lactation.
- *Mineral metabolism:* During pregnancy, the mother stores approximately 50 gm of calcium and 35-40 gm of phosphorus. Only half the calcium goes to the fetus especially during the last month, the rest being stored in the maternal tissues to be utilized during lactation.
- *Iron metabolism:* The fetus contain 375 mg of iron which accumulate at a rate of approximately 0.4 mg/day in the first 6 month of pregnancy and about 4 mg/day during last 3 months of pregnancy. A further 500-700 mg of iron is required by the mother for increased Hb synthesis and myoglobin formation in the growing fetus. The iron in the newborn child and iron removed in the blood lost during delivery amounts to 400-500 mg; this represents 1/8-1/10 of the total body iron and must be compensated by the increased dietary intake of iron during pregnancy.

Pregnancy Test

Earlier Bioassay Method (Aschheim–Zondek Test)

- The urine of the women (suspected to have developed pregnancy) will have hCG
- This hCG when injected into immature mice (the animal which do not ovulate naturally due to its immaturity) will cause ovulation, which can be detected.

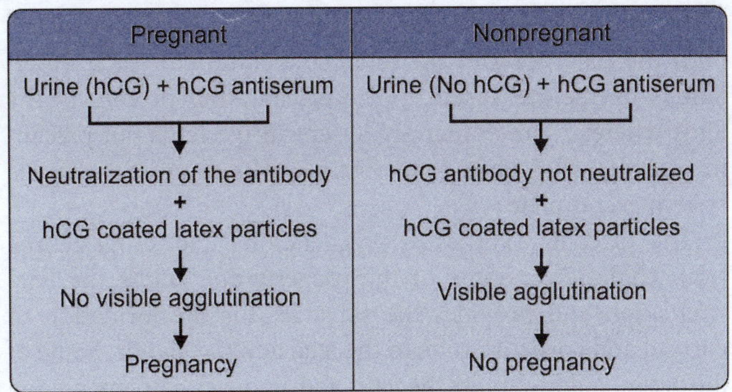

Fig. 9.14: Gravidex test

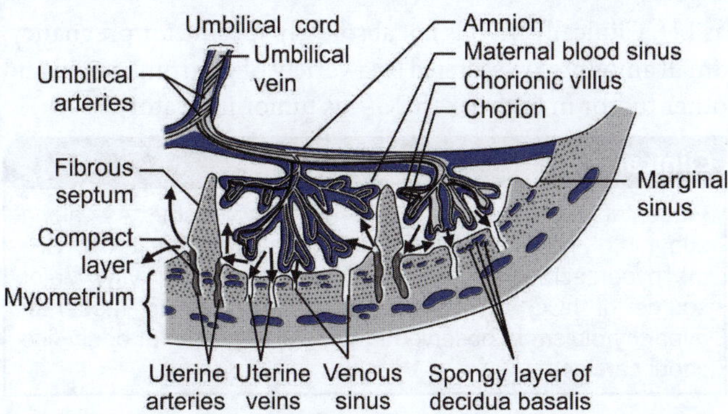

Fig. 9.15: Physiological anatomy of mature placenta. The direction of blood flow in the maternal blood sinuses is indicated by arrows

Immunological Test for Pregnancy

Gravidex test (Fig. 9.14)

Principle

a. hCG being protein in nature will cause generation of antibody when injected in suitable animal. hCG is injected in rabbit, in whom antibodies develop in the serum (called rabbit antiserum). Rabbit antiserum is then collected.
b. Small globules of latex (rubber) particles are coated with pure hCG.
c. The urine suspected to contain hCG is now treated with rabbit antiserum. If the urine contains hCG, the antibodies in the antiserum are all used up. Subsequently, when hCG coated latex particles are added to the mixture, latex particles are not agglutinated whereas, if the urine is free from hCG, the antibodies in the rabbit serum remains free. In such a mixture, (i.e. where the suspected urine contains no hCG) when the latex mixture coated with the hCG are added, antigen-antibody reaction (between hCG of latex particles and the antibodies of the serum) occur and the latex particles are agglutinated. Therefore agglutination of latex particles means that the urine is from a nonpregnant woman. Apart from diagnosis of normal pregnancy this test is also used to diagnose some diseases of the placenta.

Placenta

Placenta (Fig. 9.15) is the 'fetal lung'. It mainly consists of:

1. *Maternal part:* It is called decidua in which large blood sinuses partitioned by fibrous septa are present. Maternal blood circulates in these sinuses.
2. *Fetal part:* It consists of numerous finger-like processes called chorionic villi. These project into the maternal bloodsinuses. Chorionic villi has two layers; Cytotrophoblast and syncytiotrophoblast. Syncytiotrophoblast produces all hormones.

O_2 is taken up by the fetal blood and CO_2 is discharged into the maternal circulation across the walls of the villi in a fashion analogous to O_2 and CO_2 exchange in the lungs.

Function of Placenta

1. *Respiratory:* Diffusion of O_2 and CO_2 through placental membrane.
2. *Excretory:* Excretion of waste products.
3. *Immunological:* Many immunoglobulin molecules (IgG) from maternal circulation cross the placental barrier to confer a passive immunity in the fetus.
4. Many drugs also cross placental barrier, e.g. pethidine and anesthetics. If used in labor, these drug cause damage to fetus.
5. *Endocrine:* Fetoplacental unit produces many hormones, vital to pregnancy. Hormones produced by placenta include hCG, human chorionic somatomammotropin (hCS), human chorionic thyrotropin (hCT), estrogen and progesterone.

Placental Hormones

Hormones produced by placenta include:

1. Human chorionic gonadotropin (hCG)
2. Human chorionic somatomammotropin (hCS)
3. Human chorionic thyrotropin (hCT)
4. Estrogen and progesterone.

hCG

Human chorionic gonadotropin (hCG) is a placental hormone. It is a glycoprotein that contains galactose and hexosamine. It is produced by syncytiotrophoblast. hCG is primarily luteinizing and luteotrophic and has little FSH activity. The hCG is detected in the blood at 6th day after conception and in urine after 14 days. It appears to act on the same receptor as LH. Clinically hCG is not absolutely specific for pregnancy. Small amounts are secreted by a variety of gastrointestinal and other tumor in both sex (hCG—as tumor indicator).

Clinical Note

Placental tumors can cause hyperthyroidism. As alpha subunit of hCG is identical to the alpha-subunit of TSH, the hypersecretion of hCG stimulates thyroid activity. Major source of hCG is placenta. Therefore, mild to moderate hyperthyroidism is observed in tumors of placental origin like choriocarcinoma.

Functions

a. Maintains corpus luteum of pregnancy.
b. Increase interstitial GH, leading to testosterone secretion which promote development and descent of testis.
c. Development of stomal cells and decidual cells.

hCS

It is synthesized by placental syncytiotrophoblastic cells. It resembles GH in amino acid content. It is maternal GH of pregnancy. The amount of hCS secreted is directly proportional to the size of the placenta. Therefore, low hCS levels are signs of placental insufficiency.

hCT

It is a placental substance with properties like that of TSH.

Estrogen and progesterone

The fetus and placenta interact as a functional unit is called *fetoplacental* unit (Fig. 9.16) in the formation of estrogen and progesterone.

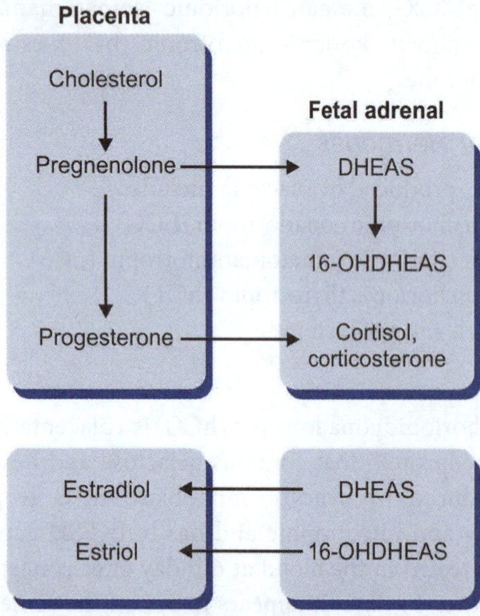

Fig. 9.16: Fetoplacental unit

In connection with estrogen synthesis during pregnancy, both the placenta and the fetus cooperate with each other. Some enzyme are absent in the placenta but present in the fetus whereas some other are absent in the fetus but present in placenta. But when two system works in unison enzyme system is complete.

The placenta synthesize pregnenolone and progesterone from cholesterol. Some of the progesterone enters the fetal circulation and provides the substrate for the formation of cortisol and corticosterone in the fetal adrenal glands. Some of the pregnenolone enters the fetus and along with pregnenolone synthesized in the fetal liver is the substrate for the formation of dehydroepiandrosterone sulfate (DHEAS) and 16-hydroxy dehydroepiandrosterone sulfate in the fetal adrenal. The DHEAS and 16-OH DHEAS are transported back to the placenta, where DHEAS forms estradiol and 16-OH DHEAS forms estriol. Since fetal 16-OH DHEAS is the principal substrate for the estrogens, urinary estriol excretion of the mother can be monitored as an index of the state of the fetus.

Note

Increase uptake of O_2 by fetal blood as it traverses the placenta due to the double Bohr's effect because, while flowing through the placenta:

- pCO_2 of fetal blood decreases and its pH increases, this shifts O_2-hemoglobin dissociation curve to left to cause increased loading of O_2.
- pCO_2 of maternal blood increases and its pH decreases, this shift O_2- hemoglobin dissociation curve to right and causes increased unloading of O_2.

Parturition

Parturition means birth of the baby. Towards the end of pregnancy, the uterus becomes progressively more excitable, until finally it develops strong rhythmic contractions so that the baby is expelled.

The process of parturition (labor) is divided into three stages (Flowchart 9.2):

1. Dilatation of cervix.
2. Expulsion of the fetus with membranes.
3. Expulsion of the placenta from the uterus.

Initiation of Labor

Initiation is usually indicated by the appearance of labor pains which are due to the conversion of slow and rhythmic uterine contractions (Braxton Hicks contraction) to strong and powerful contractions. These contractions become stronger at full term and force the baby through the birth canal thereby causing parturition. Mainly two categories of effects lead up to the intense contractions responsible for parturition: (1) Hormonal factors that increases excitability of

Flowchart 9.2: Mechanism of parturition

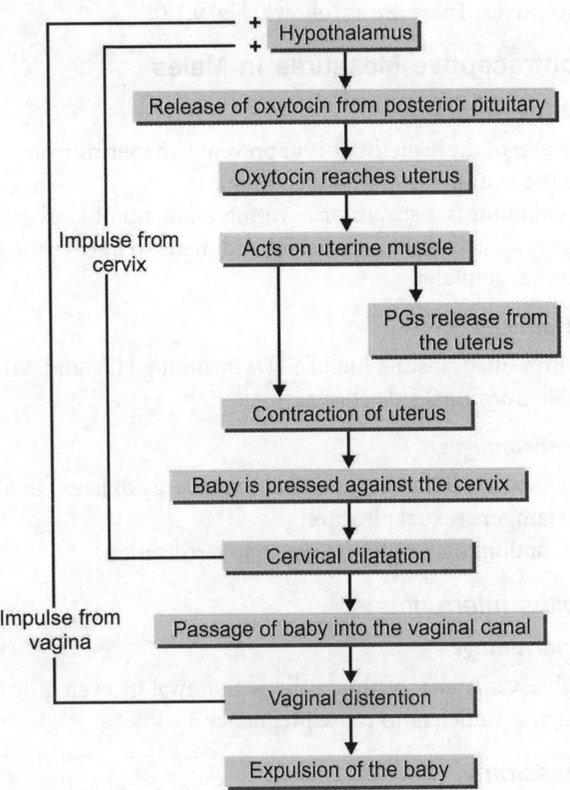

uterine musculature and (2) Mechanical factors that increases uterine contractility.

Hormonal Factors

1. *Increased ratio of estrogens to progesterone:* The high estrogen to progesterone ratio sensitizes the uterus to stretch, prostaglandins (they are released locally) and oxytocin. Estrogen has a definite tendency to increase the degree of uterine contraction as they increase the number of gap junctions between adjacent uterine smooth muscle cells. From the seventh month of pregnancy, estrogen secretion continues to increase while progesterone secretion remains constant or even decreases slightly and thereby maintaining a high E/P ratio.
2. *Effect of oxytocin on uterus:* Oxytocin appears to play a prominent role in the processs of parturition. It facilitates parturition by causing contraction of the estrogen primed uterus. The uterine muscle increases its oxytocin receptors near term and also the rate of oxytocin secretion by neurohypophysis is considerably increased at the time of labor.
3. *Effect of fetal hormones on uterus:* The fetal pituitary gland secretes increasing quantities of oxytocin which plays a role in exciting the uterus. The fetal adrenal glands secrete large quantities of cortisol which is a uterine stimulant. The fetal membranes release PGs in high concentration at the time of labor which increases the intensity of uterine contraction.

Mechanical Factors

1. *Stretch of the uterine musculature:* Uterine muscle being a visceral type of smooth muscle contracts when stretched. The sensitized uterus when stretched by the fully developed fetus brings out powerful contractions.
2. *Stretch or irritation of the cervix:* The stretching or irritation of nerves in the cervix initiates reflexes to the body of the uterus which may result in powerful uterine contractions.

Lactation

Lactation is the process of milk output from mammary gland. It is divided into two stages: (1) Secretion and (2) Ejection.

Milk Secretion

Initiation of milk secretion is called lactogenesis. After expulsion of placenta, there is decline in estrogens and progesterone. The drop in estrogen initiates lactation. Estrogen at low levels probably helps milk secretion by inhibiting prolactin inhibiting factor (PIF). Prolactin secretion increases during breastfeeding.

Maintenance of secretion is called galactopoiesis. This is the function of prolactin mainly with the aid of other hormones.

Effect of lactation on menstrual cycle

Women who do not nurse their infants have 1st menstrual cycle 6 weeks after delivery. Women who nurse regularly have amenorrhea for 25–30 weeks. Nursing stimulates the prolactin secretion, which in turn inhibits GnRH secretion and thereby ovulation is inhibited.

Milk Ejection

Expulsion of formed milk from the gland is possible due to:
1. Suckling action by the baby.
2. Contraction of myoepithelial cells by oxytoxin secreted by suckling reflex.
3. Continuous production of milk creates a positive pressure which pushes the milk out.

Suckling Reflex (Fig. 9.17)

It is a *neuroendocrine reflex.*

Due to suckling by baby → stimulation of tactile receptors in the areolor region of the breast → activate somesthetic neural pathway → transmit signal to paraventricular nuclei in hypothalamus → oxytoxin is formed and released through posterior pituitary → reach mammary gland through blood → contraction of myoepithelial cells → ejection of milk.

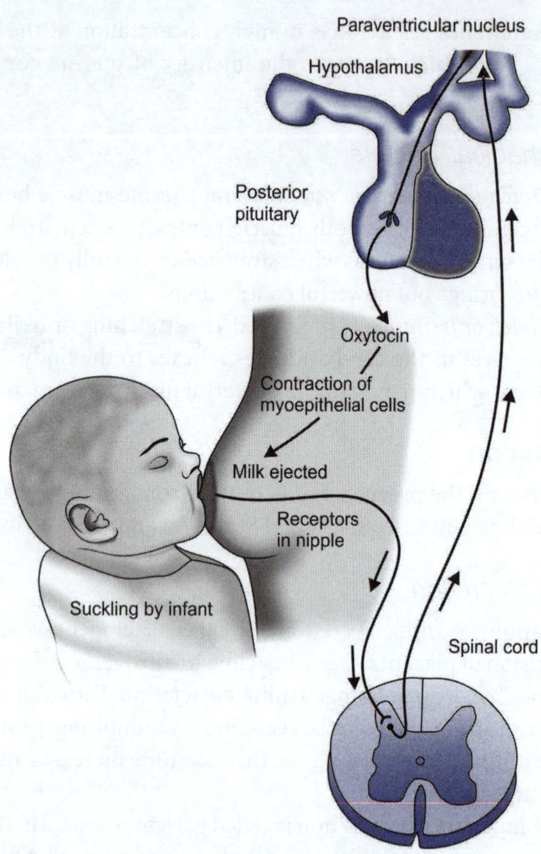

Fig. 9.17: Suckling reflex

Hormonal Changes at Puberty

Puberty is triggered by a release of gonadotropins (FSH and LH) from pituitary gland. These hormones act as signals to the gonads (testes/ovaries) that trigger the production of:

1. Estrogen, progesterone and some testosterone in women.
2. Testosterone in men. In both males and females, testosterone is responsible for development of pubic hair, accelerated bone growth, and acne during puberty. For boys, testosterone is responsible for the process of virilization, including the enlargement of the penis, increased libido and growth of facial and chest hair. Estrogen is the major hormone responsible for female pubertal development. It causes development of breast and thickening of endometrium. Progesterone causes proliferation of acne in mammary glands and converts watery cervical secretion to viscid and scanty. Leptin facilitates release of gonadotropin releasing hormone (GnRH), thereby helping in pubertal onset. Other hormones which are involved in puberty are thyroxine and growth hormone.

CONTRACEPTION

Contraception means prevention of conception (fertilization of ovum) and thus to stop reproduction.

Various methods or agents used for contraception are contraceptives. These are as follows (Fig. 9.18):

Contraceptive Measures in Males

Barrier Methods

The aim of these methods is to prevent live sperms from meeting the ovum. For example, condom.

Condom is a sheath or covering made up of latex rubber, mostly coated with spermicides and made to fit over the male external genitalia.

Advantages

- Prevents transmission of STDs including HIV and AIDS.
- No hormonal side effects.

Disadvantages

- Latex condoms can cause itching (allergy to latex) in few.
- Hampers sexual pleasure.
- Condom may rupture leading to fertilization.

Coitus Interruptus

Disadvantage

Slightest mistake in timing the withdrawal or even a drop of semen is sufficient to cause pregnancy.

Vasectomy

Advantages

It is relatively safe and convenient method.

Disadvantage

About 50% of vasectomized patients develop antibodies against sperms. So in those patients wishing to restore fertility at a later stage success rate after restoration of vas is only 50%.

Drugs: Gossypol (Spermicide)

Disadvantage

Drugs are too toxic to be used clinically.

Testosterone

Disadvantage

In such high doses testosterone causes sodium and water retention.

Contraceptive Measures in Female

Conventional Methods

Cervical diaphragm

Disadvantage

- Trained persons will be needed to demonstrate the technique of use.
- Local infection can be caused if it is left in the vagina.

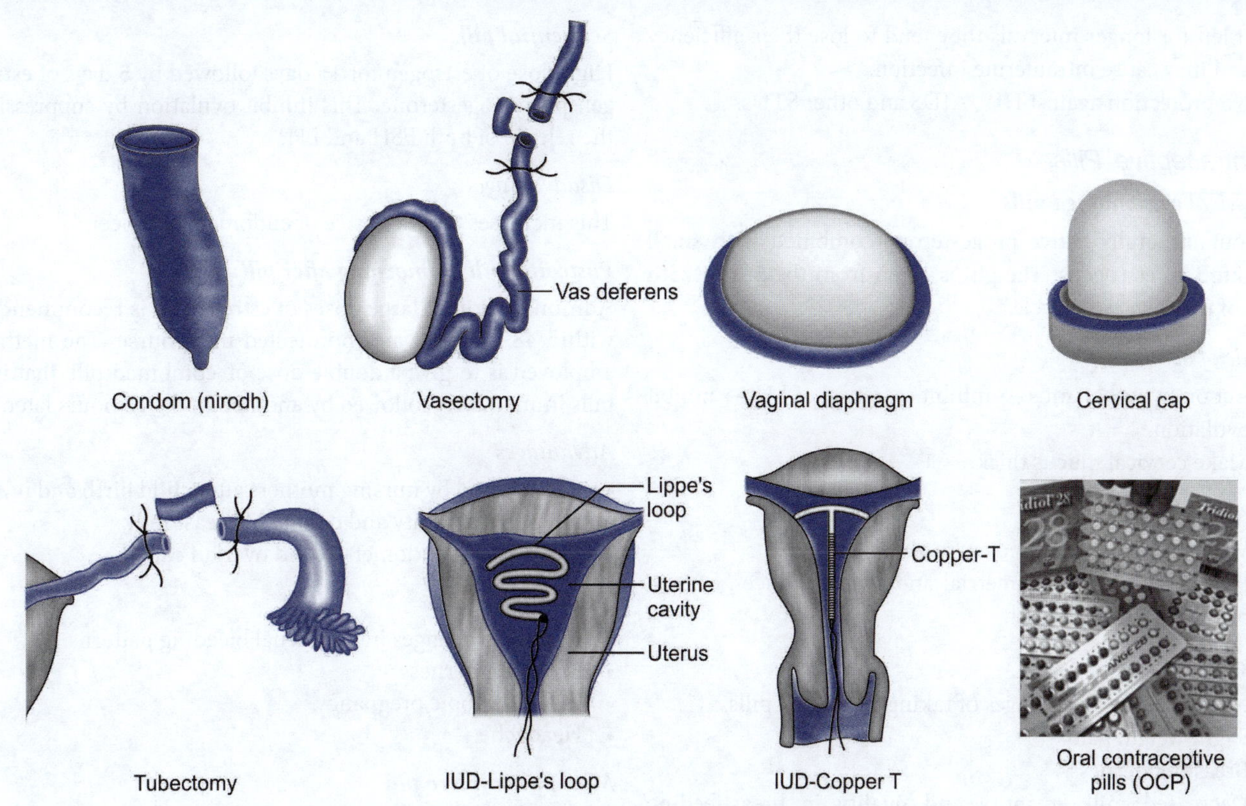

Fig. 9.18: Contraceptive measures

Douches

Disadvantage

It produces burning sensation and irritation locally besides producing messiness.

Rhythm method

It involves confinement of sexual intercourse to safe period only.

Tubectomy

Bilateral ligation of the fallopian tubes.

Advantages

It is relatively safe and permanent means of terminating pregnancy.

Intrauterine Device (IUD)

Implantation of a foreign body into the uterine cavity for contraceptive purposes. Types of IUD's are:

- *Nonmedicated IUD or inert IUD's:* These are referred to as 1st generation IUD's. It comprises of the inert or nonmedicated devices, usually made of polyethylene, or other polymers. They are available in different shapes and sizes—loops, spirals, coils, rings. The Lippes loop is the best known. The IUD causes a foreign body reaction in the uterus causing cellular and biochemical changes in the endometrium and uterine fluids that impair the viability of the gamete. They also prevent implantation.
- *Copper IUD (second generation IUD's):* By adding copper to IUD. It was found that copper has strong anti-fertility effect, e.g. copper-T. Copper seems to enhance the cellular response in the endometrium. By altering the biochemical composition of cervical mucus, copper ions may affect sperm motility, capacitation, and survival. It also affects the enzymes in the uterus.
- *Hormone releasing IUD (3rd generation):* The most widely used hormonal device is Progestasert which is a T-shaped device filled with progesterone. It acts by increasing the viscosity of cervical mucus and thereby prevent sperm from entering the cervix.

Advantages

- Long lasting and long-term prevention of pregnancy.
- Very effective and no side effects.
- No interactions with other medicines.

Disadvantages

- Chances of ectopic pregnancy very high.
- Menstrual changes in the first 3 months with occasional spotting between periods.

- If left for longer intervals they tend to lose their efficiency and may cause intrauterine infection.
- No protection against HIV, AIDS and other STDs.

Contraceptive Pills

Classical or combined pills

It contains orally active progesterone combined with small amounts of estrogens. The pill is given from the 5th to 25th day of the menstrual cycle.

Mode of action

- Act on hypothalamus → inhibit secretion of LH → inhibit ovulation.
- Make cervical mucus thick.

Advantages

- Very effective when used correctly.
- Helps to prevent endometrial and ovarian cancer, ectopic pregnancy, ovarian cyst.

Disadvantages

- Nausea in the intial stages of taking combined pills.
- Slight weight gain.
- Breast tenderness.
- Decreased milk quantity and quality in breastfeeding women.
- On long-term use of oral contraceptives there is high risk of thromboembolic phenomenon.
- Not effective unless taken every day.
- Does not provide protection against STD including AIDS.

Sequential pill

High dose of estrogen for 15 days followed by 5 days of estrogen plus progesterone. This inhibit ovulation by suppressing the release of both FSH and LH.

Disadvantage

This increases the incidence of endometrial cancer.

Postcoital pill or 'morning after pill

Administration of large doses of estrogen. It is recommended within 48 hours of an unprotected intercourse. The method employed is to give a double dose of 'combined pill' that is 2 pills immediately followed by another 2 pills 12 hours later.

Advantages

- Can be used by nursing mothers after child birth and it will not affect quantity and quality of breast milk.
- May prevent endometrial and ovarian cancer.

Disadvantages

- It leads to changes in menstrual bleeding patterns.
- Breast tenderness.
- Risk of ectopic pregnancy.
- Headache.

Mini pill or micro pill

Low dose of progesterone throughout the menstrual cycle. This prevents fertility without inhibiting ovulation.

Progesterone antagonist

Progesterone antagonists like mifepristone is helpful in producing abortion.

CHAPTER

10

Nerve and Muscle Physiology

NEURON

Structural and functional unit of nervous system is called neuron. The term neuron is used to describe the nerve cell and its processes, the dendrites and the axon (Fig. 10.1). It is specialized for the function of reception, integration and transmission of information in the body. The basic structure of neuron is best studied in a spinal motor neuron.

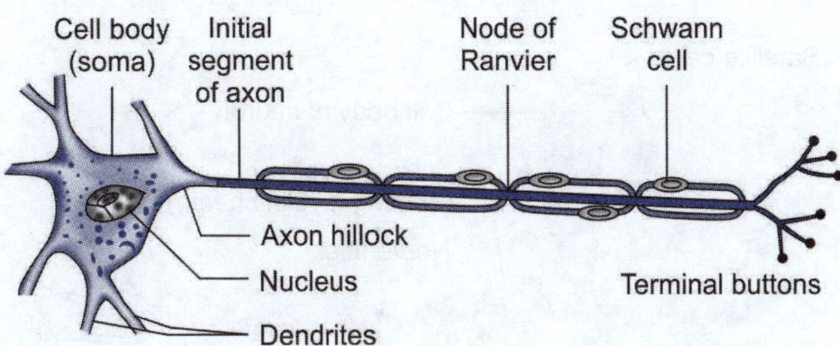

Fig. 10.1: Structure of neuron

Structure

Nerve Cell Body (Soma or Perikaryon)

They are of various size and forms: stellate, round, pyramidal, fusiform, etc. Its principal constituents are similar to a generalized cell. However, after fixation with special stains its cytoplasm also reveals the presence of:

Nissl granules/bodies

Nissl bodies are large granular body found in neuron. They are present in all over the soma (body), except in axon hillock and they extend to some extent in the dendrites, but not within the axon. These granules are rough endoplasmic reticulum (RER) with free ribosomes and are the site of protein synthesis. They are thought to be involved in the synthesis of neurotransmitter such as acetylcholine. Nissl bodies are basophilic granules. Chromatolysis (disappearance of nissl bodies) is an important histological sign of neuronal injury.

Neurofibrillae

These are fine threads 6–10 nm in diameter and of variable length. They traverse the cytoplasmic matrix forming a loose framework of fibrils in the cytoplasm.

Note

There is no centriole which indicate that the highly specialized nerve cell lost its power of division. Nerve cell once destroyed are replaced merely by neuroglia, cells which support the nerve cell.

Dendrites

These are 5–7 processes extending out from the cell body and arborize extensively after they leave the cell. They also contains nissl granule, mitochondria and neurofibrillae. They are the receptive processes of the neuron. Impulse can be transmitted from one dendrite to another in the CNS.

Axon (Axon Cylinder or Nerve Fiber)

It originates from a thickened area of the cell body called axon hillock, in which there is no nissl granules. The first portion of the axon is called initial segment. In a motor neuron, the axon hillock and the initial segment of the axon have the lowest threshold for excitation. This is because they have a much higher density of voltage gated sodium channels. The cytoplasmic fluid occupying the center of the axon is known as axoplasm. The cell membrane enveloping the cytoplasm is also continued on the axon as axolemma. Axon vary from a few microns in length to as long as 90 cm. Axon is the single elongated cytoplasmic extension with the specialized function of conducting impulses away from the cell body.

Synaptic Knobs (Terminal Buttons or Axon Telodendria)

The axon divides into terminal branches, each ending in a number of synaptic knobs. They contain granules or vesicles in which synaptic transmitter secreted by the nerve is stored.

Functionally speaking, the neuron can be divided into four zones:

1. Dendrites and Soma (cell body)—Receptor zone
2. Axon hillock of body and initial segment of axon—Generator area (Nerve impulse is generated)
3. Axon (main length)—Transmitter zone (Transmits nerve impulse).
4. The nerve terminals (Terminal knobs or buttons)—Release zone (release neurotransmitters).

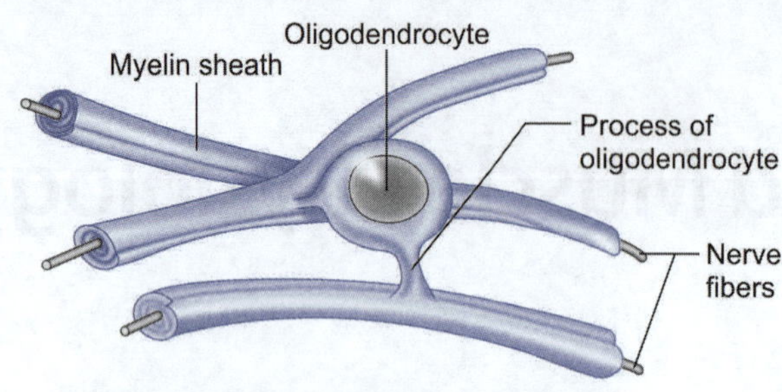

Oligodendrocytes have processes that form myelin sheaths around CNS nerve fibers

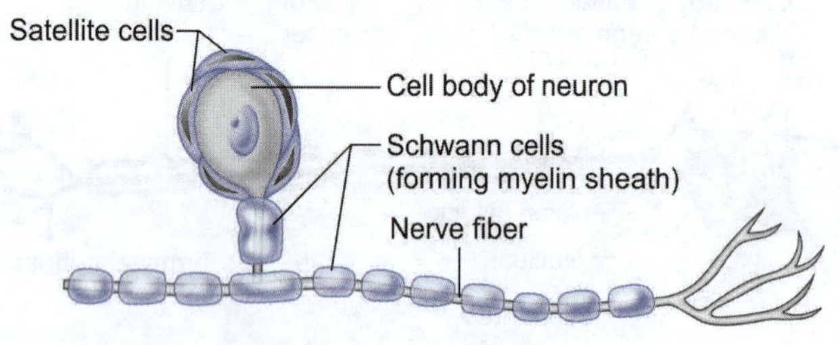

Satellite cells and Schwann cells (which form myelin) surround neurons in the PNS

Fig. 10.2: Myelinogenisis

Myelinogenesis

Neurolemma or sheath of Schwann has got a cell, Schwann cell which takes part in the deposition of myelin sheath round the axon, a process called myelinogenesis. Myelination of axons in the CNS system is by the oligodendrocytes. One oligodendrocytes sends processes to up to 40 axons (Fig. 10.2).

Schwann cells are found both in myelinated and nonmyelinated nerve fibers of peripheral nervous system (Table 10.1). In myelinated nerves, Schwann cells provide structural support and form myelin sheath, whereas in nonmyelinated nerves Schwann cells only provide structural support. Schwann cells are derived from neuroectoderm.

Glial Cell (Neuroglia)

Glial cell means glue, these are the cells which support the nerve cells. Glial cells are very numerous. There are approximate ten times as many glial cells as neurons. Unlike the neurons, the glial cells are capable of multiplying by mitosis. Glial cell are of three types:

1. ***Microglia:*** They are phagocytic cells that enter the CNS from meninges and blood vessels.
2. ***Astrocytes:*** They are found throughout the brain joining to the blood vessels and investing synaptic structures, neural bodies and neural processes.

   Function: It plays an important role in support, transport mechanisms, inflammatory and repairative reactions and also helps in forming the blood-brain barrier. They also help in maintaining optimal concentration of ions and neurotransmitter (specially glutamine) in the brain neurons.
3. ***Oligodendrolia:*** These are cells that form myelin around within CNS. The axons in the CNS do not have Schwann cells.

Table 10.1: Differences between myelinated and unmyelinated nerves

Myelinated nerves	Unmyelinated nerves
1. Multiple layers of Schwann cell membrane make myelin, formed by coiling of membrane many times round the axon.	1. Axons are simply surrounded in the Schwann cell without wrap ping of myelin.
2. Faster conduction of nerve impulse (50–100 times) than the unmyelinated fiber because of saltatory conduction, i.e. jumping of impulse from node to node over intersegmental region.	2. Slower conduction of nerve impulses as it is a continuous process due to lack of myelination.
3. For example i. All preganglionic fibers of ANS ii. Nerve fibers in somatic nervous system more than 1 mm in diameter.	3. For example i. All post-ganglionic fibers of ANS ii. Nerve fibers in somatic nervous system less than 1 mm in diameter

Orthodromic and Antidromic Conduction (Fig. 10.3)

Experimentally, an axon can conduct impulse in either direction. When an action potential is initiated in the middle of the axon, the impulse shall travel in both direction, i.e. one along the axon towards its terminal knobs and one in opposite direction, i.e. along the axon towards the cell body (soma) and dendrites. However, in the intact body, i.e. in the natural situation, the impulses are conducted in the one direction only, i.e. from synaptic junction or receptors along axons to their termination. Such conduction is called orthodromic conduction. Conduction in opposite direction is called antidromic conduction, i.e. opposite to physiological direction. However, antidromic conduction is very rare and may be seen only in muscle tissue, sensory nerve supplying the blood vessels. In nerve fibers, the propagation of action potential is unidirectional (orthodromic) because transmission across neuromuscular junction and synapses is unidirectional.

Nerve Fibers Types and Function

Erlanger and Gasser's Classification (Table 10.2)

Nerve fibers have been divided into A, B and C groups. A group is further subdivided into α, β, γ and δ fibers. Only C fibers are nonmyelinated, A and B fibers are myelinated.

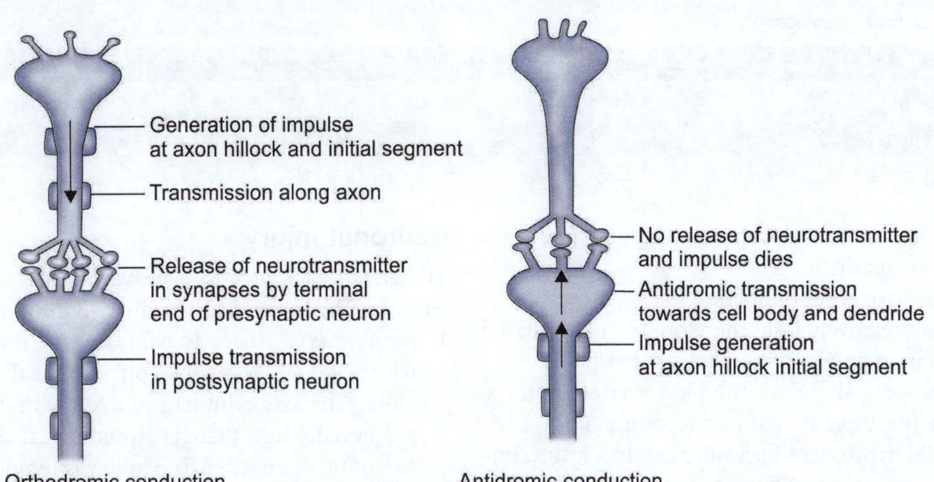

Fig. 10.3: Types of conduction

Table 10.2: Erlanger and Gassers classification

Class of nerve fiber	Diameter of fiber (in µm)	Velocity of conduction (m/s)	Function
A			
Aα	12–20 (Thickest and heavily myelinated)	70–120	Proprioception, somatic motor
Aβ	5–12 (Thinner than a; myelinated)	30–70	Touch, pressure, motor
Aγ	3–6 (Still more thin; slightly myelinated)	15–30	Motor to muscle spindles
Aδ	2–5 (Still thinner)	12–30	Pain, cold, touch
B	<3 (Myelinated)	3–15	Preganglionic fibers of ANS
C			
Dorsal root	0.4–1.2 (Unmyelinated)	0.5–2	Pain, temperature, some mechanoreception, reflex responses
Sympathetic	0.3–1.3 (Unmyelinated)	0.7–2.3	Postganglionic sympathetic

Table 10.3: Numerical classification for sensory neurons

Number	Origin	Fiber Type
Ia	Muscle spindle, annulospiral ending	Aα
Ib	Golgi tendon organ	Aα
II	Muscle spindle, flower-spray ending, touch, pressure	Aβ
III	Pain and temperature receptors, some touch, pressure	Aδ
IV	Pain and other receptors	Dorsal root 'C' fibers

Numerical Classification (Lloyed and Hunt) (Table 10.3)

This is used for sensory neurons and is based on the origin of nerve fibers.

Physio-clinical Classification (Table 10.4)

It has clinical as well as physiological significance and is based on sensitivity to hypoxia, pressure and anesthetic agents.

Important Facts

- Type A fibers have maximum velocity because they are thick and myelinated. Among A fibers, A α have maximum conduction because they are thickest and myelinated.
- Type C fibers have slowest conduction because they are thin and nonmyelinated. Type C fibers are post ganglionic autonomic fibers especially postganglionic sympathetic.
- Type B fibers are preganglionic autonomic fibers, both sympathetic and parasympathetic preganglionic.

Table 10.4: Physio-clinical classification

	Most susceptible	Intermediate	Least susceptible
Sensitivity to 'Hypoxia'	B	A	C
Sensitivity to 'Pressure'	A	B	C
Sensitivity to 'Local anesthetics'	C	B	A

- Thickest fibers are for proprioception. Thinnest fibers are postganglionic sympathetic (C).
- Pain is carried by two types of fibers:
  1. *A δ:* These are relatively fast. Therefore the pain carried by these is fast pain (epicritic pain or first pain).
  2. *C:* These are slow, therefore the pain carries by these is slow pain (protopathic pain or second pain).

Local anesthesia, hypoxia and pressure can block the conduction of nerve impulses. Different fibers have different susceptibility.

- Most susceptible fibers to pressure are A fibers and least susceptible fibers to pressure are C fibers. Amongst the A fibers, A α are most susceptible to pressure.
- Most susceptible fibers to hypoxia are B fibers and least susceptible fibers to hypoxia are C fibers.
- Most susceptible fibers to local anesthesia are C fibers and least susceptible fibers to local anesthesia are A fibers.

Neuronal (Axoplasmic) Transport System

Axoplasmic transport is the physical transport of substances in the axoplasm. Neurons are secretory cells; they release neurotransmitters at the axon terminals. Axoplasmic transport may be slow or fast. Fast transport may be antegrade or retrograde, whereas slow transport is always antegrade.

Fast Axoplasmic Transport

It may be antegrade or retrograde:

- *Fast antegrade transport (400 mm/day):* It occurs along the microtubules and is driven by kinesin. It transports membrane-bounded organelles like ER, mitochondria, golgi derived vesicles, microvesicles containing neurotransmitter, lipid, proteins, actin, myosin and the clathrin used in recycling of synaptic vesicle membrane.
- *Fast retrograde transport (200 mm/day):* It also occurs along the microtubules and is driven by the molecular motor dynein. Materials transported by retrograde transport system include empty (used) microvesicles for recycling or degradation by lysosomes, and nerve growth factors. Some toxins (tetanus toxin) and viruses (herpes and rabies) may reach the CNS by retrograde transport.

Slow Axoplasmic (Slow Antegrade) Transport

Slow transport carries tubulin of microtubules, protein subunits of neurofilaments and soluble enzyme for synthesis of neurotransmitters. Occurs at a rate of 0.5–10 mm/day. It is always anterograde. The mechanism is not clear.

Neuronal Injury

The effects of injury to a nerve depend upon the degree of damage. The injuries can be divided into three types:

1. *Neurapraxia:* There is contusion of the peripheral nerve which causes reversible physiological nerve conduction block. The axis cylinder (i.e. axon with its endoneurium) is preserved. Thus, there is physiological conduction without anatomic disruption. The injury is temporary and recovery is complete. It is seen in crutch palsy, tourniquet palsy, and saturday night palsy. Neurapraxia has best prognosis for recover.
2. *Axonotmesis:* There is injury to axon with myelin sheath, but endoneurium is preserved. Spontaneous recovery is expected in some cases. This is seen in closed fracture and dislocations.
3. *Neurotmesis:* There is complete anatomical section of nerve. No recovery is possible. It is seen in open wound.

Structure of a Peripheral Nerve (Fig. 10.4)

A peripheral nerve consists of masses of axis cylinders (axon), each with a neurilemmal tube. An individual nerve fiber is enclosed in a collagen connective tissue known as *endoneurium*. A bundle of such nerve fibers are further bound together by fibrous tissue to form a fasciculus. Binding fibrous tissue is known as *perineurium*. A number of fasciculi are bound together by a fibrous tissue sheath known as *epineurium*. An individual nerve, therefore, is a bundle of a number of fasciculi.

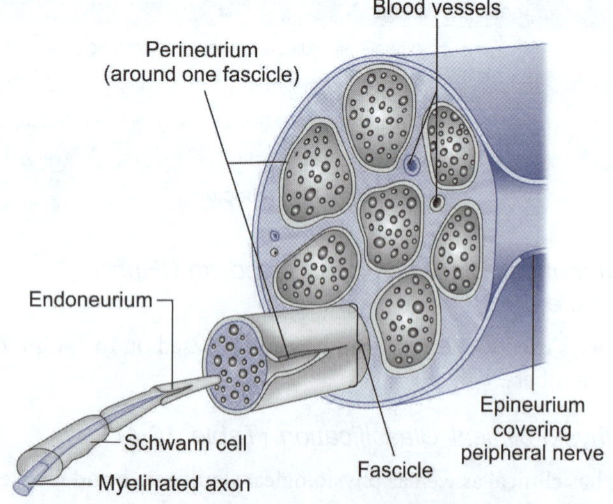

Fig. 10.4: Structure of a peripheral nerve

Degeneration and Regeneration of Nerve Fibers

When a nerve fiber is injured sufficiently, the part distal to the injury dies. Some changes in the proximal part are also seen. The entire process is known as degeneration (also called *Wallerian degeneration*, after Waller who described it).

Common causes of injury

a. Transection
b. Crushing
c. Injection of toxic or poisonous substance into the nerve.
d. Ischemia-interference in blood supply.
e. Hyperpyrexia-increase in body temperature.

Grading of injury (by 'Sunderland')

- *First degree injuries:* Most commonly seen and is secondary to ischemia caused by direct pressure to a nerve for a limited time. Ischemia produces local anoxia with temporary impairment of nerve function. It gets corrected within hours to few weeks, because the axon is not destroyed but merely loses its functional properties for a short time.
- *Second degree injuries:* Prolonged or severe pressure damages the nerve fibers at the pressure point eventually causing death of axon locally and distally.
- *Third degree injuries:* Endoneurial tubes becoming interrupted.
- *Forth degree injuries:* Fascicles becoming disorganized.
- *Fifth degree injuries:* Through and through cutting of nerve fibers, i.e. complete transection.

Degenerative changes occur at three levels

1. Changes in nerve cell body (retrograde changes)
2. Changes in the distal stump
3. Changes at the site of injury.

Series of Degenerative Changes

1. Change in nerve cell body begin within 48 hours of injury
   a. Chromatolysis: Nissl's granule disintegrate.
   b. Golgi apparatus, mitochondria, and neurofibrils are fragmented and disappear.
   c. Cell draws more fluid and become round.
   d. Nucleus increase in size and move to periphery.
2. Change in the distal stump begin within 24 hours of injury
   a. Axis cylinder breaks into short lengths and few days later little debris is left.
   b. Myelin sheath breaks up more slowly than axon into small oily droplets. It occurs in two stages: 1. Physical destruction up to 8–10 days, 2. Chemical destruction starts at 8th day and goes on till 32 days.
   c. Nucleus of Schwann cell start multiplying mitotically, which fill up the endoneurial tubes.

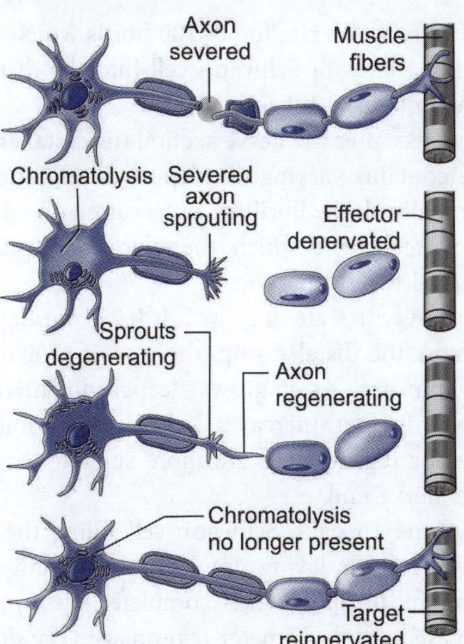

Fig. 10.5: Peripheral nerve damage and repair

   d. Macrophages from endoneurium start phagocytosing debris of axis cylinder and myelin sheath.
   e. Once the debris are cleared, Schwann cell cytoplasm starts proliferating and fills up the endoneurial tubes.
3. Changes in the site of injury
   Schwann cell differentiate into thin enlongated cells, mainly from the distal end and very little from the proximal end. It can bridge up the gap of 3 cm. Rate of progress of growth is 1–2 mm/day.

Regenerative Changes

A degenerated nerve may regenerate, provided there is neurilemmal sheath. In places where the neurilemma is absent, there can be no regeneration. Nerve fibers of CNS therefore, once degenerated, never regenerate as these nerves have no neurilemma. Degenerative and regenerative processes go side by side (Fig. 10.5).

1. **Changes in the nerve cell body**
   It begins in 20 days and is completed in 80 days. Nissl granules and Golgi apparatus gradually reappear, cell regains its normal size and nucleus returns to its central position. Repair of cell may even occur if the axon does not regenerate.
2. **Changes in the distal stump and at the site of injury**
   a. Axis cylinder from the proximal stump elongates and then grows out in all directions as rounded pseudopod like structures called fibrils towards the distal stump.

b. Each axon gives rise to 50–100 fibrils which are guided by the strands of Schwann cell into the distal ends of the endoneurial tubes.
c. 2–3 weeks after the nerve section the distal endoneurial tube contains varying number of developing fibrils.
d. Eventually all the fibrils re-innervating one tube degenerate except one which thereupon progressively gets enlarged to fill the tube.
e. To begin with, rate of growth is 0.25 mm/day, but once it enters the distal stump, the rate of growth becomes 3–4 mm/day. As it grows deeper down, the rate of growth further increases because mechanical conditions for regeneration are more suitable than those in a cut nerve end.
f. In approx 15 days, Schwann cell filling the endoneurial tube starts laying down myelin sheath round the successful fibril, which is completed by 1 year.
g. Increase in fiber diameter takes place very slowly. Final diameter attained is 80–85% of normal. It is limited by the diameter of the distal tube and the size of the parent nerve cell. Therefore, functional recovery is not full which takes longer time and may be associated with different complications if it does not reach its own cut stump. That is why, for a motor nerve, recovery may be complete but for a mixed nerve it is rarely so.

Denervation Hypersensitivity

When the motor nerve to skeletal muscle is cut and allowed to degenerate, the muscle becomes extremely sensitive to ACh. This phenomenon is referred to as denervation hypersensitivity or supersensitivity and is seen in smooth muscles also. Smooth muscles, unlike skeletal muscle do not atrophy when denervated, but it becomes hyper-responsive to the chemical mediator that normally activates it. Hypersensitivity is limited to the structure immediately innervated by the destroyed neurons. For example, the response of the denervated iris. If the postganglionic sympathetic nerves to one iris are cut in an experimental animal and after several weeks, if norepinephrine is injected intravenously, the denervated pupil dilates widely. A much smaller, less prolonged response is observed on the intact side.

Causes

a. Synthesis and activation of more receptors
b. There is an increase in the area of muscle membrane sensitive to ACh
c. ACh receptors of fetal gamma subunit appears

In orthograde degeneration (Wallerian degeneration), part distal to cut degenerates. Retrograde degeneration of axon is towards nearest collateral (Fig. 10.6).

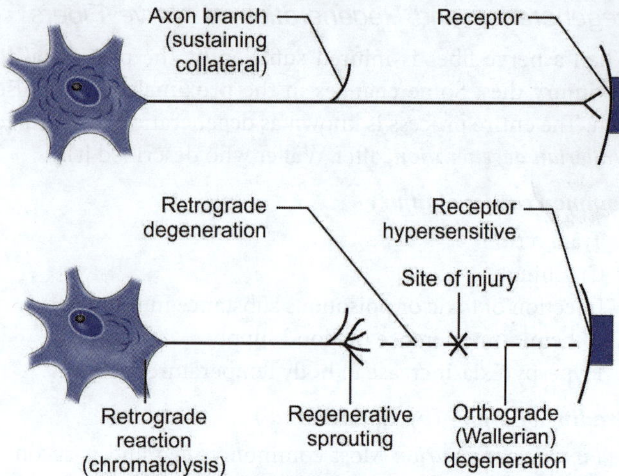

Fig. 10.6: Retrograde degeneration

Clinical Note

CNS neurons do not repair. In the case of peripheral nerves, a Schwann cell myelinates only a small segment of the axon, that is, between the two adjacent nodes of Ranvier. In the case of CNS nerves, oligodendrocytes form the myelin for these neurons; almost 20 axons are myelinated by a single oligodendrocyte. If a peripheral nerve is cut, it can regenerate and repair. The cut axon can regrow along the path that is created by the proliferating Schwann cells. In the CNS, the injured and transected axons make an attempt to regrow. However, there is no definitive path to guide them. This lack of guidance path is attributed to the fact that a single oligodendrocyte myelinates many axons in the CNS.

NEUROMUSCULAR JUNCTION (NMJ)

It is the junction between the motor nerve and skeletal muscle fiber. Nerve membrane which is in close approximation with the muscle membrane is called presynaptic membrane, while the muscle membrane is called postsynaptic membrane. The space between these membranes is called synaptic cleft (50–100 nm wide) which is filled with ECF.

Postsynaptic membrane has many folds of muscle membrane called subneural cleft which increases the surface area for the synaptic transmitter. Axon terminal has many mitochondria (for the synthesis of ACh) and minute vesicles or granules, which contain small packets of chemical transmitter, acetylcholine (ACh) responsible for synaptic transmission. An enzyme specific acetylcholinesterase is found in high concentration in postsynaptic clefts, which destroys the ACh.

Synthesis Storage and Release of ACh

Acetylcholine is synthesized within the mitochondria from 'choline' in the presence of enzyme choline acetyltransferase

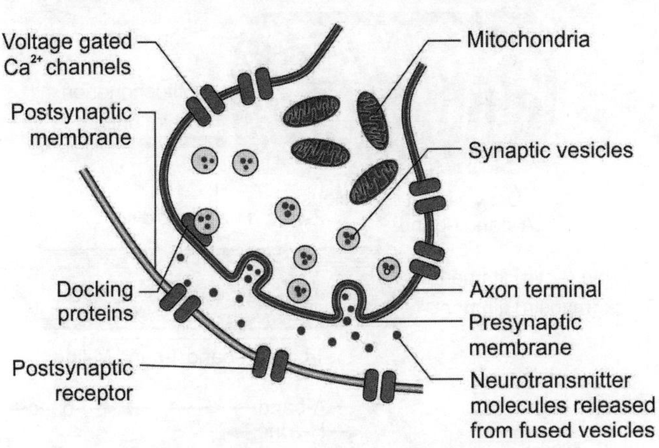

Fig. 10.7: Neuromuscular junction

(choline acetylase). In addition, it requires acetyl Co-enzyme A, ATP and glucose. With the exception of choline all components required for synthesis of ACh are present within mitochondria or gain ready access to them.

Acetylcholine once formed is temporarily stored in minute vesicles (synaptic vesicles) (Fig. 10.7). Nerve impulse causes fusion of vesicles with membrane of terminal nerve fiber by increasing permeability of Ca^{2+}. Ca^{2+} in ECF helps in fusion by changing ionic composition and thereby decreasing the flow of axoplasm, therefore, vesicles easily come in contact with the membrane. Mg^{2+} decreases this process. The amount of transmitter released is directly proportional to the Ca^{2+} influx.

Sequence of Events (Flowchart 10.1)

In response to a stimulus, sodium ions enter the axon of motor neuron leading to depolarization. This reduces the membrane potential in motor nerve axon. When the impulse reaches the end of axon, it increases the permeability to calcium ions. Calcium ions enter the axon of motor neuron through voltage gated calcium channels. It is this calcium entry that causes exocytosis of acetylcholine stored in motor nerve terminals. Acetylcholine, once released into the synaptic cleft is degraded by the enzyme acetylcholine esterase. Few molecules of Ach which escapes degradation finds its receptor, nicotinic acetylcholine receptor in the muscle. Nicotinic acetylcholine receptor in the muscle is N_M type. Binding of acetylcholine to these receptors increases influx of Na^+ ions leading to a depolarizing potential called the endplate potential. Endplate potential are local potentials. Once they cross the threshold, action potential is fired. In response to the action potential, muscle contracts.

Flowchart 10.1: Sequence of events during nerve impulse transmission

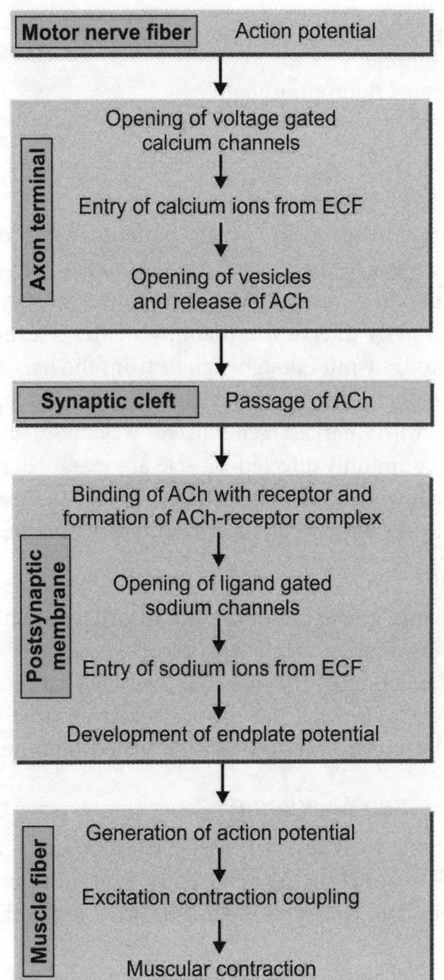

Note

It appears that vesicle breaks with the membrane when VAMP, a vesicle membrane protein connects with syntaxin, a cell membrane protein. The connection occurs in presence of G proteins—a SNAP, b SNAP, SNAP-25 and NSF.

Toxins which blocks neurotransmitter release

a. d-tubocurarine competes with ACh for same nicotinic receptors on the motor endplate.
b. Tetanus and botulinum neurotoxin-b cleaves VAMP
c. Botulinum neurotoxin-b cleave SNAP-25
(Tetanus cause spastic paralysis, botulinum cause flaccid paralysis).

Drug that stimulate neuromuscular junction by inactivating acetylcholinesterase

a. Neostigmine
b. Physostgmine
c. Diisopropyl fluorophosphate.

Disease

Myasthenia Gravis

Autoimmune disease in which patients have developed antibodies against their own ACh-activated ion channels. These antibodies destroy ACh receptors, thereby causing muscle paralysis due to the inability of the neuromuscular junctions to transmit enough signals from the nerve fibers to the muscle fibers. The disease is characterized by rapid onset of fatigue with marked generalized weakness of muscles. The most commonly affected muscle are extraocular muscle, facial, swallowing and mastication muscle. In severe form patient may die with paralysis of respiratory muscles.

Treatment

In myasthenia gravis (autoimmune disorder) antibodies are produced against nicotinic N_M receptors in the NMJ. To prevent the action of the antibody, we have to increase the release of ACh, for that the cholinesterase enzyme has to be inhibited by anticholinesterases such as neostigmine.

Lambert-eaten Syndrome

In this muscle weakness is caused by antibodies against one of the Ca^{2+} channels in the nerve endings at the neuromuscular junction. This decreases the normal Ca^{2+} influx that causes ACh release.

SKELETAL MUSCLE

Skeletal muscle is made up of many long thin cells called muscle fibers. Each muscle fiber is multinucleated, 1–40 mm long, cylindrical, 50–100 µm diameter and surrounded by a cell membrane, the sarcolemma. Muscle fibers are made up of many fibrils called myofibrils. Each myofibril is 1–2 µm in diameter. The cytoplasm in the muscle fibers is called sacroplasm.

Light Microscopic Appearance

The cross striations which are characteristic of skeletal muscle are due to difference in the refractive indices of various parts of muscle fiber. Therefore, the muscle fiber is seen to show alternate dark and light cross bands (Fig. 10.8).

1. The dark band is made of highly refractile material (anisotropic) called A-band (1.5 µm in length).

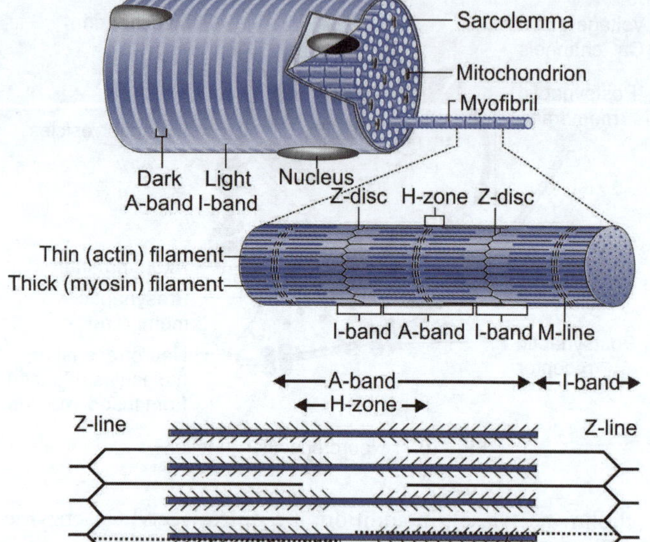

Fig. 10.8: Electron microscopic appearance of skeletal muscle

2. In the center of each A-band is found a slight less refractile region called H-band.
3. M line is seen in the middle of H-band, due to central bulge of A-band.
4. The alternate light band is made of lower refractile material (isotropic), therefore looks lighter and is called I-band (1 µm).
5. In the center of each I-band is found a narrow line of highly refractile material which looks dark called Z-line.
6. Contractile unit of the muscle is the substance between two adjacent Z-lines called sarcomere (2.5 µm).

Electron Microscopic View

The myofibrils are made up of two sets of protein filaments, thick and thin filaments.

1. *Thick filament:* Made out of myosin (cause for A-band). Myosin molecule is made up of 6 polypeptide; 2 heavy chain and 4 light chain. Myosin treated with proteolytic enzyme (trypsin) reveals 2 fragments.
   i. *Short compact head of heavy meromyosin (HMM):* It has 2 important sites: (a) Actin binding site-where myosin comes in contact with actin, (b) ATPase (catalytic) site-that hydrolyses ATP (Fig. 10.9).
   ii. *Long chain of light meromyosin:* It has only structural function and acts as backbone for HMM.
2. *Thin filament:* Made of actin, tropomyosin and troponin. They arrange themselves to form 2 chains of globular units

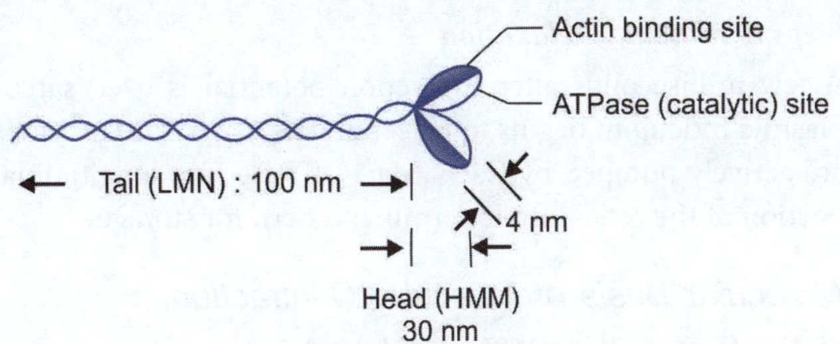

Fig. 10.9: Electron microscopic structure of thick filament

that form a double helix (responsible for I-band formation). Each thin filament contains 300–400 actin molecules and 40-60 tropomyosin molecule.

Actin

It occurs in two forms:

- *G actin:* Each molecule bind with 1 molecule of ATP firmly.
- *F actin:* Formed by polymerization of G actin.

Tropomyosin

It covers the binding site of actin where myosin head comes in contact with actin, i.e. it prevents interaction between actin and myosin.

Troponin

They are small globular proteins. It is made up of 3 subunits:

- Troponin 'T'—binds the other troponin components to tropomyosin
- Troponin 'I'—inhibits the interaction of myosin with actin
- Troponin 'C'—contains binding site for Ca^{2+} that initiates muscle contraction.

Sarcotubular System (Fig. 10.10)

Sacroplasm (cytoplasm of skeletal muscle) contains sacrotubular system. It is highly specialized system of internal conduction of depolarization within the muscle fiber. It is made T-system (transverse tubular system) and a longitudinal sarcoplasmic reticulum (LSR).

T-system

They are inwardly directed extensions of the sarcolemma into the muscle fibers at the junction between 'A' and 'I' bands (A-I junctions). Its function is the rapid transmission of the action potential from the cell membrane to all the fibrils in the muscle. The T-tubule protein is a modified voltage-sensitive Ca^{2+} channel known as the dihydropyridine receptor (so named because it binds the class of drugs called dihydropyridines). The main role of DHP receptor, however, is not to conduct Ca^{2+}, but rather to act as voltage sensor.

LSR

Longitudinally on either side of the tubular system are found the sacs of the dilated LSR. These sacs are called terminal cisternae, which are rich in glycogen and Ca^{2+}. Ca^{2+} channels in sarcotubular reticulum are not voltage gated and allow the release of Ca into the cell. These are called ryanodine receptors. In skeletal muscle, one T tubule is surrounded by two L tubules. This classical arrangement is called triad. But in cardiac muscle, one T tubule is surrounded by one L tubule. This arrangement is called dyad.

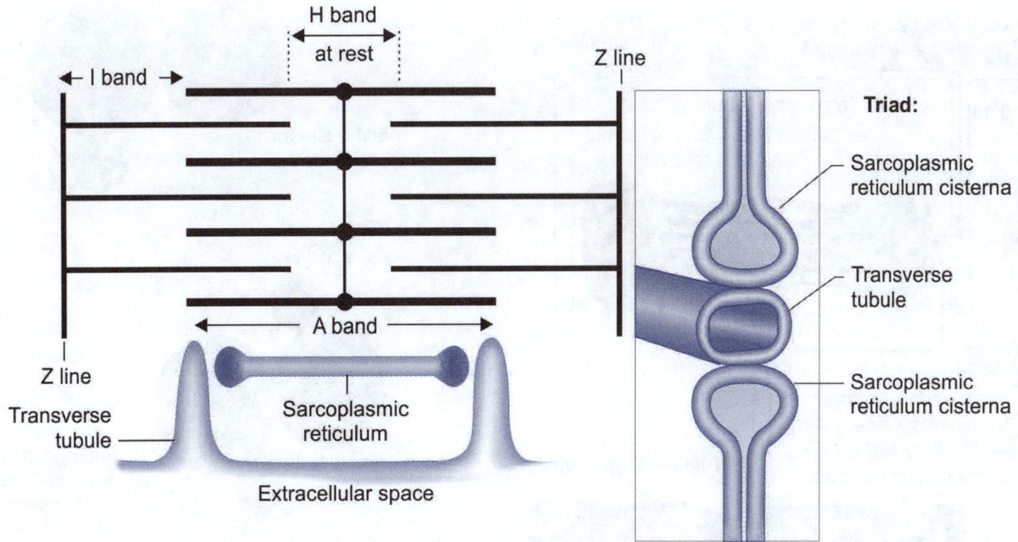

Fig. 10.10: Sarcotubular system

Action

Depolarization of T-tubule cause the DHP receptors to induce a conformational change to open the ryanodine receptors channel. Ca^{2+} is thus released from the lateral sac of sarcoplasmic reticulum. This Ca^{2+} bind with the troponin, removes blocking action of tropomyosin.

Excitation Contraction Coupling

Process by which depolarization of the muscle fiber initiates contraction. Sequence of events in excitation contraction coupling (Fig. 10.11).

Steps in muscular contraction

- Stimulation of motor neuron.
- Release of ACh into synaptic cleft causing generation of endplate potential.
- Depolarization of muscle membrane by increasing its permeability to Na^+.
- Generation of action potential in the muscle fiber.
- Inward spread of action potential along the T-system.
- Spread of depolarization to terminal cistern with release of Ca^+ in the myofibrils.
- Increase of concentration of Ca^{2+} in ICF by 2000 times.
- Muscle contraction.

Role of Ca^{2+}

- Ca^{2+} binds with troponin C causing tropomyosin to move laterally. This exposes the binding sites for the myosin heads on the actin.
- Activates prosthetic group of myosin filament which acts as enzyme (ATPase).

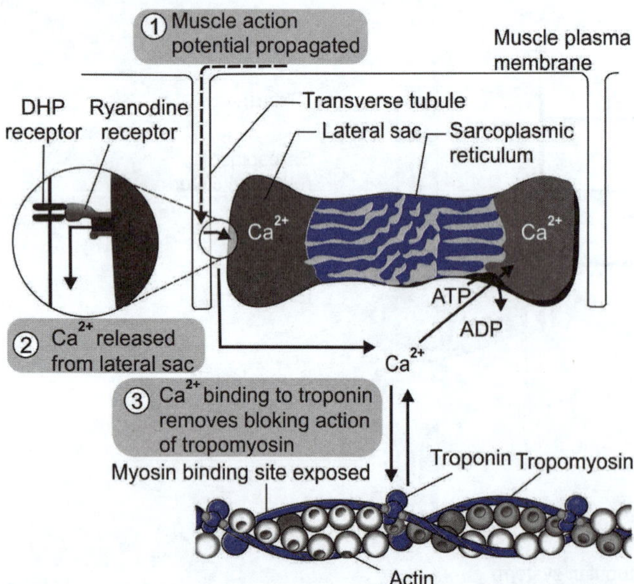

Fig. 10.11: Sequence of events in excitation contraction coupling

Steps in muscular relaxation

A few milliseconds after the action potential is over, sarcoplasmic reticulum begins to reaccumulate Ca^{2+}. The Ca^{2+} ions are actively pumped by Ca^{2+}- Mg^{2+} ATPase into longitudinal portion of the reticulum to terminal cistern for storage.

Molecular Basis of Muscular Contraction

Sliding filament theory (Ratchet theory)

The process by which the shortening of the contractile elements in the muscle is brought about is by sliding of actin filament over the thick (myosin) filaments. The sliding of filaments is brought about by formation of the cross-bridges between the head of myosin and actin molecules.

Events during formation of the cross-bridges

i. In resting muscle no cross-bridges are formed since troponin 'I' is lightly bound to actin and tropomyosin covers the actin sites where myosin bind to actin. Therefore, the troponin–tropomyosin complex constitutes a relaxing protein which inhibits the interaction between actin and myosin.
ii. Ca^{2+} released from the terminal cisterns by the action potential, binds to troponin 'C' and causes.
   a. The binding of troponin 'I' to actin is weakened, this permits tropomyosin to move laterally uncovering the binding sites for myosin heads on actin filaments (Fig. 10.12).

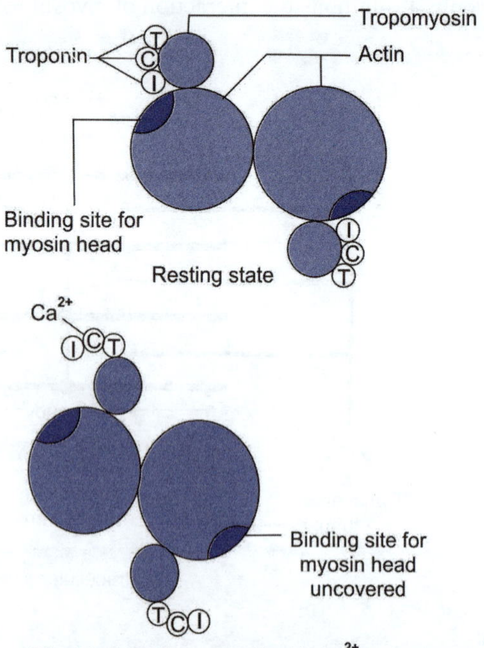

Fig. 10.12: Configurational change in thin filament

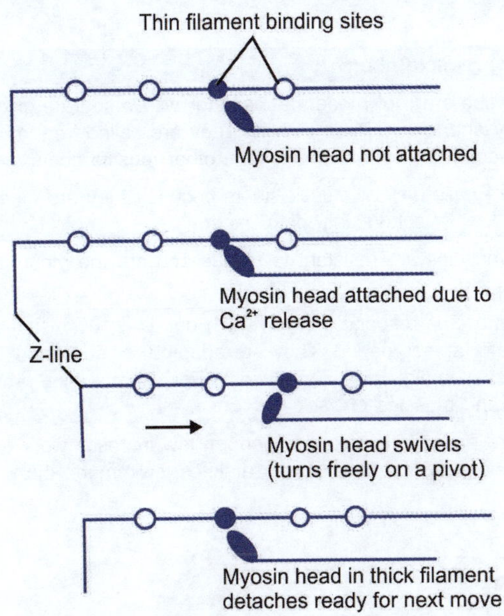

Fig. 10.13: Mechanism of formation of cross-bridges

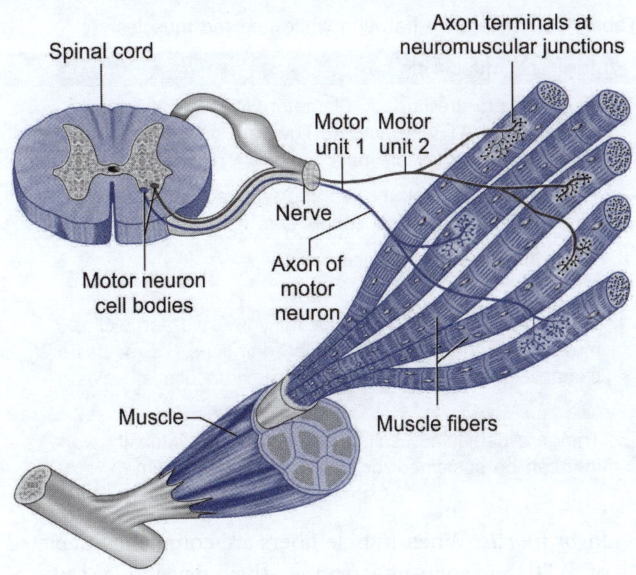

Fig. 10.14: Motor unit

b. Hydrolysis of ATP by ATPase activity in the myosin heads produces energy.

iii. Seven myosin binding sites on actin filaments are uncovered for each molecule of troponin that binds a Ca^{2+}. The heads of the myosin molecules link to the actin, produce movements of myosin on actin by swiveling.

Mechanism of sliding of thin filaments over thick filaments

- The sliding during muscle contraction is produced by breaking and re-forming of cross-bridges between actin and myosin, repeating the process in serial fashion for 5–6 times (Fig. 10.13).
- The width of 'A' bands is constant, whereas the 'Z' move closer together when the muscle contracts.

Motor Unit

Motor unit is the functional unit of muscle contraction in the intact body. It consists of the single motor neuron cell body, its axon fibers and the muscle fibers innervated by it. The cell bodies of the motor neurons supplying the skeletal muscle fibers lie in the ventral horn of the spinal cord or the motor cranial nerve nuclei (Fig. 10.14). In simple words, each single motor neuron and all the muscle fibers it supplies constitutes a motor unit.

Properties of Motor Unit

1. The number of muscle fibers in a motor unit varies inversely with the precision of movements performed by that part.
2. Each motor unit innervates only one type of muscle fiber. In other words, in a single motor unit the muscle fibers supplied by it are of the same type. These are of 2 types- 'red' (Type I) and 'white' (Type II) muscle fibers.
3. All the efferent fibers passing to skeletal muscles are excitatory. There are no efferent nerves which on stimulation produce relaxation of the muscle, i.e. there are no inhibitory efferents to skeletal muscle (as compared to cardiac and smooth muscles where the efferent supply is both excitatory and inhibitory).
4. Depending on the type of muscle fibers they innervate, motor units are of two types, 'slow' and 'fast' motor units.

Applied Aspect

1. When the motor nerve to a skeletal muscle is cut it causes:
   a. Disuse atrophy of the muscle, i.e. shrinkage of muscle fibers, which finally gets replaced by fibrous tissue (fibrous muscle)
   b. Complete paralysis of the muscle
   c. Appearance of fine, irregular contractions of individual fibers called fibrillations:
   d. *Denervation hypersensitivity:* These effects are the classical consequences of LMN (lower motor neuron), i.e. injury to the spinal/cranial motor neurons which directly innervate the muscles.
2. *Muscular dystrophy:* It is a syndrome characterized by progressive muscle weakness due to mutation in dystrophin gene, which results in congenital defect in dystrophin-glycoprotein complex. This is a large protein complex that connects the thin filaments to the transmembrane protein in the sarcolemma and thus provides support and strength to the fibers.

Table 10.5: Difference between white and red muscles

White (fast) muscle fibers	Red (slow) muscle fibers
1. Muscle fibers are large in diameter with high glycogen capacity and ATPase activity. They are called 'white' muscle fibers because they are pale	1. Muscle fibers are of moderate diameter with moderate glycogen capacity and low ATPase activity. They are called 'red' muscle fibers because they are darker than other muscle fibers
2. They are called 'fast' muscle fibers because they are innervated by large, fast conducting motor neurons	2. They are called 'slow' muscle fibers because they are innervated by small, slow conducting motor neurons
3. These muscles get fatigued easily	3. These muscles are resistant to fatigue and are the most used muscles
4. These muscles are specialized for fine rapid and skilled movements and have short twitch durations (7.5 sec). For example, muscles of the hand and extraocular muscles	4. These muscles respond slowly (which duration 100 msec) and have long latency period. They are adapted for sustained, slow and posture maintaining contractions. For example, long muscles of limb and muscles of back
5. They are particularly suited to perform high intensity work that can be sustained for only short period of time	5. They are particularly suited to perform low intensity work over long periods of time such as for athletes, swimmers, etc.

3. *Rigor mortis:* When muscle fibers are completely depleted of ATP and phosphocreatine, they develop a state of extremely rigidity called rigor. When this occurs after death, the condition is called rigormortis. In rigor, almost all of the myosin heads attach to actin but in an abnormal, fixed and resistant way.
4. *Myotonia:* A condition characterized by difficulty and slowness in relaxing muscle after voluntary effort. Various forms of myotonia defined clinically are due to abnormal genes on 7, 17 or 19 chromosomes, which results in abnormalities of Na^+ on Cl^- channels.

Types of Muscle Fibers

Muscles can be divided into two types: 1. Fast muscles (white muscles), and 2. Slow muscles (red muscles). Fast muscles are pale looking, whereas slow muscles are more red (Table 10.5). This is so because, the slow muscles have greater capillary network. In human beings, most muscles contain a variable mixture of fast and slow muscle fibers. The postural muscles are largely slow muscles.

White Muscles

White muscles constitute 3/4th of the total muscle mass and have greater speed of contractions. They have a resting blood flow of 3 ml/min/100 gm, which may increase to 60–70 ml/min/100 gm in maximal exercise. These muscles are prone to O_2 debt.

Red Muscles

They comprise 25% of the total muscle mass and are concerned with maintenance of posture. Their activity is of the steady prolonged type which requires a relatively low O_2 usage. Their resting blood flow is 20–30 ml/min/100 gm due to low basal myogenic tone. They have vascular bed 3 times the size of white muscles with high flow capacity, approx. 150 ml/min/100 gm. Because of greater surface area of the capillary bed and their lower O_2 requirement, these muscles are unlikely to be exposed to O_2 debt.

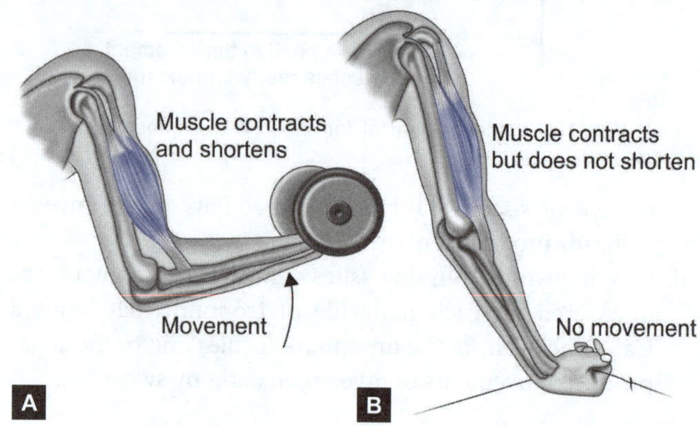

Figs 10.15A and B: Isotonic vs isometric contraction

Isotonic Contraction (Fig. 10.15A)

When muscle contraction is associated with change in length at constant tension. The tension is equal to the weight lifted during contraction of the muscle. Here external work is performed, greater amount of energy is used than isometric contraction. Therefore, muscle strength is best increased by isotonic exercise. Exercises one does in the gym are isotonic exercises as muscle length changes in each step but not tension.

Isometric Contraction (Fig. 10.15B)

When muscle contraction is associated with no apparent change in muscle length, but there is increase in tension, the phenomenon is called isometric contraction. The muscle develops tension (tension is the force of the contracting muscle acting on the object), but does not shorten or lengthen; for example, when somebody is trying to lift a heavy object (when the object is not lifted actually). According to the law of physics, if displacement is zero (position of the object does not change), the work done (force x displacement) is also nil, though force is generated and energy is spent. Thus, in isometric contraction no external work is done.

SMOOTH MUSCLE

Smooth muscle is distinguished anatomically from skeletal and cardiac muscle because it lacks visible cross striations. Actin and myosin-II are present and they slide on each other to produce contraction. However, they are not arranged in regular arrays, as in skeletal and cardiac muscle, and so the striations are absent. Smooth muscle is involuntary. Troponin is absent. Z lines are not there, instead there are dense bodies in the cytoplasm. Actin filament is attached to dense bodies by a protein called α-actinin. T tubules are also absent. Sacroplasmic reticulum is not well-developed. It is rudimentary to moderately developed.

Types

There is considerable variation in the structure and function of smooth muscle in different parts of the body. In general, smooth muscle can be divided into visceral/unitary smooth muscle and multiunit smooth muscle (Table 10.6 and Fig. 10.16).

1. **Single unit (visceral) smooth muscle:** This type of smooth muscle behaves as if the entire muscle mass as single unit, i.e. syncytium. The gap junctions between muscle fibers are so generous that the impulse of activation can spread rapidly from one cell to another. Gap junctions are responsible

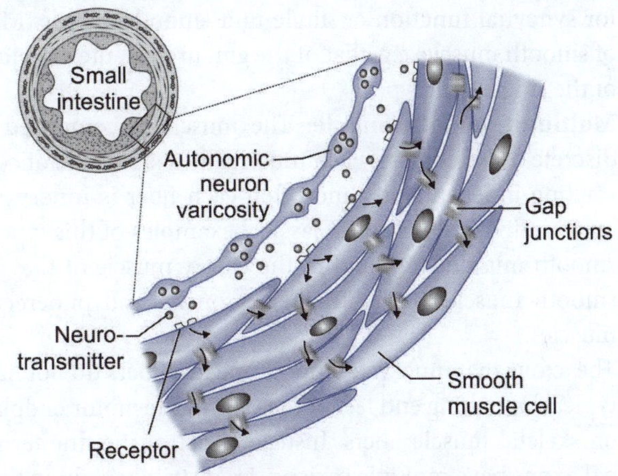

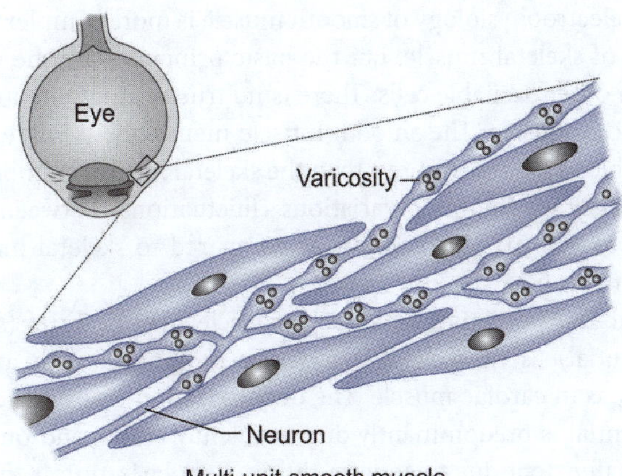

Fig. 10.16: Morphology of smooth muscle fiber

Table 10.6: Difference between single unit and multiunit muscle

Single unit/Visceral smooth muscle	Multiunit smooth muscle
1. It is called single unit smooth muscles because it functions in a syncytial fashion. It occurs in large sheets and has low resistance fashion. Single unit smooth muscles have low resistance bridges between individual muscle cells	1. It is called multiunit smooth muscle because it is made up of individual units without interconnecting bridges, i.e. non-syncytial in character. So its contractions are discrete, fine and localized
2. Location: Wall of hollow viscera, i.e. GIT, ureters, bronchi, uterus and urinary bladder	2. Location: Ciliary muscles of eye, iris, pilomotor muscle of skin and muscles of blood vessels
3. In certain areas the muscles are characterized by appearance of spontaneous activtiy, so called	3. Each muscle fiber of multiunit smooth muscle has its own nerve supply
4. Rhythmic contraction and relaxation of these muscles is independent of their innervation. Innervation has role only in modulating its activity	4. These muscles are sensitive to chemical mediators at the nerve endings (ACh or NE) in response to which muscle contracts. Single stimulus to the nerve causes repeated firing of action potential which produces irregular tetanic contractions rather than a single muscle twitch as seen in skeletal muscle
5. Active tension is produced when the muscle is stretched	5. No response by the muscle to stretch

for syncytial function of single unit smooth muscle. Most of smooth muscle, e.g. that of the gut, ureters, uterus, etc. is of the single-unit type.

2. **Multiunit smooth muscle:** The muscle is composed of discrete muscle fibers. Each muscle fiber is capable of contracting independently and often each fiber is innervated by an individual neuron. Classical examples of this type of smooth muscle are found in the ciliary muscle of the eye; smooth muscle of iris, trachea, bronchi; and piloerector muscles.

The axons that innervate smooth muscle fibers do not have typical branching end feet of the type in the motor endplate on skeletal muscle fibers. Instead, most of the fine terminal axons have multiple varicosities distributed along their axes.

Electrical and mechanical activity

The electrophysiology of smooth muscle is more complex than that of skeletal muscle, but the basic principles are the same as in other excitable cells. There is no true resting potential in smooth muscle. The smooth muscle membrane is more permeable to ions even at rest than the skeletal muscle membrane. RMP shows rhythmic variations (fluctuations) between –60 mV to –50 mV. RMP is low as compared to skeletal muscle and neuron.

Action potentials in smooth muscle may be brief (spike potential) as in skeletal muscle, or prolonged, with a plateau, as in cardiac muscle. The depolarization phase of action potential is predominantly due to calcium influx and only to a small extent due to sodium influx. Repolarization is due to decrease in the influx of calcium and sodium, and efflux of potassium ions. The entry of calcium during depolarization not only makes a significant contribution to the depolarization but also switches on the contractile process.

Molecular Basis of Smooth Muscle Contraction

Ca^{2+} is involved in the initiation of contraction of smooth muscle. However, visceral smooth muscle generally has a poorly developed sarcoplasmic reticulum and the increase in intracellular Ca^{2+} concentration that initiates contraction is primarily due to Ca^{2+} influx from the ECF via voltage-gated and ligand-gated Ca^{2+} channels.

In addition, the myosin in smooth muscle must be phosphorylated for activation of the myosin ATPase. In smooth muscle, Ca^{2+} binds to calmodulin and the resulting complex activates calmodulin-dependent myosin light chain kinase. This enzyme catalyzes the phosphorylation of the myosin light chain on serine at position 19. The phosphorylation allows the myosin ATPase to be activated and actin slides on myosin, producing contraction. This is in contrast to skeletal and cardiac muscle, where contraction is triggered by the binding of Ca^{2+} to troponin C. Myosin is dephosphorylated by myosin light chain phosphatase in the cell. This enzyme is inhibited when it is phosphorylated and activated by dephosphorylation. It is dephosphorylated by a rho-associated kinase that is activated by ligands which produce inhibition of smooth muscle activity. However, dephosphorylation of myosin light chain kinase does not necessarily lead to relaxation of the smooth muscle. Various other mechanisms such as latch bridge mechanism by which myosin cross-bridges remain attached to actin for sometime after the cytoplasmic concentration falls. This produces sustained contraction with little expenditure of energy, which is especially important in vascular smooth muscle. Relaxation of the muscle presumably occurs when there is final dissociation of the Ca^{2+}-calmodulin complex or when some other mechanism comes into play. The events leading to contraction and relaxation of visceral smooth muscle are summarized.

1. Binding of acetylcholine to muscarinic receptors
2. Increased influx of Ca^{2+} into the cell
3. Ca binds with calmodulin
4. Activation of calmodulin-dependent myosin light chain kinase
5. Phosphorylation of myosin
6. Increased myosin ATPase activity and binding of myosin to actin
7. Contraction
8. Dephosphorylation of myosin by myosin light chain phosphatase
9. Relaxation or sustained contraction due to the latch bridge and other mechanisms.

Note

Latch mechanism facilitates prolonged holding of contraction of smooth muscles. Once smooth muscle contracts, it can maintain its contraction for a prolonged period of time with minimal expenditure of energy. This is because myosin hold on actin filaments like a latch.

CARDIAC MUSCLE

Cardiac muscle fibers are striated like skeletal muscle fibers but the most characteristic histological feature of the cardiac muscle is a syncytium like appearance. But it should be kept in mind that, it looks like a syncytium from a histological point of view, but the heart muscle is not a syncytium. A syncytium is a multinucleated mass of cytoplasm which is

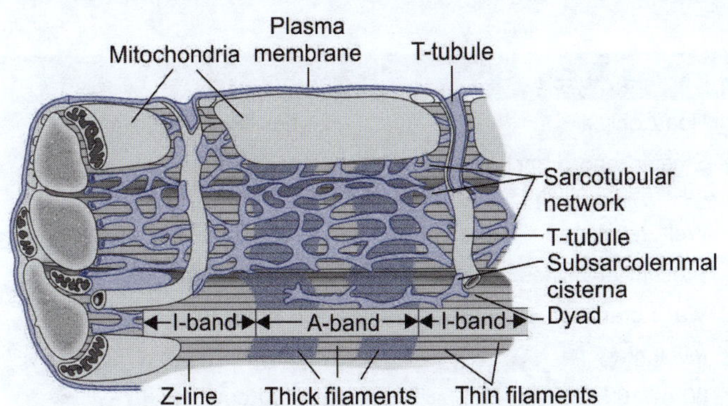

Fig. 10.17: Morphology of cardiac muscle fiber

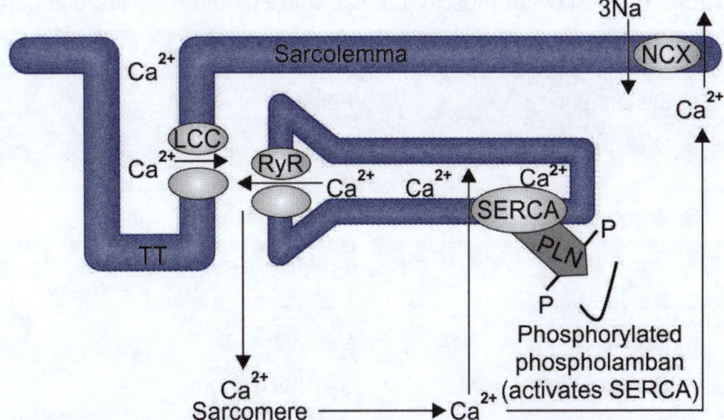

Fig. 10.18: Contraction of cardiac muscle

PLN = Phospholamban; NCX = Na^+ – Ca^{2+} exchanger; LCC = L-type calcium channels; RyR = Ryanodine receptors; TT = T tubule; SERCA = Sarcoendoplasmic reticulum Ca^{2+} – ATPase

not divided by end-membranes into individual cells. Cardiac muscle fibers branch and interdigitate, but each is a complete unit surrounded by cell membrane with a centrally located single nucleus. So, cardiac muscle look like syncytium but histologically is not syncytium (Fig. 10.17).

Each muscle fiber at its end joins with the next cell by intercalated disc. These discs are actually end membranes that separate one muscle cell from another. At the outer border of the intercalated disc, there are gap junctions (connexons) because of which cardiac muscle behaves as a functional syncytium as these gap junctions provide low-resistance bridges for spread of excitation from one fiber to other. So, from a histological point of view, cardiac muscle is not a syncytium. But functionally (electro physiologically) cardiac muscle behave as syncytium.

Contraction of Cardiac Muscle

The cardiac muscle cell contains actin, myosin, the sarcotubular system and other organelles seen in skeletal muscles. However, the T system of cardiac muscle is located at Z lines rather than at A-I junction, where it is located in skeletal muscles. Electrical property (action potential, RMP etc.) of cardiac muscle is explained in cardiovascular system.

Similar to smooth muscles, cardiac muscle contraction is started by Ca^{2+}, i.e. excitation-contraction coupling is caused by Ca^{2+}. In skeletal muscle, intracellular calcium stores are sufficient for contraction. But in cardiac muscle cells, to release calcium from intracellular stores, some calcium must enter cardiac muscle cell to trigger intracellular calcium release. Increase in cytoplasmic (sarcoplasmic) Ca^{2+} cause contraction, similar to smooth muscles. As the action potential develops, it causes Ca^{2+} influx within the cardiac cell via L-type of Ca^{2+} channels in the sarcolemma. This influx of Ca^{2+} ions triggers the release of Ca^{2+} ions from sarcoplasmic reticulum to sarcoplasm via ryanodine receptors. Increase in intracellular Ca^{2+} causes contraction of cardiac muscles, by almost similar mechanism as in smooth muscles. During relaxation, cytoplasmic (sarcoplasmic) Ca^{2+} is lowered by two mechanisms (Fig. 10.18):

1. Sarcoplasmic reticulum calcium pump (SR Ca^{2+} ATPase or SERCA): It pumps back the sarcoplasmic (cytoplasmic) Ca^{2+} into SR.
2. Ca^{2+} $3Na^+$ antiport in sarcolemma: Pumps out the cytoplasmic (sarcoplasmic) Ca^{2+}.

The protein phospholamban is a protein associated with SERCA. Phospholamban typically inhibits SERCA activity. This activity of phospholamban is inhibited by its phosphorylation. Increased level of adrenal medullary epinephrine or increased norepinephrine from sympathetic nerve endings activates β adrenergic receptors on cardiac muscle cells. This in turn activates adenylyl cyclase enzyme resulting in an increase in cAMP. This causes phosphorylation of phospholamban. Phosphorylation of phospholamban by a cAMP dependent protein kinase inhibits the activity of phospholamban. Inhibition of phospholamban causes increased activity of SERCA.

Increased activity of SERCA facilitates: 1. Relaxation of heart because of rapid calcium uptake by SERCA, 2. Increased force of contraction, because more calcium is available for release during the next contraction, and 3. Decreased duration of contraction because of rapid reaccumulation of calcium by sarcoplasmic reticulum.

The features of skeletal muscle, cardiac and smooth muscles are compared in Table 10.7.

Table 10.7: Skeletal muscle, cardiac and smooth muscles compared

Characteristics	Skeletal muscle	Cardiac muscle	Smooth muscle
1. Distribution	Fixed to skeleton	Heart only	Two types: Single and multi
2. Structure	Striated; multi-nucleated; non-syncytial	Striated and branched; single nucleus; syncytial	Unstriated; single nucleus; both synctial and non-syncytial
3. Sarcoplasmic reticulum	Well developed	Well developed	Poorly developed
4. Sarcotubular system	Present at A-I junction	Present at Z-lines	Present but not so characteristic
5. Nerve supply	Via somatic nerve	Via 2 branches of ANS	Via two branches of ANS
6. Control	Voluntary	Involuntary	involuntary
7. Blood supply	3–4 ml/100 gm	80 ml/100 gm/min	1.4 ml/100 gm/min
8. RMP	-90 mV	-80 mV	-55 mV unstable
9. Action potential i. Duration ii. Amplitude	 30-40 msec 120 mV	 250 msec at HR 75 bpm 100 mV	 50 msec 60 mV
10. Absolute refractory period	1–3 msec	180–200 msec	Not defined
11. Phenomenon of tetanus	Present	Not seen	Seen
12. Muscle twitch duration	7.5 msec (fast muscle) 100 msec (slow muscle)	1 1/2 times the total duration of action potential	100 msec
13. Excitation contraction coupling	Rapid process	More rapid process	Very slow process
14. All or none law	Application for single muscle fiber	True for whole of artria or ventricles	True for single muscle fiber
15. Length tension relationship	Maximum active tension at the optimal length	Similar to skeletal muscle	Shows property of plasticity
16. Phenomenon of fatigue	Possible	None	Possible

CLINICAL QUESTIONS

1. **A soldier after death was found in a rigid posture and his limbs could not be disengaged.**
   a. What is the condition called?
   b. What is the cause of the condition?
   c. What is its importance?
2. **A patient came with the complaints of progressive paralysis in muscles. He also had ptosis. On giving injection Neostigmine, patient showed improvement.**
   a. Identify the condition.
   b. What is the cause?
   c. Discuss the action of Neostigmine.
3. **An axon was stimulated with a suprathreshold stimulus within 1 msec and then after 3 msec of firing of the action potential. Response was not observed in the first case but was present in the second case.**
   a. What is this phenomenon known as?
   b. What are the two types?
   c. What is the ionic (molecular) basis of each?
4. **An arrow hit a tourist wandering through the African jungle and he developed skeletal muscle paralysis.**
   a. Which drug may be present in the arrow tip?
   b. What is the mechanism of action of the drug?
5. **A person was brought to the hospital with history of snakebite. On examination patient had ptosis, was unable to lift his neck and his respiratory rate was decreased.**
   a. What is the cause of this condition?
   b. Explain the effects.

Answers for Clinical Questions are given in the Appendix

CHAPTER

11

Central Nervous System

INTRODUCTION

Nervous system is divided into central nervous system and peripheral nervous system. The central nervous system consists of brain and spinal cord. Peripheral nervous consists of the nerves extending outside the CNS. It is divided into somatic and autonomic nervous system.

Brain

The brain has three parts:

1. Forebrain (Prosencephalon) comprises:
   i. Telencephalon—consists of cerebrum and their inter connections.
   ii. Diencephalon—thalamus plus hypothalamus.
2. Midbrain (Mesencephalon)
3. Hindbrain (Rhombencephalon) comprises:
   i. Pons
   ii. Medulla oblongata
   iii. Cerebellum.

Spinal Cord

Spinal cord lies in the spinal canal and ends at the lower border of the first lumbar vertebra. The lowermost three segments of the spinal cord (S3, 4, 5) are known anatomically as the conus medullaris, while the above four segments (L4, 5, S1, 2) are known anatomically as epiconus. It is formed of gray matter (cells) surrounded by white matter. In a transverse section, the gray matter resembles the letter H (2 anterior and 2 posterior horns). The white matter contains ascending and descending nerve fibers arranged into tracts.

A cross-section of spinal cord (Fig. 11.1) shows the following structures: (a) Anterior median fissure, (b) Posterior median fissure, (c) Central canal, (d) Anterior horn, (e) Posterior horn, (f) Anterior gray commissure, (g) Posterior gray commissure, (h) Anterior white column, (i) Posterior white column, (j) Lateral white column.

SYNAPSE

Information about external environment is sensed by receptors which acts as transducer. They convert sensations to action potential which travel via nerve fibers to the center. Hence, there is a series of nerve fiber to the center. The junction between different neuron is known as synapse. It may be a junction between:

- Two neurons
- Neuron and a muscle
- Neuron with different glands of the body.

Terminal part of axon (which is involved in the formation of synapses) is divided into several terminal branches and each terminal branch has an enlargement at the end called synaptic knob. These synaptic knobs contain synaptic vesicles (presynaptic vesicles) containing a chemical transmitter (neurotransmitter). The part of cell membrane of axon of presynaptic neuron which is involved in formation of synapse is called presynaptic membrane. Similarly, part of cell membrane of postsynaptic neuron at synapse is called postsynaptic membrane. The presynaptic membrane (presynaptic terminal) is separated from the postsynaptic membrane by a space called synaptic cleft, which is 20–50 nm wide. The postsynaptic membrane contains appropriate receptors for the chemical transmitter present in presynaptic vesicle.

Types of Synapse (Fig. 11.2A)

- Axodendritic-axon of one neuron with dendrite of other.
- Axosomatic-axon of one neuron with soma of other.
- Axoaxonal-axon with axon.

Physiological Classification of Synapse (Table 11.1)

- Chemical synapse
- Electrical synapse

Process of Synaptic Transmission

The brief sequence of events at a synapse is as follow (Fig. 11.2B):

- An action potential arrives at the presynaptic nerve terminal and depolarizes presynaptic membrane due to sodium influx.
- When presynaptic membrane depolarizes to –40 to –20 mV, the voltage-gated Ca^{2+} channels in the presynaptic terminal open up, resulting in an influx of free Ca^{2+} into the nerve terminal.

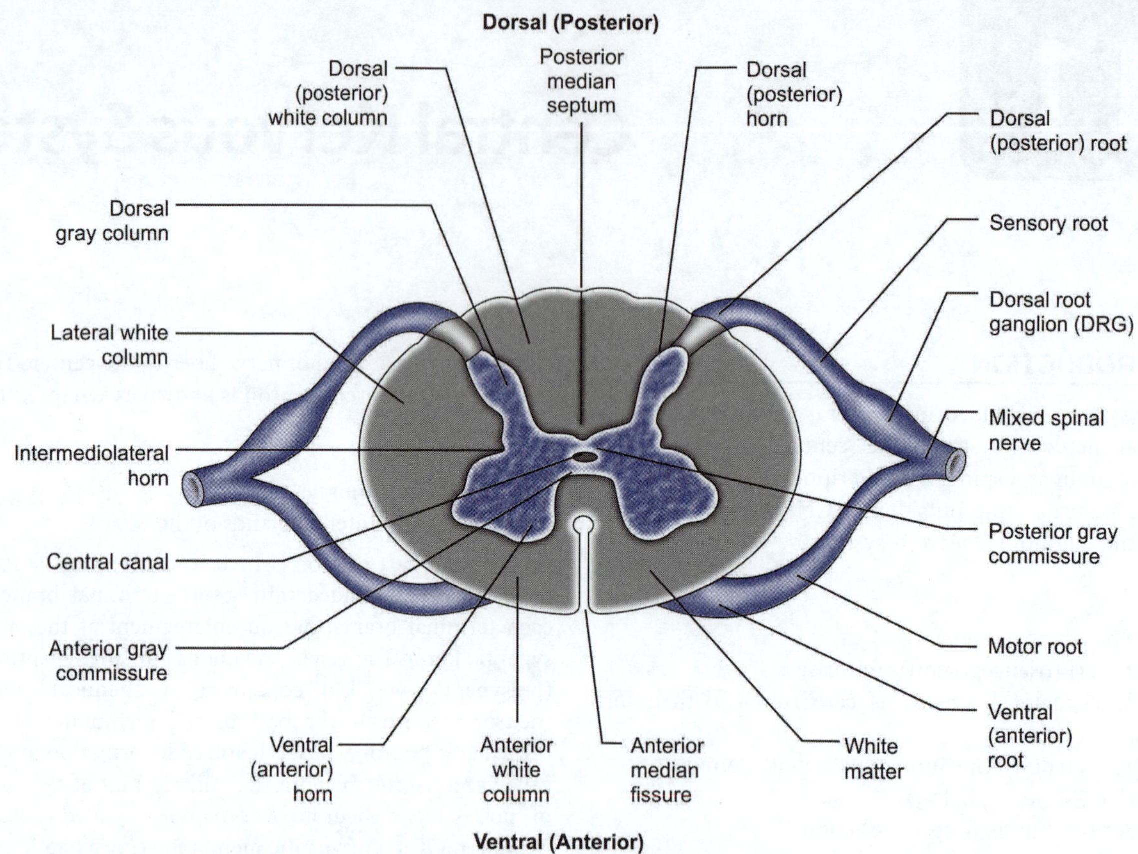

Fig. 11.1: Cross-section of spinal cord

Table 11.1: Difference between chemical and electrical synapse

Chemical synapses	Electrical synapses
1. Transmission of impulses from pre to postsynaptic site occurs due to release of chemical mediators	1. Gap junctions which are formed by the close approximation of pre and postsynaptic membranes act as low resistance bridges through which ions pass easily
2. Seen at most of the synaptic junctions in the nervous system. Unidirectional transmission of signals, i.e. from presynaptic to postsynaptic neuron	2. Seen at some of the synaptic junctions in the nervous system and can transmit signals in either direction, e.g. Lateral vestibular nucleus, cerebral cortex, hippocampus
3. Presence of synaptic cleft	3. Synaptic cleft is replaced by low resistance bridges
4. Synaptic delay present	4. Synaptic delay absent due to low resistance bridges
5. Sensitive to hypoxia	5. Insensitive to hypoxia
6. Infinite processing of information possible as it allows for large number of synapses per neuron and a large variety of neurotransmitters. This is of immense help in the processing of learning and memory	6. Transmission across it is rapid and efficient as there are not too many synapses on the same neuron

- The rise in intracellular Ca^{2+} stimulates exocytosis of neurotransmitter of synaptic vesicle into the synaptic cleft.
- The released neurotransmitter binds to receptors on postsynaptic membrane.
- Binding of neurotransmitter on postsynaptic membrane receptors opens up the ion channels, and depending upon the type of neurotransmitter and synapse, postsynaptic membrane becomes depolarized or hyperpolarized. If the depolarization reaches to threshold level, action potential is developed which gets transmitted along the axon of postsynaptic neuron.

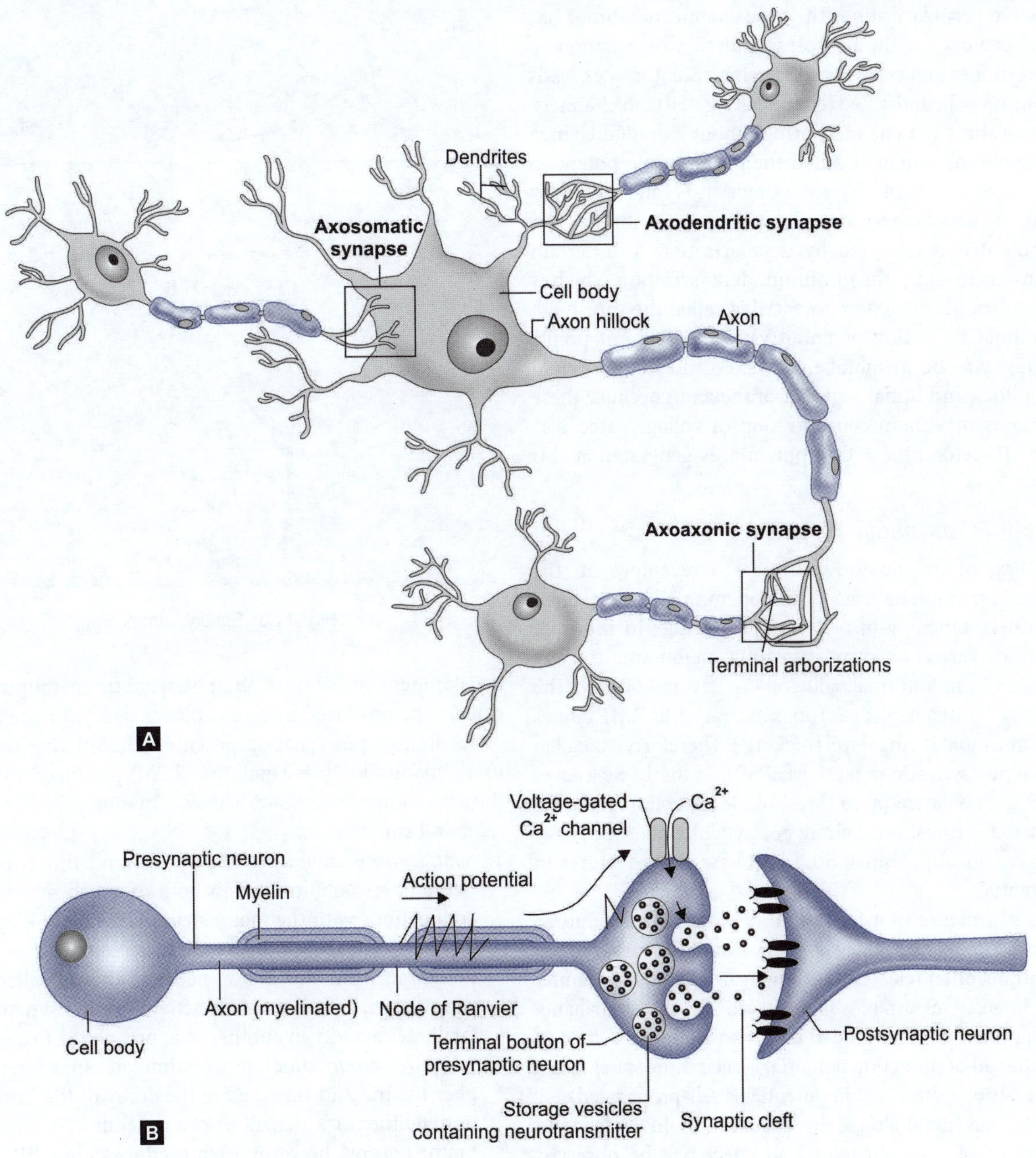

Figs 11.2A and B: **A.** Types of synapse; **B.** Chemical transmission at synapse

- The neurotransmitter released is cleared from the synaptic cleft quickly through reuptake into presynaptic terminals (most common), rapid enzymatic degradation or quick diffusion away from the synaptic cleft.

Time taken for the impulse to cross the synapses is called synaptic delay, i.e. the interval between the arrival of impulse at presynaptic terminal and development of potential in post-synaptic membrane. It is due to the time required for the release and action of the chemical transmitter. At a synapse, the synaptic delay is approximately 0.5 ms. Therefore, number of neurons (synapses) involved in a reflex action can be calculated from the latency of response because at each synapse the latency would increase by 0.5 ms.

Electrical Events at Synapses

Single stimulus applied to the sensory nerves, does not lead to the formation of a propagated action potential. In a postsynaptic neuron, rather it produces a transient partial depolarization or a transient hyperpolarization. The postsynaptic membrane has specific receptors for the neurotransmitter. Combination of neurotransmitter molecules with specific receptor sites leads to opening up of ligand-gated (chemically-gated) ion channels. Opening of these ion channels brings about a graded change in the membrane potential called the postsynaptic potential. If the summated postsynaptic potential is an excitatory potential, it depolarizes the postsynaptic membrane. An action potential is triggered by depolarization of a certain minimum magnitude. The minimum depolarization which is essential to trigger an action potential is called the threshold. The threshold for action potential varies at different points on the postsynaptic membrane. The site of lowest threshold is axon hillock and initial segment of the axon because these area contains maximum concentration of voltage gated Na^+ channels. Therefore, the action potential is generated at this area.

Excitatory Postsynaptic Potential

The binding of the neurotransmitter to receptors on the postsynaptic membrane triggers the opening of ligand-gated Na^+ channels. Opening of Na^+ channels results in influx of Na^+ and depolarization of postsynaptic membrane, e.g. say RMP comes from a normal value of –70 mV to –60 mV. The excitability of postsynaptic neuron is increased, as RMP comes closer to threshold (firing) level (–55 mV). Therefore, it is called excitatory postsynaptic potential (EPSP). If the EPSP causes the RMP to depolarize up to threshold level, action potential develops and is transmitted along postsynaptic neuron.

EPSP is a local potential. So, EPSP has all the features of local potential:

- Graded in nature (not follows all or none). Its magnitude depends upon the intensity of stimulus, (amount of neurotransmitter released), i.e. it increases in graded manner if the intensity of stimulus is increased. On the other hand, action potential is not-graded and is an all or none change, i.e. either all of the action potential is seen or not at all.
- Not self-propagated (action potential is self-propagated).
- May or may not followed by an effect: If EPSP leads to generation of action potential an effect will be observed (e.g. contraction of a muscle). If EPSP does not shoot up to firing (threshold level), no action potential develops and no effect is seen. On the other hand, action potential once developed always has an effect.

Ionic Basis of Development of EPSP

AP come → Synaptic transmitter released → Synaptic transmitter combines with the receptors of postsynaptic membrane and this combining causes opening of Na^+ Ca^{2+} ion channels in the postsynaptic membrane → entry of Na^+ and other cations inside the cell from the ECF → hypopolarization and development of EPSP in the postsynaptic membrane. EPSP can also be produced by agents that close K^+ channels.

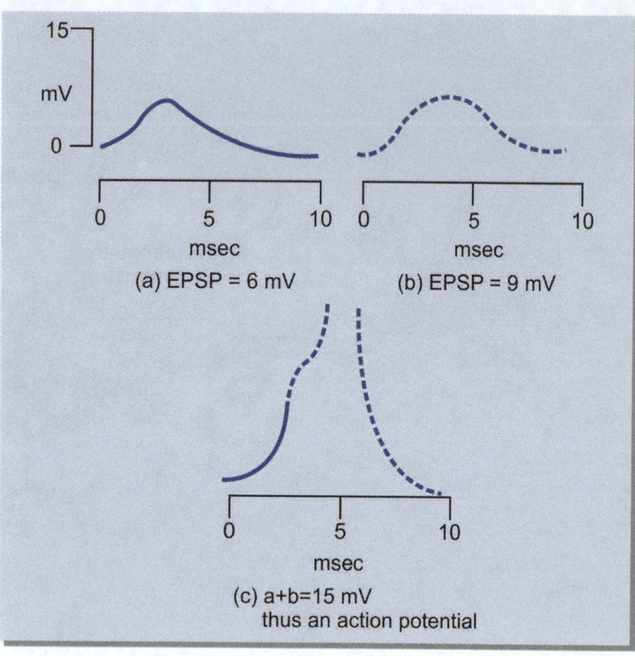

Fig. 11.3: Spatial summation

Excitatory postsynaptic potential (EPSP) due to activity in 1 synaptic knob is small, but EPSP produced by each of the active knobs summate. This summation may be spatial or temporal summation.

1. *Spatial summation (Fig. 11.3):* On stimulating two afferent nerve fibers simultaneously, both of which make synaptic connections with the motor neuron, their EPSP's get summated to the critical level and thus may produce a 'spike' discharge from the motor neuron. This is called spatial summation. In other words activity in one synaptic knob facilitates activity in another to approach the firing level.
2. *Temporal summation:* If we stimulate an afferent nerve fiber for the 2nd time before the decay of the 1st stimulation, neither of which alone can generate a 'spike' from the motor neuron; however, each produces some EPSP which get summated to the critical level necessary for the initiation of a 'spike' potential. This is called temporal summation (Fig. 11.4).

Inhibitory Postsynaptic Potential

Sometimes the combination of chemical transmitter (like GABA, Glycine in brainstem and spinal cord) with the receptor makes the postsynaptic membrane hyperpolarized (For example, the RMP of –80 mV becomes –90 mV). This difference (–10 mV in this case) is called inhibitory postsynaptic potential (IPSP). The excitability of postsynaptic

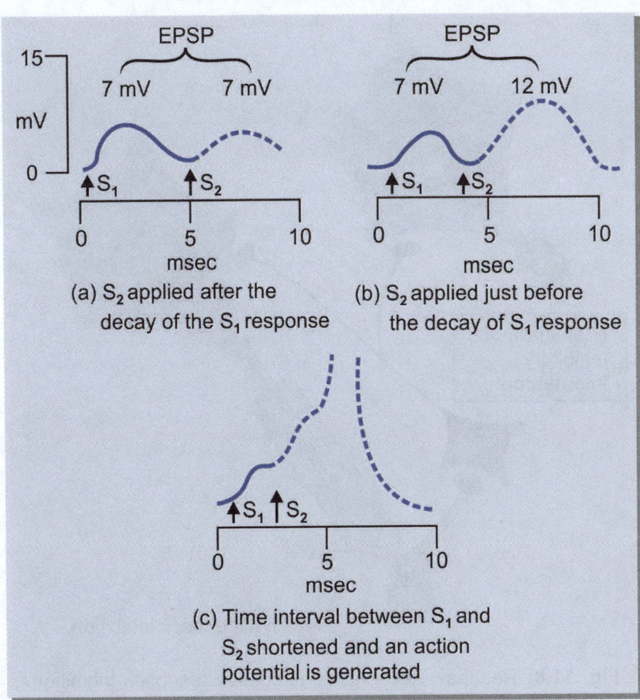

Fig. 11.4: Temporal summation

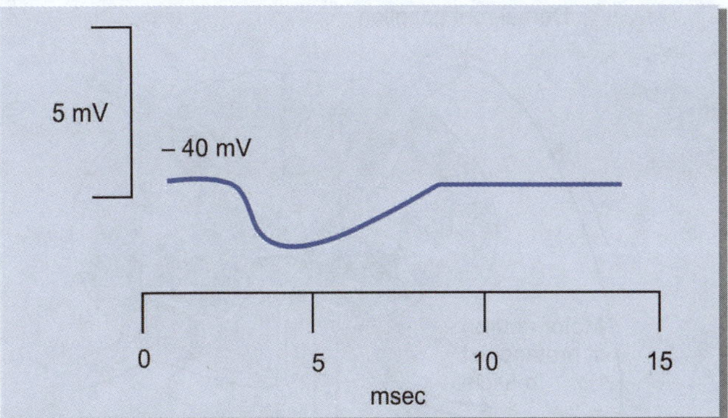

Fig. 11.5: Inhibitory postsynaptic potential

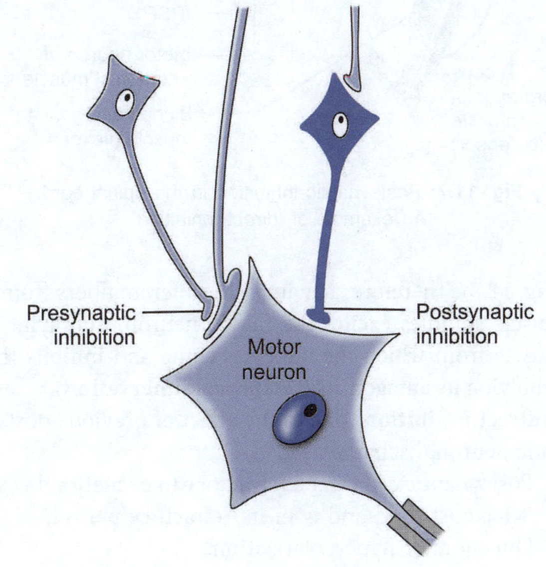

Fig. 11.6: Presynaptic and postsynaptic inhibition

neuron is reduced, as RMP moves away from firing (threshold) level. Therefore, it is called inhibitory postsynaptic potential. IPSP is also a local potential with all features of local potential. Besides opening of ligand-gated Cl^- channels, IPSP can also be produced by opening of ligand-gated K^+ channels which causes efflux of K^+ and hyperpolarization. Hyperpolarization begins at 1–1.5 msec after the entry of afferent impulse into the spinal cord and rises to peak in 1–5 -2 msec after its onset and declines exponentially with a time constant (time to decay to 1/e, or 1/2.718 of maximum) of about 3 msec. During this potential, the excitability of the neuron to other stimuli is decreased; consequently, it is called an IPSP.

Ionic Basis of Development of IPSP

Inhibitory postsynaptic potential (Fig. 11.5) is due to inhibitory chemical transmitter liberated on the subsynaptic membrane, therefore it becomes permeable to K^+ and Cl^- but retains a high degree of impermeability to Na^+. This results in hyperpolarization of the whole postsynaptic membrane. IPSPs can also be produced by opening of K^+ channels, with movement of K^+ out of the postsynaptic cell. In addition, they can be produced by closure of Na^+ or Ca^{2+} channels.

Synaptic Inhibition

The transmission at synapses can be inhibited by naturally existing mechanism. It is of two types: postsynaptic and presynaptic (Fig. 11.6).

Postsynaptic Inhibition

It depends upon the delivery of an inhibitory chemical by the incoming axons which hyperpolarize the subsynaptic membrane. It is subdivided into direct and indirect inhibition:

- **Direct inhibition (by development of IPSP):** Afferent fibers from muscle spindle (stretch receptors) in skeletal muscle are known to pass directly to the spinal motor neuron of the motor unit supplying the same muscle. Impulses in this afferent supply cause EPSP which summate to produce propagated response in postsynaptic motor neurons. At the same time, IPSP's are produced in motor neurons supplying the antagonist muscles. This later response is mediated by branches of afferent fibers that end on golgi bottle neurons. These interneurons, in turn, secrete the inhibitory transmitter glycine at synapses on the proximal dendrites or cell bodies of the motor neurons that supply the antagonist

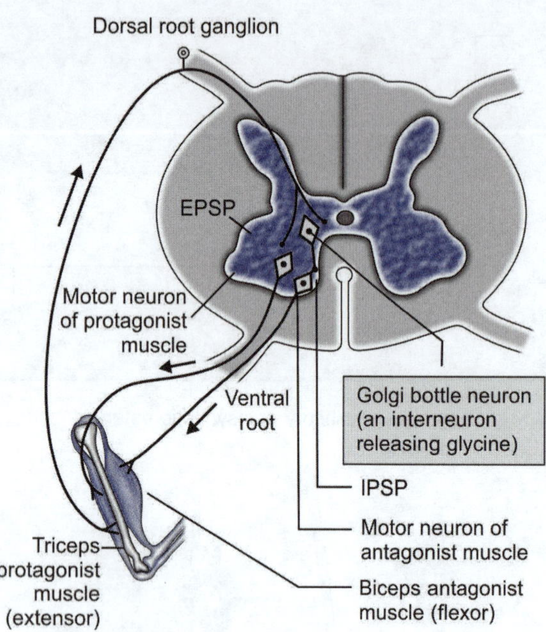

Fig. 11.7: Postsynaptic inhibition in the spinal cord: An example of 'direct inhibition'

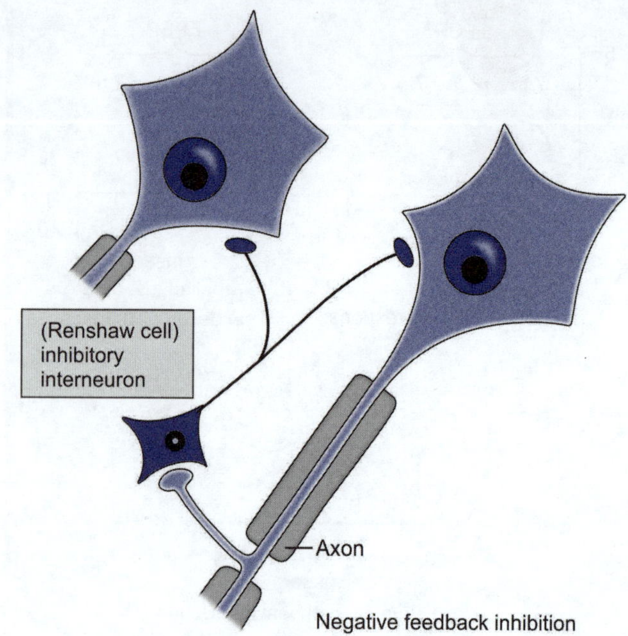

Fig. 11.8: Renshaw cell inhibition/negative feedback inhibition

(Fig. 11.7). Therefore, activity in the afferent fibers from the muscle spindles excites the motor neurons supplying the muscle from which the impulses come and inhibits those supplying its antagonists **(reciprocal innervation)**.

- **Indirect inhibition** (due to the effect of previous postsynaptic neuron discharge), e.g.
  - Postsynaptic cell can be refractory to excitation because it has just fired and is in its refractory period.
  - During after hyperpolarization.
  - Renshaw cell inhibition or negative feedback inhibition.

Renshaw Cell Inhibition

In this inhibition, motor nerve gives off some collateral branches as they traverse the spinal cord towards the ventral root and these collaterals make excitory synaptic connections with interneurons, called Renshaw cell situated in the ventromedial part of ventral horn (Fig. 11.8). These Renshaw cell in turn send axons which make inhibitory synaptic connections with the motor neurons. Renshaw cell are stimulated by ACh.

Presynaptic Inhibition

This type of inhibition occurs at the presynaptic terminals before the signal ever reaches the synapse. Presynaptic inhibition occurs because of failure of the release of excitatory neurotransmitter substance from the presynaptic axon terminal. This occurs in synapses where an inhibitory neuron (C in Fig. 11.9) synapses with the afferent fibers of an excitatory neuron (A in Fig. 11.9) before the later synapses with the efferent neuron (B in Fig. 11.9). In other words the presynaptic inhibition occurs because of axo-axonal synapse.

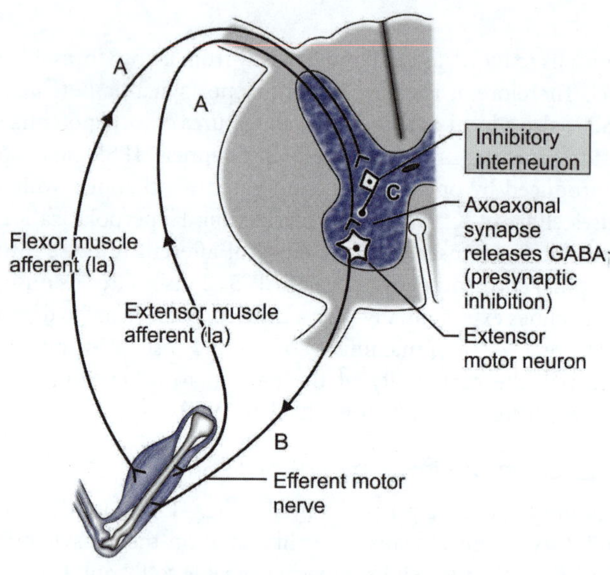

Fig. 11.9: Presynaptic inhibition

Activation of presynaptic receptors reduces the opening of Ca^{2+} channels directly or increases Cl^- and or K^+ conductance (which indirectly reduces Ca^{2+} entry), and this decrease the size of the action potential reaching the excitatory ending. So the amount of excitatory transmitter released is reduced. The inhibitory transmitter at the axo-axonal synapse is GABA. Acting via GABA A receptors, it increases Cl^- conductance, whereas GABA B receptors via G protein, produces an increase in K^+ conductance. Other transmitters also mediate presynaptic inhibition by G protein-mediated effects on Ca^{2+} channels and K^+ channels.

Note

1. Presynaptic facilitation is produced when the action potential is prolonged and the Ca^{2+} channels are open for a longer period. Therefore, repolarization gets delayed, allowing depolarization to continue. It is mediated by serotonin (Serotonin released at an axo-axonal ending increases intraneuronal cAMP levels, and the resulting phosphorylation of one group of K^+ channels closes the channels, slowing repolarization and prolonging the action potential).
2. *Feed forward inhibition:* It is seen in cerebellum. In this type of inhibition a neuron is connected through two pathways: One excitatory and other inhibitory. For example, in cerebellum the stimulation of Basket cells (BC in Fig. 11.10) produces IPSPs in the Purkinje cells (PC in Fig. 11.10). However, the basket cells and the Purkinje cells are excited by the same parallel-fiber excitatory input. This arrangement is called feed forward inhibition and helps to prevent the duration of the excitation produced by any given afferent impulse.

Properties of Synapse

1. *Convergence and divergence:* Many presynaptic neurons meet on a common focus on any single postsynaptic membrane called convergence. For example in spinal motor neuron, some inputs come directly from the dorsal root, some from the long descending spinal tracts, and many from interneurons.

   The axon of most presynaptic neurons divide into many branches that separate out in different direction to end on many postsynaptic neurons called divergence.
2. *One way conduction:* Synapses permits conduction of impulses in one direction only, i.e. from the presynaptic to postsynaptic neuron. This is because the chemical mediator at the synaptic junction is located in the synaptic knob of the presynaptic fibers but not in the postsynaptic membrane.
3. *Synaptic delay:* When an impulse reaches the presynaptic terminals, there is a gap of about 0.5 msec before a response is obtained in the postsynaptic neuron called synaptic delay. This is due to the time it takes for the synaptic mediator to be released and to act on the postsynaptic membrane.

   Significance

   a. Conduction along a chain of neurons is slow if there are many synapse in the chain.
   b. It is possible to determine whether a given synapse is mono or polysynaptic.
4. *Synaptic fatigue/Habituation:* Repeated stimulation of presynaptic neuron lead to gradual decrease and finally disappearance of the postsynaptic response, e.g. epilepsy
5. *Summation (Fig. 11.11):* Hypothetic nerve neuron A and B converge on X.B diverges on X and Y.A stimulus applied to A or B will set-up an EPSP in X.
   - If A and B are stimulated at the same time, two areas of depolarization will be produced in X and their action will sum up called spatial summation.

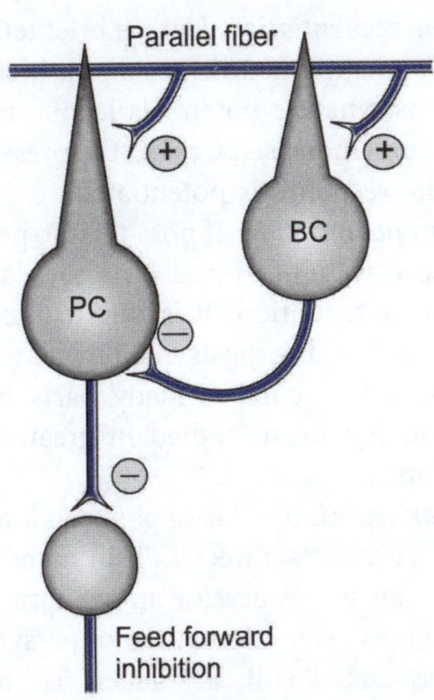

Fig. 11.10: Feed forward inhibition

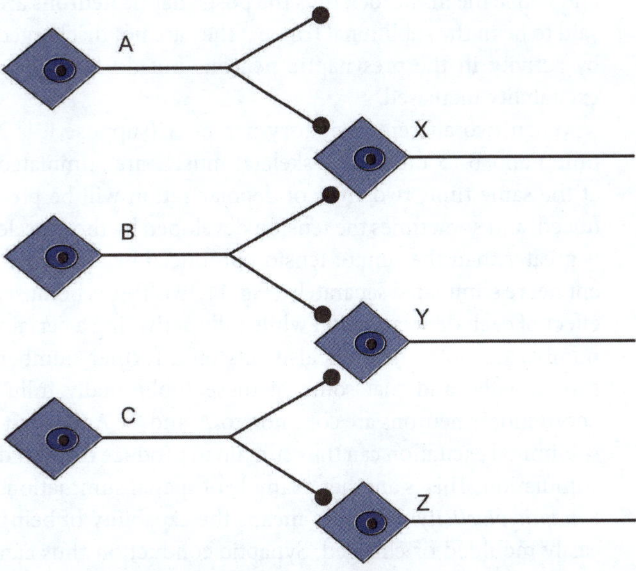

Fig. 11.11: Summation

PHYSICON—The Reliable Icon in Physiology

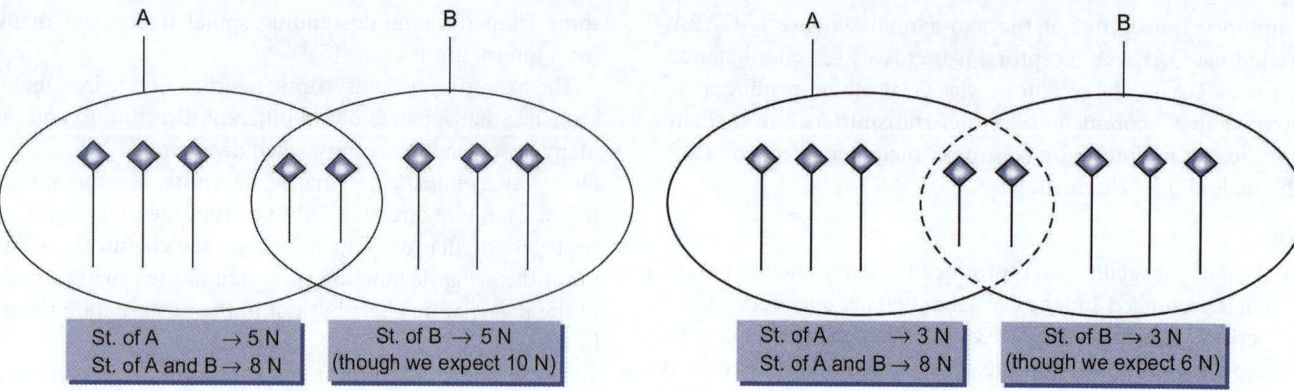

Fig. 11.12: Occlusion

Fig. 11.13: Subliminal fringe

- If neuron B is stimulated repeatedly, X and Y will discharge called temporal summation.

6. *Occlusion (Fig. 11.12):* When two afferent nerves A (suppose it is 5 units) and B (5 units) to a skeletal muscle are simultaneously stimulated, it is sometimes seen that the tension developed by the muscle under observation is less than the sum of tension produced by each afferent nerve stimulated separately. This phenomenon is called occlusion. This is because some of the motor neurons which are common to both, are excited maximally when either A or B is stimulated separately; they give no greater response when A or B are stimulated together. This decrease in response is due to presynaptic fibers sharing postsynaptic neurons (refer the figure given for summation). Thus, occlusion is due to afferent fibers overlapping in their central distribution.
7. *Subliminal fringe:* Subliminal means below the threshold, and fringe means border, thus the postsynaptic neurons are said to be in the subliminal fringe if they are not discharged by activity in the presynaptic neurons but do have their excitability increased.

   When two afferent excitatory nerves A (suppose it is 3 units) and B (3 units) to a skeletal muscle are stimulated at the same time, two areas of depolarization will be produced, and sometimes the tension developed by the muscle is greater than the sum of tension produced by each afferent nerve stimulated separately (Fig. 11.13). This is because, effect of each depolarization while fully activating a certain number of motor neurons also acts on a further number subliminally; and that some of these subliminally influenced motor neurons are common to 'A' and 'B'. As a result, subliminal excitation can thus sum up to produce threshold stimulation. This is another example of spatial summation.
8. *Synaptic plasticity:* Plasticity means the capability of being easily moulded or changed. Synaptic conduction thus can be increased (strengthened) or decreased (weakened) on the basis of past experience. These changes can be presynaptic or postsynaptic and play an important role in learning and memory. There are five forms of synaptic plasticity (Fig. 11.14):

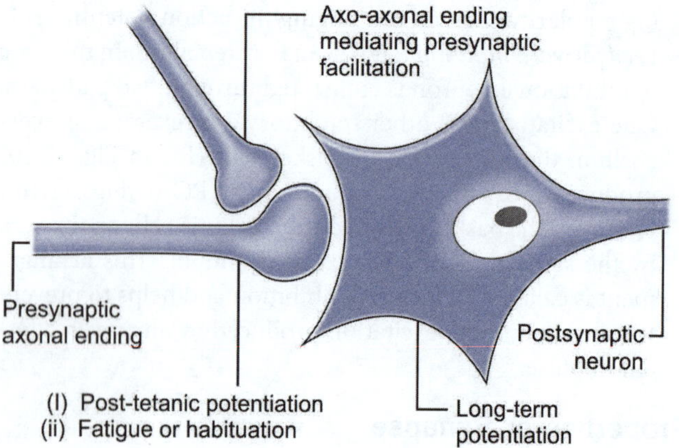

Fig. 11.14: Synaptic plasticity

1. *Post-tetanic potentiation:* Here, a brief tetanizing stimuli in the presynaptic neuron results in increased production of postsynaptic potentials lasting up to 60 sec. It occurs due to increased Ca^{2+} in the presynaptic neuron. Hence, the response is potentiated.
2. *Long-term potentiation:* If post-tetanic potentiation gets much more prolonged and lasts for days, it is called long-term potentiation. It is due to increase in intracellular Ca^{2+} in the postsynaptic neuron rather than presynaptic. It occurs in many parts of the nervous system but has been studied in greatest detail in the hippocampus.
3. *Long-term depression:* It is opposite to long-term potentiation (LTP). It resembles LTP in many ways, but it is characterized by a decrease in synaptic strength. It is produced by slower stimulation of presynaptic neurons and is associated with a smaller rise in intracellular Ca^{2+} than occurs in LTP. This phenomenon commonly occurs in the hippocampus and the cerebellum.

4. *Habituation:* When a same stimulus occurs again and again, the response to stimulus decreases referred to as habituation.
5. *Sensitization:* It is the prolonged occurrence of increased postsynaptic responses after a stimulus (to which an animal is habituated) is paired once or several times with a noxious stimulus. It is due to presynaptic facilitation. Sensitization may occur as a transient response, or if it is reinforced by additional pairings of the noxious stimulus and the initial stimulus. It is due to a Ca^{2+} mediated change in adenylyl cyclase that leads to a greater production of cAMP.

Note

Effect of pH

- *Alkalosis:* When pH is increased the neuronal excitability is markedly elevated.
- *Acidosis:* When pH is decreased the neuronal excitability is decreased. For example in diabetic ketoacidosis neuronal excitability decreases.

RECEPTORS

Receptors (Fig. 11.15) are transducers that converts various forms of energy into action potential and nerve impulses. Sensory system starts with receptors. Information about various internal and external environment reaches nervous system via various receptors. Sensory receptors may be a part of a neuron or a specialized cell that can generate action potential in afferent neuron. Receptors along with the surrounding nonneural cells are called sense organs. Sensory receptors can be divided into:

- *Exteroreceptors:* These provide information about external environment, like touch, pressure, temperature, light, sound, taste, smell etc.
- *Proprioceptors:* These provide information about the position of the body or limbs in the space. They are present in muscle, tendons and joints, and also in the vestibular apparatus.
- *Interoreceptors (visceroreceptors):* They sense the state of the viscera or the internal environment, e.g. receptors sensing BP (baroreceptors), chemoreceptors, osmoreceptors, etc.

There are five basic types of receptors:

1. *Mechanoreceptors:* Mechanical compression and stretching of receptors are detected. For example, tactile receptors, pacinian corpuscles, muscle spindles, Golgi tendon organ, proprioceptors.
2. *Thermoreceptors:* Detect changes in warm and cold temperature.
3. *Nociceptors:* Detect damages occuring in tissues like pain.
4. *Electromagnetic receptors:* For example, rods and cones.

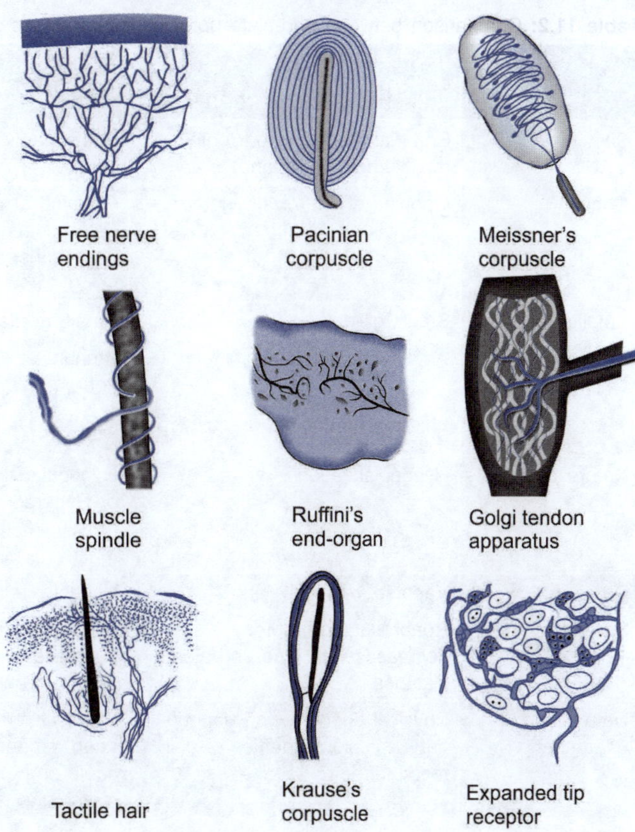

Fig. 11.15: Cutaneous receptors

5. *Chemoreceptors:* For example, taste and smell, carotid body and aortic body, chemoreceptors in hypothalamus, osmoreceptors in hypothalamus.

Properties of Receptors

1. *Adequate stimulus:* Receptors in each of the sense organs are adapted to respond to one particular form of energy (stimulus) at a much lower threshold than other receptors respond to this form of energy which is called adequate stimulus. For example, touch for tactile receptors, light for rods and cones.
2. *Receptor/generator potential:* Whatever be the strength of stimulus that excites the receptor, its immediate effect is to change the membrane electrical potential of the receptor. The receptor converts mechanical energy into electrical response called sensory transduction.

   Small depolarizing potential developed in receptors is called receptor/generator potential. It is a nonpropagated local graded potential, i.e. magnitude is proportionate to the strength of stimulus (does not obey all or none law). It depolarizes the nerve at 1st node of Ranvier. Once the firing level is reached, an action potential is developed and

Table 11.2: Comparison between end-plate potential, postsynaptic potential, receptor potential and action potential

	End-plate potential (EPP)	Postsynaptic potential (PSP)	Receptor potential (RP)	Action potential (AP)
Site	End-plate (specialized region on muscle cell membrane)	Postsynaptic membrane	Receptor nerve ending	Axons
Origin	Opening of chemically gated channels by neurotransmitters	Opening of chemically gated channels by neurotransmitters	Opening of ionic channels by adequate stimulus (e.g. touch or temperature)	Suprathreshold depolarization by EPP, PSP, RP or AP in nearby segment of axon
Amplitude	Small, graded	Small, graded	Small, graded	Large, all or none
Determinants of amplitude	Amount of neurotransmitter	Amount of neurotransmitter	Stimulus intensity	Amplitude fixed for a given set of conditions, can vary if the condition change
Nature of signal	Hypopolarization	Hypopolarization (EPSP) or Hyperpolarization (IPSP)	Hypopolarization (Exception-Hyperpolarization occurs in visual receptors)	Hypopolarization
Duration	Variable, relatively long	Variable, relatively long	Variable, relatively long	All or none, short
Spread	Nonpropagated, spread decreases with time and along distance	Nonpropagated spread decreases with time and along distance	Nonpropagated, spread decreases with time and along distance	Propagated with decrement
Nature of phenomenon	Physical phenomenon dependent on cable properties of cell membrane	Physical phenomenon dependent on cable properties of cell membrane	Physical phenomenon dependent on cable properties of cell membrane	Uniquely biological phenomenon

is propagated. If the receptor potential is great enough, the neuron fires again and again as soon as it repoarizes and it continues to fire as long as the generator potential is at the threshold level of excitation. Thus, the node converts graded response of receptor potential into action potential. The frequency of action potential in the sensory nerve is proportionate to the strength of stimulus (Table 11.2).

Mechanism of Generation

The basic cause of receptor potential is change in membrane permeability. This is explained below by taking the case of pacinian corpuscle. In pacinian corpuscle the central fibers are surrounded by capsule of multiple layer of connective tissue. Compression anywhere in capsule deform the membrane of nerve fiber. Tip of nerve which is inside the capsule is demyelinated. 1st node of Ranvier is inside the capsule.

Ionic Basis

Compression on the capsule → nerve endings deformed → sodium channels open → depolarization → receptor potential generated → action potential at 1st node of ranvier → propagated along sensory nerve fibers.

3. *Adaptation:* When a sustained stimulus of constant strength is applied, the frequency of action potential in its sensory nerve declines gradually. Based on degree, there are two types of adaptations:

   Rapidly adapting. For example, touch receptors.

   Slowly adapting. For example, pain receptors, chemoreceptors, baroreceptors, stretch receptors.

4. *Intensity discrimination/Sensory coding:* Information about intensity of stimulus (e.g. whether touch is fine or crude) to brain is transmitted by two mechanisms:
   a. By variation in frequency of action potential generated in the sensory nerve. This depends on the magnitude of receptor potential. As receptor potential increases, frequency of action potential increases.
   b. By variation in number of receptors stimulated.

   According to **Weber-Fechner law**, magnitude of sensation (S) felt is proportional to the logarithm of intensity (I) of stimulus.

   $S = k \log I + C$, where k and C are constants.

5. *Labelled line principle:* In the normal course, a touch or pain or temperature receptor is connected to a specific series of neurons which carry the message up to the cerebral cortex where it is interpreted. It is interesting to question whether the perceived modality of a stimulus depends on the receptor, or on the pathway through which it travels. But the modality actually depends upon the pathway. To understand better let as consider an example (though impractical), if the retina where connected to the auditory nerve, stimulation of the retina by light would evoke a

sensation of sound. That is, we would be able to 'hear a torch'. This concept of the modality being dependent on the pathway has been termed as the labelled line principle. That is the pathways (or lines) are labelled as touch lines, temperature lines, etc. Thus, a labelled line sensory channel consists of a set of neurons devoted to carry particular sensory modality.

6. *Muller's doctrine of specific nerve energy:* Nerve fibers transmit only nerve impulse or action potential, but we experience different sensations. For example, the action potential produced in a nerve fiber from a thermoreceptor is identical to that produced in a tactile receptor. There are separate pathway for each sensation. Each nerve tract terminate at a specific point in CNS. The type of sensation felt when nerve fiber is stimulated is determined by the point in the nervous system (cortex), where the fibers ends. When the nerve pathway from a particular sense organ is stimulated, the sensation is produced for which the receptor is specialized, no mattter how or where along the pathway it is stimulated. This principle is called Muller's doctrine of specific nerve energy. For example if the sensory nerve from a pacinian corpuscle in the hand is stimulated by pressure at the elbow or by irritation from a tumor in the brachial plexus,the sensation evoked is touch.
7. *Law of projection:* If we stimulate anywhere in the pathway, the sensation produced is projected to the area where receptors are located. This explains the phantom limb phenomenon.

Phantom Limb

If a person's limb is amputated, ends of nerve cut at the time of amputation form nerve tangles or neuromas. These are hypersensitive. These neuromas are stimulated with minimum stimulus or discharge spontaneously. This generates impulses in nerve fiber that previously came from the receptors in the removed limb and the sensation produced are projected to where the receptors used to be located.

REFLEXES

Reflex is an involuntary (automatic) response to a stimulus. It depends on integrity of reflex pathway, i.e. the reflex arc. Here, a sensory impulse is automatically converted into a motor effect through the involvement of central nervous system. When a person walks bare footed and he steps over a thorn he withdraws his affected limb while extends his other limb (to support the body weight), the whole action is reflex and does not require the presence of will.

Reflex Arc

It consist of a receptor, an afferent neuron, an efferent neuron and an effector organ (Fig. 11.16). The number of synapses

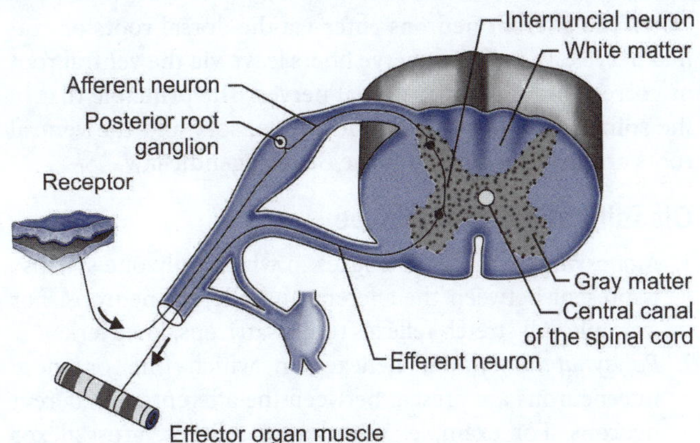

Fig. 11.16: Reflex arc

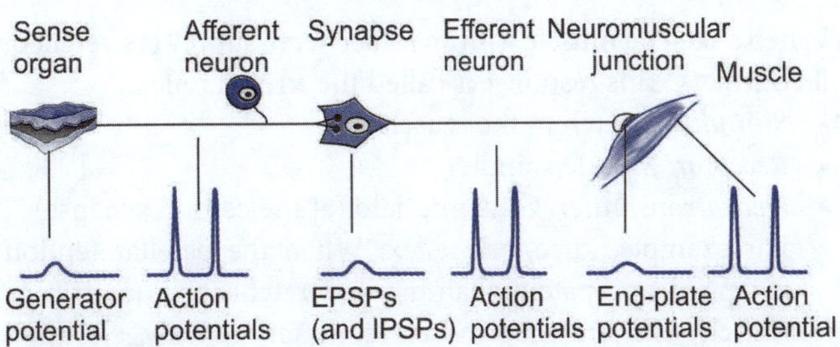

Fig. 11.17: Relative strength of various potentials

(connection between afferent and efferent neurons) vary from one to many hundred. These synapses are located in the brain or spinal cord.

Activity in the reflex arc starts in a sensory receptor with a receptor potential, which is a nonpropagated graded response whose magnitude is proportionate to the strength of the stimulus. This generates all-or-none action potentials in the afferent nerve, the number of action potentials being proportionate to the size of the generator potential. In the CNS, the responses are again graded in terms of EPSPs and IPSPs at the synaptic junctions. All-or-none responses are generated in the efferent nerve. When these reach the effector, they again set up a graded response (end-plate potential). When the effector is smooth muscle, responses summate to produce action potentials in the smooth muscle, but when the effector is skeletal muscle, the graded response is always adequate to produce action potentials that bring about muscle contraction (Fig. 11.17).

From above it is clear that in the portions of the arc specialized for transmission (afferent and efferent axons, muscle membrane), the responses are all-or-none action potentials. It should be emphasized that the connection between the afferent and efferent neurons is usually in the CNS, and activity in the reflex arc is modified by the multiple inputs converging on the efferent neurons.

Note: The afferent neurons enter via the dorsal roots or cranial nerves. The efferent nerve fibers leave via the ventral root or corresponding motor cranial nerves. The principle that in the spinal cord, the dorsal roots are sensory and the ventral roots are motor is known as the Bell-Magendie law.

Classification of Reflexes

1. *Monosynaptic reflexes:* Reflexes in which only one synapse is present between the afferent and efferent neurons. For example, All stretch reflexes (biceps, triceps, knee jerks).
2. *Polysynaptic reflexes:* Reflexes in which one or more interneurons are present between the afferent and efferent neurons. For example, Withdrawal reflexes, gross flexor reflex, gross extensor reflex.

Monosynaptic Reflexes (Stretch Reflexes)

When a skeletal muscle with an intact nerve supply is stretched, it contracts. This response is called the stretch reflex.

- *Stimulus*: Stretch to the muscle
- *Receptor:* Muscle spindle
- *Neurotransmitter:* Glutamic acid (at the central synapse)
  For example, knee-jerk reflex: When the patellar tendon is tapped by a patellar hammer, it stretches the quadriceps muscle, the stretched muscle contracts reflexly, elevating the leg.
- *Reaction time:* The time between the application of the stimulus and the response is called the reaction time. For example, For knee jerk it is 19–24 msec.
- *Central delay:* It is the time taken for the reflex activity to traverse the spinal cord. The central delay for the knee jerk is 0.6–0.9 msec.
  Since, the minimum synaptic delay is 0.5 sec, therefore only one synapse could have been traversed for this reflex activity, stretch reflexes are thus called monosynaptic reflexes.

Muscle Spindle

Muscle spindles are located within the muscle, intermingled with the muscle fibers. Within the spindle, a few specialized muscle fibers are present. These fibers are called intrafusal fibers (because they are within the spindle), to distinguish them from fibers of muscle itself which are called extrafusal fibers.

1. *Extrafusal fibers:* They are regular contractile units of the muscle.
2. *Intrafusal fibers:* They are muscle fibers in the muscle spindle which is the sense organ for stretch reflex. Each muscle spindle consists of 10 muscle fibers. These fibers are enclosed in a connective tissue capsule. These fibers are more embryonic in character. The fibers in the spindle have less distinct striations than rest of the fibers in spindle. The ends of the capsule of the spindle are attached to the tendons at either end of the muscle (or to sides of extrafusal fibers). Only the ends of intrafusal fibers are contractile. There are two types of intrafusal fibers in mammalian muscle spindles:

Nuclear Bag Fibers

They contain many nuclei in a dilated central area and so called nuclear bag fibers. There are two nuclear bag fibers per muscle spindle. Nuclear bag fibers are of two types:

a. *Nuclear bag fiber-1:* With low level of myosin ATPase activity.
b. *Nuclear bag fiber-2:* With high level of myosin ATPase activity.

Nuclear Chain Fibers

They are thinner and shorter and lacks a definite bag. There are four or more nuclear chain fibers per muscle spindle. Their ends connect to sides of nuclear bag fibers.

Sensory Innervation

Sensory innervations is through group Ia and group II sensory fibers. Sensory nerve (afferent) endings in each spindle are of two types:

1. *Primary (annulospiral) endings:* They are the terminations of rapidly conducting group Ia afferent fibers. One branch of the Ia fibers innervates nuclear bag fiber 1, another branch innervate nuclear bag fiber 2 and nuclear chain fibers.These sensory fibers wrap around the center of nuclear bag and nuclear chain fibers.
2. *Secondary (flower spray ending):* They are the terminations of group II sensory fibers and are located nearer the ends of the intrafusal fibers but only on nuclear chain fibers.

Motor Innervation

Muscle spindle (Fig. 11.18) is the only organ receiving motor innervation. Motor innervation comes from:

i. γ efferents of Leksell (small motor neurons)
   They go exclusively to muscle spindles. The ending of γ efferent fibers are of two types:
   a. Plate ending on nuclear bag fibers (γ_1).
   b. Trail ending on nuclear chain fibers (γ_2).

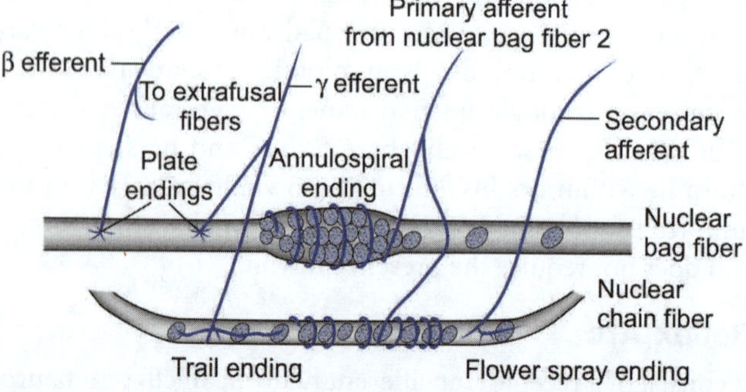

Fig. 11.18: Muscle spindle and its neural connections

ii. β motor neurons (larger motor neurons)
They innervate both intrafusal and extrafusal fibers.

Response of Muscle Spindle to Stretch

Functionally muscle spindle shows two types of responses:

1. *Dynamic (by nuclear bag fibers):* Here primary sensory nerve ending discharge impulse at rapid rate when the muscle is rapidly stretched. They fire less rapidly if stretch is continued. The discharge of impulses start only if there is change in the degree of stretching of muscle. Thus, the response depends upon the rate of change in the length of the muscle.
2. *Static (by nuclear chain fibers):* When stretch is continuing, static responses comes into play. Thus muscle spindle gives response to change in the length of the muscle as well as rate of change in length.

Mechanism of Activation of Muscle Spindle

a. Intrafusal fibers are parallel to extrafusal fibers. When the extrafusal fibers (muscle fibers) are passively stretched, stretch is transmitted to the intrafusal fibers → stimulation of Ia fibers → stimulation of α motor neuron → contraction of extrafusal fibers (stretch reflex) → shortening of muscle belly.
b. Stimulation of γ efferents produces contraction of intrafusal fibers → stretches nuclear bag portion of spindles → stimulation of Ia sensory fibers → stimulation of α motor neuron → contraction of extrafusal fibers (stretch reflex) → shortening of muscle belly.

Thus, the muscle can be made to contract via stimulation of α motor neuron that innervate the extrafusal fibers directly or stimulation of γ motor neurons that initiate contraction indirectly via stretch reflex. Stretching causes contraction of extrafusal fibers and shortening of muscle. Thus, spindle discharge decreases. The spindle and its contraction constitute a feedback circuit thus maintaining the length of the muscle.

Functions

1. *Maintenance of our posture:* Maintaining posture (e.g. standing) or changing the posture are effected by appropriate adjustment of γ motor activities of different groups of muscles.
2. Role of muscle spindle in voluntary motor activity. Normally for initiation of skeletal muscular contraction, stimulation of α motor neurons are neccessary. Along with α motor neuron firing, the γ motor neuron also fire concomitantly, so that a skeletal muscle contraction can be made effective (α - γ linkage).

   Imagine what would have happened if this do not occur: Stimulation of the α motor neuron → initiation of contraction of extrafusal fibers; but this contraction will cause (as there is now a shortening of the extrafusal fibers), relieving of stretch of the nuclear bag region, causing the Ia afferents to stop its discharge. This in turn will lead to lengthening of the extrafusal fibers, i.e. cancellation of the α motor stimulation effect. The concomitant firing of the γ efferent prevents this.
3. *Damping function:* An important function of stretch reflex is its ability to prevent oscillation or jerkiness of body movements. This effect can also be called as signal averaging function of muscle spindle.
4. It plays a role in the maintenance of muscle tone.

Inhibition of Stretch Reflexes

Because of it is monosynaptic pathway, the inhibition of stretch reflexes is produced by pathways that end with inhibition of α-motor neurons. This is brought out by two mechanisms:

Reciprocal Innervation

When stretch reflex occurs, the muscle that antagonizes the action of the muscle involved relaxes, i.e. when the agonist contracts the antagonist is relaxed (Fig. 11.19). This is due to reciprocal innervation.

- Receptor—muscle spindle
- Afferent nerve—Ia
- Center—spinal cord
- Efferent nerve—a motor neuron to antagonist muscle.

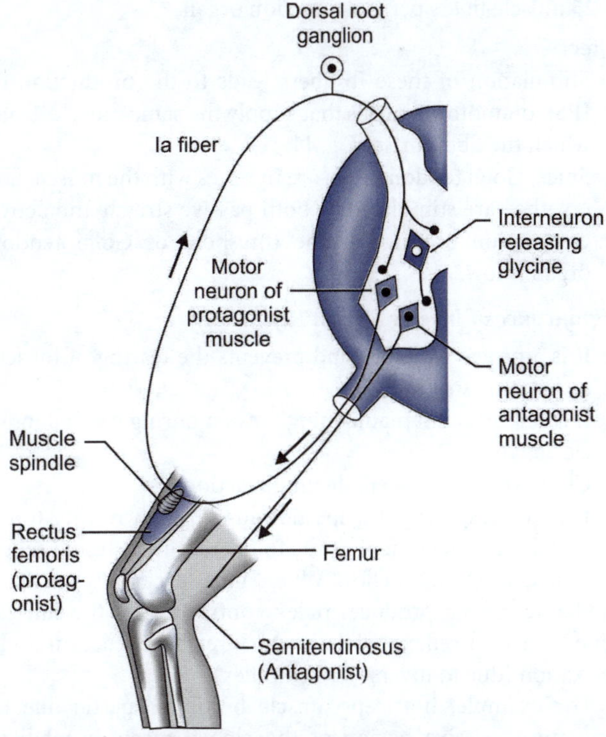

Fig. 11.19: Reciprocal innervation

In the spinal cord a collateral branch from Ia fibers arises. It synapses with an inhibitory interneuron (Golgi bottle neuron) that synapses directly on motor neuron supplying the antagonist muscle. The pathway mediating this effect is bisynaptic, i.e. two synapses are involved. This is an example of postsynaptic inhibition.

Significance

Reciprocal innervation ensures that the movement of the 'agonist' muscle is not obstructed by contraction of the 'antagonist' muscles.

Inverse Stretch Reflex/Autogenic Inhibition

As the strength of the stretch increases, the reflex contraction also increases. But after a certain extent, as the strength of stretch increases contraction ends and muscle relaxes. This relaxation in response to strong stretch is called inverse stretch reflex.

- Receptor—golgi tendon organ.
- Afferent—Ib myelinated nerve fibers
- Center—spinal cord, the Ib fibers end on inhibitory interneurons that inturn end directly on the motor neurons
- Efferent—α motor neurons to muscle fiber.

Golgi Tendon Organ

This organ consists of a net-like collection of knobby nerve endings among the fascicles of a tendon (Fig. 11.20). There are 3–25 muscle fibers per Golgi tendon organ.

Effect

- Stimulation of these Ib fibers leads to the production of IPSP on motor neurons that supply the same muscle, from which the fibers arise (Fig. 11.21).
- Since, Golgi tendon organ are in series with the muscle fibers, they are stimulated by both passive stretch and active contraction of muscle. The threshold of Golgi tendon organ is low.

Significance of Inverse Stretch Reflex

1. It is a protective reflex and prevents the tearing of muscle by extreme stretch.
2. It is important in maintaining tension during normal muscle activity.
3. Clasp-knife effect/Lengthening reaction.

It is the response of a spastic muscle (high resting tone) to stretching or lengthening due to operation of stretch reflex and inverse stretch reflex. When muscles are hypertonic, moderate stretch produces reflex contraction of the muscle (due to stretch reflex), while strong stretch produces muscle relaxation (due to inverse stretch reflex).

For example, if triceps muscle becomes spastic due to any cause, passive flexion of the elbow, meets immediate resistance due to initiation of the stretch reflex in the triceps muscle. Further stretch activates inverse stretch reflex, as a result the resistance to flexion suddenly collapses and arm flexes. However, continued passive flexion stretches the muscle again, and the sequence may be repeated. This sequence of resistance followed by relaxation when a limb is moved passively is known as the clasp-knife effect because of it's resemblance to the closing of a pocket knife. It is known as the lengthening reaction because it is the response of a spastic muscle to lengthening.

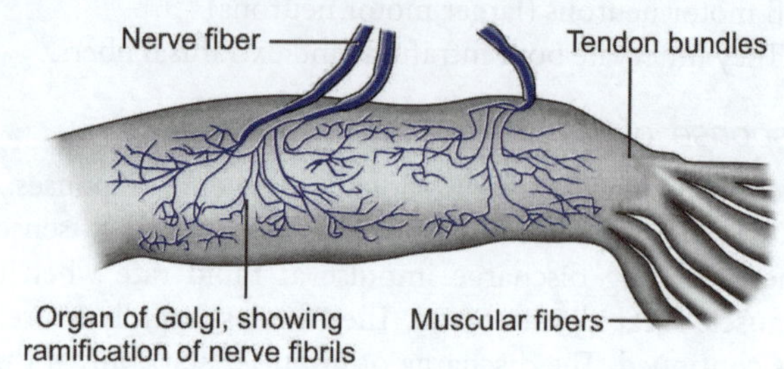

Fig. 11.20: Golgi tendon organ

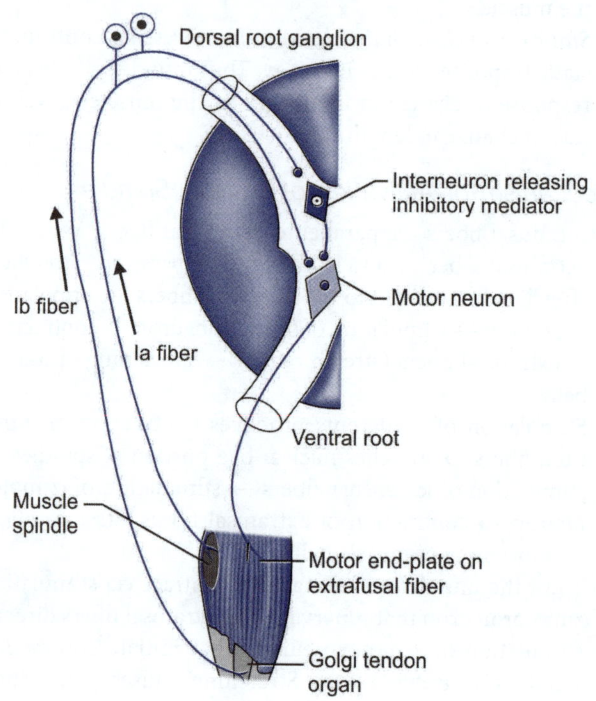

Fig. 11.21: Pathway responsible for stretch and inverse stretch reflex

Polysynaptic Reflexes (Withdrawal Reflexes)

When more than one synapse is involved in the reflex pathway, it is called polysynaptic reflexes (Fig. 11.22). The reflex path branches in a complex fashion. Because of the difference in the

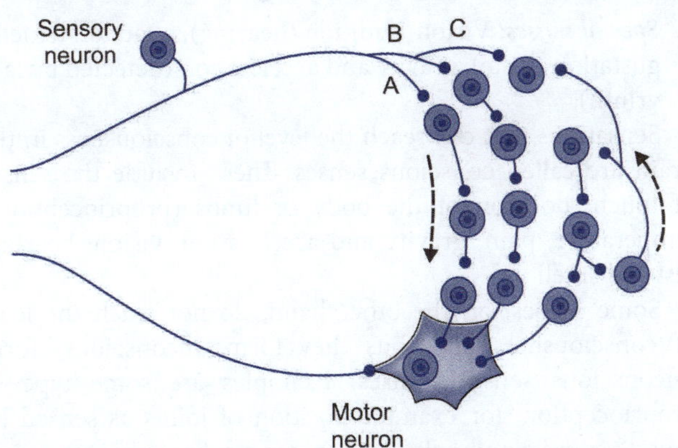

Fig. 11.22: Polysynaptic connections between afferent and efferent neurons in the spinal cord. The dorsal root fiber activates pathway A, pathway B and pathway C. Note that one of the interneurons in pathway C connects to a neuron that doubles back to other interneurons, forming reverberating circuits

number of synapses, the synaptic delay varies. The activity in the branches with fewer synapses reaches the motor neurons first followed by the activity in the longer pathways. This will lead to prolonged response in motor pathways.

Some of the branched pathways turn back on themselves, permitting activity to reverberate until it becomes unable to cause a propagated trans-synaptic response. Such circuits are called reverberating circuits. These are common in brain and spinal cord, e.g. withdrawal reflex.

Withdrawal Reflex

It is a typical polysynaptic reflex.

- *Stimulus:* It occurs in response to a noxius and usually painful stimulation of the skin, subcutaneous tissue or muscle.
- *Response:* Contraction of the flexor and inhibition of extensor.
- *Effect:* The part stimulated is flexed and withdrawn from the stimulus (flexor response).
  If stimulus is still stronger, the response includes flexion and withdrawal of that limb and extension of opposite limb. This is called crossed extensor response (Fig. 11.23).

Mechanism

If the strength of stimulus is more, the excitatory impulse spread up and down the spinal cord to more and more motor units, a phenomenon called irradiation of stimulus and the increase in the total motor units is called recruitment of motor units.

Importance

It is a protective reflex. Flexion of the stimulated limb gets it away from the source of irritation and extension of the other limb supports the body. The pattern assumed by all the 4 limbs

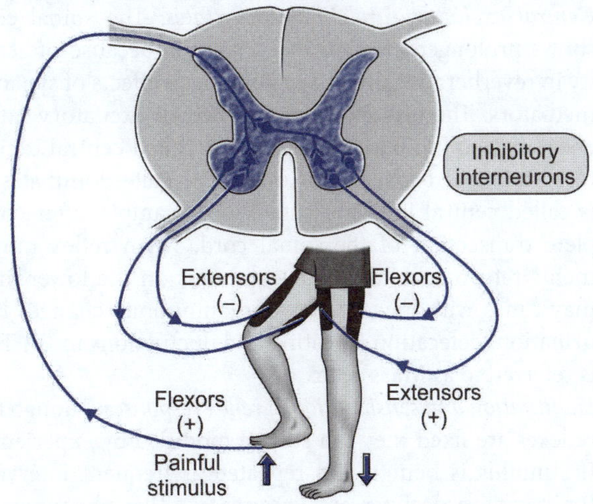

Fig. 11.23: Withdrawal reflex

puts the animal in a position to run away from the offending stimulus.

Characteristic Features

1. Withdrawal reflexes are prepotent, i.e. they prevent the spinal pathways from any other reflex activity taking place at the moment.
2. A weak stimulus causes quick flexion movement whereas a strong stimulus causes prolonged flexion and sometimes a series of flexion movements. The prolonged response is due to prolonged repeated firing of motor neurons. The repeated firing is called after discharge, which is due to continued bombardment of motor neurons by impulses arriving by complicated and circuitous polysynaptic paths (reverberating circuits).
3. *Local sign:* It refers to the ability of the reflex to confine the withdrawal exactly to the portion of the body affected by the noxious stimulus. For example, if the medial surface of the limb is stimulated, the response will include some abduction with flexion, whereas stimulation of the lateral surface will produce some adduction with flexion. This dependence of the exact response on the location of the stimulus is called local sign.

General Properties of Reflexes

1. *Adequate stimulus:* The stimulus that produces a reflex is very precise, as the receptors respond maximally only when an appropriate specific stimulus is applied. It is called adequate stimulus for the particular reflex.
2. *Final common pathway:* The α motor neurons that innervate the extrafusal fibers are the final common pathway over which the neural control system coordinates the activity of skeletal muscle fibers. It serves both as the integrating center and efferent pathway.

3. *Central excitatory and inhibitory states:* The spinal cord shows prolonged changes in excitability because of activity in reverberating circuits or prolonged effects of synaptic mediators. The prolonged state in which excitatory influences exceed inhibitory influences is called central excitatory state and conversely if inhibitory state dominates, it is called central inhibitory state. For example, after complete transection of the spinal cord, when reflex movements return, a mild noxious stimulus on the lower limb may cause withdrawal reflex and autonomic changes like urination, defecation, sweating and fluctuations in BP. This is referred to as **Mass reflex.**
4. *Habituation and sensitization of reflex responses:* Though the reflexes are fixed they can still be modified by experience. If stimulus is benign and repeated at frequent intervals, the response declines and disappears. This phenomenon is called habituation. It is due to synaptic fatigue which is due to exhausation of chemical transmitter, as its synthesis is not as rapid as its release. The decrease in release of neurotransmitter can also be due to gradual inactivation of Ca^{2+} channels at presynaptic terminal. This decreases intracellular Ca^{2+} and release of neurotransmitter.

SENSORY SYSTEM

The sensory system brings information from the periphery to the CNS. Sensory mechanisms within the human nervous system may be classified into two categories:

1. *General senses:* Somesthetic sensations (touch, pressure, pain, temperature, proprioception) and visceral sensations (visceral pain, baroreception, chemoreception).
2. *Special senses:* Vision, audition (hearing), olfaction (smell), gustation (taste), gravity and acceleration (detected by labyrinth).

Sensations that can reach the level of consciousness in the brain are called conscious senses. These include the senses of touch, position of the body or limbs (proprioception), temperature, pain, gravity and acceleration, vision, hearing, test and smell.

Some senses, on the other hand, do not reach the level of consciousness and thus they form unconscious (form unconscious senses) senses. Examples are some type of proprioception, for example position of joints as sensed by muscle spindle and golgi tendon organs, baroreceptor reflex, chemoreceptor reflex, etc.

Sensory Cortex

Both the lemniscal and anterolateral systems ultimately convey impulses to the sensory cortex.

Primary Sensory Area (S1)

1st somatic sensory area, located in postcentral gyrus containing the Brodmann's area 3, 1, 2.

- Area 3-respond to light touch
- Area 1 and 2 respond to deep stimuli such as pressure and joint movement.

It is supplied by afferents from both side of face and opposite side of the body.

Sensory Homunculus

The different areas of body have a topographical representation in the postcentral gyrus. The representation is such that the

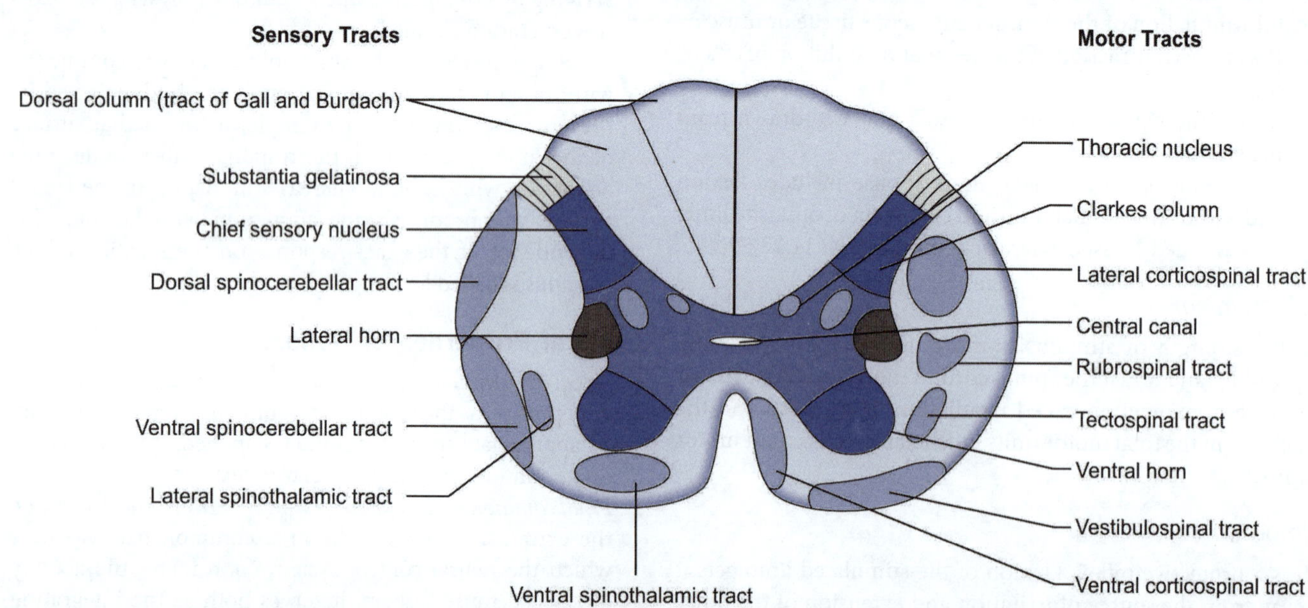

Fig. 11.24: Cross-section of spinal cord showing location of major sensory and motor tract

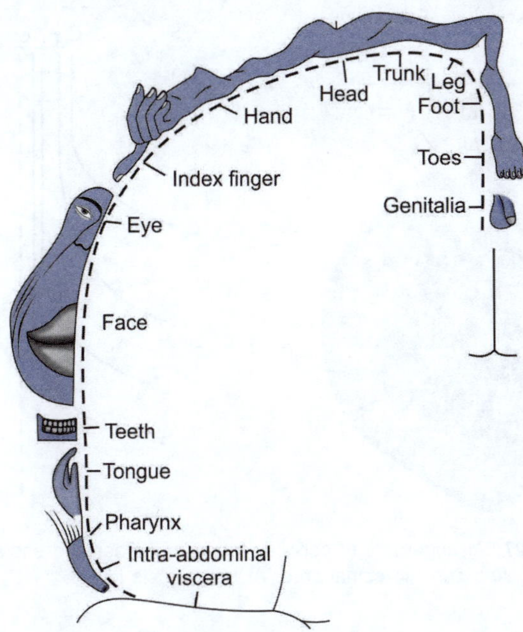

Fig. 11.25: Sensory homunculus

body appears upside down. Thus, foot area occupies the most medial part of the gyrus, (which is on the medial side of the cerebral hemisphere) and face area is situated in lateral part of the gyrus. Tongue occupies a position further down than that of the face. However, the parts of the face are not represented in an inverted manner (Fig. 11.25).

Areas of the body, which are very sensitive (that is, where the population of receptors is very high), occupy a bigger space irrespective of the actual size of the organ. The sensory homunculus represents the opposite half of the body as both the lemniscal and anterolateral system have crossed the midline to end on the opposite half of the cortex.

Functions of S1

Widespread bilateral excision of somatosensory area I causes loss of the following types of sensory judgment:

1. The person is unable to localize discretely the different sensations in the different parts of the body. However, he or she can localize these sensations crudely, such as to a particular hand, to a major level of the body trunk, or to one of the legs. Thus, it is clear that the brainstem, thalamus, or parts of the cerebral cortex not normally considered to be concerned with somatic sensations can perform some degree of localization.
2. The person is unable to judge critical degrees of pressure against the body.
3. The person is unable to judge the weights of objects.
4. The person is unable to judge shapes or forms of objects. This is called astereognosis.
5. The person is unable to judge texture of materials because this type of judgment depends on highly critical sensations caused by movement of the fingers over the surface to be judged.

Clinical Note

Cortical lesions do not abolish all the somatic sensations. Cortical anesthesia mainly involves loss of proprioception and tactile sensations (fine touch, two point discrimination), astereognosis or stereoanesthesia). Pain and temperature are least affected, but they are poorly localized. This is because pain and temperature are primarily appreciated by thalamus, only their localization requires the help of somatosensory area I. For other forms of sensation, like tactile sensations and proprioception, thalamus is unable to analyze the details of sensations.

Secondary Sensory Area (S2)

Located in parietal cortex in lateral cerebral sulcus, removal of it produces deficits in discrimination power.

Plasticity of Sensory Cortex (Cortical Plasticity)

The afferent connections of the sensory cortex can change with extensive use or total disuse of the senses. Extensive or rigorous sensory use of a particular part of the body leads to an increase in the area representation of that part in the sensory cortex. Similarly, if a particular part of body is not used, (e.g. a part of body is ablated), sensory afferents from the neighboring part establish connections with area of the unused part. For example, if a digit is amputated, the cortical representation of the neighboring digits spread into the cortical area that was formerly occupied by the representation of amputated digit. This results in feeling that the sensation (pain) is arising from the amputated digit, when the neighboring digits are stimulate. Cortical plasticity may be one of the theory to explain phantom limb pain.

Ascending (Sensory) Tracts (Fig. 11.24)

1. Tracts in dorsal white column (Medial lemniscal system/ Tract of Gall and Burdach).
   a. Fasciculus gracilis
   b. Fasciculus cuneatus.
2. Tracts in lateral white column
   a. Lateral spinothalamic tract
   b. Dorsal spinocerebellar tract
   c. Ventral spinocerebellar tract.
3. Tract in ventral white column
   a. Ventral spinothalamic tract.

Always for any sensory pathway there are three order neurons:

i. 1st order neuron-from receptors to spinal cord or to medulla (in case of dorsal column pathway).

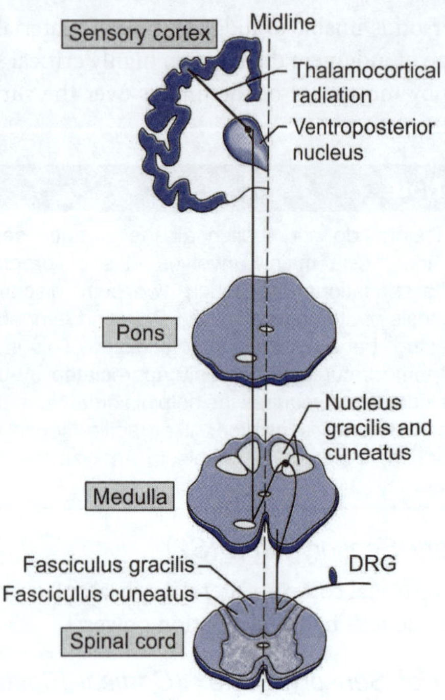

Fig. 11.26: Dorsal or posterior column pathway

ii. 2nd order neuron from the spinal cord or at the level of medulla to thalamus.
iii. 3rd order neuron from thalamus to sensory cortex.

Tracts in Dorsal White Column

It conveys the following information from various part of the body (Fig. 11.26)—fine touch, tactile localization and two point discrimination, pressure, vibration, proprioception, kinesthetic sensation and some unconscious kinesthetic impulses to cerebellum (via external arcuate fibers), some superficial reflexes.

Fine touch pathway

Receptors (for both fine and crude touch)—Meissner's corpuscle, Merkle's corpuscle, Pacinian corpuscle.

1st order neuron

Impulse is carried from receptors to spinal cord (to fasciculus gracilis and cuneatus) by A β fiber. Some touch impulses are also conducted via C fibers. They do not relay there. Fasciculus gracilis receives afferents from lower half (lumbar and sacral segments) (Fig. 11.27). Fasciculus cuneatus receives afferents from upper half (cervical and thoracic segments). Above the midthoracic region the fibers from spinal cord are represented as sacral to cervical segment from medial to lateral in the spinal cord.

Majority of fibers end in medulla in nucleus gracilis and nucleus cuneatus respectively (1st relay station).

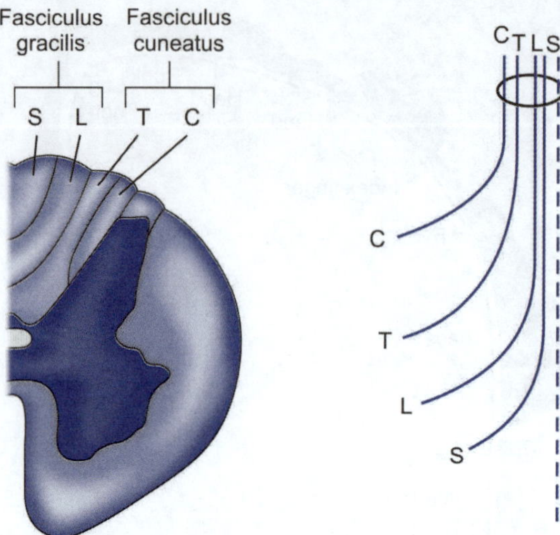

Fig. 11.27: Arrangement of cervical, thoracic, lumbar and sacral fibers in the spinal cord: At Midthoracic level

2nd order neuron

2nd order neuron arise from nucleus gracilis and nucleus cuneatus. They are divided into two groups:

1. External arcuate fibers-dorsal and ventral group
   a. Dorsal fibers via inferior cerebellar peduncle of same side to end in cerebellum
   b. Ventral fibers via opposite side to cerebellum.
2. Internal arcuate fiber-cross to opposite side and pass through midbrain in the medial lemniscus to end in specific relay nuclei of thalamus (ventroposterior nuclei) this forms the 2nd relay station.

3rd order neuron

Axons of 3rd order neurons pass via posterior limb of internal capsule to end in the sensory cortex.

Lateral Spinothalamic Tract

It carries fibers of all types of pain, temperature, itch and tickle sensation.

Pathway of pain

Receptors-free nerve endings.

1st order neuron

Impulse is carried from receptors to spinal cord by:

- *A δ (fast pain):* The neurotransmitter is glutamate.
- *C-slow pain:* The neurotransmitter is substance P.
  On entering the spinal cord pain signal take two pathway to the brain, through:
  i. *Neospinothalamic pathway for fast pain:* A δ terminate mainly in lamina 1 of dorsal horn cells.

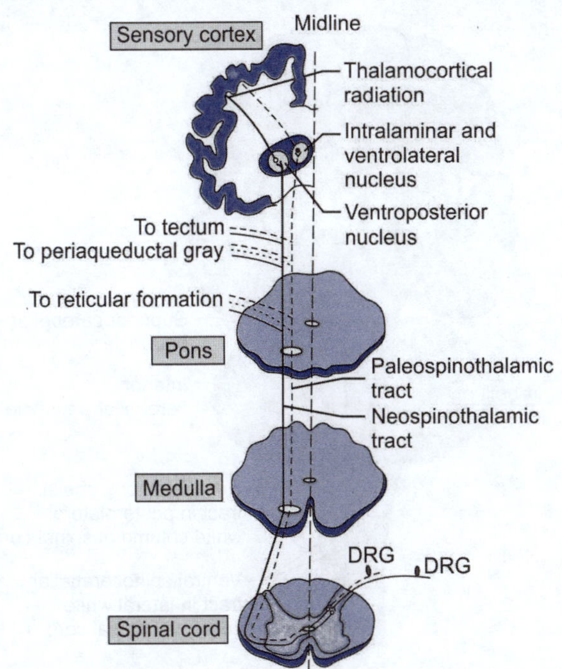

Fig. 11.28: Lateral spinothalamic pathway

ii. *Paleospinothalamic pathway for slow pain:* C fiber terminates on lamina 2 and 3 (lamina 2 and 3 together called as substantia gelatinosa).

2nd order neuron

2nd order neurons arise at the level of spinal cord. Most of axons of 2nd order neurons cross in anterior white commissure obliquely to opposite side of the same segment. They ascend in the lateral spinothalamic tract. Fibers from neospinothalamic tract end in the ventroposterior nuclei of thalamus. Fibers from paleospinothalamic pathway end in intralaminar and ventrolateral nuclei of thalamus (Fig. 11.28).

On their way to thalamus these fibers send collaterals to reticular formation, periaqueductal gray, tectum. Paleospinothalamic fibers give off much more collaterals than the neospinothalamic tract (only 1/10th to 1/4th of the fibers pass to the thalamus).

Axons from the sacral and lumbar segments of body are pushed laterally by axons crossing midline at successive higher levels. Therefore the fibers are represented as cervical to sacral segments from medial to lateral in the spinal cord.

A lesion in cervical region situated close but outside the spinal cord (e.g. tumor) will cause loss of pain sensation in the sacral or lumbar segments as they are most superficial. But sensation of cervical region persists (Fig. 11.29).

3rd order neuron

In thalamus 3rd order neuron starts and ends in sensory cortex.

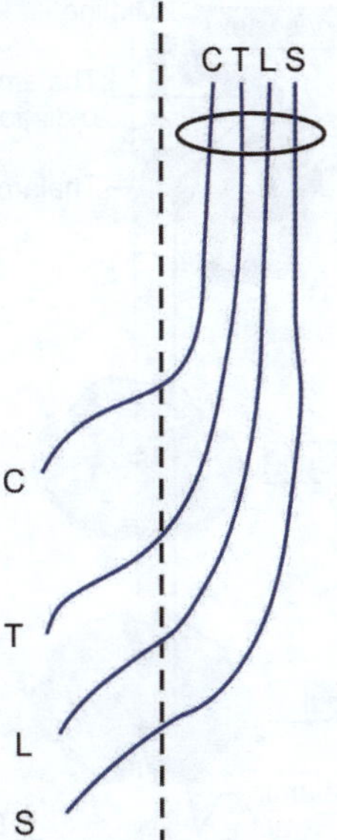

Fig. 11.29: Sacral and lumbar segment pushed laterally by axons crossing midline at successive higher level

Ventral (Anterior) Spinothalamic Tract

It conveys crude touch.

Crude touch pathway

1st order neuron

Impulse is carried from receptors to spinal cord by A β fibers. Some touch impulses are also conducted via C fibers. After entering the spinal cord the fibers end round the cells which are situated at the median part in the dorsal horn (1st relay station), from where 2nd order neuron arises (Fig. 11.30).

2nd order neuron

2nd order neuron cross in anterior white commissure obliquely to opposite side of same segment to end in ventroposterior nucleus of thalamus. Small number of axons of 2nd order neurons are uncrossed and may ascend homolaterally as anterior spinothalamic tract.

While ascending, the ventral spinothalamic tract runs in parallel with the lateral spinothalamic tract and together constitutes the spinal lemniscus or anterolateral system of ascending fibers. At higher brainstem level, this tract sends several collaterals into the reticular formation and tegmentum.

3rd order neuron

In thalamus 3rd order neurons starts and ends in sensory cortex.

Dorsal (Posterior) Spinocerebellar Tract

Functions: It carries 'unconscious' kinesthetic impulses to the cerebellum which are essential for the regulation of body posture.

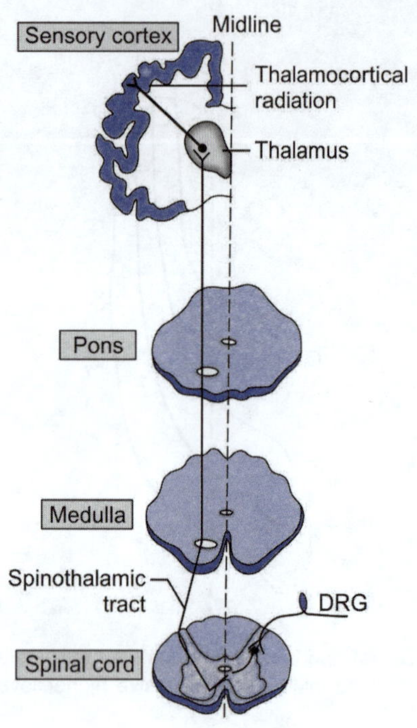

Fig. 11.30: Ventral (anterior) spinothalamic tract

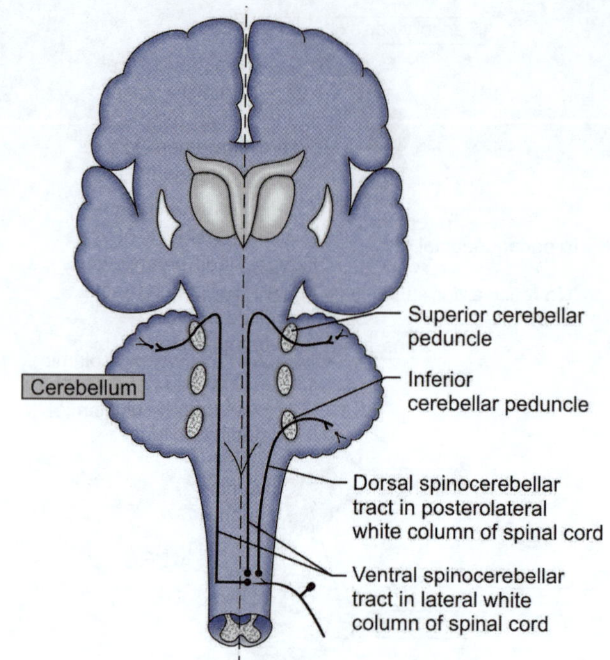

Fig. 11.31: Ventral (anterior) spinocerebellar tract

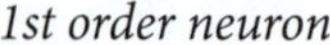

1st order neuron

The 1st order neuron arises from the muscle spindle, joints and the skin. It enters the spinal cord via the DRG and makes a short ascent in the dorsal funiculus of the same side, then terminate in the Clarke's column of cells (nucleus dorsalis).

2nd order neuron

2nd order neuron arises from the Clarke's column and it proceeds up through the dorsal spinocerebellar tract of the same side and reaches medulla. In medulla, fibers enter the inferior cerebellar peduncle of the same side and end in 'vermis of cerebellum' from where the 3rd order neurons arise.

3rd order neurons

3rd order neurons arise from the vermis of cerebellum and its axons passes to the anterior and posterior lobes of the cerebellar cortex.

Ventral (Anterior) Spinocerebellar Tract

Functions: Same as that of dorsal (posterior) spinocerebellar tract.

1st order neuron

The 1st order neuron arises from the muscle spindle, joints and the skin. It enters the spinal cord via the DRG and terminate in the Clarke's column of cells (nucleus dorsalis).

2nd order neuron

2nd order neuron arises from the Clarke's column of cells. Most of the 2nd order neuron cross to the opposite side (some remain uncrossed) and it proceeds up via the ventral spinocerebellar tract of the same side and extends up to the level of red nucleus (in midbrain). At red nucleus, fibers turn sharply backwards and downwards and then enter the superior cerebellar peduncle of same side and end in 'vermis of cerebellum' from where the 3rd order neurons arise (Fig. 11.31).

3rd order neurons

3rd order neurons arise from the vermis of cerebellum and goes to the anterior lobe of the cerebellar cortex.

Somatosensory pathways are summarized in Table 11.3.

Sensation from Face

Sensation from face are carried by sensory root of trigeminal nerve. Peripheral processes of neurons in the trigeminal ganglion pass through the ophthalmic, maxillary, mandibular divisions of trigeminal nerve. Trigeminal sensory nucleus has three components (Fig. 11.32).

a. Principal/chief/main sensory nucleus—located in pons.
b. Spinal nucleus—extend down to upper spinal cord.
c. Mesencephalic nucleus—extend from pons into midbrain.

1st order neuron: Located in trigeminal ganglion.

2nd order neuron: Located in the three components of the sensory trigeminal nucleus.

3rd order neuron: Located in VPM nucleus of thalamus.

Fibers conveying touch, tactile sensations, pressure terminate in the principal nucleus. Fibers arising from the

Table 11.3: Somatosensory pathways summary

Sensation	1st order neuron	2nd order neuron	3rd order neuron	Pathway	Destination
Temperature and pain	Posterior root ganglia	Substantia gelatinosa	Ventral posterior lateral nucleus of thalamus	Lateral spinothalamic tract, spinal lemniscus	Somatosensory cortex
Crude touch (light touch) and pressure	Posterior root ganglia	Substantia gelatinosa	Ventral posterior lateral nucleus of thalamus	Anterior spinothalamic tract, spinal lemniscus	Somatosensory cortex
Discriminatory touch (fine touch), vibration, proprioception	Posterior root ganglia	Nuclei gracilis and cuneatus	Ventral posterior lateral nucelus of thalamus	Fasciculi gracilis and cuneatus, medial lemniscus	Somatosensory cortex
Unconscious proprioception	Posterior root ganglia	Nucleus dorsalis (Clarke's column)		Anterior and posterior spinocerebellar tract	Cerebellar cortex

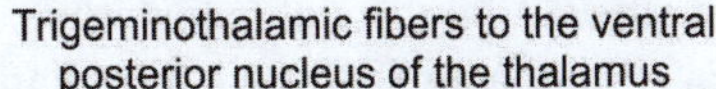

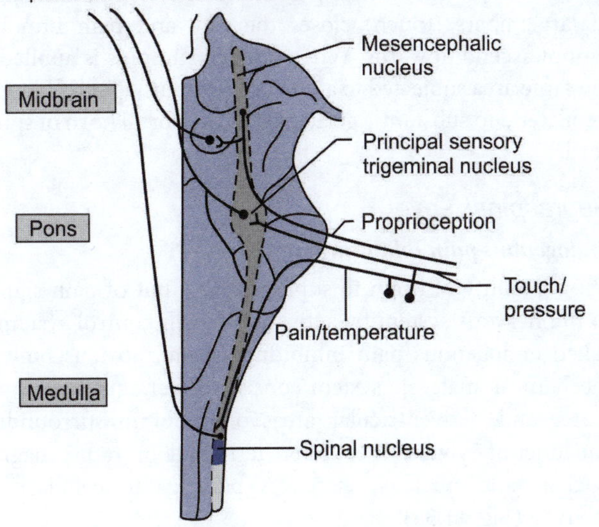

Fig. 11.32: Sensory supply of face

principal sensory cross to the opposite side and ascend up to terminate in ventroposterior nucleus of thalamus. From here, the fibers are send to the sensory cortex.

Fibers carrying pain and temperature from face, after reaching trigeminal ganglion descend from the pons through the medulla and spinal cord to end in the spinal nucleus. Fibers from the spinal nucleus cross to opposite side, ascend up in the spinal cord and medulla to the ventroposterior nucleus of thalamus. From here the fibers are send to the sensory cortex.

Proprioceptive impulses from the muscles of mastication and from the facial and extraocular muscles enter the pons and ascend to the mesencephalic nucleus. They are the only primary afferents to have their cell bodies located within the CNS. From the mesencephalic nucleus fibers leave, cross to opposite side to terminate in the ventroposterior nucleus of thalamus. From the ventroposterior nucleus of thalamus, the fibers are send to the sensory cortex.

Pain Sensation

Pain refers to an unpleasant sensory and emotional experience associated with actual or potential tissue damage.

Visceral Pain

Pain sensation from visceral organs can arise due to conditions like ischemia (e.g. cardiac pain), obstruction of hollow viscous, inflammation, distention, severe vasodilatation, etc.

Characteristic features of visceral pain

1. It is referred.
2. It is poorly localized.
3. Accompanied by autonomic symptoms like nausea, vomiting and fall of BP.
4. Pain of hollow viscous is often felt as colic, i.e. it comes and goes to reappear again.
5. Visceral pain initiates reflex spasm (contraction) of skeletal muscle in the abdominal wall and makes it rigid. Clinically this reflex spasm is called *guarding*. It is a protective reflex.

Referred Pain

Irritation of a viscus frequently produces pain that is felt not in the viscus, but in some somatic structure that may be considerable distance away. Such a pain is said to be referred pain. For example:

a. Cardiac pain is referred to inner aspect of left arm.
b. Pain in tip of shoulder caused by irritation of central portion of diaphragm.
c. Pain in testicle due to distention of ureter.

When visceral pain is both local and referred, it seems to spread from local to distant site-radiating pain. For example, in appendicitis pain starts in the right iliac fossa and radiates towards center of abdomen.

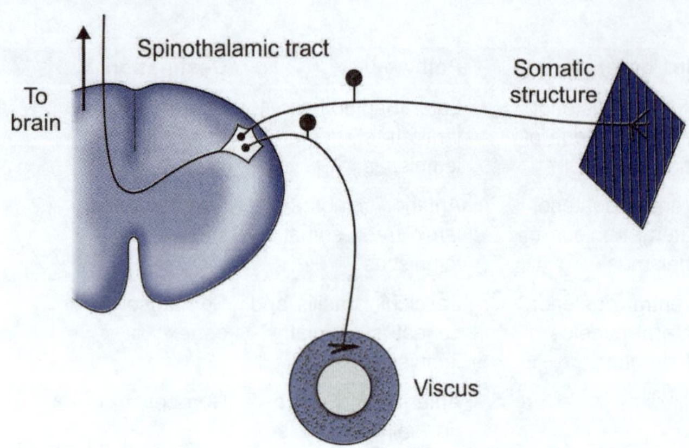

Fig. 11.33: Convergence theory

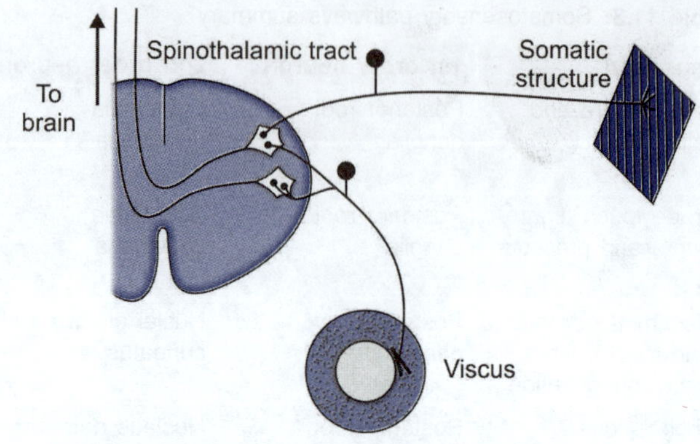

Fig. 11.34: Facilitation theory

Basis

Pain is referred, usually to a structure that developed from the same embryonic segment or dermatome. This principle is called dermatomal rule. For example, heart and the arm have the same segmental origin, testicle has migrated with its nerve supply from the primitive urogenital ridge from which kidney and ureter developed.

Theories of referred pain

1. *Convergence theory:* It holds that somatic and visceral afferents converge on the same spinothalamic neurons (Fig. 11.33).
2. *Facilitation theory:* The afferent impulses from visceral structures produce subliminal fringe effects that lower the threshold of spinothalamic neurons. Therefore, any slight activity in the pathways transmitting pain impulses from somatic regions and which normally would die out with in the spinal cord is facilitated (Fig. 11.34).

Modulation of Pain

Noxious stimuli of comparable intensity may produce varying degrees of pain in same individual under different circumstances. For example, injury acquired by an individual in sports field is less painful than comparable injury in road accidents. This is due to modulation of pain. Modulation of pain occurs at spinal and supraspinal level.

Spinal Level

Gate control theory

According to this theory, the dorsal column acts as gate for the transmission of pain sensation. It has been observed that the activation of large myelinated touch fibers reduces pain. Touch fibers give collateral (directly or through interneurons) in the substantia gelatinosa of the dorsal horn of the spinal cord. These collaterals inhibit the pain fiber presynaptically. So pain is not transmitted to higher centers.

Thus, the dorsal horn is the GATE through which the pain impulses reach the lateral spinothalamic system. Stimulation of large fibers (touch) closes the gate and pain impulses cannot ascend upwards. When a touch stimulus is applied to the same area subjected to a noxious stimulus, touch fiber give a collateral to substantia gelatinosa of the dorsal horn of spinal cord.

Supraspinal Level

Endogenous pain inhibiting system

The capability of brain to suppress the input of pain signals to the nervous system by activating a pain control system is called endogenous pain inhibiting system. So it is built in mechanical analgesic system consists of periaqueductal gray mater and periventricular areas of midbrain surrounding aqueduct of Sylvius. These fibers terminate on raphe magnus nucleus and nucleus reticularis paragiganto cellularis in medulla (Fig. 11.35).

Periaqueductal gray area in the midbrain

It inhibits pain by stimulating the raphe magnus nucleus. Neurons of periaqueductal gray (PAG) have opioid receptors on the surface membranes. When opioid receptors are stimulated by exogenously administrated opiod compounds (analgesics) or by endogenous opioid neurotransmitters (enkephalins), the pain suppression mechanism is activated leading to reduced pain.

Raphe Magnus Nucleus

The seratonergic neurons of the raphe magnus nucleus (RMN) and nucleus reticularis paragiganto cellularis (NRPC) descend and end on interneurons in posterior horn of spinal cord. These neurons secrete serotonin (Serotonin stimulate interneurons in spinal cord). These interneurons produce neurotransmitter enkephalin. The interneurons synapse with A δ and C fibers of first order.

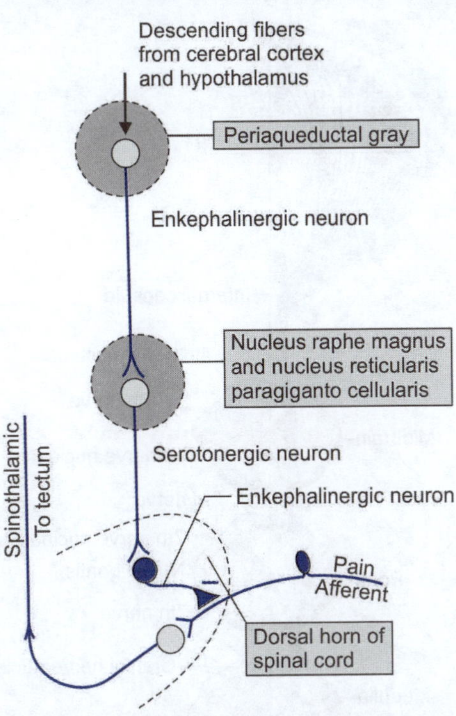

Fig. 11.35: Endogenous pain inhibiting pathway

Substance P is released during the stimulation of afferent A δ and C fibers. These afferent neurons possess opiate receptors on the membrane surface. Opiate peptides like enkaphalins and endorphins produced endogenously binds to these receptors and decrease the release of substance P. Thus the transmission of pain is inhibited. These cause mainly presynaptic inhibition on pain pathway.

Note

- Fibers from the limbic system supply the PAG. This explains why a soldier wounded in the battle field feel no pain during the heat of battle.
- Collaterals from spinothalamic tract stimulate descending inhibitory pathway.

Revised Gate Control Theory

Pain modulation theory is revised to form revised gate control theory. According to this, the touch fibers while ascending to the thalamus give off collateral fibers to reticular formation, nucleus raphe magnus and nucleus reticularis paraganto cellularis. These collaterals activates descending fibers (from NRM and NRPC) which inhibit pain pathway.

Clinical application

1. Gate control theory explains the relief of pain by rubbing skin near painful areas and relief of pain by balm and by counter irritants.
2. In acupuncture, introduction of sharp needles in selected spots cause local pain and it activates endogenous pain inhibiting system and give relief to pain anywhere in the body.

MOTOR SYSTEM

Most voluntary movements depend ultimately on the pattern and rate of discharge of the spinal motor neuron (α motor neuron) and homologous neurons in the motor nuclei of the cranial nerves. These neurons (α motor neurons) are the final common pathway (efferent) for skeletal muscle contraction. Their discharge depends upon two factors:

1. Descending pathways from brain which effect the discharge of α motor neuron either directly or through interneurons or through γ motor neuron—Voluntary activity.
2. Afferent from muscle spindle or golgi tendon organ—Reflex activity (involuntary activity).

Reflex activity (stretch reflex etc.) has been explained in this book. Here we will concentrate on voluntary activity. Voluntary movements are initiated in the cerebral cortex and the movements are achieved when descending pathways regulate the discharge of α motor neuron either directly through the descending pathway from cerebral cortex to spinal cord (pyramidal tract) or indirectly through the pathway which first descend from cortex to lower brain area (brainstem) and then from brainstem to spinal cord (extrapyramidal system). The motor cortex is the name given to parts of the cerebral cortex which on electrical stimulation, promptly result in discrete movements in the body. The fundamental impulses for muscle contraction originate from the motor cortex. The motor control of body has a three tier system:

1. *Target identification:* This is determining the goal or purpose of movement, i.e. command for motor action. It is originated in cortical association areas.
2. *Plan of action:* It is programing the sequence of movement. Once the goal of movement is made in association area, the command for action is given to the areas, where the programing the sequence of movement to achieve the goal is planned. These areas are cortex itself, basal ganglia and lateral part of cerebellar hemisphere.
3. *Execution:* It is the actual performance of the movement. Once the sequence of movements is planned, this information is conveyed to motor cortex. The fundamental impulses for the muscle contraction originate in the motor cortex. From motor cortex, the descending pathway terminate on spinal cord (directly or indirectly through brainstem pathways) and the planned movement is executed by regulation of α motor neuron discharge.

Motor Cortex

Primary Motor Area (Area 4)

Located in the precentral gyrus. Area of cortex representing a part of body is not proportional to the size of the part, but rather to intricacy of movements in the region. Thus relatively large areas of cortex are responsible for movements in the hands or in the lips. In the precentral gyrus, the body is represented in the upside manner-Motor homunculus.

Motor Homunculus

The various parts of the body are topographically represented in the precentral gyrus based on the motor projections from the motor cortex. The feet is represented at the top of the gyrus and the face at the bottom. The facial area is represented bilaterally, but the rest of the representation is generally unilateral. Stimulation of different areas produce response on muscles of opposite half of the body. The cortical representation of each body parts is proportionate in size to the skill with which the part is used in fine, voluntary movement. The area involved in speech (lowermost part of face) and hand movements (fingers) are especially large in the cortex (Fig. 11.36). An individual neuron in the primary motor cortex does not control an individual muscle. Rather, they simultaneously stimulate a set of synergistic muscles such that a single joint on contralateral side moves in particular direction. Additional motor areas are primarily:

a. *Premotor area (area 6):* Lies anterior to the precentral gyrus. Its functions are programming of motor activity and postural support for wide variety of detailed movement.

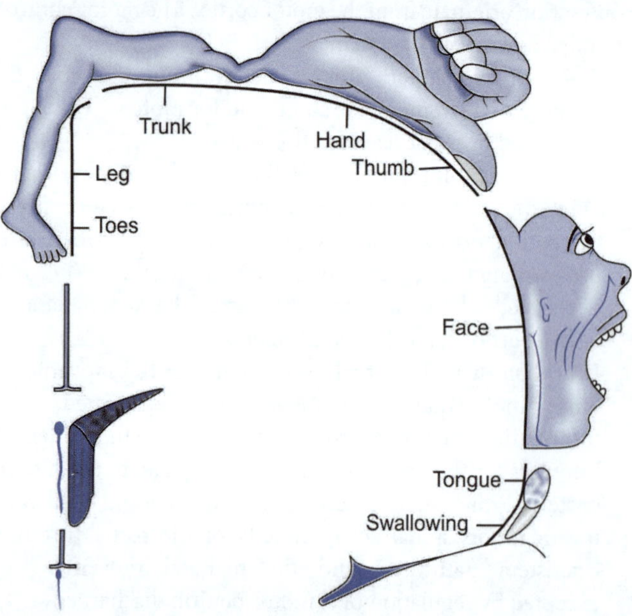

Fig. 11.36: Motor homunculus

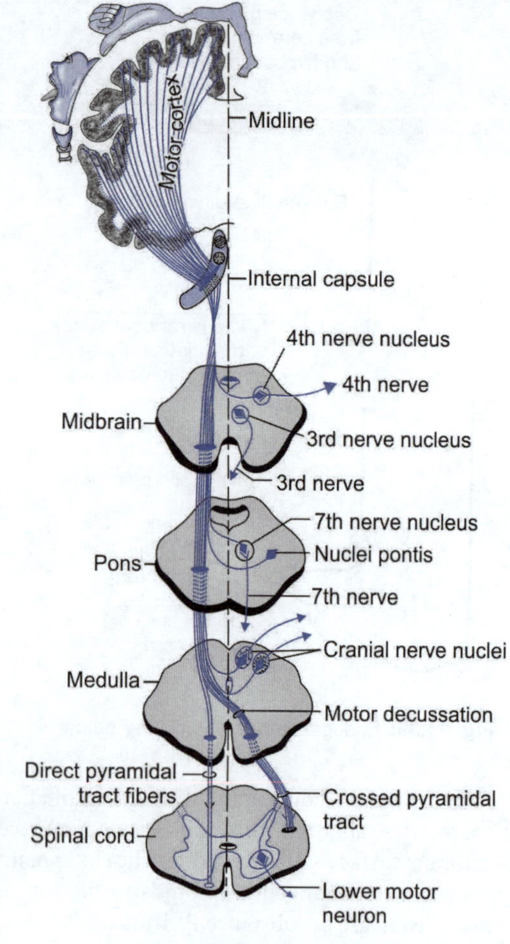

Fig. 11.37: Pyramidal tract

b. *Supplementary motor area:* Primarily involved in voluntary movement which are complex and involve planning.
c. Frontal eye field (area 8)
d. Occipital eye field (area 19).

Pyramidal Tract

This is the longest tract starting from the motor cortex and reaching the last segment of the spinal cord. The pyramidal (PT) fibers pass from the motor area to the spinal ventral horn cells and to motor nuclei of opposite side (Fig. 11.37).

1. The pyramidal tract fiber to the spinal ventral horn cells constitute the ***corticospinal tract***.
2. The pyramidal fiber to the motor cranial nuclei (3 and 4 in the midbrain, 5, 6, 7 in the pons, 9 to 12 in medulla) constitute the ***corticobulbar tract***.

Origin

- 30% from motor cortex, area 4 in precentral gyrus
- 30% from premotor cortex, area 6
- 40% from somatosensory area 1 and 2.

Course of Pyramidal Tract

The pyramidal tract fibers arise from Betz cells of cerebral cortex. They converge towards the brainstem as a radiating mass of fibers called corona radiata to reach the internal capsule.

- *In internal capsule:* It lie in the bend (genu), and the anterior 2/3 of the posterior limb. In internal capsule the PT fiber get intermingled with extrapyramidal fibers (EPT). Therefore lesion in this region includes both PT and EPT fibers.
- *In midbrain:* It lie ventral to the substantia nigra, occupying the middle 3/5 of this region.
- *In pons:* They occupy the most ventral aspect in front of trapezium. Here the compactness of bundle is loosened.
- *In medulla:* In the medulla scattered fibers are reunited to a compact bundle. This compact bundle now produce an elevation called pyramid.
  - In the lower part of medulla 80–85% fiber cross to the opposite side, enters the lateral white column called lateral corticospinal tract(crossed/indirect). It extends throughout the cord.
  - About 15–20% fiber do not cross and enter anterior white column near the median fissure called anterior corticospinal tract (uncrossed/direct). Through interneurons they cross the midline, when it reaches the level of muscles it controls. It does not extend beyond the lower cervical or midthoracic region.

In the brain stem, some of the descending pyramidal fibers seperate to supply the motor nuclei of the cranial nerves of both sides except the lower half of facial nucleus and the hypoglossal nucleus which are supplied only from the opposite pyramidal tract. These fibers are known as corticobulbar as they do not reach the spinal cord.

Functions of Pyramidal Tract

1. Lateral corticospinal tracts convey motor impulses to the spinal cord for controlling voluntary movements, specially the fine and precise movements of fingers and hands to carry out skilled work.
2. Anterior corticospinal tract control the muscles of trunk and proximal portion of limb to carry out postural adjustments and gross movements.
3. Corticospinal fibers arising from the somatic sensory area (1 and 2) and parietal lobe association cortex are concerned with sensory-motor coordination.
4. Some corticospinal fibers end at excitatory synapses on α and γ motor neurons, whereas others end on interneuron that may excite or inhibit the α motor neurons and thus controlling α motor neuronal activity.
5. Corticobulbar fibers are responsible for voluntary control of muscle of larynx, pharynx, palate, upper and lower face, jaw and eye.

Extrapyramidal System/Tract

The part of descending brainstem and spinal pathways which do not pass through the pyramids and are concerned with postural control are referred to as extrapyramidal system. The various extrapyramidal tracts includes:

Medial Longitudinal Fasciculus

It arises from the medial vestibular nucleus, reticular formation, superior colliculus and interstitial nucleus of Cajal. The tract descends uncrossed up to upper cervical region.

Functions

- Coordination of reflex ocular movements
- Integration of movements of eyes and neck.

Lateral Vestibulospinal Tract

It arises from lateral vestibular nucleus of same side, runs uncrossed and ends at various levels of spinal cord.

Functions

- Maintenance of muscle tone and posture.
- Maintenance of position of head and body during acceleration.

Medial Vestibulospinal Tract

It arises from the medial and inferior vestibular nuclei on both sides, descends uncrossed and ends at various levels of spinal cord.

Function

Maintenance of equilibrium and muscle tone.

Reticulospinal Tract

It arises from the reticular formation of pons and medulla, descends mostly uncrossed and extends up to the thoracic segments.

Functions

- Coordination of voluntary and reflex movements
- Control of muscle tone.

Rubrospinal Tract

It arises from the red nucleus, crosses to the opposite side and extends up to the thoracic segments.

Function

The tract has a facilitatory influence on flexor muscle tone.

Tectospinal Tract

Fibers arise from superior colliculus in the midbrain, cross to the opposite side in the tegmentum and descend up to the lower cervical region.

Functions

This tract indirectly connects retina with spinal motor neuron and coordinates retinal impulses with body movements.

Olivospinal Tract

Fibers arise from inferior olivary nucleus of medulla, crosses to opposite side and descends up to cervical region. It is less developed and less important in mammals.

Functions

Control of movements due to proprioception.

Disease or lesion of extrapyramidal tract causes difficulty in initiating the voluntary movements.

Difference between pyramidal and extrapyramidal tracts are given in Table 11.4.

Applied Aspect

Upper Motor Neuron Lesions

Paralysis that results from lesion of descending fibers between their origin from cortical motor areas and their termination on anterior horn cells in the spinal cord is called as upper motor neuron paralysis.

So, upper motor neurons include corticospinal, corticobulbar and extrapyramidal tracts and the cell whose axons form these pathway (Betz cells of primary motor cortex).

Lower Motor Neuron Lesions

Lower motor neurons (LMN) paralysis occurs in diseases that cause destruction of anterior horn cells or their axons in dorsal root, nerve plexuses or the peripheral nerves. The examples

Table 11.4: Pyramidal and extrapyramidal tracts compared

Pyramidal tracts	Extrapyramidal tracts
1. Phylogenetically it is a newer motor system developed recently	1. It is an old motor system
2. Its axons pass without relay to the spinal segments where they form synapses with either interneurons in the dorsal horn or directly with the motor neuron themselves	2. Discharges is through several tracts. Polysynaptic and multi-channel pathway
3. They have greater influence over motor neurons that control muscles involved in fine movements, particularly those of the fingers and hand	3. They are involved with coordination of the large muscle groups used in the maintenance of upright posture, in locomotion and in head and body movements when turning towards a specific stimulus
4. Lesions of these tract produces 'spasticity' (Table 11.5) in the muscles involved	4. Its lesion produces 'rigidity' of the muscles involved
5. The tract start functioning after the completion of myelination at the second year after birth	5. The tract starts functioning from before birth
6. Slower rate of conduction	6. Faster rate of conduction
7. Only facilitatory fibers are present	7. Both facilitatory and inhibitory fibers present

Table 11.5: Difference between rigidity and spasticity

Spasticity	Rigidity
1. Seen following the lesion of pyramidal tract (corticospinal tract), the most common site being the internal capsule	1. Seen following the lesion of basal ganglia and therefore called extrapyramidal rigidity
2. Involves only one group of the muscle either agonist or antagonist. Antigravity muscles are usually involved	2. Involves both the agonist as well as the antagonist muscle, therefore more uniform hypertonia and often it is so distributed as to produce a general attitude of flexion of the limbs and trunk
3. A state of increased tone which is described as clasp knife type	3. Hypertonia described here is of two types: i. *Lead pipe rigidity:* Passive movement of an extremity meets with a plastic dead feeling resistance as though bending a lead pipe ii. *Cogwheel rigidity:* Resistance to passive movement of an extremity is regularly or irregularly variable. There will be series of catches during passive movement of the extremity. This is described as like a lever rubbing on the teeth of a cogwheel
4. It is form of spasticity which is stretch sensitive. The degree of increased tone developed during any passive stretch is proportional to the speed of the applied stretch	4. No similar phenomenon seen here

of LMN disease are nerve lesion as occurs in nerve injury or diseases of the nerve, poliomyelitis and lesion of nerve roots.

The motor nuclei of the cranial nerves are similar in function to the AHC, as they form the cell bodies of the LMN of the cranial nerves. Thus, lesion of a cranial nerve nucleus, like lesion of an AHC is a LMN lesion.

For spinal cord

UMN: Corticospinal and extrapyramidal tract

LMN: From α motor neuron (AHC) to peripheral nerve carrying motor impulse to the muscle.

For brainstem

UMN: Corticobulbar tract

LMN: Motor cranial nerves with their nuclei

Facial Palsy

Symptoms of facial nerve palsy depend on the location of injury. The motor nucleus of CN VII has upper and lower divisions that supply the upper and lower face, respectively. There is bilateral innervation of the upper division but only contralateral innervation of the lower division (Fig. 11.38). UMN lesions (above facial nerve nucleus, i.e. cerebral cortex, internal capsule) results in facial palsy that affects the contralateral lower face but spares the forehead and brow muscles (as upper part of face receives fibers from same side also). LMN lesions (including facial nerve nucleus and the cranial nerve) affects the ipsilateral upper and lower face (see Page 368).

Some Popular Clinical Terms

1. *Hemiplegia:* Paralysis of one half of the body. There are two types of hemiplegia—dense hemiplegia and crossed hemiplegia.

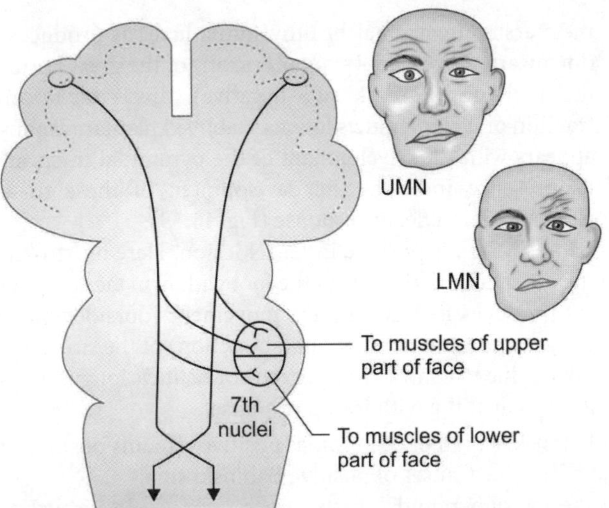

Fig. 11.38: Pyramidal supply to the facial nucleus

   a. *Dense hemiplegia*: Here the lesion occurs at internal capsule. There is weakness of whole opposite side of the body including face. This is a type of UMN type of lesion affecting the whole opposite of the body.
   b. *Crossed hemiplegia:* Here the site of lesion is in the brainstem. Cranial nerve involvement depends on the level of lesion. There is ipsilateral cranial nerve involvement (LMN type of cranial nerve lesion) and contralateral weakness of body (UMN type).

   The patient walks on a narrow base, has a difficulty in bending his knees and drags his feet along as if they are glued to the floor this is referred as spastic or hemiplegic gait.
2. *Paraplegia:* Paralysis of both the lower limbs.
3. *Monoplegia:* Paralysis of single limb.
4. *Quadriplegia:* Paralysis of all the four limbs.

Difference between upper motor neuron lesions and lower motor neuron lesions is given in the Table 11.6.

Effects of Lesions at Various Levels of CNS

Pyramidal system (PS) can be injured by cerebrovascular accidents (CVA). The CVA is the major cause of pyramidal lesions. Two major forms of CVA are: (1) Infarction (2) Hemorrhage. In the brain, an artery can be blocked by thrombosis or embolism. The CVA can damage the pyramidal system at various places like internal capsule, motor cortex and brainstem.

1. When the injury is located at internal capsule then hemiplegia (contralateral side) is the rule. This is because pyramidal tract fibers are so crowded here that even a slight injury will cause damage to large number of fibers. In severe lesions, sensory and visual tracts are involved, so hemianesthesia and homonymous hemianopia develop. The usual cause of capsular lesion is the rupture of Charcot's artery (lenticulostriate branch of middle cerebral artery; this is also called the artery of cerebral hemorrhage as it accounts for more than 60% of the causes of intracerebral hemorrhage).
2. When there is a damage of area 4, monoplegia (contralateral side) or localized lesion (e.g. in the face) is the general rule. This is because the PT fibers are very scattered here. Therefore to cause hemiplegia, lesion in area 4 has to be very extensive. Morever in cortical lesions, there will be other signs, e.g. convulsive seizures, astereognosis, aphasia, etc.
3. Brainstem lesions can be often diagnosed by reference to the gross anatomy. For example:
   a. In lesions of midbrain, there will be signs of 3rd nerve paralysis on the side of lesion and spastic hemiplegia on the other (contralateral) side (Weber's syndrome).
   b. When the lesion is lower down in the brainstem, there will be, symptoms depending on the exact site of injury.

Table 11.6: Differences between lower and upper motor neuron lesion

Lower motor neuron lesion (LMNL)	Upper motor neuron lesion (UMNL)
1. It is due to the lesion of the lower motor neurons (LMNs), i.e, the spinal and cranial motor neurons that directly innervate the muscle	1. It is due to the lesion of the upper motor neurons, i.e. the neurons that originate in the brain and spinal cord that can influence the activity of LMNs; lesion of the pyramidal tracts being the major cause
2. Usually single or individual muscle is affected	2. It involves a group of muscles
3. Flaccid paralysis occurs, i.e. the muscles becomes completely paralyzed (hypotonia). This is due to complete loss of muscle tone as the integrity of reflex arc is it lost.	3. Spastic paralysis occurs, i.e. affected muscles become hypertonic. It is due to: i. Release phenomenon, i.e. loss of higher inhibitory control ii. Denervation hypersensitivity of centers below the transaction
4. All reflexes superficial and deep are lost as the motor pathway is damaged	4. Superficial reflexes are lost but the deep reflexes are exaggerated. Deep reflexes are exaggerated because of increased γ motor discharge
5. Gross muscle wasting occurs as all muscles are paralyzed. Disuse atrophy of muscle occurs, i.e. shrinkage of muscle fiber occurs and is finally replaced by fibrous tissue	5. Minimal wasting of occurs, i.e. minimal disuse atrophy occurs because muscles though not used in voluntary movements are continuously in action to maintain posture by reflexes.
6. Fasciculation and fibrillation present	6. No fasciculation and fibrillation
7. Babinski sign/Plantar reflex not elicited	7. Babinski sign positive (abnormal)

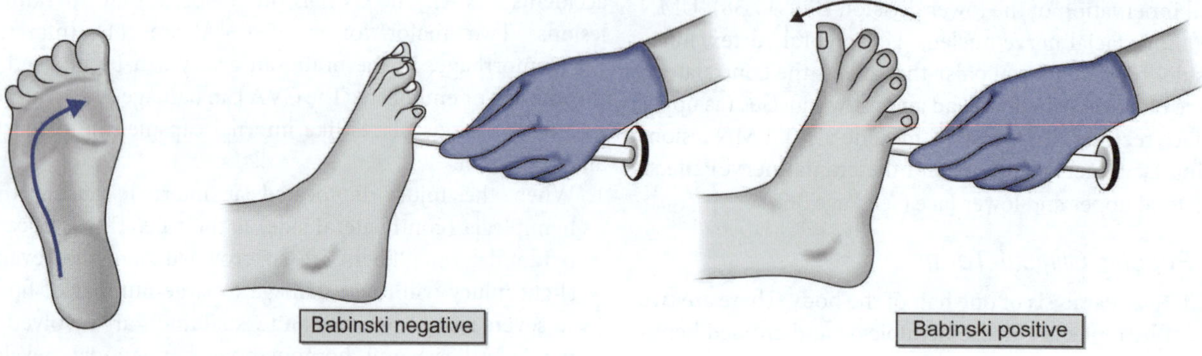

Fig. 11.39: Babinski response

There will be signs of injury of 7th, 9th, 10th or even hypoglossal (12th) nerve injury on the side of lesion and spastic hemiplegia on the contralateral side.

4. Upper level of spinal cord—quadriplegia + respiratory paralysis.
5. Thoracic and lumbar—paraplegia, respiration remains normal.

Note

1. Cerebrovascular accident induced damage of PS is called stroke or apoplexy. Onset of stroke is usually sudden. In the initial phase there will be usually signs of shock. After a few days, provided the patient survives, the shock passes off and the stage of chronic pyramidal lesion appears.
2. Babinski's response is obtained by stroking (to pass gently in one direction) outer edge of the sole of the foot with firm tactile stimulus. The direction of stroke is from the heel towards the little toe and then medially across the metatarsus. In normal healthy individuals, it produces a downward movement (plantar flexion) of the great toe and the small toes (Babinski sign-negative). This is due to contraction of flexor hallucis longus. Babinski plantar response appears with the development of the pyramidal tracts and its presence indicates the development of these tracts. Normally it is a flexor response (Fig. 11.39).
3. Babinski sign is positive in UMN lesion. Here on stroking the outer edge of the sole of the foot with firm tactile stimulus produces first an upward movement (dorsiflexion) of the great toe and fanning out (abduction) of the small toes. This is due to contraction of extensor hallucis longus; physiologically it is a withdrawal response.

Babinski sign if once becomes positive remains positive for rest of the life. Causes of positive Babinski sign:

i. Lesion of pyramidal tracts
ii. Infants (below 1year) as the pyramidal tracts are not well developed

Table 11.7: Differences between somatic and autonomic nervous system

	Somatic nervous system	Autonomic nervous system
Efferent neuron	Single efferent neuron between CNS and effector organ	Two efferent neuron (pre and post ganglionic)
Ganglia	No ganglia in efferent pathway	Ganglia is the site of synapse between two efferent neurons
Neurotransmitter	Always acetylcholine	Acetylcholine or epinephrine/norepinephrine
Innervates	Skeletal muscle	Smooth, cardiac muscle and glands
Effect of stimulation	Always causes excitation (inhibition occurs centrally through inhibitory interneurons)	Either excitation or inhibition according to receptor (inhibition is peripheral)
Spinal column pathway	In anterior horn cells	In autonomic ganglia
Synapse	Well defined	Not well defined
Function	Controls voluntary movements	Controls involuntary movements
Miscellaneous	1. Skeletal muscle activity is entirely dependent on its nerve supply 2. Activity is confined to certain muscle groups	1. Activities controlled by ANS shows considerable autonomy 2. Activity is more generalized

iii. During deep sleep
iv. Cheyne-Stokes respiration due to hypoxia.

Release Phenomenon

Some features are not normally seen in healthy persons because they are suppressed by the CNS. Some particular damages of CNS cause release of it and the feature, uptill now suppressed, become manifested. In the newborn Babinski's sign is normally +ve: when PT develops fully, Babinski's sign is suppressed and flexor plantar response appears. The UMN lesions causes, the release and Babinski's sign appears again. Common examples of release phenomenon are Babinski's sign, decerebrate rigidity and cerebellar tremor.

Note

1. Babinski's sign is a release phenomenon.
2. Spasticity or spastic paralysis usually means a combination of following signs:
   a. Clasp-knife rigidity.
   b. Presence of Babinski's sign.
   c. Loss of voluntary power.
   d. Exaggereated reflex.

AUTONOMIC NERVOUS SYSTEM

The portion of nervous system that controls the body. Most striking feature of the system is rapidity and intensity of action.

Classification

Anatomical

Craniosacral outflow: Cranial outflow supplies the visceral organs via 3, 7, 9, 10 cranial nerves and sacral outflow supplies pelvic viscera via pelvic branches of S2-S4. They are parasympathetic fibers.

Thoracolumbar outflow: T1-T12 and L1-L3 (mainly L1, L2). They are sympathetic fibers.

Physiological (Table 11.7)

- Sympathetic (thoracolumbar)
- Parasympathetic (craniosacral).

Chemical

i. *Cholinergic:* Release acetylcholine. The neurons that are cholinergic are:
   a. All the preganglionic.
   b. The anatomically parasympathetic postganglionic neurons.
   c. The anatomically sympathetic postganglionic neurons that innervate sweat glands.
   d. Anatomically sympathetic neurons that end on blood vessels in skeletal muscles and produce vasodilation.

ii. *Adrenergic:* Producing epinephrine (adrenalin) or norepinephrine (noradrenaline) at neuroeffector junction. They are found in sympathetic postganglionic fibers except sweat glands, piloerector muscles, some blood vessels of skeletal muscle and adrenal medulla.

ANS includes the following:

1. Areas controlling visceral function located in cerebral hemispheres including part of cerebral cortex, limbic system and hypothalamus.
2. Autonomic centers in brainstem and in reticular formation contains cardiovascular, respiratory centers and cranial nerve nuclei (3, 7, 9, 10).

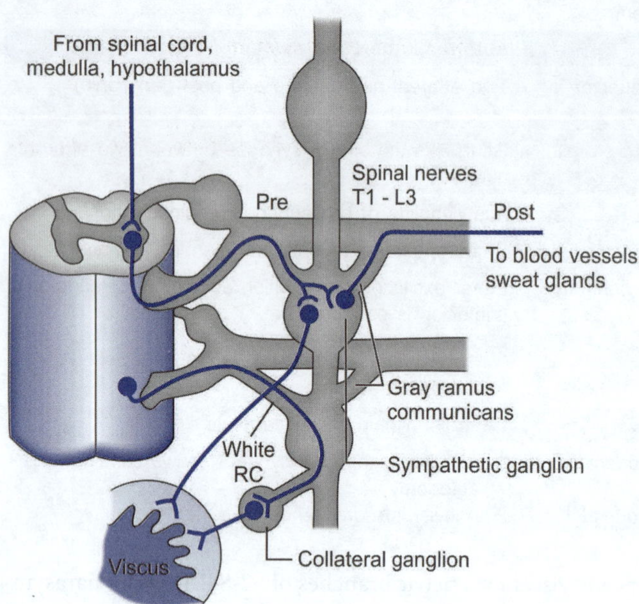

Fig. 11.40: Sympathetic division of nervous system

3. Autonomic center in spinal cord-in lateral horn (sympathetic; thoracolumbar and parasympathetic; sacral).
4. Peripheral part of ANS—autonomic nerves and ganglia.

Sympathetic Nervous System

Sympathetic fibers originate in spinal cord along the spinal nerve where its cell body is located. From there they first go to paravertebral sympathetic ganglion chain and then to tissues and organs that are stimulated by sympathetic nerve. Preganglionic fibers (myelinated 'B' fibers) originate from lateral horn and pass through anterior route immediately after the spinal nerve leaves the spinal canal. These fibers then leave the spinal nerve and pass through the white ramus into one of the ganglia (Fig. 11.40). From the ganglia the course of fibers can be one of the following:

a. Most of them end on the cell bodies of the postganglionic neurons.
b. Some fibers pass upwards or downwards in sympathetic chain and synapse with ganglia at higher or lower level.
c. Some end in peripheral sympathetic ganglia other than preganglionic and postganglionic.

Postganglionic fibers originating from the ganglia innervate various organs. Some of the postganglionic fibers pass back from sympathetic chain and enter spinal nerve as gray ramus communicans (unmyelinated 'c' fibers). These fibers enter all parts of body through spinal nerves and supplies blood vessels, piloerector muscles, etc.

Note: Sympathetic nerves also extends to adrenal medulla. Preganglionic fibers originating from lateral horn pass through sympathetic chain into splanchnic nerves (here there is no synapse). Splanchnic nerve enter adrenal medulla. In adrenal medulla, they end directly on modified neuronal cells. They secrete epinephrine or norepinephrine directly into blood stream. Postganglionic neurons are modified into secretory cells. Eighty percent secretion of adrenal medulla is epinephrine and 20% is norepinephrine.

Parasympathetic Nervous System

Seventy-five percent of all parasympathetic fibers are from vagus nerve. Vagal fibers supply heart, lungs, esophagus, stomach, entire small intestine, poximal large intestine, liver, gallbladder, pancreas and upper portion of ureters. Occulomotor fibers supply pupillary sphincter and cilliary muscle. Facial nerve supply lacrimal glands and submandibular glands. Glossopharyngeal supply parotid gland. Sacral fibers are through pelvic nerve. From sacral plexus S2, S3, S4 supply portion of large intestine, external genitalia and lower portion of ureter (Fig. 11.41). In parasympathetic system, ganglia is located in or near the organs. So preganglionic fibers are long and postganglionic fibers are short.

Neurotransmitters of ANS

1. Acetylcholine all ganglia, in adrenal medulla (preganglionic sympathetic), postganglionic parasympathetic endings, sympathetic cholinergic nerve endings.

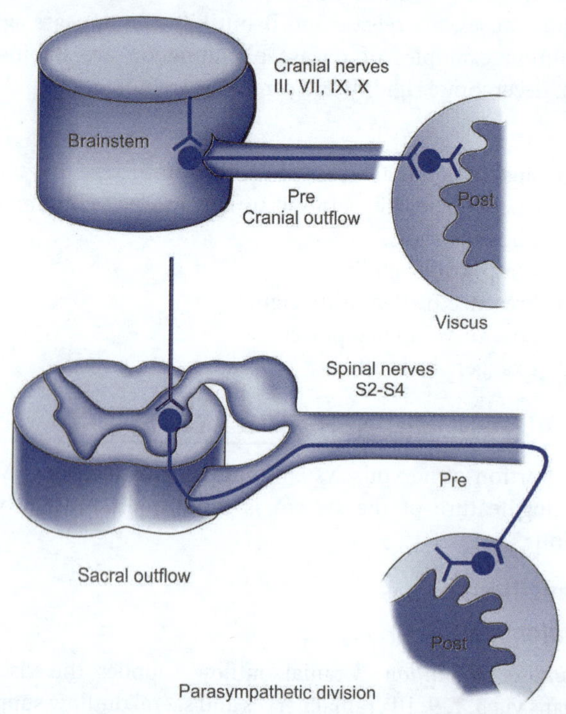

Fig. 11.41: Parasympathetic division of nervous system

2. Adrenaline and noradrenaline: Postganglionic sympathetic nerve endings (mainly noradrenaline), adrenal medulla (postganglionic sympathetic; mainly adrenaline).

Synthesis of Neurotransmitters

1. Acetylcholine

Site: Terminal ends of nerve fibers and it is stored in vesicles.

Steps:

$$\text{Acetyl CoA} + \text{Choline} \xrightarrow{\text{choline acetyl transferase}} \text{ACh}$$

Fate:

$$\text{ACh} \xrightarrow{\text{cholinesterase}} \text{Acetate} + \text{Choline}$$

2. Epinephrine and norepinephrine

Site: Axoplasm of terminal nerve ending.

Steps:

In vesicles:

$$\text{Tyrosine} \xrightarrow{\text{hydroxylation}} \text{DOPA} \xrightarrow{\text{decarboxylation}}$$

$$\text{Dopamine} \xrightarrow{\text{hydroxylase}} \text{Norepinephrine}$$

In adrenal medulla:

$$\text{Norepinephrine} \xrightarrow{\text{methylation}} \text{Epinephrine}$$

Fate of noradrenaline:

Reuptaken into terminal nerve endings and are diffused into surrounding tissue fluids. Some of them are destroyed by catechol-o-methyltransferase.

Difference between sympathetic and parasympathetic nervous system is given in the Table 11.8.

Table 11.9: Difference between α and β receptor

α receptor	β receptor
Vasoconstriction	Vasodilation (β_2)
Iris dilatation	Cardio acceleration (β_1)
Intestinal relaxation	Intestinal relaxation (β_2)
Intestinal sphincter contraction (α_1)	Uterus relaxation (β_2)
Piloerector contraction	Bronchodilatation (β_2)
Bladder sphincter (α_1) relaxation	Calorigenesis (β_2)
	Bladder sphincter relaxation (β_2)

Adrenergic and cholinergic receptors

Seen on effector organs.

1. Adrenergic receptors: (Table 11.9)
   - α_1 and β_1 causes excitation
   - α_2 and β_2 causes inhibition.
2. Cholinergic receptors:
   - *Nicotinic:* In all autonomic ganglia and NMJ of skeletal muscle
   - *Muscuranic:* In neuroeffector junction of smooth muscles and glands.

SPINAL CORD LESIONS

Spinal cord transections can be divided into three types: complete, incomplete and hemisection of spinal cord.

Complete Transection of Spinal Cord

The complete transection of spinal cord occurs due to:

a. Bullet injury which causes dislocation of spinal cord.
b. Accidents which cause dislocation of spinal cord/occlusion of blood vessels.

Table 11.8: Differences between sympathetic and parasympathetic nervous system

	Sympathetic	Parasympathetic
Nerve fibers	Thoracolumbar (T1-L2/L3)	Craniosacral outflow (CNS 3, 7, 9, 10)
Preganglionic fibers	Short	Long
Postganglionic fibers	Long	Short
Sympathetic ganglia	Close to vertebral column	Lies in/close to organ supplied
Function	Prepare the individual to face emergency situation	Concerned in vegetative aspect of day-to-day living, i.e. digestion, absorption, sexual erectile function
Actions	Causes dilatation of pupil, increased heart rate, increased BP, provide better perfusion, constrict cutaneous vessels to limit bleeding, decreases threshold in reticular formation hence increases alertness, increase blood glucose, free fatty acid to provide more energy	Decreased heart rate, decrease SV, favors storage of absorbed nutrients
Known as	Catabolic nervous system	Anabolic nervous system
Neurotransmitter	At ganglia: Acetylecholine At organ: Adrenaline/noradrenaline	At ganglia as well as postganglia: Acetylcholine

The complete transection causes immediate loss of sensation and voluntary movement below the level of lesion. Even though the higher centers remain unaffected, the spinal centers below the level of injury loose the function. The effects occur in three stages:

Stage of Spinal Shock

It is the first stage of effects that occurs immediately after injury. It is also called the stage of flaccidity. Patient feels as if he is cut into two portions. The various signs and symptoms that develop during this stage are:

1. *Paralysis of limbs:* Depending on the level of lesion the paralysis of limbs can be of the following types:
   - Hemiplegia (paralysis of one-half of the body)
   - Quadriplegia (paralysis of all the 4 limbs)
   - Paraplegia (paralysis of both the lower limbs).
2. *Flaccid paralysis:* Because of the transection, the iso-lated segments of the spinal cord have lost their power of mediating reflex functions, therefore the muscles are completely paralyzed (Flaccid paralysis)
3. *Loss of reflexes:* All the spinal reflexes are markedly decreased or lost because of the injury to anterior and posterior nerve roots.
4. *Loss of sensations:* All the sensations below the transection is lost because of the injury to posterior nerve roots and sensory neurons in the posterior gray horn.
5. *Effect on visceral organs:* The urinary bladder and rectum become paralyzed. Detrusor muscle becomes atonic. There will be retention of urine and constipation. The penis is flaccid and erection is not possible.
6. *Venous return:* Venous return is very much decreased. Venous return depends on the muscle tone during resting condition. During activity it depends upon contraction of skeletal muscle (muscle pump). But in complete transection of spinal cord, muscle tone is lost and flaccid paralysis occurs, leading to decreased venous return.

   In addition, the limbs are immobile and smooth muscles of blood vessels loose tone. So blood accumulates in the lower limb, becomes cold and blue (cyanotic) due to accumulation of blood in the lower limb.
7. *Effect on blood pressure:* The effect on BP depends upon the level of injury.

   Lesion anywhere below L2 segment: The blood pressure is not affected much because the sympathetic vasoconstrictor fibers leave the spinal cord between T1 and L2 segments.

   Lesion at or above T1 segment: All the sympathetic vasoconstrictor fibers leaving the spinal cord from T1 and L2 segments are transected, i.e. completely cut off from higher medullary cardiovascular center regulating BP. So the BP falls drastically. The mean arterial BP falls below 40 mm Hg.
8. Skin becomes dry and scaly and bed sores may develop.
9. No sweating in the region affected by vasomotor paralysis.

Note: Severity of complete transection depends upon the level of lesion. The complete transection at the cervical region can be very fatal, because the diaphragm and other respiratory muscles are cut off from the respiratory centers. This leads to paralysis of these muscles leading to sudden arrest of breathing.

In humans stage of spinal shock usually last for a period of at least two weeks. There is functional depression of the nervous system, a phenomenon called ***diaschisis.***

Stage of Reflex Activity

This stage is also called stage of recovery. After 3 weeks period, depending largely upon the general health of the patient, the reflex activity begins to return to the isolated segments of the spinal cord.

i. First the functional activities return to the smooth muscle. Urinary bladder becomes automatic. Similarly reflex defecation also occurs.

ii. Next sympathetic tone of blood vessels is regained. As a result:
   a. Blood pressure is restored to normal at rest, but precise feedback regulation is absent and wide fluctuations in BP are common.
   b. The skin which has become dry and scaly now shows sweating again and it becomes more healthy.
   c. Bed sores heal up rapidly.
   d. Because of accompanying return of reflex activity to the skeletal muscle, circulation through the limbs is greatly improved and they become warm and of good color.

iii. *Muscle tone:* Tone in the skeletal muscle returns slowly after 2 or 3 weeks. The tone of flexor muscles return first, so that now even though both the flexors and extensors are hypotonic, the flexors are less hypotonic than extensors. The limbs in this condition adopt a position of slight flexion and the paralysis is therefore called ***paraplegia in flexion.***

iv. *Reflex activity:* Reflex activity begins to return after few weeks of return of muscle tone. The flexor reflexes appear first. The first reflex, which usually appears is the Babinski's reflex. Babinski's sign is +ve.

   Mass reflex can be elicited in some cases by scratching the skin over the lower limbs or the anterior abdominal wall. This reaction constitutes the spasm in flexor muscles of both the lower limbs, evacuation of urinary bladder and profuse sweating.

   Tendon jerks begin to appear. Initially the knee jerk returns then the ankle jerk.

Note: The mass reflex can be utilized to provide paraplegic patients a degree of bladder and bowel control. Patients can be trained to initiate urination and defecation by intentionally producing mass reflex with the help of a stroke or a pinch on their thighs.

Stage of Failure of Reflex Activity

As the stage of reflex activity continues, a time comes when the reflex activities of stage II fails because of the degeneration of neural tissue of spinal cord below the lesion and intercurrent infections. Once again there develops hypotonicity of muscles, mass reflex disappears, bed sores appears and the patient dies.

Though the reflex movements return, the muscles below the level of injury have less power and less resistance.

a. Usually the general condition of the patient starts detiorating.
b. In general, malnutrition, infection or toxemia causes failure of reflex function.
c. The reflexes becomes more difficult to elicit.
d. The threshold for stimulus increases.
e. Mass reflex is abolished.
f. The muscles become extremely flaccid and undergo wasting.

Hemisection of Spinal Cord (Brown-Sequard Syndrome)

The lesion involving one lateral half of the spinal cord is called hemisection of the spinal cord (Figs 11.42 and 11.43). It can occur due to injury during accidents, gun shot injuries, tumor, etc.

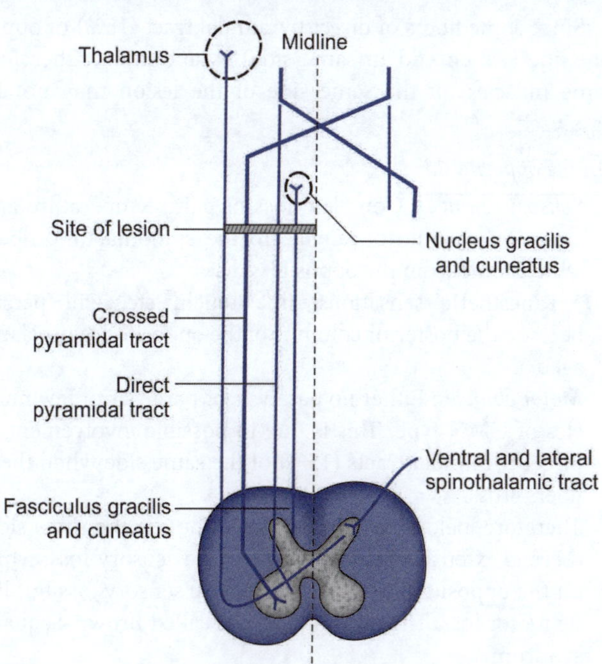

Fig. 11.42: Hemisection of spinal cord

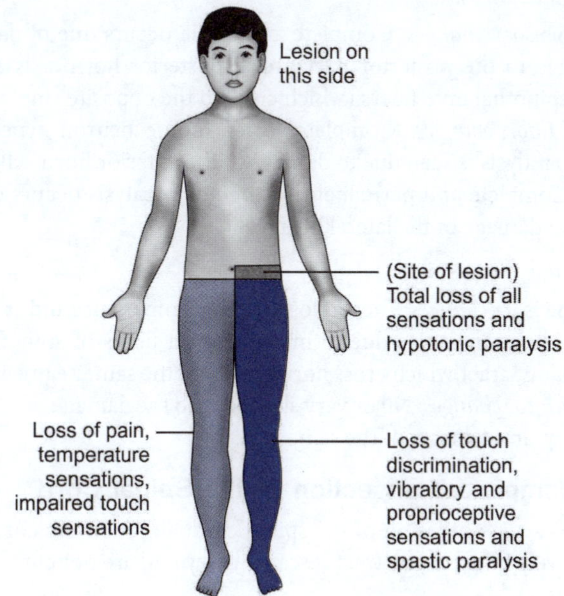

Fig. 11.43: Clinical features of Brown-Sequard syndrome

Symptoms of Hemisection of Spinal Cord

Here autonomic functions are usually normal. The other functional changes that take place can be divided into three categories:

1. Changes below the level of lesion
2. Chages at the level of lesion
3. Changes above the level of lesion.

The effects in these places differ on the same side and on the opposite side. There are changes in sensory and motor function.

Changes below the level of lesion

On the same side

1. *Sensory changes:* Fine touch, tactile localization and tactile discrimination, stereognosis, vibration sense and kinesthetic sense (sense of movement and position) is lost due to damage to uncrossed fibers of dorsal column tract.

   Pain, temperature and crude touch remain unaffected as the spinothamalic tracts (anterior and lateral) carrying these sensations cross to the opposite side and escape injury.

2. *Motor changes:* The motor changes resembles the effects of UMN type of lesion, due to damage of the crossed pyramidal tracts. These include spastic paralysis, +ve Babinski's sign, loss of superficial reflexes, exaggerated deep reflexes.

   Temporary loss of vasomotor tone due to damage of the descending fibers from the VMC in the medulla to the lateral horn cells. This leads to the dilation of blood vessels and fall in BP.

Since some fibers of direct pyramidal tract (15%) of opposite side (which end in same side) escape injury, therefore some muscles on the same side of the lesion may not be paralyzed.

On the opposite side

1. *Sensory changes:* Complete loss of pain, temperature and crude touch due to damage to the spinothalamic fibers which come from the opposite side.

   Kinesthetic sensations, fine touch, etc. will persist because the posterior columns of the opposite are not damaged.
2. *Motor changes:* Either no paralysis or paralysis of few muscles of UMN type. This is due to possible involvement of direct pyramidal tracts (15%) of the same side when these fibers cross.

   Therefore, below the level of the lesion, on the same side, there is extensive motor loss but little sensory loss; while on the opposite side there is extensive sensory loss but little motor loss. This phenomenon is called Brown-Sequard syndrome.

Changes at the level of lesion

On the same side

1. *Sensory changes:* Complete anesthesia occurs due of damage to the posterior nerve root, posterior horn cells and spinothalamic fibers (which cross to the opposite side).
2. *Motor changes:* Complete lower motor neuron type of paralysis is seen due to damage to the anterior horn cells. Complete and permanent vasomotor paralysis occurs due to damage of the lateral horn cells.

On the opposite side

1. *Sensory changes:* There is loss of pain, temperature and crude touch sensations due to injury of pain fibers of spinothalamic tract which cross horizontally in the same segment.
2. *Motor changes:* Nil or very slight due to the damage of some pyramidal tract of the same side.

Incomplete Transection of the Spinal Cord

In this type of lesion of the spinal cord, although the cord is severely injured, few tracts escape injury and are not cut.

Stage of Spinal Shock

It is identical with that of complete transection of the spinal cord.

Stage of Reflex Activity

Transection of the spinal cord is irregular. Therefore some of the descending tracts in the ventrolateral columns of spinal cord (especially vestibulospinal and reticulospinal) may escape injury and some connections persist between the brain and spinal cord. These tracts mainly reinforce the activity of the extensor motor neurons producing extensor hypertonia (Paraplegia in extension), i.e. the legs lie extended at hip and knee with toes pointing slightly downwards.

Characteristic Features

1. All features of upper motor neuron lesion is seen.
2. Involuntary movements are relatively infrequent, but when they occur, involve an increase of extensor tone, producing downward movement of feet and toes.
3. *Reflex movements:* The stretch reflex reappears first, then the flexor reflexes appear.

Sensory Disturbances

1. *Tabes Dorsalis:* In this condition degeneration of dorsal (sensory) nerve roots occurs. It affects the fibers specially in dorsal columns and fibers which convey pain. The disease is usually caused by syphilis.

   Characteristic features: In tabesdorsalis both sensory and motor functions are affected.
   - Numbness or paresthesia and lightning pains
   - Atonicity of bladder
   - Loss of position sense, vibration sense, passive movement.
   - Deep tendon reflexes like knee, ankle, biceps, triceps jerks are lost
   - Marked disturbance of voluntary movements
   - Loss of pain sensations particularly in the joints lead to deformities of the joints. There is no proper support and movements at the joint become uncontrolled is called Charcot's joint.
2. *Syringomyelia:* In this condition the gray matter around the central canal of spinal cord shows excessive growth of neuroglial tissue with cavity formation.

VESTIBULAR APPARATUS

Vestibular apparatus is the sensory organ for detecting sensation of equilibrium. It is encased in a system of bony tubes and chambers located in the petrous portion of the temporal bone, called the bony labyrinth. Within this system are membranous tubes and chambers called membranous labyrinth. The membranous labyrinth is the functional part of the vestibular apparatus. It consists of: (1) Three semicircular canal, (2) The otolith organ—saccule and utricle (the two sac like organ) (Fig. 11.44).

Semicircular Canal

Semicircular canals are the tubular structures placed at right angles to each other. Because of this type of arrangement, the semicircular canals represent the three axis of rotation: vertical, anteroposterior and transverse axis. The three membranous

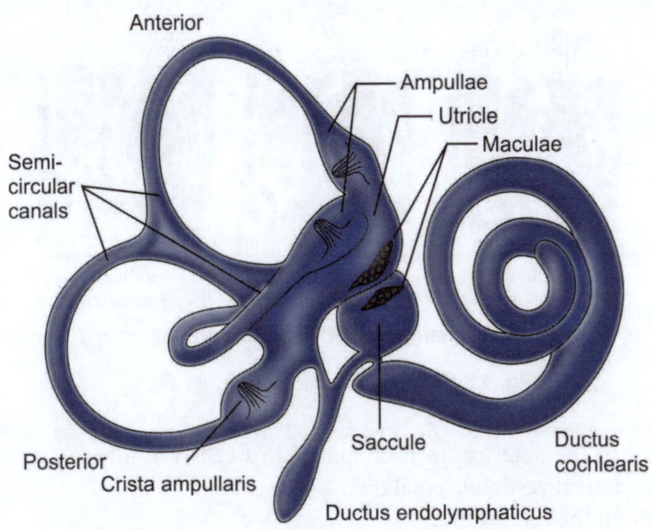

Fig. 11.44: Membranous labyrinth showing semicircular canals

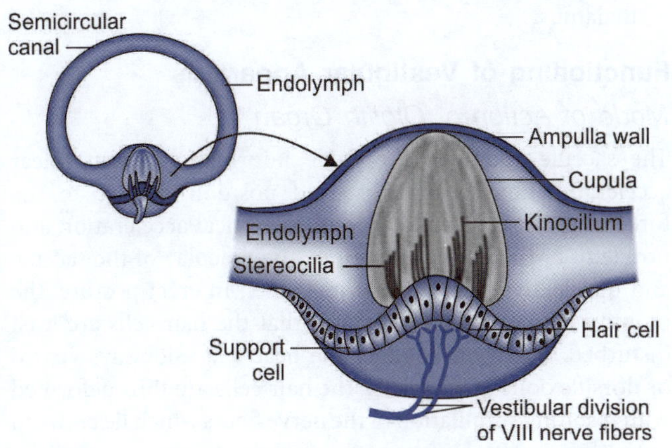

Fig. 11.45: Structure of crista (of semicircular canals) and macula (of Otolith organ)

canals are: horizontal (lateral), superior (anterior) and inferior (posterior). They contain endolymph and are separated from bony canal by the perilymph. Each canal begins as a dilation (or ampulla), containing a projecting ridge (on its inner aspect), called crista ampullaris (Fig. 11.45). Cristae are the receptors in the semicircular canals.

Each crista consists of hair cells and sustentacular cells (supporting cell) surmounted by a gelatinous partition (cupula) that closes off the ampula. The processes of the hair cells are embedded in the cupula, and the bases of the hair cells are in close contact with the afferent fibers of the vestibular division of the vestibulocochlear nerve.

Otolith Organ—Utricle and Saccule

The otolith organ is formed by utricle and saccule. The utricle communicates with the saccule by means of the ductus

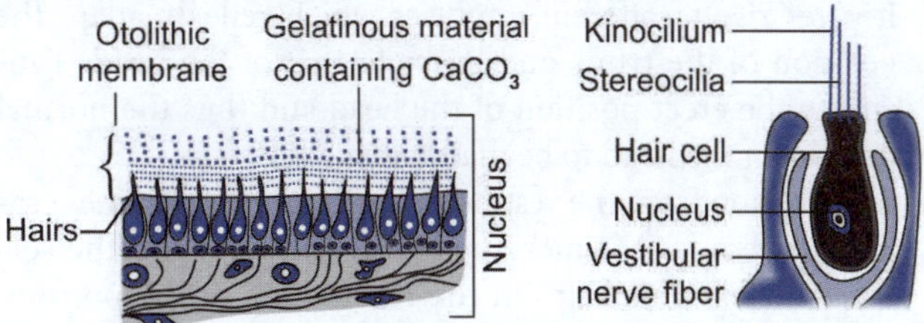

Fig. 11.46: Hair cell showing kinocilium and stereocilia

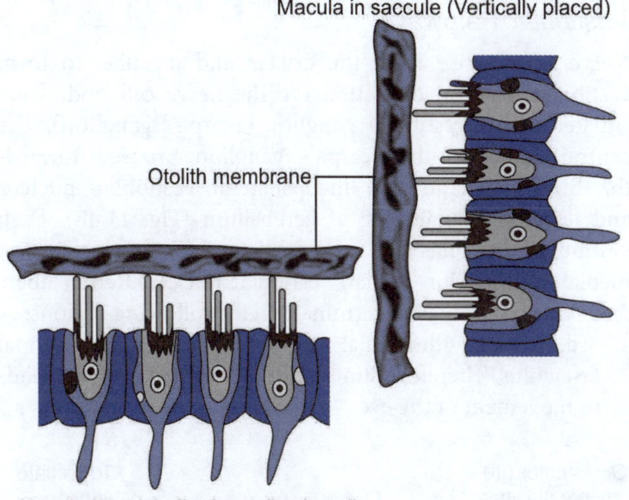

Fig. 11.47: Otolith organ (utricle and saccule with position of macula)

endolymphaticus. Both utricle and saccule contains a projecting ridge called the macula (like cristae, they are the receptors in otolith organ). Like crista, macula is also formed by hair cells and supporting cells which project into a firm gelatinous material, the cupula.

A large nonmotile hair called kinocilium (Fig. 11.46) is located at one end of hair cells. In the remaining hair cells, small cilia with progressive increase in height are present, called stereocilia. Between the hair cells lie the fibers of origin of vestibular division of VIII nerve. In the saccule and utricle, the cupula contains many chalky ($CaCO_3$) particles called otoliths (or otoconia) hence the name otolith organ. The hairs plus gelatinous materials containing $CaCO_3$ is called otolith membrane.

When head is in the normal erect position:

- The macula of each utricle is in horizontal plane
- The macula in each saccule is in vertical plane (Fig. 11.47).

Functions

The vestibular apparatus plays an important role in postural activity. The otolith organ (saccule and utricle) is stimulated by gravity and the semicircular canals activated by rotational movements. It plays an important role in postural activity.

1. It gives rise to afferent impulses which reflexly adapt the position of the trunk and limbs to that of the head. Thus enable the erect position of the head and thus the normal posture of the head to be maintained.
2. Information from the vestibular apparatus also reaches cranial nerve nuclei (which supply eye muscles) and the cerebral cortex. This helps in the recognition of the position and the movements of the head. As a result the position of the eyes is held approximately constant allowing visual fixation on moving objects.

Vestibular Pathways

Nerve fibers arise from the cristae and maculae to form vestibular division of VIII nerve.The nerve cell bodies are situated at the vestibular ganglion (Scarpa's ganglion). The central axons of the Scarpa's ganglion proceed towards the brainstem and end in ipsilateral vestibular nucleus and flocculonodular lobe of cerebellum (Fig. 11.48). Each vestibular nuclei has four subparts: lateral (Deiters), superior, medial and inferior (spinal) vestibular nuclei. Efferent fibers from vestibular nucleus terminate in the following regions:

1. 3rd, 4th and 6th cranial nuclei, via median longitudinal fasciculus. Therefore stimulation of vestibular nuclei leads to movement of the eyes.

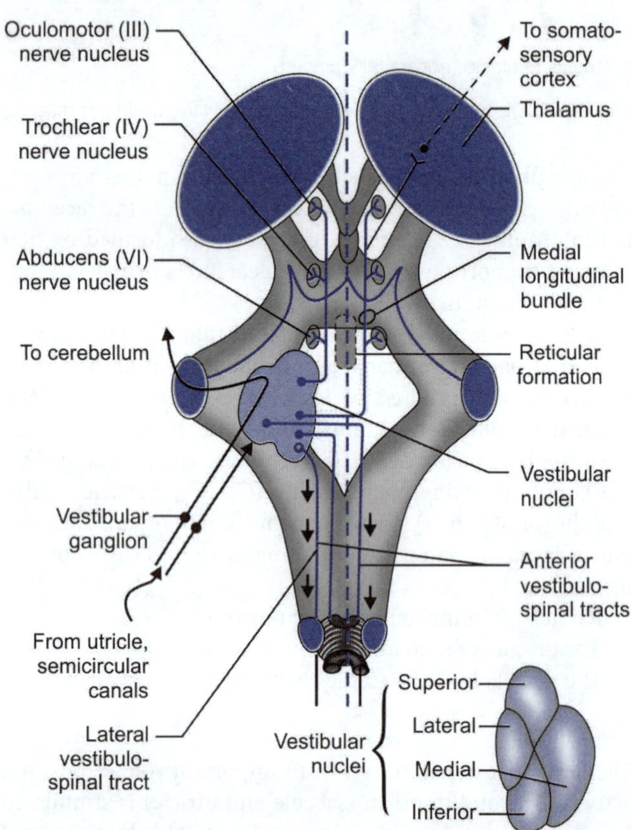

Fig. 11.48: Vestibular pathway

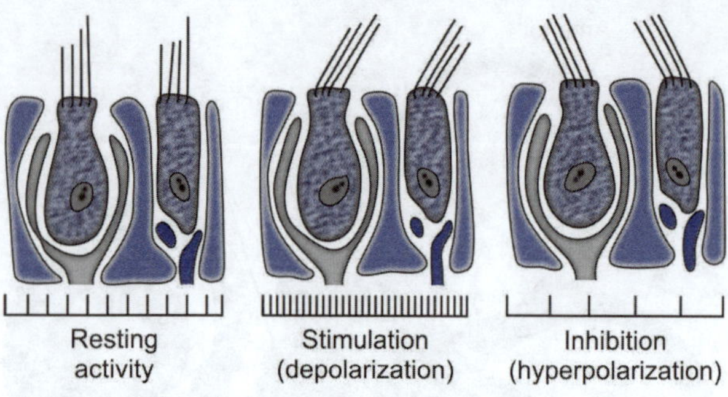

Fig. 11.49: Mode of action of Otolith organ

2. In the anterior horn of spinal cord cells via anterior and lateral vestibulospinal tract.
3. In the cerebellum.
4. In the nuclei of reticular formation.
5. In the primary somatosensory cortex via the opposite thalamus.

Functioning of Vestibular Apparatus

Mode of Action of Otolith Organ

The saccule and utricle provide information about linear acceleration and change in head position relative to the force of gravity. Saccule respond to vertical acceleration and utricle to horizontal acceleration. The maculae of the saccule and utricle are stretch receptors. When in erect posture, the otolith membranes are so placed that the hair cells are least disturbed. Based on bending the head (e.g. sideways/ventro or dorsiflexion) gravity acts. The hair cells are thus deformed with resulting stimulation of the nerve fibers which lie between them (Fig. 11.49).

1. Saccule is stimulated when there is sideways flexion of neck. If head is tilted to right:
   - Cupula of right saccule hangs downwards and pulls on its macula; thus maximally stimulated.
   - In left saccule there is upward movement of cupula to produce minimal stimulation.
2. The utricular macula are stimulated when there is ventro- or dorsiflexion of neck.
   - Head erect (upright)-minimal stimulus.
   - Head is bend forward or backward-maximal stimulation.

For this reason, the maculae of saccule and utricle are called gravity receptors. The receptors of vestibular apparatus show little or no adaptation.

Mode of Action of Semicircular Canals

The semicircular canal detects angular action during rotation of head along three perpendicular axis. When a person rotates in clockwise direction, i.e. in vertical axis, horizontal canal moves in clockwise direction. But there is no corresponding

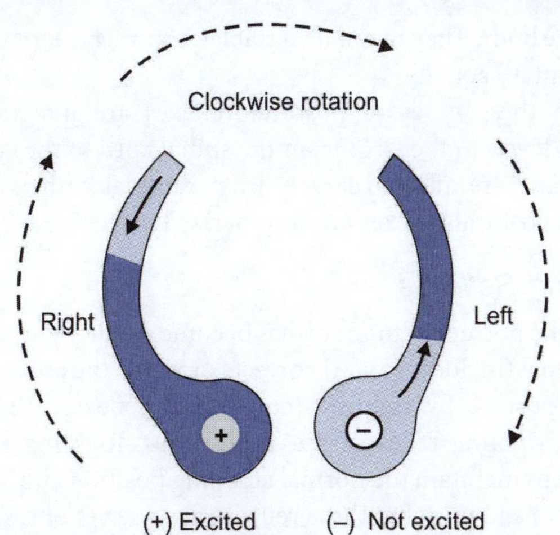

Fig. 11.50: Mode of stimulation of semicircular canals

movement of endolymph inside the canal at the beginning of rotation due to inertia. This phenomenon causes relative displacement of endolymph in the direction opposite to that of the rotation of head. That is, fluid is pushed in anticlockwise direction.

Thus in the right semicircular canal, the endolymph flows towards the ampulla (stimulation) and in left canal fluid moves away from the ampulla (decreased impulse discharge). The combination of increased discharge from one ampulla and decreased discharge from other form the basis of detection of direction of movement (Fig. 11.50).

The movement of endolymph in semicircular canal, in turn causes corresponding movement of gelatinous cupula causing cilia of hair cell to bent leading to stimulation of hair cells. Thus at the beginning of rotation in clockwise direction around vertical axis, the hair cells at ampulla of horizontal canal in right ear are stimulated. But, the hair cells in horizontal canal of left ear are not stimulated. Because of stimulation, the hair cells in right horizontal canal send information (impulses) through sensory nerve fibers to vestibular, cerebellar and reticular centers. Now, these centers send proper instructions to various muscles of the body to maintain equilibrium of the body during angular acceleration (rotation). On the other hand, rotation in anticlockwise direction causes stimulation of hair cells in ampulla of horizontal canal in left ear only.

Adaption of Receptors in Semicircular Canal During Rotation

The hair cells of crista ampullaris generate impulse (50–100 impulse/min) at rest. At the beginning of rotation discharge increases to 600–800 impulse/min. However, rapid discharge of impulses lasts only for first 20–25 sec of rotation. Afterwards during continuous rotation, the frequency of impulses falls back to resting level as endolymph starts moving along with semicircular canal at the same speed. This causes adaption of the hair cells.

Role in Regulation of Posture

1. The tract that descends from the vestibular nuclei into the spinal cord maintains tone in antigravity muscle and coordinates the adjustments made by the limbs and eyes in response to the change in body position. The vestibular apparatus thus plays a role in the support of the head during movement, orientation of the head in space and in reflexes (tonic labyrinthine and righting reflexes) accompanying locomotion. That is why the vestibular apparatus is sometimes called the sense organ of balance (equilibrium).
2. It controls eye movements via its ascending connections to the cranial nerve nuclei. Therefore, in spite of changes in head position the eye can remain fixed on the same point (***vestibulo-ocular reflex***). For example, if the head is rotated to the left, the eyes move towards right in order to prevent an image from moving off the fovea.
3. Orientation in space: Orientation, i.e. relative position of various body parts in space depends on four inputs:
   a. From vestibular receptors.
   b. From visual information.
   c. By impulses from proprioceptors in joint capulse.
   d. By impulses from cutaneous exteroceptors.

Vestibular Dysfunctions

Motion sickness: When a person, traveling by ship, rides a rough sea, he is expected to develop sea sickness; similar symptoms can develop when traveling by air or in a rough bus journey. All such sickness are called motion sickness. It is due to excessive and repeated stimulation of vestibular apparatus.

Symptoms

Nausea, vomiting, sweating, diarrhea, pallor, salivation, discomfort, headache, disorientation and lack of emotion.

Prevention

- Avoiding greasy and bulky food before travel
- Taking antiemetic drugs (drug preventing nausea and vomiting).

REGULATION OF POSTURE

Posture refers to the static position of any part of the body. Movements are the transition from one posture to another. Physiologically maintenance of posture refers to subconscious adjustment of tone in different muscles so as to maintain balance during displacement of the body caused by gravity or acceleration. A particular posture is produced through one or more reflexes. In a particular posture, some muscles are in a state of contraction and others are relaxed. Regulation of posture can be studied under two headings:

1. Mechanisms involved in maintenance of posture.
2. Role of different regions of nervous system in maintenance of posture.

Mechanisms Involved in Maintenance of Posture

The two main mechanisms involved in the maintenance of posture are:

a. Muscle Tone

i. *In upright posture:* The muscle tone is maintained through reflex adjustments of tone in the antigravity muscles (flexors of arm and extensors of leg). The center of gravity of the head passes in front of the atlanto-occipital joint. Thus the head has always got a tendency to roll forwards. To hold the head in erect position, cervico-occipital muscles are to be maintained in a state of constant tension.

ii. *Lean forward:* Here there is increased tone in extensors of trunk and flexors of leg.

iii. *Lean backward:* Here there is increased tone in rectus abdominis and extensors of leg.

iv. *Lean sideways:* Contralateral extensor oblique muscle has increased tone.

Maintenance of muscle tone: Stretch reflex plays the main role in maintenance of muscle tone. The center for muscle tone lies in the α-motor neurons of spinal cord, which are stimulated through a constant γ-motor neuron discharge. The activity of α and γ motor neurons is modified by both extrapyramidal and pyramidal fibers which terminate on them.

b. Postural Reflexes

The postural reflexes help to maintain the body in balanced and upright position.

Reflex Pathway

- Afferent organ: Eyes, vestibular apparatus and proprioceptors
- Center: Neuronal networks in brainstem and spinal cord.
- Efferent organ: Various skeletal muscles, supplied by α motor neurons.

Posture gives steady background for different movement mainly by two type of reflexes:

1. *Static reflexes:* These are elicited by gravitational pull and involve sustained contraction of muscles.
2. *Statokinetic reflexes:* These reflexes, also called phasic reflexes and they are elicited by acceleratory displacement of the body. They maintain a stable postural background for voluntary activity.

Both these types of postural reflexes are integrated at various levels in the CNS from the spinal cord to the cerebral cortex and are affected largely by pyramidal pathways. The various postural reflexes are summarized in Table 11.10.

Righting Reflexes

When the posture of the body has become suddenly abnormal, the animal (including man) corrects or rights the abnormality of the posture by righting (correcting) reflexes. There are various righting reflexes (see Table 11.9). Righting reflexes operate to maintain the normal standing position and keep an animal's head upright. These reflexes are a series of responses integrated for the most part in the nuclei of the midbrain.

Labyrinthine righting reflexes

When the midbrain animal is held by its body and tipped from side-to-side, the animal keeps its head in level (former position). This head reflex is known as labyrinthine righting reflexes. The stimulus is tilting of the head, which stimulates the otolithic organs; the response is compensatory contraction of the neck muscles to keep the head level.

Body on head righting reflex

If the animal is laid on its side, the pressure on that side of the body initiates reflex righting of the head even if the labyrinths have been destroyed. This is the body on head righting reflex. Pressure on the side of the body may cause body righting even if the head is prevented from righting.

Neck righting reflexes

If the head is righted by either of these mechanisms and the body remains tilted, the neck muscles are stretched. Their contraction rights the thorax and initiates a wave of similar stretch reflexes that pass down the body, righting the abdomen and the hindquarters.

Optical righting reflexes

In cats, dogs and primates, visual signs can initiate optical righting reflexes that right the animal in the absence of labyrinthine or body stimulation. Unlike the other righting reflexes, these responses depend upon an intact cerebral cortex. In intact humans, the operation of these reflexes maintains the head in a stable position and the eyes fixed on visual targets despite movements of the body and the jerks and jolts of everyday life. The responses are initiated by vestibular stimulation, stretching of neck muscles and movement of visual images on the retina and the responses are the vestibulo-ocular reflex (VOR) and other remarkably precise reflex contractions of the neck and extraocular muscles.

Table 11.10: Various righting reflexes

Reflex	Stimulus	Response	Receptor	Integrated in
Stretch reflexes	Stretch	Contraction of muscle	Muscle spindles	Spinal cord, medulla
Positive supporting (magnet) reaction	Contact with sole or palm	Foot extended to support body	Proprioceptors in distal flexors	Spinal cord
Negative supporting reaction	Stretch	Release of positive supporting reaction	Proprioceptors in extensors	Spinal cord
Tonic labyrinthine reflexes	Gravity	Contraction of limb extensor muscles	Otolithic organs	Medulla
Tonic neck reflexes	Head turned 1. To side 2. Up 3. Down	Change in pattern of extensor contraction 1. Extension of limbs on side to which head is turned 2. Hind legs flex 3. Forelegs flex	Neck proprioceptors	Medulla
Labyrinthine righting reflexes	Gravity	Head kept level	Otolithic organs	Midbrain
Neck righting reflexes	Stretch of neck muscles	Righting of thorax and shoulders, then pelvis	Muscle spindles	Midbrain
Body on head righting reflexes	Pressure on side of body	Righting of head	Exteroceptors	Midbrain
Body on body righting reflexes	Pressure on side of body	Righting of body even when head held sideways	Exteroceptors	Midbrain
Optical righting reflexes	Visual cues	Righting of head	Eyes	Cerebral cortex
Placing reactions	Various visuals, exteroceptive and proprioceptive cues	Footing placed on supporting surface in position to support body	Various	Cerebral cortex
Hopping reactions	Lateral displacement while standing	Hops, maintaining limbs in position to support body	Muscle spindles	Cerebral cortex

Role of Different Regions of Nervous System in Posture Maintenance

This can be experimentally investigated (usually in a cat) by producing transection in the neural axis at various levels.

Spinal Animal

The role of spinal cord in the maintenance of posture can be studied in a spinal animal. The spinal animal can be produced by a transection in the spinal cord at cervical region and respiration is maintained artificially by respiratory pump.

The posture in spinal animal during the stage of reflex activity

Except the basic stretch reflex and supporting reflexes which are integrated in spinal cord, all the other postural reflexes are absent. This is because all the postural reflexes require the integrity of UMN coming from various levels of neural axis.

Note

i. Though stretch reflex and supporting reactions are present, they are very weak and cannot support the weight of the animal. Therefore the animal cannot stand on its legs.

ii. Muscle tone returns first in flexor muscles, therefore flexors become less hypertonic than extensors producing paraplegia in flexion (both lower limbs are in state of flexion).

Decerebrate Animal

Decerebrate animal is one in whom the brainstem is transected at intercollicular level between superior and inferior colliculi. The intercollicular section causes total loss of the communications between the cerebral cortex and brainstem (that is why the name decerebration, i.e. removal of cerebrum is given to this operation, this is not to be confused with decortication). So this preparation can be used to study the role of brainstem in maintenance of posture.

Explanation

i. The medullary inhibiting area having no intrinsic activity of its own, now becomes greatly (but not totally) non-functioning. This center, however, continues to receive some impulses from the cerebellum.

ii. The brainstem facilitatory areas, having intrinsic activity of its own, continue to discharge the facilitatory impulses and

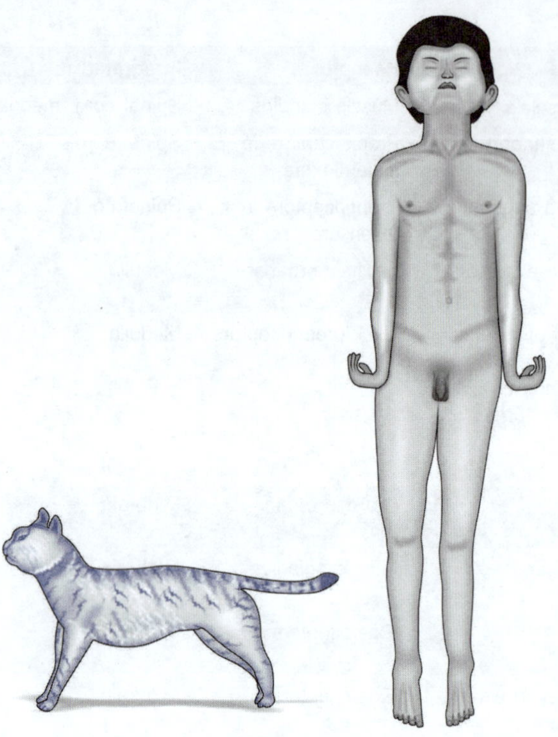

Fig. 11.51: Decerebrate rigidity

now this impulses remain unopposed (as the inhibitory areas are now largely silent).

iii. The vestibular nucleus normally sends facilitatory impulses to the spinal center. In a decerebrate preparation, such facilitatory impulses are exaggerated.

Decerebrate Rigidity

Decerebrate rigidity refers to the marked increase in the tone (hypertonia) of extensors, i.e. antigravity muscles occurring, immediately after decerebration of the animal.

Characteristic features of decerebrate rigidity (Fig. 11.51):

a. Hyperextension of all the four limbs.
b. Dorsiflexion (hyperextension of tail and head)
c. Extreme hyperextension of the spine (opisthotonos) which produces concave configuration of the back.
d. The animal can be made to stand on four limbs but is easily toppled by a slight push.
e. Postural reflexes which can be elicited in a decerebrate animal are stretch reflexes, positive supporting reaction, negative supporting reaction, crossed extensor reflex, tonic neck and labyrinthine reflexes.
f. Righting reflexes are absent, therefore decerebrate animal can stand on its four legs but slight displacement causes the decerebrate animal to topple over.

So the conclusion is, in decerebrate rigidity, there is a great preponderance of facilitatory influences reaching the spinal center from above. Experiments have established that these facilitatory influences cause stimulation of the γ efferent and thus increase the tone. Viewed in another way, the decerebrate rigidity is due to the release of the brainstem centers from the influences of the cerebral cortex, red nuclei and the basal ganglia. Lacking this input, the medullary reticular inhibitor system becomes nonfunctional; full overactivity of the pontine excitatory system occurs, and rigidity develops. The decerebrate rigidity therefore is another example of release phenomenon.

Note

Tonic labyrinthine reflexes

This reflex is best studied in decerebrate animal. In the decerebrate animal, the pattern of rigidity in the limbs varies with the position. No righting responses are present, and the animal stays in the position in which it is put. If the animal is placed on its back, then there is profound extension of all four limbs, but if the animal is turned to either side, the rigidity decreases. Rigidity is minimum when the animal lies at prone position. These changes in rigidity are due to the action of gravity on the otolithic organs and are effected via the vestibulospinal tracts. This reflex rigidity is known as the tonic labyrinthine reflexes. These reflexes are abolished by removal of the labyrinth (Fig. 11.52).

Tonic neck reflexes

The reflexes are set up from neck muscles. If the head of a decerebrate animal is turned to side, up or down, changes in the pattern of rigidity occur. If the head is turned to right, the right limb is extended and the left limb is relaxed. This is the position often assumed by a normal animal looking to one side. Flexion of the head (head turned down) causes flexion

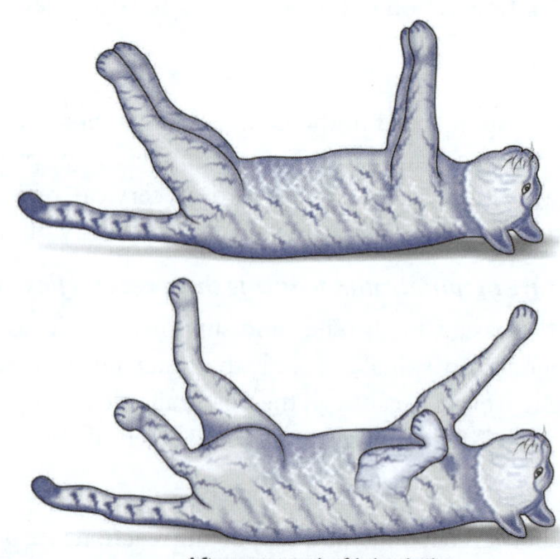

Fig. 11.52: Tonic labyrinthine reflex

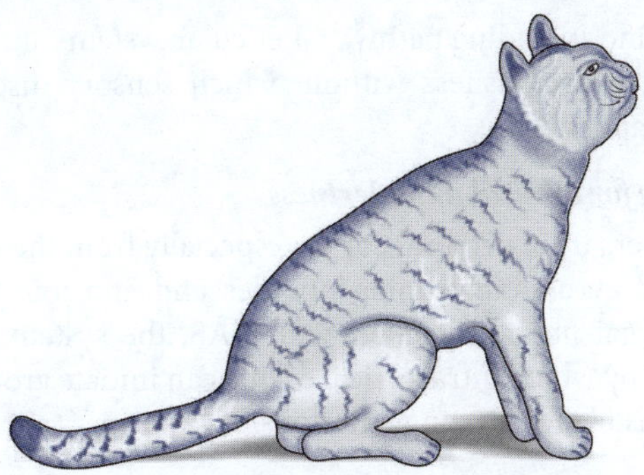

Fig. 11.53: Tonic neck reflex

of the forelimbs and continued extension of the hind limbs, the posture of an animal looking into a hole in the ground. Extension of the head (head turned up) causes flexion of the hind limbs and extension of the forelimbs, the posture of an animal looking over an obstacle. These responses are the tonic neck reflexes (Fig. 11.53). They are initiated by stretch of the proprioceptors in the upper part of the neck and they can be sustained for long periods.

Midbrain Animal

Midbrain animal is prepared by the section of the neural axis at the superior border of the midbrain. So this preparation can be used to study the role of midbrain in maintenance of posture.

Characteristic features

- Midbrain animal has extensor rigidity similar to that of a decerebrate animal only when the animal lies quietly on its back. The rigidity disappears when the limb is performing a reflex activity.
- No spinal shock is present.
- Righting reflexes, having integration center in the midbrain are present. These include labyrinthine righting reflex, neck righting reflex, body on head righting reflex and body on body righting reflex.

Decorticate Animal

Decorticate animal is one in which only the superficial few millimeters of cerebral cortex alone is removed with the basal ganglia and brainstem remaining intact. So this preparation can be used to study the role of basal ganglia in maintenance of posture. Postural characteristics of a decorticate animal:

a. *Moderate rigidity:* Moderate rigidity is present due to loss of the cortical area that inhibits spinal γ-motor neurons discharges via reticular formation. It is seen only when the animal is at rest. This is because the basal ganglia which are intact in decorticate animal activate the descending inhibitory reticular formation and thereby prevent hypertonia.

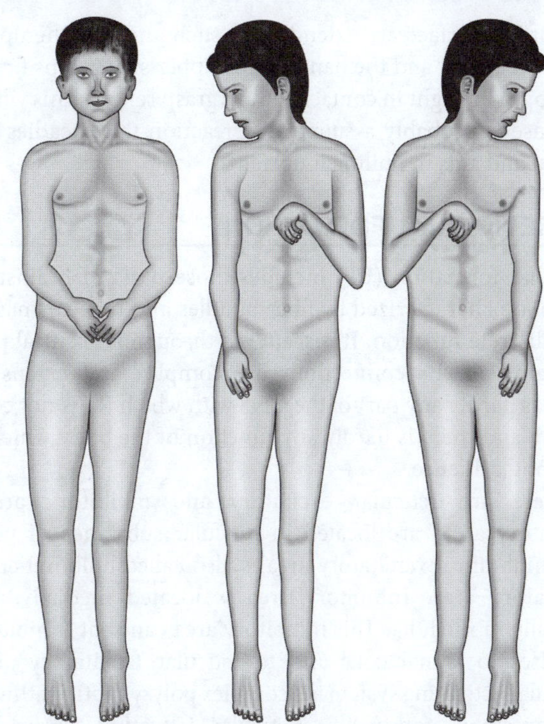

Fig. 11.54: Typical posture of a decorticate man

b. *Typical posture:* The typical posture in a decorticate man consists of full extension of legs, arms lying across the chest, with some semiflexion at the elbow, slight pronation of forearm and flexion of wrist and fingers (Fig. 11.54).
c. *Postural reflexes:* In decorticate man or animal following reflexes like typical neck reflexes, righting reflexes can be elicited. Postural reflexes which are seriously disrupted by decortication are the hopping and placing reactions.

Note

Two types of postural reactions, the hopping and placing reactions, are seriously disrupted by decortication.

Hopping reaction

When a standing animal is pushed laterally, hopping movements keep the limbs in position to support the body. This response is called hopping reaction.

Placing reaction

If one limb of a standing animal is pushed out from under it, the limb is promptly replaced on the supporting surface in position to support the body. This response is known as placing reaction. Placing reactions are usually abolished on one side by unilateral decortications.

Grasp reflex

If brain tissue in primates above the thalamus is removed and the animal is allowed to lie on one side, the limbs next to the supporting surface are extended. In such animals, the upper limbs are flexed and the hand on the upper side grasps firmly any object brought in contact with it (grasp reflex). This whole response is probably a supporting reaction that steadies the animal and aids in pulling it upright.

RETICULAR FORMATION

Reticular formation (RF) includes those parts of brainstem which are characterized by fiber bundles and nuclear masses with discrete function. It is scattered throughout central part of brainstem. Its connections are complex and extensive. There is hardly any part of the CNS with which RF is not connected, and there is hardly any function of the body which it does not influence.

There are reticular excitatory and inhibitory areas. Excitatory areas are located in reticular substance of pons and midbrain. Excitatatory area is also called bulboreticular facilitatory area. Inhibitory area is located medially and ventrally in medulla. This inhibitory area can sent inhibitory impulses to spinal cord and to reticular facilitatory area. Reticular activating system is a complex polysynaptic pathway. The system is nonspecific. Reticular activating system has ascending and descending fibers. It is essential for life because:

- Vital centers such as CVS, respiratory, swallowing, vomiting, etc. are located in reticular formation.
- It receives and integrates information from all parts of CNS.
- Its neurons send axons to most regions of brain and spinal cord. Thus, it influence all parts of CNS.

Type of Reticular System

Pathways that convey information from the reticular formation are divided into two systems—ascending and descending reticular system.

Ascending Reticular System

The ascending reticular pathway (Fig. 11.55) is also called reticular activating system (RAS).

1. It is a complex polysynaptic pathway whose fibers extend from brainstem to thalamus.
2. It receives afferent collateral from:
   - Specific sensory pathways
   - Trigeminal, auditory, olfactory, visual pathway.
3. A single peripheral stimulus gives rise to impulses which ascend to cerebral cortex via two pathways:
   - Specific sensory pathways which are responsible for sensory discrimination.
   - Collateral branch given to reticular formation.

From reticular formation, impulses reach nonspecific nuclei of thalamus and from there to cerebral cortex through nonspecific ascending pathway. Reticular system functions by arousing consciousness without which sensory discrimination is impossible.

Pathway for arousal and alertness

Some fibers from cerebral cortex, especially from the superior temporal gyrus and frontal lobe descend and join to form corticofugal fibers. Together with RAS, the system provide pathway by which intracortical events can initiate arousal and is responsible for alerting emotions.

Descending Reticular System

The reticular fibers that descend to the spinal cord form the reticulospinal tracts. It modifies the activities of spinal motor neurons. This system comprises the descending inhibitory reticular system and descending facilitatory reticular system.

Functions of Reticular Formation

1. The RAS and related components are concerned with alertness, maintenance of attention and wakefulness that make perception possible.
2. Control of muscle tone and regulation of postural reflexes.
3. Role in the integration of autonomic activity through connections to ANS.
4. Conditioning and learning.
5. Reticular formation is connected to hypothalamus and limbic system. Hence it plays an important role in emotional reactions.

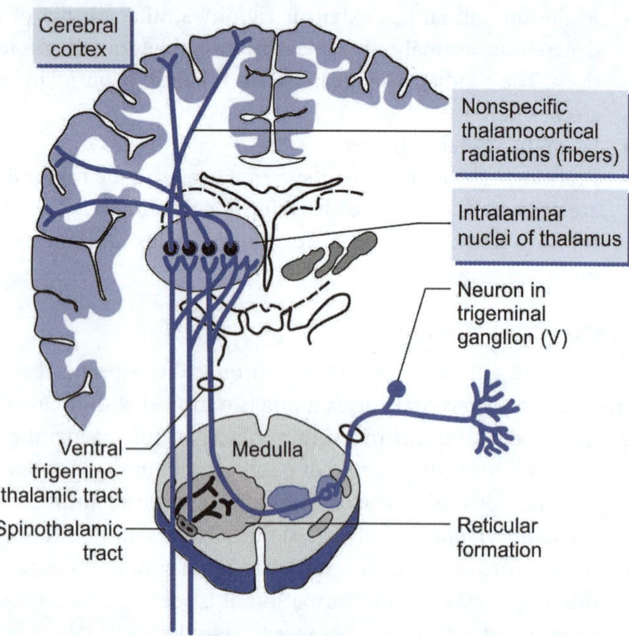

Fig. 11.55: Reticular activating system

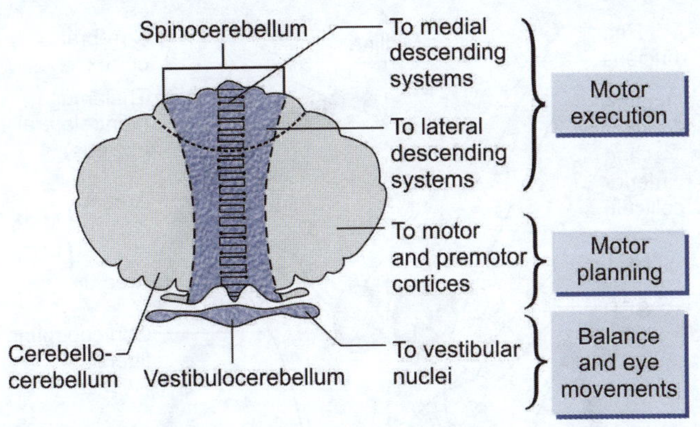

Fig. 11.56: Functional division of cerebellum

CEREBELLUM

Cerebellum is situated posterior to the brainstem. It influences motor functions. Cerebellum receives copy of motor plan from motor cortex. It also receives information from periphery regarding the ongoing movements. It projects to almost all areas of brain that are involved in control of motor activities. Therefore, cerebellum strongly influences all aspects movement starting from rate, range, force and direction to the termination of movement. Hence, damage to cerebellum results in severe incoordination of movement.

Anatomical Divisions

The cerebellum is divided into three parts by two transverse fissures. The posterolateral fissure separates the medial nodulus and the lateral flocculus on either side from rest of the cerebellum. The primary fissure divides the remainder into an anterior and posterior lobe.

Functional Divisions

Functionally the divisions/lobes are named according to the connections they make with other components of the motor control system (Fig. 11.56).

a. *Flocculonodular lobe:* It is functionally related to the vestibular apparatus and therefore also called the vestibulocerebellum. It is concerned with control of body posture. It is also called vestibulocerebellum.
b. *Spinocerebellum:* The entire anterior lobe and parts of the posterior lobe that receive information from the spinal cord, are called spinocerebellum. It occupies the median portion of the cerebellar cortex and receives proprioceptive input from the body. It is concerned with control of axial (trunk) and limb muscles and postural reflexes.
c. *Neocerebellum:* The remaining part of the posterior lobe (lateral portions of cerebellar hemispheres) forms the neocerebellum. It receives information from the cerebral cortex and pons. It is concerned with skilled voluntary movements. It is also called cerebrocerebellum.

Note

On each side cerebellum is connected to the brainstem by three peduncles:

a. Superior cerebellar peduncle-connects midbrain to cerebellum.
b. Middle cerebellar peduncle-connects pons to cerebellum.
c. Inferior cerebellar peduncle-connects medulla to cerebellum.

Organization

The cerebellum has an external cerebellar cortex separated by white matter from the deep cerebellar nuclei. The primary afferent inputs; the mossy and climbing fibers send collaterals to the deep nuclei and pass to the cortex. There are four deep nuclei: Dentate, globose, emboliform and the fastigial nuclei.

Cerebellar Cortex

Microscopically the gray matter of cerebellar cortex consists of five main types of neurons:

1. Stellate cells
2. Basket cells
3. Purkinje cells
4. Granule cells
5. Golgi cells

Purkinje cells are one of the largest neurons in the body. These five types of neurons are arranged in three layers:

1. *Molecular layer:* This layer is most superficial and is composed of two types of neurons (Stellate and basket cells) and unmyelinated nerve fibers.
2. *Purkinje cell layer:* It is composed of a single layer of large flask-shaped Purkinje cells and dendrites of Purkinje cells.
3. *Granule cell layer:* It consists of granule and Golgi cells with their processes and sensory mossy fibers with their synaptic glomeruli.

Neuronal Circuits and Neuronal Activity in Cerebellum

Cerebellum executes its functions through excitatory output of the deep cerebellar nuclei to the brainstem and thalamus. Neural connections (Fig. 11.57) within the cerebellar cortex is basically concerned with modulating or timing the excitatory output of the deep cerebellar nuclei via the fibers of Purkinje cells. This is done in accordance with the signals received by the cerebellar cortex from different parts of the brain and body. Neuronal activity in cerebellum involves three processes:

Afferents to Cerebellar Cortex

Afferents to cerebellar cortex reach via two types of fibers:

i. Climbing fibers

These fibers represent terminations of axons reaching the cerebellum from the inferior olivary nucleus. The climbing fibers

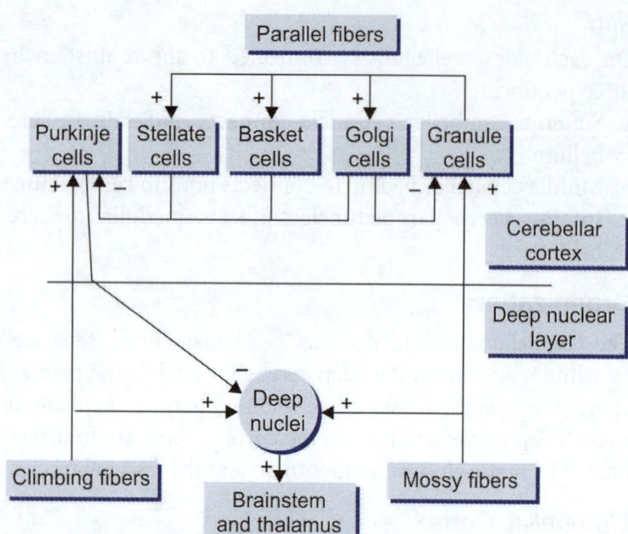

Fig. 11.57: Diagram of neural connections in the cerebellum + and – signs indicate whether endings are excitatory or inhibitory

excite Purkinje cells and the deep cerebellar nuclei, Purkinje cells and the deep cerebellar nuclei directly.

ii. Mossy fibers

Originates from cell bodies in the spinal cord and brainstem (spinocerebellar). They terminate on granule cells and indirectly influence Purkinje cells. The mossy fibers excites granule cells and the deep cerebellar nuclei.

Neuronal Activity of Intrinsic Cerebellar Circuitry

- Climbing fibers directly excite cerebellar deep nuclei initially and later they travel up in cerebellum and excite purkinje cells.
- Purkinje cells in turn inhibit deep nuclei. So, there is strong excitation to deep nuclei followed later by inhibition.
- Mossy fiber directly excites cerebellar deep nuclei initially and later they travel up in cerebellum and excite granule cells.
- Granule cells in turn excite stellate, basket and Golgi cells. This is called feed forward activation.
- Stellate, basket and Golgi cells inhibit Purkinje cells. This is called feed forward inhibition.
- To regulate granule cell output, Golgi cells inhibit granule cells back. This is called feedback inhibition.

Neuronal Activity of Deep Cerebellar Nuclei

The deep cerebellar nuclei receive excitatory inputs via collaterals from the mossy fibers, climbing fibers and also other excitatory inputs. The neuronal activity in the cerebellar cortex plays an important role in modulating the excitatory signals of the pathways from the deep cerebellar nuclei to thalamus, cerebral cortex and to brainstem nuclei. Because of this modulating or timing effect the cerebellar cortex is able to well organize and coordinate the different movements of the body.

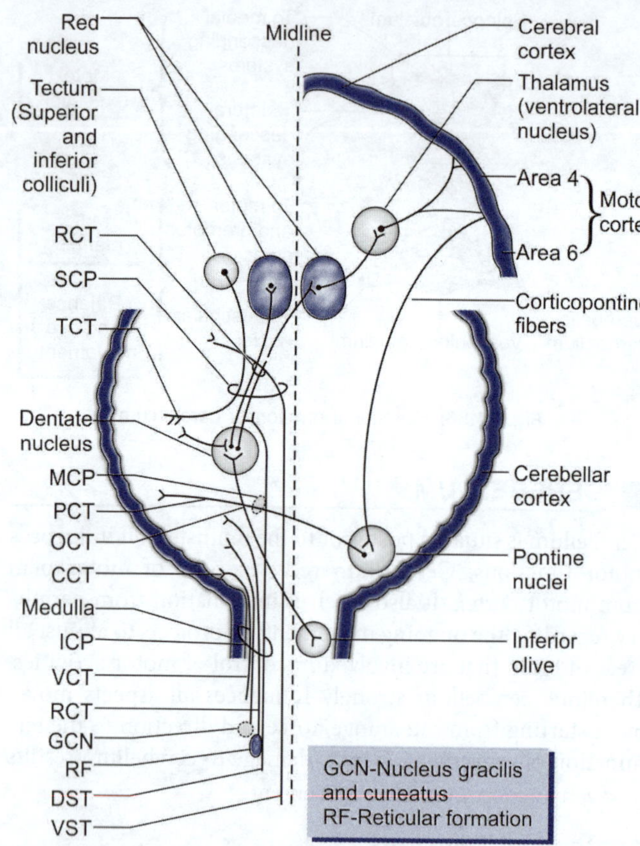

Fig. 11.58: Afferent cerebellar connections

Connections of the Cerebellum

Afferent Connections (Fig. 11.58)

Tracts through superior cerebellar peduncle

1. *Ventral spinocerebellar tract (VST):* It carries a large portion of extroceptive (cutaneous) and proprioceptive fibers from all parts of the body. The fibers enter the cerebellum via the ipsilateral superior cerebellar peduncle and is distributed mainly to the vermis and anterior lobe.
2. *Tectocerebellar tract (TCT):* It arises from the superior and inferior colliculi which relays fibers respectively from the eye and ear. This tract carries visual impulses from superior colliculus and auditory impulses from the inferior colliculus to spinocerebellum through the superior cerebellar peduncle (SCP).

3. *Rubrocerebellar tract (RCP):* It arises from the red nucleus, may be both crossed and uncrossed. It enters via the superior cerebellar peduncle (SCP) and is distributed mainly to the dentate nucleus. It transmits impulses which have originated from the motor cortex and relays in the red nucleus.
4. *Olivocerebellar tract (OCT):* This tract is formed by the climbing fibers arising from the inferior olivary nucleus in medulla. After taking origin, these fibers cross the midline and reach the spinocerebellum through the superior cerebellar peduncle of the opposite side. It carries proprioceptive inputs from whole body via relay in inferior olive. The inferior olivary nucleus receives afferent fibers from three sources:
   a. Brainstem nuclei of the same side.
   b. Spinal cord through spino-olivary tract of same side.
   c. Cerebral cortex of opposite side.

Tracts through middle cerebellar peduncle

Cortico-ponto-cerebellar tract: It arises in the motor cortex (areas 4 and 6) and other parts of cerebral cortex. It ends in the nuclei pontis. From the nuclei pontis the pontocerebellar fibers cross to enter the opposite side in the middle cerebellar peduncle (MCP) and are distributed to all parts of the cerebellar cortex (except flocculonodular lobe).

Tracts through inferior cerebellar peduncle

1. *Dorsal spinocerebellar tract (DST):* It carries mainly extroceptive (cutaneous) and proprioceptive impulses from the trunk and leg. It is an uncrossed tract, and reaches the spinocerebellum through the inferior peduncle of the same side. It is distributed to the anterior lobe, pyramis, uvula and the median part of the paramedian lobe.
2. *Vestibulocerebellar tract (VCT):* It arises in the vestibular nuclei. It passes through the inferior cerebellar peduncle (ICP) of the same side and reach the deep cerebellar nuclei. It supplies mainly the flocculonodular lobe and uvula.
3. *Cuneocerebellar tract (CCT):* This tract arises from the external arcuate nucleus. It reaches the spinocerebellum through the inferior cerebellar peduncle of the same side to anterior lobe, pyramis and uvula. It carries proprioceptive impulses from the arm and neck muscles to spinocerebellum.
4. *Reticulocerebellar tract (RCT):* It arises in the lateral reticular nucleus and is uncrossed. It is distributed via the inferior cerebellar peduncle of the same side to the whole of cerebellar cortex.

Efferent Connections

Purkinje cell axons pass to the deep cerebellar nuclei in an orderly manner. Their influence on these nuclei is purely inhibitory via release of GABA.

Functions of Cerebellum

The cerebellum controls the motor activities both voluntary (via pyramidal system) as well as nonvoluntary, like tone, posture and equilibrium (via the extrapyramidal system).

1. *Control of body posture and equilibrium:* The flocculonodular lobe (vestibulocerebellum) is concerned with the control of body posture and equilibrium. Afferents from the vestibular apparatus pass directly or after relay in the vestibular nuclei to the flocculonodular lobe. The efferents from them return back to the vestibular nuclei. From these nuclei the vestibulospinal tract connects with spinal motor neurons.
2. *Control of muscle tone and stretch reflexes:* Spinocerebellum regulates the postural reflexes by modifying the muscle tone. It facilitates the γ motor neurons in the spinal cord. The γ motor neurons reflexly modify the activity of the motor neurons and thus regulate the muscle tone. Thus, cerebellum forms an important site of linkage of α-γ systems responsible for muscle tone.
3. *Control of voluntary movements:* Cerebellum is not able to initiate any motor activity, but coordinates the movements initiated by motor cortex. Coordination of movements is the result of appropriate regulation of time, rate, range (extent), force and direction of muscular activity. This is made possible because the cerebellum establishes reciprocal connections with most regions of CNS to which it is connected.
4. *Control of eyeball movements:* The oculomotor, trochlear and abducent nuclei which supply the extraocular muscles of eye movements are brought under cerebellar control by vestibular nuclei. Pyramis is concerned with the movement of eyeball because its stimulation causes upward eye movement to ipsilateral side. It also has a role in the judgment of distance.

Cerebellar Lesions

The cerebellar lesion of one hemisphere produces dysfunction on the same side of the body whereas the lesions of the vermis affect both the sides (due to double crossing, each cerebellar hemisphere influences the opposite cortex; which in turn influences the motor cortex via the corticospinal tracts which controls the movement of the opposite side of the body. Because of the double decussation each cerebellar hemisphere controls the voluntary movements on its own side of the body).

Characteristic Features

Disturbance of posture

a. *Atonia or hypotonia:* The muscle tone is either completely lost (atonia) or markedly decreased (hypotonia) on the affected side due to loss of facilitatory effect of the neocerebellum. Therefore, the muscles feel soft and the limb moves to and fro slowly.

b. *Attitude:*
   i. Trunk is bent with concavity towards the affected side. This is because the weight of the body is thrown on the unaffected leg.
   ii. Face is rotated towards the opposite side (pulled by the healthy muscles).
   iii. The homolateral shoulder is lower than the opposite normal shoulder.
   iv. The leg is abducted and rotated outwards.
c. *Spontaneous deviation:* If the eyes are closed and the arms are held straight out in front of the body, homolateral arms bend laterally.
d. *Nystagmus:* It is a tremor of the eyeballs which occurs when the patient attempts to fix his eyes on an object. It consists of a slow to and fro movement on looking to the affected side due to hypotonia and a rapid to and fro movement on looking to the opposite side.
e. *Deep/Tendon reflexes:* The deep reflexes become weak and pendular. For example, pendular knee jerk, i.e. after the initial reflex response, the leg on falling continues to swing freely to and fro. This is due to hypotonia of quadriceps muscle.

Disturbance of voluntary movements

a. *Ataxia:* It is the lack of coordination of movements due to errors in the rate, range, force and direction of movement. It is the hallmark of cerebellar disorder and characterized by:
   i. *Decomposition of the movement:* The movement seems to occur in stages. The patient cannot easily combine the movements of several joints into a single smooth, coordinated motion. For example, to move the arm, they might first move the shoulder, then the elbow and finally the wrist.
   ii. *Asynergia:* There is lack of coordination between protagonists, antagonists and synergists.
   iii. *Dysmetria*: The movement is poorly carried out in direction, range and force, therefore, the movements overshoot their intended mark, i.e. post pointing (hypermetria) or fall short of it (hypometria). There is inability to control range of motion. For example, while reaching for a glass of water, his hand either stops in the midway or overshoots. It results from the loss of the neural circuit required to control the duration and strength of a movement.
b. *Intention tremor:* It is a common remarkable feature of cerebellar lesions. There is no tremor at rest. Such patients cannot perform movements smoothly. If they reach for an object, their movements are jerky and accompanied by oscillating, to and fro tremors that become more marked as the hand approaches the object. The tremors are coarse and they occur at a frequency of 4–6/sec. Clinically these disturbances can be demonstrated by finger nose test, rebound phenomenon, adiadochokinesis and heel-knee test.
c. *Gait:* Patients walk in a clumsy manner, with their feet wide apart (wide-based gait). They have such difficulty in maintaining balance that their gait appears drunken, called ***drunken gait.*** The patient walks in a zig-zag line and deviates to the affecters side due to hypotonia.
d. *Speech:* Slurred, scanning type of speech results. It is also slow and lalling (like a baby) due to imperfect use of the movements of the laryngeal muscles and tongue.

THALAMUS

Thalamus is a part of diencephalon which processes all the sensory information (except olfaction) that reaches the cortex. The two thalami are ovoid masses of grey matter lying close together rostrally and joined in the midline by the mass intermedia and separated only by the third ventricle. The thalamus is a sensory relay and integrative center connecting with many areas of brain, including the cerebral cortex, basal ganglia, hypothalamus and brainstem. Ascending sensory fibers, ascending through the brainstem, synapse in the thalamus and then relayed to the cerebral cortex via the internal capsule. Motor fibers descending from cerebral cortex pass to brainstem via the internal capsule but without synapsing in the thalamus.

Anatomical Classification of Thalamic Nuclei

The thalamus is divided into three nuclear groups (Fig. 11.59) by the internal medullary lamina (consists of white matter).

1. *Anterior group of nuclei:* The mass of gray matter enclosed within the bifurcation of the internal medullary lamina is called anterior nucleus.

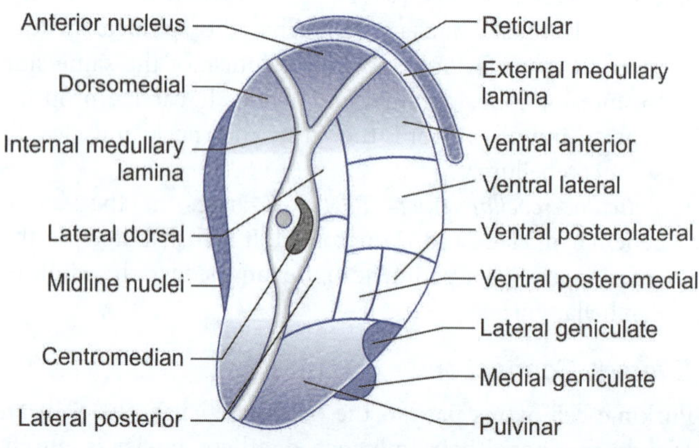

Fig. 11.59: Nuclei of thalamus

2. *Lateral group of nuclei:* The mass of gray matter present in the lateral part of the thalamus is subdivided into ventral and dorsal group of nuclei.
   a. The ventral group of nuclei contains:
      i. Ventral anterior nucleus
      ii. Ventral lateral nucleus
      iii. Ventral posterior nucleus
      iv. Medial geniculate body
      v. Lateral geniculate body.
   b. The dorsal group of nucleus contains:
      i. Pulvinar (cluster of neurons lying most posteriorly)
      ii. Lateral posterior
      iii. Lateral dorsal.
3. *Medial group of nuclei:* It includes the following nuclei:
   i. Centromedian and other intralaminar nuclei
   ii. Dorsomedial nucleus.
   iii. Midline nucleus.

Functional Classification of Thalamic Nuclei

Functionally the thalamic nuclei can be grouped under 2 divisions:

Nonspecific Projection Nuclei

They receive afferents from RAS and project diffusely to neocortex. Impulse in them is responsible for diffuse secondary response and the alerting effect of RAS. Nuclei involved are:

a. Anterior group of nuclei

Afferent - From mammillary body of hypothalamus via mammillothalamic tract
Efferent - To cingulate gyrus
Function - Part of Papez circuit
- Associated with limbic system
- Concerned with recent memory and emotion.

b. Midline nucleus

Afferents - Spinothalamic
- Trigeminothalamic
- Medial lemniscus
- Reticular formation
- Hypothalamus
- Other thalamic nuclei

Function - Center for integrating 'crude' visceral and somatic sensations.

c. Intralaminar nuclei

Afferents - RAS
- Basal ganglion
- Other thalamic nuclei.

Function - Integrates somatic and visceral sensory impulses before projecting this information to cortex. It is also responsible for alerting affects of RAS.

d. Dorsomedial nucleus

Afferents - Hypothalamic nuclei
Efferents - Prefrontal cortex (8, 9, 10, 11)
Function - Association center for synthesis of crude and somatic sensation.

Specific Projection Nuclei

Specific projection nuclei are classified as part controlling motor, sensory and integrative functions.

Motor function

a. Ventral lateral

Afferents - Cerebellum (dentate nucleus), globus pallidus
Efferents - Premotor area
Functions - Relay proprioceptive information and voluntary motor function, i.e. motor control and planning, programing.

b. Ventral anterior

Afferents - Basal ganglia (substantia nigra and globus pallidus)
Efferents - Area 6
Functions - Motor controlling, planning and programing.

Sensory function

a. Ventroposterolateral nucleus

Afferents - Spinothalamic tract, medial leminscus (ML)
Efferents - Postcentral gyrus (3, 1, 2).

b. Ventroposteromedial

Afferents - Trigeminal and ML (face and taste fibers)
Efferents - Postcentral gyrus (3, 1, 2).

Integrative functions

a. Lateral dorsal nucleus

Afferent - Superior colliculus
Efferent - Cingulate gyrus and hippocampal area.

b. Lateral posterior: Has reciprocal connection with areas 5 and 7 of parietal association area.

c. Pulvinar

Afferent - Thalamic nuclei and cortex
Efferent - Cortex (parietal, temporal and occipital areas)
Function - Integrates auditory, somatic and visual information.

d. Medial geniculate body: Concerned with audition.

e. Lateral geniculate body: Concerned with vision.

Functions of Thalamus

1. The thalamus is a great sensory relay station and integrating center for most inputs before relaying them to the cerebral cortex.
   i. Relay station in the pathway of somesthetic sensation coming from opposite side of the body.

ii. Relay station for impulses coming from opposite side of cerebellum on their way to motor cortex.
iii. Relay station for impulse from RF.
iv. Relay station in the auditory and visual pathways.
v. Relay station for autonomic and emotional reactions due to its connections with the hypothalamus and limbic lobe.

2. It is responsible for maintenance of conscious and alerting responses of RAS.
3. It is responsible for subcortical perception of sensations particularly that of pain.
4. It is concerned with control of muscular movements via its connections with basal ganglia, cerebellum and motor cortex.

ELECTROENCEPHALOGRAM

The record of electrical activity of the brain (cerebrum) is called electroencephalogram (EEG). It can be recorded by placing two electrodes on the scalp and connecting them via a suitable amplifier to a cathode ray oscilloscope (CRO). It was first introduced by Hans Berger. EEG obtained by placing the electrodes directly on the exposed surface of cerebral hemisphere (pial surface of the cortex) called electrocorticogram (ECoG).

Normal EEG

The EEG can be recorded by using two methods: Bipolar and unipolar.

1. *Bipolar method:* It is a record of potential difference between two cortical electrodes. For example, frontal area, occipital area, etc.
2. *Unipolar method:* It is a record of potential difference between an active electrode and an indifferent electrode applied on some part of the body distant from the cortex such as ear lobe. The waves of EEG are classified according to the frequency and voltage (Table 11.11).

α-Rhythm

They are present at rest (physical as well as mental) when the eyes are closed and form the most prominent component of the EEG (Fig. 11.60). Its frequency is decreased by low blood glucose, low body temperature high arterial pCO_2 and sleep; also its frequency is increased by high blood glucose, rise in body temp, low arterial pCO_2 alerting states. The α-waves are associated with decreased levels of attention and when α-rhythms are being generated subjects report that they feel relaxed and happy.

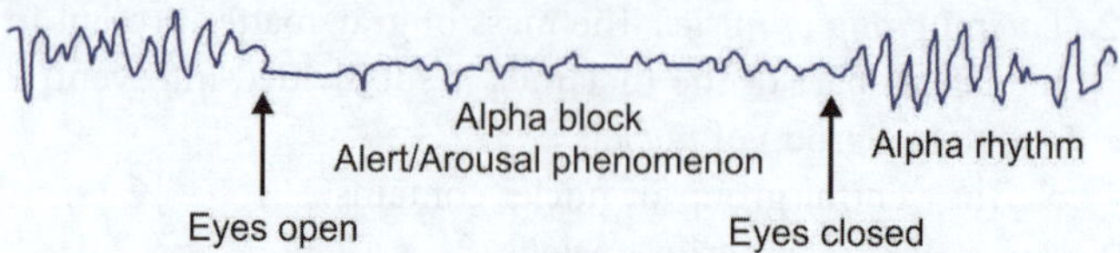

Fig. 11.60: Replacement of alpha rhythm by an asynchronous, low voltage beta rhythm when the eyes are opened

The replacement of regular α-rhythm with fast, high frequency, irregular low amplitude (voltage) activity is called α block/desynchronization of EEG. It represents a breaking up of the synchronized activity of the cortical neurons responsible for the α-wave pattern. A break up of the α-pattern is produced by any form of sensory stimulation such as opening of the eyes or mental concentration.

Uses of EEG

1. Localization of pathological condition
   - Subdural hematoma/fluid collection is associated with decreased EEG activity over that area.
   - Lesion in the cortex causes local formation of irregular or slow waves in EEG.
2. *Diagnosis of epilepsy:* Epilepsy is due to excessive discharge of cerebral neurons. Epileptic foci generate high voltage (amplitude) waves in the EEG, which can be localized.

Forms of Epilepsy

Epilepsy describes a condition in which a person has recurrent seizures. A seizure occurs due to abnormal excessive neuronal activity in the brain. Depending on the distribution of discharges, this abnormal brain activity can have various manifestations ranging from dramatic convulsive activity (like vigorous shaking) to brief periods of loss of consciousness.

Table 11.11: Main features of normal EEG rhythm

EEG rhythm	Frequency (Hz)	Amplitude (μV)	Associated features
1. Alpha (α)	8–12	50–100	Present maximally in the occipital and parieto-occipital areas when the eyes are closed
2. Beta (β)	14–30	5–10	Generally seen in frontal region (normal awake pattern); commonly seen in infants
3. Theta (θ)	4–7	10	Often found over the parietal and temporal areas (normal in children and in early sleep)
4. Delta (δ)	1–4	20–200	Usually appear during sleep; can be produced by over breathing or evidence of organic brain diseases when seen in awake state

Grandmal Epilepsy

It is characterized by loss of consciousness without aura (warning sign). This is followed by generalized convulsions with tonic muscle contractions and clonic jerks. Here, EEG shows high voltage (up to 1000 μV) activity during the tonic phase, slow waves each preceded by a spike at the time of each clonic jerk and slow wave over sometime even after the attack is over.

Petit Mal Epilepsy

It is a form of epilepsy in children characterized by abrupt loss of consciousness without falling or incontinence, and lasting for a few seconds. Here, EEG shows 3 doublets per second each consisting of typical spike and rounded waves.

SLEEP

Sleep is defined as unconsciousness from which the person can be aroused by sensory or other stimuli. It is a physiological process by which bodily functions are periodically rested. It is to be distinguished from coma, which is unconsciousness from which the person cannot be aroused.

Physiological Changes During Sleep

1. *CVS:* Heart rate, cardiac output, vasomotor tone and BP decrease.
2. *Respiratory system:* Tidal volume, respiratory rate, pulmonary ventilation decreases:
3. BMR decreases.
4. Urine volume decreases while phosphate content and specific gravity increases. Therefore, more concentrated urine is formed.
5. *Secretions:*
   a. Salivary and lacrimal secretion decreases
   b. Sweat secretion increases
   c. Gastric secretion either remains unaltered or increases.
6. Muscles are completely relaxed and the tone is minimum.
7. *Eye:*
   a. Eyeballs roll up and out due to flaccidity of external ocular muscles
   b. Eyelids come closer due to drooping of the upper eyelid
   c. Pupils constrict.
8. Blood volume increases resulting in the dilution of the plasma.
9. *Nervous system:*
   a. EEG shows appearance of δ waves.
   b. Deep reflexes are reduced.
   c. Superficial reflexes remain unchanged.
   d. Light reflex is retained.

Types of Sleep

1. **NREM (Nonrapid eyeball movement sleep/Slow wave sleep):** In NREM sleep (Table 11.12) is divided into 4 stages each successive stage will have an EEG pattern with slower frequency and high voltage than the preceding one. Initially there is a considerably tone in postural muscle and it progressively decreases. The eyes begin slow, rolling movements until they finally stop in stage 4 (deep sleep) with the eyes turned upwards. During NREM sleep there is release of both growth hormone and gonadotropins from the pituitary. Body metabolism is lowered. Also there is decrease in BP, heart rate and respiratory rate. When awakened, person does not report dreaming. After a person has been in NREM (slow wave) sleep for about an hour, the sequence of sleep stages is repeated in reverse order, i.e. the person passes from stage 4 to 3, 2 and 1; then he finally enters into the REM sleep.
2. **REM (Rapid eyeball movement sleep)/Paradoxical sleep:** During REM sleep, the eyeballs move frequently (saccadic eye movements). Saccadic eye movements are small jerky, fast movements that rapidly bring the eye from one fixation point to another and may be associated with watching visual images of dreams. Here, EEG shows desynchronized pattern. Dreaming is closely associated with this sleep. When awakened the persons report that 80–90% of the time they had been dreaming. REM sleep is associated with increase and irregularity in BP, heart rate and respiratory rate. The skeletal muscle tone is markedly reduced. This is responsible for snoring during sleep as relaxed tongue in supine posture partially obstructs the air passage.

REM sleep is associated with large phasic potentials in groups of 3–5. They originate in the pons and pass rapidly to the lateral geniculate body and thence to the occipital cortex, therefore called ponto-geniculo-occipital (PGO) spikes. This activates the reticular inhibiting area in the medulla, producing the hypotonia.

Teeth grinding (bruxism) in children, erection of penis, engorgement of clitoris, and twitches of the facial or limb muscles may occur in REM sleep.

Sleep Cycle

A sleep cycle consists of two phases: NREM sleep followed by REM sleep. Continuous recordings of adults show that the average total sleep period comprises of 4 or 5 such cycles, each lasting 90–100 minutes. In a typical 90 minute sleep cycle NREM sleep occupies the 1st 70 minutes and REM the last 20 minutes.

Table 11.12: Behavioral and EEG changes in two types of sleep

Stage	Behavioral observation	EEG changes
NREM (slow wave sleep)		
Stage 1	This is the stage of drowsiness and falling asleep (light sleep). It is characterized by: i. Easily aroused by moderate stimuli or even by neck muscle jerks ii. Continuous lack of awareness	α-waves reduced in frequency and amplitude
Stage 2	True sleep and there is further lack of sensitivity to activation and arousal	Characterized by the appearance of sleep spindles (due to reverberating activity between the thalamus and the cerbral cortex). These are bursts of regular alpha like waves (10–14 Hz, 50 mV). Appearance of α rhythm is between b rhythm is known as sleep spindles
Stage 3	Sleep deepens	Sleep spindles are occasional and are now superimposed on a background of waves of δ type
Stage 4	Stage of deep sleep in which, it is difficult to arouse the person. Arousal occurs only with vigorous stimulation and when awakened, person does not report dreaming	Slow high voltage d waves
REM (Paradoxical) sleep	Deepest sleep • REM sleep is also called paradoxical sleep because the sleeping person is difficult to arouse despite having a desynchronized EEG that is characteristic of alert, awake state • Skeletal muscle tone is markedly reduced except in the eye where REM occurs • REM sleep and dreaming are closely associated. REM sleep is more towards morning and hence dreams are more frequent towards waking hours	EEG becomes desynchronized, i.e. low voltage fast activity seen (resembling awake state with eyes open) Large spikes are seen in the EEG called PGO spikes (ponto-geniculo-occipital) which are characteristic of REM sleep

Genesis of Sleep

Genesis of NREM Sleep

1. Inhibition of RAS inputs by the descending pathways which arise from preoptic and diagonal band of Broca.
2. Stimulation of sleep promoting mechanism (i.e. the rhythmic discharge from the thalamus). These mechanisms get influenced by:
   a. **Diencephalic sleep zone:** Present in posterior hypothalamus, intralaminar and anterior thalamic nuclei.
   b. **Medullary synchronizing zone:** It is present in the reticular formation of the medulla oblongata.

Mechanism that Can Cause Sleep

The most important stimulation area for sleep is the raphe nuclei in the lower half of pons and in the medulla. Nerve fibers from this nuclei spread locally in the brainstem reticular formation and also upward into the thalamus, hypothalamus, most areas of the limbic system, and even the neocortex of the cerebrum. In addition, fibers extend downward into the spinal cord, terminating in the posterior horns where they can inhibit incoming sensory signals, including pain. Nerve ending of fibers from the raphe neurons secretes serotonin. When a drug that block the formation of serotonin is given, then the sleep is deprived for several days. Therefore it is assumed that serotonin is a transmitter substance associated with production of sleep.

Stimulation of some areas in the nucleus of the tractus solitarius also cause sleep. Stimulation of several regions in the diencephalon can also promote sleep, including rostral part of hypothalamus and an occasional area in the diffuse nuclei of the thalamus.

Genesis of REM Sleep

Genesis of REM sleep is due to two factors:

1. Discharge of NE (Norepinephrine) from the neurons located in the pontine reticular formation and locus coeruleus.
2. The cholinergic system is necessary for shifting NREM to REM sleep.

Note

- Resperine, which depletes the serotonin and catecholamines, block the slow wave sleep.
- Barbiturates decrease the amount of REM sleep.

Table 11.13: Differences between NREM and REM sleep

NREM	REM (Paradoxical sleep)
1. Hypotonia	1. More hypotonia
2. Slow-high voltage 'd' waves	2. Fast low voltage 'b' rhythm waves
3. No rapid movement of the eyeballs	3. Rapid movement of the eyeballs
4. Dreams cannot be recalled or vague recalling	4. Dreams can be recalled easily
5. No ponto-geniculo-occipital spikes (PGO)	5. PGO spikes are present. These can be recorded from the occipital cortex. PGO spikes take origin from the pontine RF
6. Pulse, BP, respiration are lowest and regular	6. Pulse, BP, respiration increased and are irregular
7. Serotonin content of the Raphe nucleus is associated with SWS (slow wave sleep)	7. Noradrenaline content of the locus-coeruleus is associated with paradoxical sleep
8. Threshold for arousal by the sensory stimulus is elevated	8. Threshold for arousal by the sensory stimulation is further elevated
9. 75% of total sleep	9. 25% of total sleep
10. Brain activity is less	10. Brain activity is more
11. O_2 consumption is less	11. O_2 consumption is more

Sleep Disorders

1. *Insomnia:* It is a condition of being unable to sleep.
2. *Somnambulism or sleep walking:* It is more common in children and may last several minutes. Such individuals walk with their eyes open and avoid obstacles, but when awakened they cannot recall the episode.
3. *Nocturnal enuresis:* Involuntary voiding of urine during sleep at night.
4. *Narcolepsy:* It is a disease of unknown cause in which there is an uncontrollable urge to sleep during day time activities.

Difference between NREM and REM sleep is given in Table 11.13.

BASAL GANGLIA

The basal ganglia like cerebellum constitute another accessory motor system that function not by itself, but in close association with the cerebral cortex and corticospinal motor control system. Infact, the basal ganglia receive most of their input signals from the cerebral cortex itself and also return almost all their output signals back to the cortex.

The term basal ganglia (BG) is applied to group of nuclei (mass of gray matter) in the forebrain and upper part of the brainstem that have motor activity of great importance (Table 11.14). It influences the pyramidal system activity. The basal ganglia differ from the cerebellum in the way they regulate motor activity. Unlike the cerebellum, the basal ganglia does not receive input from the spinal cord, but they do receive direct input from the cerebral cortex. The main action of basal ganglia is on the motor area of the cortex by the way of the thalamus. In addition to the role in motor control, basal ganglia also contributes to affective and cognitive function. The lesions of basal ganglia produce abnormal movement and posture.

Table 11.14: Basal ganglia

	1. Caudate nucleus	Striatum
Lenticular nucleus {	2. Putamen	
	3. Globus pallidus (pallidum)	
	4. Subthalamic nucleus (body of Luys)	
	5. Substantia nigra	

Caudate Nucleus

It possesses a head and tail (terminating at the amygdaloid nucleus). The caudate nucleus and putamen are together called the corpus striatum or neostriatum.

Putamen and Globus Pallidus

Putamen and globus pallidus are together called lenticular nucleus. Globus pallidus (GP) is also called paleostriatum. Globus pallidus is subdivided into external (ES) and internal segment (IS) by medial medullary lamina. Substantia nigra is subdivided into two parts: Pars compacta and pars reticularis. It is particularly rich in copper content.

Note

In basal ganglia three biochemically distinct pathways normally operate in a balanced fashion

1. Nigrostriatal dopaminergic system
2. Intrastriatal cholinergic system.
3. GABA ergic system that project from striatum to GP and SN.

Neural Pathways through Basal Ganglia

The inputs, interconnections and outputs constitute two important neural pathways through the basal ganglia that are involved in control of motor activities—the direct pathway and the indirect pathway. Ventral anterior (VA) nucleus of thalamus is the major motor nucleus of thalamus. Thalamus must activate motor cortex for all voluntary movements to occur. But, at rest thalamus is inhibited by the output nuclei of basal ganglia namely globus pallidus internus (GPi) (Fig. 11.61A).

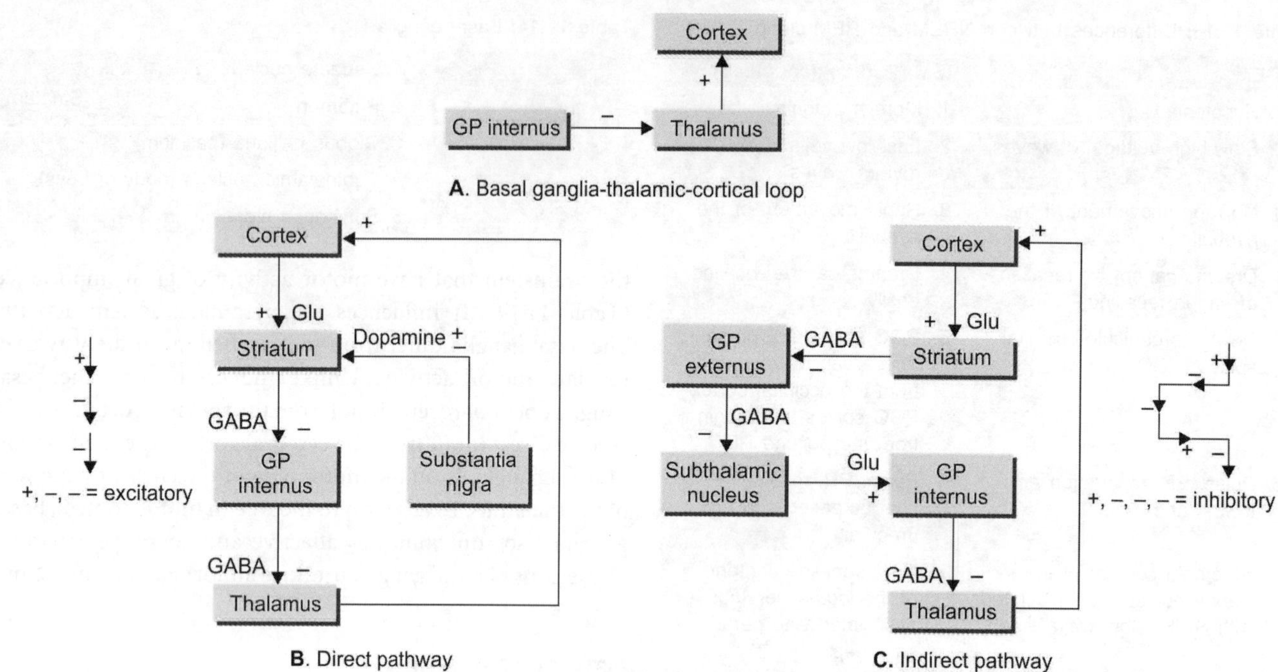

Fig. 11.61A to C: Neural pathways through basal ganglia

Direct Pathway

The direct pathway is stimulated during movement. Cortex projects to striatum. Striatum projects to globus pallidus internus (GPi), which projects to thalamus and thalamus in turn projects to motor cortex. This is the direct pathway (Fig. 11.61B). The projection of cortex to striatum is excitatory (glutaminergic). Projection of striatum to globus pallidus internus is inhibitory (GABAergic), and projection from globus pallidus internus to the thalamus is inhibitory (GABAergic).

How the voluntary movements are initiated?

- To initiate voluntary movements, motor cortex must inhibit basal ganglia.
- Motor cortex does this through activating the input nuclei of basal ganglia namely striatum.
- Striatum inhibits globus pallidus internus (GPi) by releasing the neurotransmitter GABA. Since the globus pallidus internus (GPi) is inhibited, it can't inhibit the thalamus. Therefore, activation of striatum finally excites the thalamic neurons (disinhibition).
- Consequently, thalamus can now activate the target neurons in the motor cortex for all voluntary movements to occur via thalamocortical projection. Now the complete loop is called cortical-basal ganglia-thalamic-cortical loop. This is called the ***direct pathway.***

Indirect Pathway

This involves connection from striatum to the external segment of globus pallidus (GPe), which project to subthalamic nucleus. Subthalamic nucleus projects to internal segment of globus pallidus, which in turn projects to thalamus (Fig. 11.61C). In this pathway, striatum inhibits globus pallidus externus, which inhibits subthalamic nucleus. Subthalamic nucleus activates globus pallidus internus.

Now, how to terminate the motor movement once it is initiated?

- The answer is simple. Globus pallidus internus (GPi) have to be activated again.
- Globus pallidus internus (GPi) is activated by subthalamic nucleus.
- But, subthalamic nucleus is tonically inhibited by globus pallidus externus (GPe).
- Now to inhibit globus pallidus externus (GPe), motor cortex activates striatum.
- Striatum inhibits globus pallidus externus (GPe). Now, the subthalamic nucleus is activated.
- Subthalamic nucleus activates globus pallidus internus (Gpi) which further inhibits thalamus.
- Therefore, stimulation of striatum activates globus pallidus internus through this indirect pathway. The final output of striatum through this indirect pathway is inhibitory (as globus pallidus internus activation inhibits thalamocortical projections).

In Essence

The direct and indirect pathways have opposite effects. Normally, there is a balance between these two pathways.

Alteration of activity in either of the pathways leads to imbalance in motor output from basal ganglia. Therefore, in basal ganglia disorders, both hypo- and hyperkinetic features are observed.

Direct pathway: Direct pathway is mainly to initiate voluntary movements. Globus pallidus interna (GPi) is inhibited in direct pathway. Disinhibition of motor thalamus → promotes movement. Lesions causes difficulty in initiating movements (e.g. Parkinson disease).

Indirect pathway: Indirect pathway is to terminate the initiated movement. Globus pallidus interna (GPi) is activated in indirect pathway. Inhibition of motor thalamus → inhibits movement. Lesions causes unintentional or spontaneous movements (e.g. Huntington disease).

Modulation by Nigrostriatal Projections

Another important connection of these pathways is the nigrostriatal projections. The dopaminergic projections from pars compacta of substantia nigra to the striatum appear to have an excitatory influence on the direct pathway and inhibitory influence on the indirect pathway. This is primarily due to the differential expression of dopamine receptors in basal ganglia. Dopamine activates direct pathway through D1 receptor. Dopamine inhibits indirect pathway through D2 receptor. Ultimately, by doing this, dopamine facilitates voluntary motor movements. Therefore, projection from substantia nigra to striaturn is important physiologically. The neurons in the striatum are cholinergic. In striatum, the ratio of acetylcholine and dopamine keeps the striatal neurons active. Alteration in this ratio results in abnormalities in motor activities.

Functions of Basal Ganglia (BG)

1. *Role in planning and programming of motor activity:* It is process by which an idea of involuntary movement is converted into precise action.
   Mechanism: Activity in the circuit between subthalamic nuclei and globus pallidus is an important regulator of basal ganglia output that in turn maintains movements in a smooth and appropriate state.
2. *Control of muscle tone:* Basal ganglia inhibits the stretch reflex (muscle tone) by stimulation of caudate nucleus and by the stimulation of inhibitory motor cortex as well as inhibitory reticular formation. This is why damage to BG cause rigidity.
3. *Cognitive function:* Caudate nucleus plays a role in cognitive processes (thinking process of brain, using both sensory inputs to the brain plus information already stored in memory). Lesion of head of the left caudate nucleus associated with dysarthric aphasia (difficulty in articulating words).
4. *Subconscious execution of some movements:* Basal ganglia is responsible for control of normal automatic and associated movements such as swinging of arms during walking. These movements are initiated by motor cortex.
5. Neostriatum regulates subconscious gross movements occurring in group of muscle.
6. The activity of basal ganglion increases during slow, steady damp movement and is silent during rapid, saccadic movement.
7. Globus pallidus provide muscle tone for performance of skilled movements.
8. Substantia nigra is center for coordination of impulses essential for skilled movements.

Diseases of the Basal Ganglia

Parkinson's Disease (Paralysis Agitans/Shaking Palsy)

It is caused due to degeneration of substantia nigra or globus pallidus or both and usually occurs in late middle age. Therefore, concentration of dopamine in this region, i.e. nigrostriatal system is reduced. Hence the balance between the excitatory discharge of cholinergic interneurons and inhibitory dopaminergic input in the neostriatum is disrupted.

Parkinsonism occurs in:
- Primary or idiopathic, i.e. condition occuring without apparent cause.
- Cerebral arteriosclerosis.
- Complication of encephalitis.
- Complication of drugs such as phenothiazine which blocks the dopamine (D2) receptors.

  Symptoms appear when 60–70% of nigrostriatal dopaminergic neurons are lost.

Characteristic features

It has both hyperkinetic and hypokinetic features (Fig. 11.62).

1. *Rigidity (Hyperkinetic):* Due to increased discharge of γ efferents supplying the muscle spindle.
   - It affects mainly large proximal group of muscle of limbs involving both antagonists and protagonists (biceps, knee flexors, sternomastoids).
   - Here posture is that of flexion attitude. The back is flexed, the arms adducted and flexed and the knees are bent (stooped posture).
     Rigidity may be:
   - *Cogwheel type:* Here resistance is intermittently released.
   - *Lead pipe type:* Here resistance is through out movement.

   Mechanism: Activity of neostriatum is influenced by excitatory effect on cholinergic fibers and inhibitory influence of the dopaminergic fibers. Normally there exists a balanced effect of these two opposite innervations on the neostriatum activity. Lack of dopaminergic activity due to degeneration

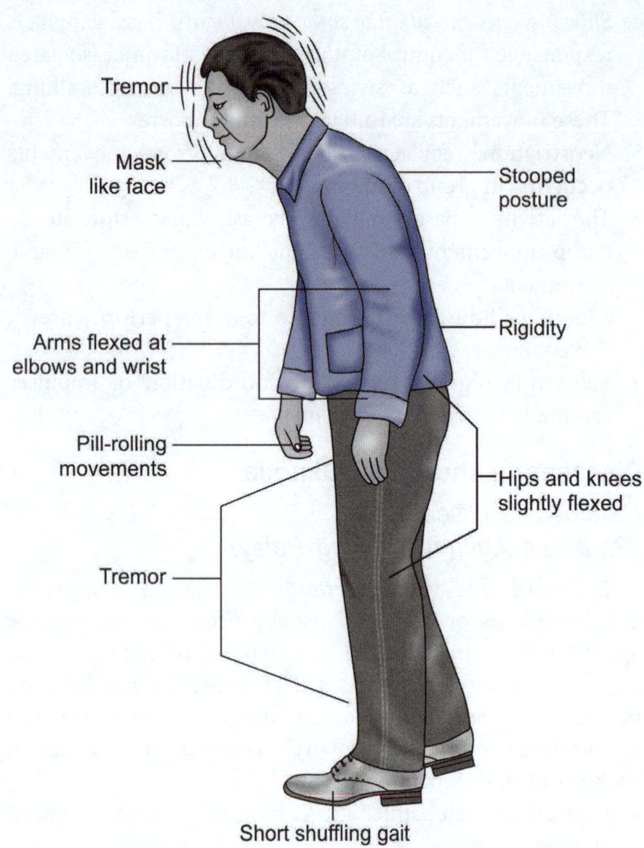

Fig. 11.62: Clinical features of Parkinson's diseases

of substantia nigra shifts the balance towards the excitatory cholinergic fibers.

2. *Tremor (Hyperkinetic):* It consists of regular, rhythmic, alternate contraction of antagonist and agonist muscle at 6–8 times/sec. It is commonly seen as pill-rolling movements, i.e. rhythmic contraction of thumb over 1st two fingers. As it is present during rest and disappears during activity it is called resting (static) tremor. It increases in emotional states, excitement or anxiety due to secretion of epinephrine, which in turn excites RAS. The tremor disappears during sleep (due to decreased activity of RAS). *Cause:* Due to degenerative lesions in reticular formation and its ascending connections.
3. *Weakness and poverty of movements (Hypokinesia):*
   - Difficulty in initiating voluntary movements (akinesia). This produces defects in fine movements of fingers.
   - Defects in fine variations of speech.
   - Mask like facial expression due to decrease in movements of facial muscles.
   - Loss of normal subconscious associated movements. For example, swinging of arms during walking.
   - Tendon reflex is more difficult to elicit as rigidity increases.
4. *Gait:* Festinant type (shuffling gait)—Patient is bent forward and walks quickly with short steps as if trying to catch up the center of gravity or preventing himself from falling down.
5. *Retropulsion:* If the patient is suddenly pulled backwards, he begins to to walks backwards and is unable to stop himself.
6. *Tendon jerks:* Tendon jerks become progressively difficult to elicit as the rigidity increases.

Treatment

1. Administration of the drug L-dopa. It can cross blood-brain barrier and reach the brain tissue where it is converted to dopamine.
2. Transplantation of dopamine secreting cells (cells obtained from brains of aborted fetuses) into caudate nucleus and putamen has been used with some short term success to treat Parkinson's disease.
3. Surgical treatment by making lesions in the internal segment of the globus pallidus (pallidotomy) or in the subthalamic nucleus helps to restore the output balance towards the normal.

Chorea, Athetosis and Ballism

These three disorders are characterized by spontaneous involuntary movements due to the interruption of the inhibitory pathway from area cortex via the caudate nucleus to the thalamus:

1. *Chorea:* It is mainly due to involvement of caudate nucleus and is characterized by rapid irregular involuntary 'dancing' movements of short duration. It is also associated with decreased muscle tone and muscular weakness.
2. *Athetosis:* It is due to lesion of lenticular nucleus and is characterized by continuous slow twisting/writhing movements.
3. *Ballism:* Involuntary flailing, intense and violent movements occur.

Hemiballism

It is due to damage of the subthalamic nucleus and is characterized by spontaneous attacks of incoordinated movements affecting whole of the opposite side of the body.

Wilson's Disease/Hepatolenticular Degeneration

It is an autosomal recessive disease. Here copper content of substania nigra is high. In this condition the ceruloplasmin (plasma copper binding protein) is low. Thus copper accumulation causing degeneration of lenticular nucleus with cirrhosis of liver. The condition is characterized by muscular rigidity, tremor, cirrhosis of liver and emotional disturbances.

Huntington's Disease

It is a autosomal dominant inherited disorder. The abnormal gene responsible for the disease is located in the short arm of chromosome 4. It usually occurs between 30 and 50 years of age. It is due to the damage to GABA-ergic and cholinergic neurons that projects to the putamen. Damage to this inhibitory pathway results in hyperkinetic features, which include:

- Hyperkinetic choreiform movements.
- Slurred speech.
- Progressive loss of memory (dementia).

It is a gradually progressive disease with no effective treatment which eventually leads to death.

HYPOTHALAMUS

Hypothalamus is the principal autonomic center of the brain. Mainly concerned with maintenance of homeostasis through its control of visceral functions and endocrine functions. Hypothalamus is the integrating center where several neural and endocrine influences originating throughout the brain converge. It is then processed and the processed outputs are diverged to all parts of the body. Thus, it acts like a funnel (Fig. 11.63) which transmits the influences of the brain on several homeostatic mechanisms to the body.

Nuclei of Hypothalamus (Fig. 11.64)

It is divided into three groups:

Anterior or Preoptic Group

1. Preoptic nucleus
2. Paraventricular nucleus
3. Anterior nucleus
4. Supraoptic nucleus

Middle or Tuberal Group

1. Dorsomedial group
2. Ventromedial group

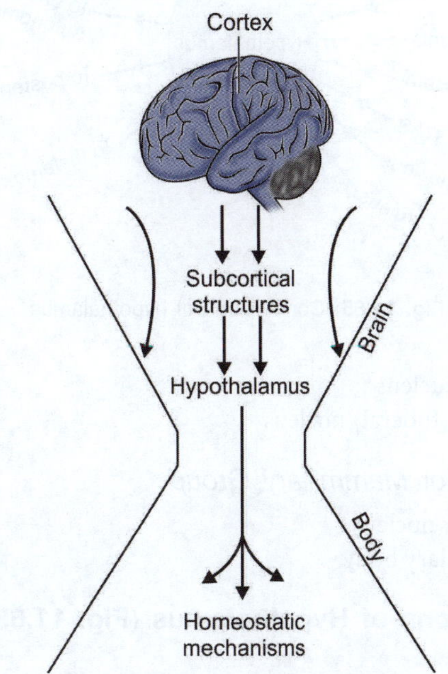

Fig. 11.63: Hypothalamus as an integrating center

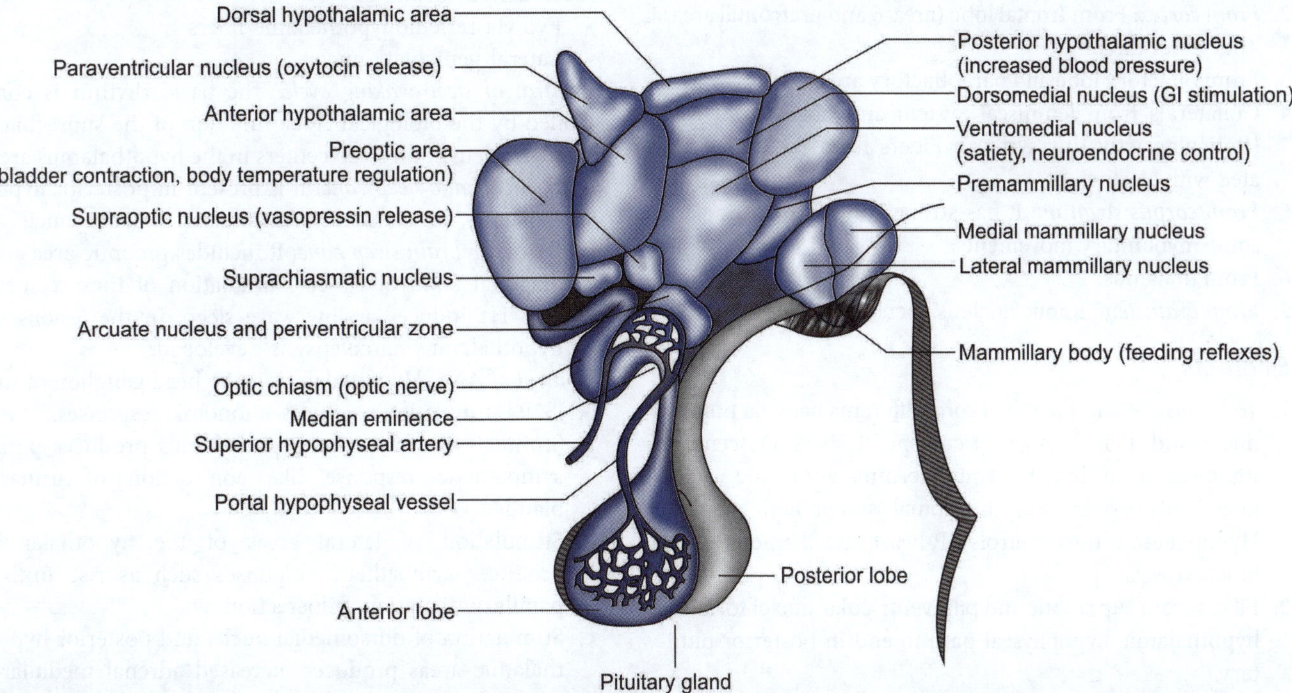

Fig. 11.64: Nuclei of hypothalamus

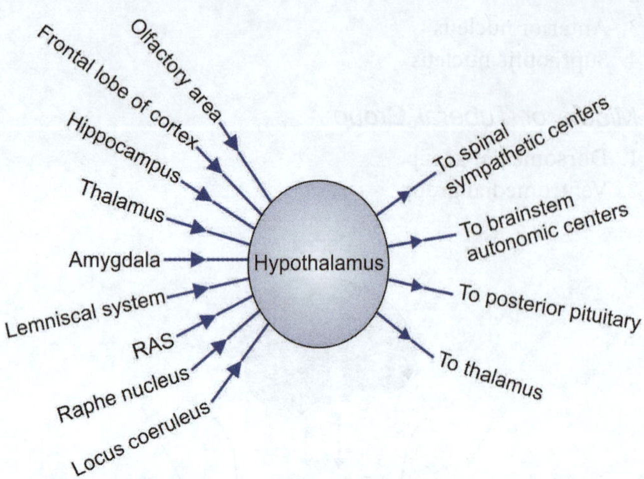

Fig. 11.65: Connections of hypothalamus

3. Lateral nucleus
4. Arcuate (tuberal) nucleus

Posterior or Mammillary Group

1. Posterior nucleus
2. Mammillary body

Connections of Hypothalamus (Fig. 11.65)

Afferents

1. *From limbic system:* Hippocampus and amygdala. They are concerned with emotion and behavior.
2. *From cortex:* From frontal lobe (area-6 and prefrontal area). They enter directly.
3. From olfactory lobe and paraolfactory area.
4. Collaterals from lemniscal system and fibers from RAS (Reticular activating system). Fibers from RAS is associated with alertness.
5. *From corpus striatum:* It has strong control over tone and some involuntary movements.
6. From thalamus.
7. *From brainstem:* Raphe nucleus, locus coeruleus, medulla.

Efferents

1. *To brainstem and the spinal cord:* Efferents pass via pontine nuclei and then through reticulospinal fibers. Descending impulses from hypothalamus terminate on the lateral horn cells, controlling the spinal sympathetic centers. Hypothalamus thus controls BP, heart rate, diameter of the blood vessels.
2. Fibers from supraoptic and paraventricular nuclei form the hypothalamic hypophyseal path to end in posterior pituitary.
3. To thalamus.
4. To midbrain.

Functions of Hypothalamus

1. *Regulation of body temperature:* The anterior portion of the hypothalamus, especially the preoptic area is concerned with regulation of body temperature. An increase in temperature of the blood through this area increases the activity of the temperature sensitive neuron, while a decrease in temperature decreases the activity.
   Anterior hypothalamus: Response to heat
   Posterior hypothalamus: Response to cold.
2. *Regulation of anterior pituitary activity:* Through the release of releasing and inhibiting factors into hypothalamo-hypophysial portal system.
3. *Regulation of postpituitary hormones:*
   - ADH: Synthesis from supraoptic nucleus
   - Oxytoxin: From paraventricular nucleus.
4. *Control of circadian rhythm:* A person's circadian rhythm is an internal biological clock that regulates a variety of biological processes according to an approximate 24 hour periods. Several body functions show a circadian (24 hour) rhythm. These functions include feeding, drinking, locomotor activity, sleep, corticosteroid secretion, body temperature and melatonin secretion by the pineal. Most of these functions are regulated by the hypothalamus.
   Neural basis of circadian rhythm: The suprachiasmatic nuclei are the main site for circadian rhythm. These nuclei receive inputs from:
   - Eye via reticulohypothalamic fibers
   - Lateral geniculate nuclei.
5. *Control of sleep-waking cycle:* The basic rhythm is controlled by the biological clock function of the suprachiasmatic nucleus. Two sleep centers in the hypothalamus are:
   a. *Diencephalic sleep zone:* It is present in posterior hypothalamus, intralaminar and anterior thalamic nuclei.
   b. *Basal forebrain sleep zone:* It includes preoptic area and diagonal band of Broca. Stimulation of these centers at 8 Hz induces a slow wave sleep. In the lesions of hypothalamus narcolepsy is developed.
6. *Control of ANS:* Hypothalamus is the head ganglion of the ANS. Its stimulation produces autonomic responses.
   a. Stimulation of anterior hypothalamus produces parasympathetic response like contraction of urinary bladder.
   b. Stimulation of lateral areas of the hypothalamus produces sympathetic responses such as rise in BP, papillary dilatation, piloerection, etc.
   c. Stimulation of dorsomedial nuclei and posterior hypothalamic areas produces increased adrenal medullary

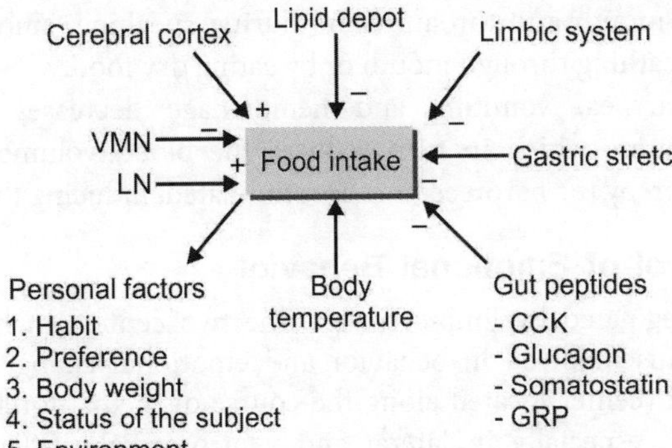

Fig. 11.66: Factors influencing food intake

secretion which is one of the physical changes associated with rage and fear.

7. *Control of hunger and feeding (Fig. 11.66):* Two centers are connected with it:
   a. Ventromedial nuclei (VMN) act as a satiety center and its bilateral lesions causes hyperphagia (hypothalamic obesity).
   b. Lateral nucleus (LN) acts as a feeding center. Its lesion cause anorexia (loss of appetite especially when prolonged) and animal dies of starvation.

Mechanism

Satiety center is the primary center that controls the food intake. It functions by inhibiting the feeding center. Thus VMN inhibit food intake and LN stimulate food intake.

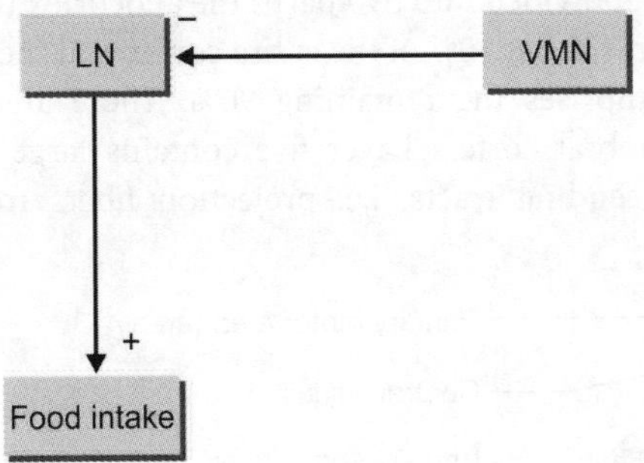

Glucostastic Theory

The cells of VMN acts as glucoreceptors. Thus activity of satiety center is governed by the level of glucose utilization within the cell. An increase in blood glucose level increases the activity of VMN. A decrease in blood glucose level decreases the activity of VMN.

Note: Deficient glucose utilization in the cells of the satiety area (VMN) of hypothalamus is the probable cause for hyperphagia in diabetes mellitus. This decreases its inhibitory effect on feeding center (LN) and thus food intake is increased.

Role of Hypothalamic Peptides

Important hypothalamic peptides that seem to plays an important role in regulation of food intake are:

i. Food intake is increased by:
   a. Neuropeptide Y (synthesized by neurons in arcuate nucleus of hypothalamus)
   b. Orexin-A and Orexin-B (synthesized by lateral hypothalamic neurons)
   c. Ghrelin (secreted by stomach and hypothalamus)
ii. Food intake is decreased by:
   a. CART (cocaine and amphetamine regulated transcript)
   b. CRH (corticotropin releasing hormone).

Lipostatic Hypothesis

According to this hypothesis the adipose tissue produces a hormone leptin, the production of which is proportional to the amount of fat. This acts on hypothalamus to decrease the food intake.

Gut Peptide Hypothesis

According to this hypothesis, presence of food in the GIT causes the release of gut peptides. These are glucagon, somatostatin, CCK which acts on the brain to cause satiety.

Thermostatic Hypothesis

According to this, the body temperature influences the food intake. Appetite is stimulated and the food intake increases when the body temperature goes below a given set point and is inhibited when the body temperature rises above a set point.

Role in Regulation of Water Balance

Hypothalamus regulates body water in two ways:

a. Creating the sensation of thirst
b. By controlling excretion of water into the urine.

Hypothalamic Mechanism

Creating the sensation of thirst: Hypothalamus contains osmoreceptors which can detect changes in osmolality of the ECF. Thus, if there is lack of water, the osmolality of ECF rises → osmoreceptors of hypothalamus are stimulated → thirst develops → drive for water intake develops.

A second hypothalamic mechanism is as follows: In conditions, where the kidneys produce renin (hemorrhage/hypovolemia), renin converts the plasma angiotensinogen to angiotensin II. Apart from its normal actions, angiotensin II also acts on the hypothalamus → development of thirst → development of thirst behavior. Cardiovascular shock therefore is associated with thirst, as this condition generates angiotensin in high quantity.

By controlling excretion of water into the urine: The increased plasma osmolarity stimulates osmoreceptors in supraoptic

Flowchart 11.1: Role of hypothalamus in regulation of water balance

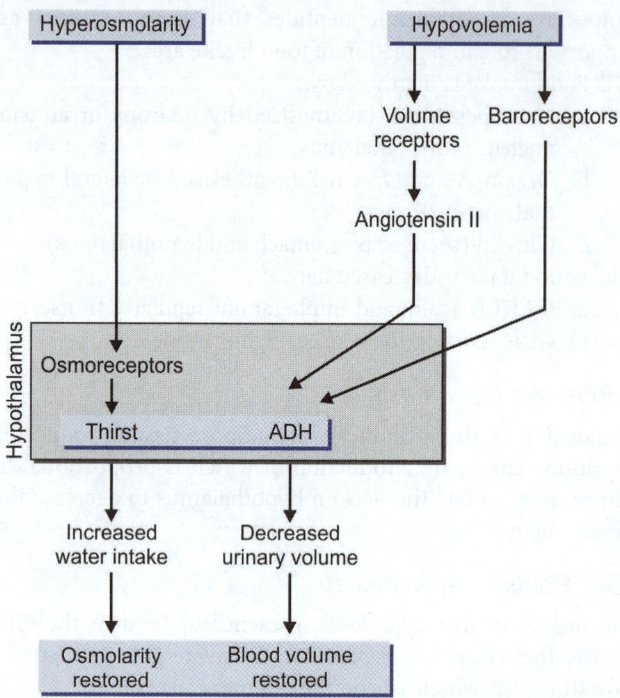

nucleus (SON). The stimulated neurons of SON in turn send impulses to postpituitary to secrete hormone ADH. ADH is also seceretед in response to angiotensin II (when fluid volume is low). Secretion of ADH increases water absorption from the collecting ducts of the kidney (Flowchart 11.1).

Note: Apart from the hypothalamus the regulation of water balance is also controlled by the following mechanisms:

i. *Buccal mucosal mechanism:* If the mucous membrane of buccal cavity becomes dry, there develops thirst. Drying of mouth and throat occurs during speaking, smoking, breathing through mouth or by eating dry food.
ii. Diarrhea, vomiting and hemorrhage decreases ECF volume which in turn reduces the blood volume and thereby the baroreceptors are stimulated, inducing thirst.

Control of Emotional Behavior

It is regulated by limbic cortex. The two centers in hypothalamus involved in behavior and emotional changes are reward (center located along the course of medial forebrain bundle, especially in lateral and ventromedial nucleus of hypothalamus) and punishment center (located in medial hypothalamus and paraventricular zone).

Sexual Behavior

Controlled by anterior ventral hypothalamus and male piriform cortex.

CORTICAL AREAS

Electrostimulation of different areas of cortex (Figs 11.67 and 11.68) was performed to study their functions. This test was performed in conscious human beings, in whom brain has been exposed for some purpose and effects studied. The cerebral cortex is a layer of gray matter, less than 4 mm thick, present on the surface of the cerebral hemispheres. It is thrown into folds which increase its surface area many times. The surface elevations created by these folds are called gyri and the grooves separating them are called sulci. Phylogenetically, the cortex is subdivided into two parts: the allocortex (old cortex) which forms about 10% of the entire cortex and the neocortex which comprises the remaining 90%. There are six layers in the cerebral cortex. Layer five contains large pyramidal cells. Descending tracts, i.e. projection fibers from cortex

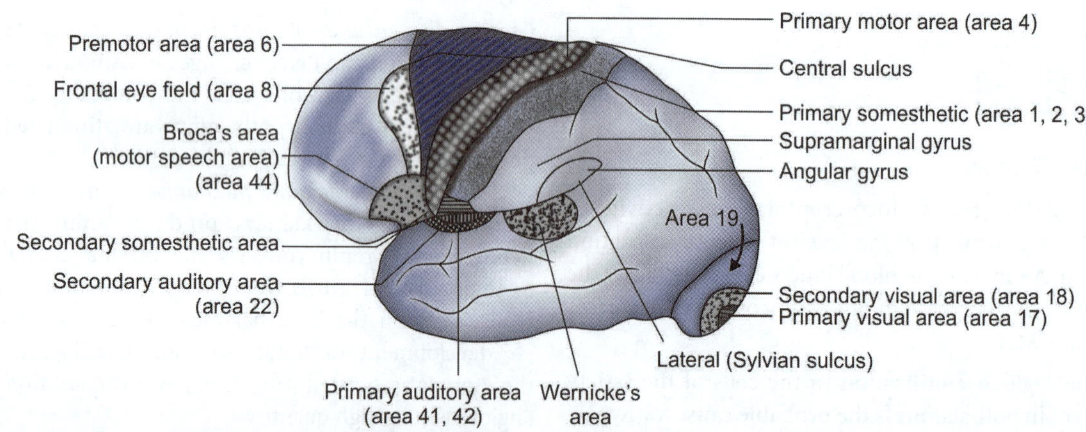

Fig. 11.67: Lateral view of cerebral cortex (left lobe)

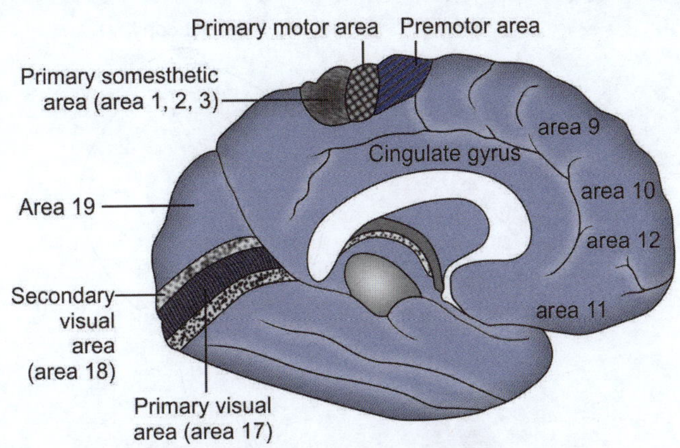

Fig. 11.68: Medial view of cerebral cortex (left lobe)

(corticospinal tract, corticobulbar tract) are the axons of these pyramidal cells.

Cerebral cortex is divided functionally into primary cortical areas (sensory and motor) and association areas:

- *Sensory area:* It also includes primary visual cortex, primary auditory cortex, primary olfactory and gustatory areas.
- *Motor area.*
- *Association area:* Most higher functions are related to the association areas. The sensory association areas provide meaning of the sensation perceived. If one holds an object in one's hand, the sensation of touch would be perceived in the hand of the somatosensory cortex. However, the nature of the object would be interrupted by the somatosensory association area.

The human brain appears fairly symmetrical anatomically between the left and right hemisphere and many basic sensory and motor functions in the brain are distributed symmetrically. Homologous regions of cerebral cortex on either side of the brain are connected to each other via long association fibers carried by the corpus callosum. For some unknown reasons, however there are marked asymmetry in several brain functions. The most obvious asymmetry in the cerebral function is the language. In most individuals, the language function depends predominantly on the left hemisphere. The left hemisphere is dominant for the language in over 95% of right handers and in over 60–70% of left handers therefore it is called the dominant hemisphere. The core structures associated with language situated in the left hemisphere are Wernicke's area and Broca's area. Other important functions associated with the dominant hemisphere (left) are detailed analytical abilities and complex motor planning activities (praxias). The right hemisphere is the nondominant hemisphere of the brain as it does not play dominant role in language.

Frontal Lobe

The major areas in this lobe are:

i. *Area 4 (primary motor area):* This area is situated in the precentral gyrus (in front of central sulcus) of frontal lobe of this area. The body is represented upside down from medial to lateral surface. The lower parts of the body are represented in medial surface and upper parts of the body. The order of representation from medial to lateral surface- toes, ankle, knee, hip, trunk, shoulder, arm, elbow, wrist, hand fingers and face. The size of representation is directly proportional to skill of the part. However, the parts of the face are not represented in an inverted manner.

   Functions: This area is concerned with contraction of discrete muscles. It sends motor signals to the facial muscles of both sides (bilateral) and to the other muscles of the opposite side. Many of the fibers of pyramidal tract arise from the motor cortex (area 4).

   Note: There is another area called suppressor area (Area 4S). This area lies anterior to area 4 and inhibits the movements initiated by area 4 thus preventing the exaggeration of actions.

ii. *Area 6 (premotor area):* Premotor area lies in front of area 4. It contributes to both pyramidal and extra-pyramidal fibers.

   Functions: It is concerned with coordination of movements initiated by area 4. It is believed to be the cortical center for extrapyramidal system.

iii. *Area 8 (frontal eye field):* This lies anterior to area 6 in the precentral cortex. Its stimulation causes conjugate deviation of eyes to the opposite side, e.g. while reading, the action of passing from the end of one line to the beginning of the next line.

   Functions: Area 8 appears to be mainly responsible for voluntary eye movements. This area is also concerned with accommodation reflex mechanism.

iv. *Supplementary motor area:* It is situated in medial surface of frontal lobe rostral to primary motor area.

   Functions: The exact function is not clearly known but it is suggested that it is concerned with coordinated skilled movements.

v. *Prefrontal cortex (areas 9, 10, 11 and 12):* This is the anterior part of frontal lobe of cerebral cortex, in front of areas 8 and 44.

   Functions: It forms the center for higher functions like emotional, learning, memory and social behavior. Short-term memories are registered here. It is the center for planned actions. This area is also concerned with intelligence.

vi. *Broca's area (area 44):* It is the motor speech area. It lies anterior to the primary motor cortex and above the sylvian fissure in the dominent hemisphere.
vii. *Exners area (area 45):* Site adjacent to area 44 in dominant hemisphere. It is the center for writing
viii. *Paracentral lobule:* It is the cortical inhibition (control) of bladder and bowel. Located on the medial surface of the superior frontal gyrus, adjacent to the foot and leg area. Lesion here can cause incontinence of urine and feces.

Parietal Lobe

The major areas in this lobe are:

i. *Primary sensory area (somesthetic area I):* It is also called Brodmann's area 3, 1, 2. Fibers conveying impulses by spinothalamic tract, lemniscal system (touch, pain, temperature senses, etc.), after relaying in the thalamus end here and thus we become aware of the specific senses.
Functions: It is the highest area of general, conscious, sense perception.
ii. *Somesthetic area II:* It lies below the area of somesthetic area I, so that it is buried in the lateral (Sylvian) sulcus. This area receives sensory impulses from somesthetic area I and from the thalamus directly.
Function: It is concerned with perception of sensation.
iii. *Somsthetic association area:* It includes area 5 and 7 of Brodmann. It lies posterior to somesthetic area I in the parietal lobe.
Functions: This area is concerned with the synthesis of various sensations perceived by somesthetic area I. Thus, this area forms the center for combined sensations like stereognosis.

Note

Sensory motor area

The sensory area of cortex is not limited to postcentral gyrus in parietal lobe. It extends anteriorly into motor area in precentral gyrus of frontal lobe. Similarly the motor area is extended from the precentral gyrus posteriorly into post- central gyrus. Thus, the precentral and postcentral gyri are combined together by association neurons and they are functionally interrelated. So, this area is called sensory motor area.

Clinical Note

Lesion of parietal lobe results in hemineglect. Patients neglects contralateral parts of the body and contralateral portion of the external world. In extreme cases, they do not dress half their body, eat only from half of the plate or even read half of each page (Fig. 11.69).

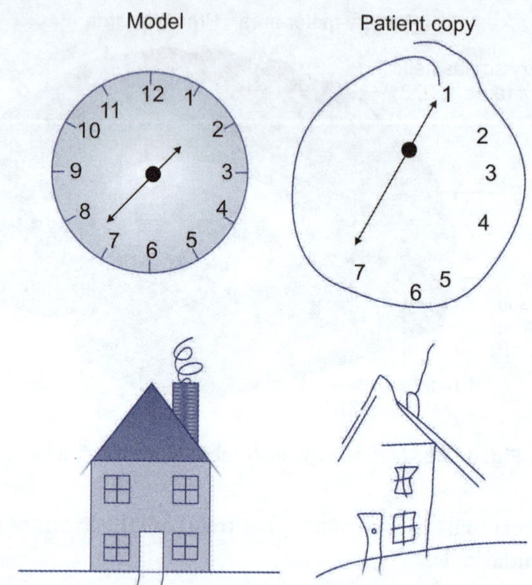

Fig. 11.69: Hemineglect. Illustration of drawings made by a person who has neglect syndrome caused by severe damage in his or her right posterior parietal cortex compared with the actual drawing the patient was requested to copy

Temporal Lobe

Major areas in this lobe are:

1. *Primary auditory area:* This includes areas 41, 42 and Wernicke's area (area 22). Areas 41, 42 are situated in the anterior transverse gyrus and lateral surface of superior temporal gyrus. Wernicke's area is located in the upper part of superior temporal gyrus posterior to areas 41 and 42.
Functions: This area is concerned with perception of auditory impulses, analysis of pitch and determination of intensity, source of sound.
2. *Auditopsychic area (areas 20, 21):* This occupies the superior temporal gyrus.
Functions: This area is concerned with interpretation of auditory sensation along with Wernicke's area. Lesion here produces auditory agnosia, the patient hears but does not understand (recognize) what he hears.

Occipital Lobe

Major areas in this lobe are:

i. *Primary visual area (area 17):* It is concerned with perception of visual impulses.
ii. *Visual association area (area 18):* It is concerned with interpretation of visual impulses.
iii. *Occipital eye field (area 19):* It is concerned with the movement of the eyes.

LIMBIC SYSTEM

The term limbic has been derived from the word 'limbus' which means a ring. Thus the limbic system is applied for that parts of the cortex (limbic cortex or limbic lobe) and subcortical structures that form a ring around the brain stem.

Limbic cortex/limbic lobe surrounds the subcortical structures of the limbic system (Fig. 11.70). Phylogenetically, limbic cortex is an older part of the cerebral cortex (allocortex) having primitive histological structures.

Limbic cortex is composed of:

a. Orbitofrontal cortex
b. Subcallosal gyrus
c. Cingulate gyrus
d. Parahippocampal gyrus
e. Uncus

Subcortical structures included under the limbic system are:

a. Hypothalamus
b. Septum
c. Paraolfactory area
d. Anterior nucleus to thalamus
e. Amygdala
f. Portions of basal ganglia
g. Hippocampus.

Connections

Papez Circuit

Papez circuit refers to a closed circuit formed by connections between the cingulate gyrus (located in the prefrontal lobe), hippocampus, mammillary bodies and anterior nucleus of thalamus (Fig. 11.71). It links limbic lobe with hypothalamus and thalamus. This circuit is responsible for resting EEG and plays an important role in control and genesis of emotions.

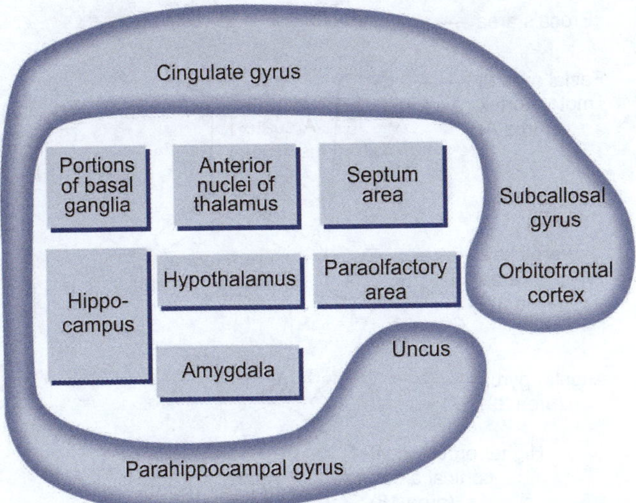

Fig. 11.70: Limbic system, showing the key position of hypothalamus

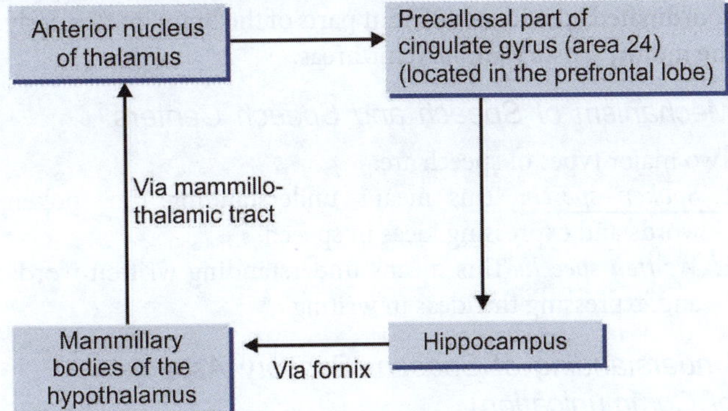

Fig. 11.71: Papez circuit

Information passes from the cingulate gyrus to hippocampus and from there via the fornix to the mammillary bodies in the hypothalamus. The mammillothalamic tract then connects the hypothalamus with the anterior thalamic nuclei, which project back to cingulated gyrus.

Functions of Limbic System

1. *Autonomic functions:* Stimulation of many parts of the limbic system specially that of amygdala produces autonomic responses such as changes in cardiovascular, respiratory and gastrointestinal system through hypothalamus.
2. *Regulation of feeding behavior:* Limbic system regulates feeding behavior mainly through hypothalamus and amygdala.
3. *Emotional behavior:* Limbic system is concerned with various emotions including various emotions of fear, rage, reward-punishment, etc.
4. *Regulation of sexual behavior:* Sexual behavior, the basic sex drive is a function of limbic system and hypothalamus which in turn are influenced by gonadal hormones and cerebral cortex.
5. *Motivational behavior:* Motivational behavior is also an important function of limbic system.

HIGHER FUNCTIONS OF NERVOUS SYSTEM

The higher functions of the nervous system include: Language (speech) and other intellectual functions like learning, memory and judgment. In general, higher functions of the nervous system in humans depend more on one cerebral hemisphere (dominant/categorical hemisphere) than on the other.

Language (Speech)

Language refers to the faculty of nervous system which enables the human to understand the spoken and printed words and to express ideas in speech and writing. It is brought about by coordinated activity of different parts of the brain, particularly the motor, sensory and psychic areas.

Mechanism of Speech and Speech Centers

Two major types of speech are:

1. *Spoken speech:* This means understanding the spoken words and expressing ideas in speech.
2. *Written speech:* This means understanding written words and expressing the ideas in writing.

Understanding of Speech (Sensory Aspects of Communication)

Understanding of spoken speech

- *Hearing of the spoken words:* To hear a sound we require an intact auditory pathway from the ears to the primary auditory center (areas 41, 42).
- *Understanding of the spoken words:* For understanding a sound, there must be activity of the adjacent auditory-psychic areas (areas 20, 21).
- *Interpretation and comprehension of speech ideas:* In order to express the ideas in speech, the activity of sensory speech center, called Wernicke's area (area 22) is essential. Wernicke's area is located in the region at the posterior end of the superior temporal gyrus in the dominant (categorical) hemisphere. It is concerned with comprehension, i.e. interpretation and understanding of auditory and visual informations.

Understanding of written speech

- *Perception of written words:* In order to see the words it requires an intact visual pathway from the eyes to the primary visual cortex (area 17).
- *Interpretation of written speech:* Inorder to interpret the written symbols (of past experience), it requires the activity of visuo-psychic areas (areas 18, 19).
- *Generation of ideas in response to written speech:* To express the ideas in writing, it involves the activity of visual speech center, called the *Dejerine area (area 39)*.Dejerine area is located in the angular gyrus behind the Wernicke's area in the dominant hemisphere. It processes informations from printed words in such a way that they can be converted into the auditory forms of the words in the Wernicke's area (internal speech). Sensory speech centers include Wernicke's and Dejerine areas.

Expression of Speech (Motor Aspect of Speech)

Expression of speech requires the skilled use of many muscles, such as muscles of the lip, tongue, larynx, hand or fingers. There is a motor speech center for both spoken and written speech in the prefrontal lobe in the dominant (categorical) hemisphere. Motor speech centers include Broca's and Exner's areas:

1. *Expression in the form of spoken speech:* Expression in the form of spoken speech involves the activity of motor speech (Broca's area) area.
   Broca's area (area 44): It is located in the inferior frontal gyrus, in the region of the anterior and ascending rami of the lateral sulcus in the dominant (categorical) hemisphere. It processes the information received from sensory speech centers into a detailed and coordinated pattern for vocalization. (Wernicke's area projects via the arcuate fasciculus to Broca's area). This pattern is then projected to the motor cortex which initiates the appropriate movements of the lips, tongue and larynx to produce speech.
2. *Expression in the form of written speech:* Expression in the form of written speech is the function of Exner's area.
   Exner's area (motor writing center): It is located in the middle frontal gyrus in the dominant (categorical) hemisphere anterior to motor cortex (i.e. in the premotor cortex). It processes the informations from Broca's area into detailed and coordinated pattern, which then along with motor cortex initiates the appropriate movements of the hands and fingers to produce written speech.
3. *Expression of both spoken and written speech:* Suppose somebody is reading a book aloud and then wishes to write what he has read, the sequence will be as follows (Fig. 11.72):
   1. The printed words will be seen first by the primary visual area (area 17), highest area for perception of visual sense.

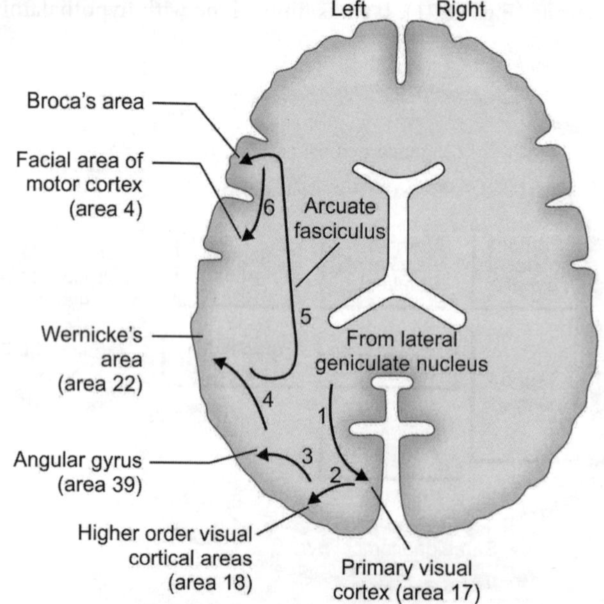

Fig. 11.72: Path taken by impulses when a subject names a visual object

2. The printed words seen are properly interpreted and understood by the visual association area (area 18).
3. The printed words which are understood are converted into internal speech by the Dejerine area (in angular gyrus).
4. The Wernicke's area (area 22) then interprets and understands the internal speech.
5. This in turn sends the information to the Broca's area for pattern coordination.
6. The Broca's area (area 44) sends detailed pattern coordination information to:
   a. Motor area (area 4) for the spoken speech.
   b. Exner's area for the written speech (motor writing center), the Exner's area along with motor area (area 4) initiates appropriate muscle movements of hand and fingers to produce written speech.

Development of Speech

For better understanding, we will now see how speech is developed in children. When the baby is born he receives sensations from the surrounding environment, which at first are meaningless, but with further development begin to acquire a meaning.

- The objects seen are received as simple meaningless images in the visual sensory area (area 17) in the occipital lobe. Repetition of the same images leads to their insertion, storage and subsequent recognition and recall in the visual psychic areas (areas 18 and 19) around area 17 in the occipital lobe.
- Similarly, the newborn child receives auditory impulses in the primary auditory sensory area (areas 41, 42 and 22) in the temporal lobe as meaningless sounds. With repetition of the sounds, they become inserted and stored for subsequent recognition and recall in the auditory psychic area (areas 20, 21) in the temporal lobe just adjacent to the auditory sensory area.
- So, when the child sees his mother by area 17, he recognizes her in area 18, and can recall her image even in her absence in area 19. He also hears her voice in area 41 and 42 and recognizes it as being hers even if he does not see her in areas 20, 21).
- Later on, the child tries to imitate the sounds he has perceived. This process needs the development of a cortical motor speech center known as Broca's area (area 44) in the frontal lobe, which is achieved by the age of 1 to 1.5 years.
- When the child goes to school and starts to learn letters and numbers he begins to develop a special visual speech center/visual psychic area (area 39) in the angular gyrus in the parietal lobe for storage, recognition and recall of their images. Areas 20, 21 also serves for the storage, recognition and recall of how they sound when spoken. When he comes to write, he imitates the images of letters and numbers stored in area 39. The execution of this process of writing requires the development of a special cortical motor center for writing (Exner's area) adjacent to Broca's area in the frontal lobe of the dominant hemisphere.
- Association fibers between the visual and auditory psychic areas allow the child to correlate between the images he sees and the sounds related to them, e.g. the sight of his mother is correlated with the word mama and vice versa. This process of correlation requires the development of an associative area (area 37) in the parietal lobe. This area also sends association fibers to Broca's and Exner's areas.
- Whether in spoken or written speech, impulses from the Broca's area or from Exner's area reach the motor area (area 4) descend in the pyramidal tract to reach the nuclei of the cranial nerves (supplying the muscles of articulation), and the AHC (supplying the muscles concerned with writing).
- Impulses from the cerebellum and extrapyramidal system share in the production of property executed speech.

Speech Disorders

Aphasia

Aphasias are abnormalities of language functions (inability to understand spoken or written speech or inability in expressing the spoken or written speech) that are not due to defects of vision or hearing or due to motor paralysis. They are caused by lesions in the categorical hemisphere. The most common cause is embolism or thrombosis of a cerebral blood vessel. The aphasia may be (Fig. 11.73):

i. **Sensory aphasia:** Sensory aphasia also known as Wernicke's aphasia is the result of lesion in the Wernicke's area.
   Characteristic features:
   a. Difficulty in understanding the meaning of the speech.
   b. Motor speech area is intact, and the patients talk very fluently that is why it is also called fluent aphasia. However, the speech does not make any sense.
ii. **Motor aphasia:** Motor aphasia, also known as Broca's aphasia results from lesions involving the Broca's motor speech area (area 44) in the frontal lobe.
   Characteristic features:
   a. Speech is slow, and words are hard to come and are limited to two or three words with which the whole range of meaning and emotion is to be expressed.
   b. Speech is nonfluent (nonfluent aphasia).
   c. Inability to write (agraphia).
iii. **Global aphasia**: Global aphasia refers to the total inability to use language communication. This condition is produced as a result of loss of both Wernicke's and Broca's areas. In this situation, speech is scant as well as nonfluent.

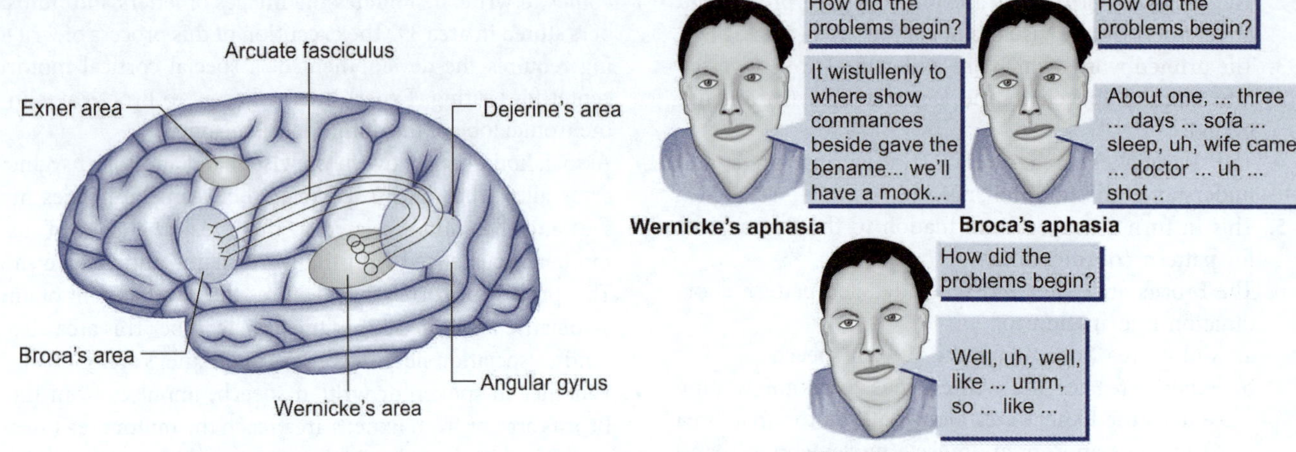

Fig. 11.73: Areas in the brain concerned with language functions and speech disorders

Dissociative Language Syndromes

Dissociative language syndromes refer to language deficit that do not result from lesion of cortical language areas, but from disruption of pathways joining them (arcuate fasciculus).

Conduction aphasia: Occurs due to separation of auditory and motor language areas without damaging these areas. Since Wernicke's area is intact, the patient understands what he hears or reads. But because of the lesion in arcuate fasciculus, he cannot use this understanding while speaking or writing as information cannot be transmitted from Wernicke's area to Broca's area. The result is that he produces fluent but faulty speech and makes plenty of mistakes in what he writes. Thus, the patient may seem to have sensory aphasia. In sensory aphasia, the patient cannot understand speech, while in conduction aphasia, he can understands spoken as well as written speech.

Anomic aphasia: When there is a lesion damaging the angular gyrus (Dejerine area) in the categorical hemisphere without affecting Wernicke's or Broca's areas, there is no difficulty with speech or the understanding of auditory information, but there is trouble in understanding written language or pictures, because visual information is not processed and transmitted to Wernicke's area. The result is a condition called anomic aphasia.

Dysarthria

It is a disorder of speech in which articulation of words is impaired, but the comprehension of spoken and written speech is not affected.

LEARNING AND MEMORY

Learning and memory are closely related. Learning is impossible without memory and memory has no meaning without learning.

Learning

Learning refers to a natural mechanism by which the individual changes his or her behavior on the basis of past experience. Learning is of two types:

a. *Nonassociative learning:* In nonassociative learning the subject learns about the properties of a single stimulus. It results when an animal or a person is repeatedly exposed to a single type of stimulus. Two forms of nonassociative learning are common in everyday life-habituation and sensitization.
b. *Associative learning:* In associative learning the subject learns about the relationship between two stimuli or between a stimulus and a behavior. Two forms of associative learning have been distinguished based on the experimental procedures used to establish the learning-classical conditioning and operant conditioning.
   i. *Classical conditioning:* Classical conditioning involves learning a relationship between two stimuli. It is also termed as Pavlovian conditioning or conditioned reflex type I (Fig. 11.74).
   Characteristic features
      1. A conditioned reflex is a reflex response to a stimulus that is acquired by repeatedly pairing the stimulus with another stimulus that normally does produce the response. It depends for its appearance on the formation of new functional connections in CNS.
      2. *Reinforcement:* It is a process of following a conditioned stimulus with a basic unconditioned stimulus which is a must for retaining a conditioned reflex otherwise it will extinct.

   Pavlov's Experiment: This experiment demonstrates classical conditioned reflex.
      a. When food, i.e. an unconditioned stimulus is presented to a hungry dog, it produces salivation (an unconditioned response).

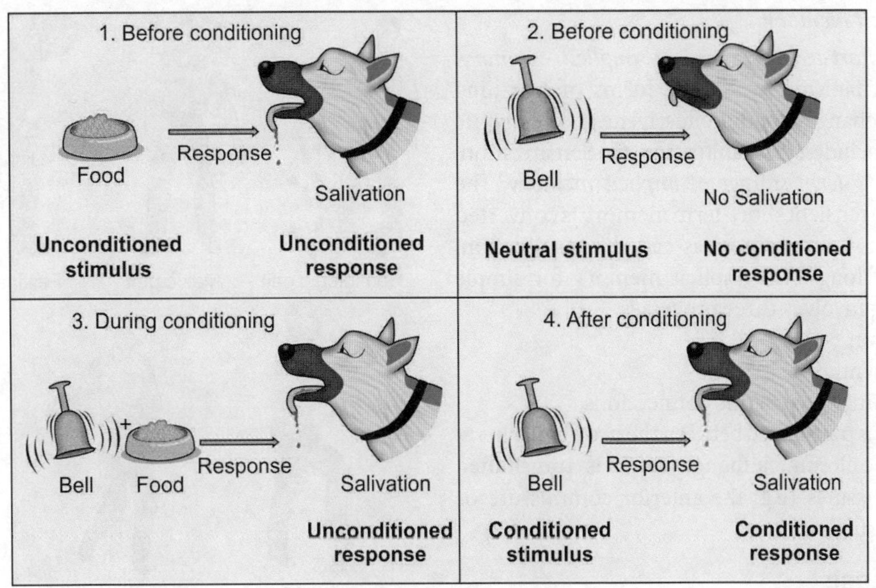

Fig. 11.74: Classical conditioning

b. If a bell is rung (a conditioned stimulus), just before the food is presented, the dog learns to associate the bell with the food.
c. Eventually, ringing the bell (a conditioned stimulus), alone causes salivation.

Note: If the food fails to appear consistently when the bell is rung, the conditioned response fades away, a process called extinction or internal inhibition. Therefore a conditioned reflex needs to be reinforced frequently, otherwise it dies out.

Physiologically the occurrence of conditioned reflex is explained by the formation of a new functional connection in the nervous system.

ii. *Operant conditioning:* Operant conditioning is a form of conditioning in which the animal is taught to perform some task ('operate on the environment') in order to obtain a reward or avoid punishment. Operant conditioning is of two types:
a. *Reward conditioning:* In it a naturally occurring response is strengthened by positive reinforcement (reward).
b. *Adverse conditioning:* In it a naturally occurring response is weakened by a negative reinforcement (punishment).

Memory

Memory is the ability to recall the past events at the conscious or unconscious level. It is the relatively permanent storage form of learned information. They can be either declarative or nondeclarative.

- *Declarative/explicit/recognition memory:* It is associated with consciousness or at least awareness. It is dependent on the hippocampus and other parts of the medial temporal lobes of the brain for its retention. Explicit memory is divided into the memory for events (episodic memory) and the memory for words, rules and language, etc. (semantic memory).
- *Nondeclarative/implicit/reflexive memory:* It does not involve awareness. Its retention does not involve processing in the hippocampus (in most instances) and includes skills, habits, conditioned reflexes, etc.

Explicit memory and many forms of implicit memory involve:
- *Short-term memory,* which lasts seconds to hours, during which processing in the hippocampus and elsewhere lays down long-term changes in synaptic strength.
- *Long-term memory,* which stores memories for years and sometimes for life. During short-term memory, memory traces are subject to disruption by trauma and various drugs, whereas long-term memory traces are remarkably resistant to disruption.

Mechanism of Memory (Physiological and Cellular Basis)

Studies of memory retention and disruption of memory have revealed that both explicit and implicit memory are stored in stages by different mechanisms. Input to the brain is processed into short term memory before it is transmitted through one or more stages (intermediate long-term memory) into more permanent long-term storage.

Mechanism of implicit memory

i. *Mechanism of short-term storage of implicit memory:* The various mechanisms for simple forms of lear-ning result from the changes in the effectiveness of synaptic transmission. It includes: (a) Habituation, (b) Sensitization.
ii. *Mechanism of long-term storage of implicit memory:* The process by which transient short-term memory is converted into a stable long-term memory is called consolidation. Consolidation of long-term implicit memory for simple forms of learning involves three processes:
   a. Gene expression
   b. New protein synthesis
   c. Growth (pruning) of synaptic connections

Much information is transferred between the two hemispheres through the corpus callosum, although some is transmitted through other commissures (e.g. the anterior commissure or hippocampal commissure).

Alzheimer's Disease

It is characterized by progressive loss of memory and cognitive function in middle aged individuals. Thus, the condition is frequently associated with:

a. Memory failure for recent events
b. Lack of spontaneous activity and initiative with loss of intellectual functions
c. Extrapyramidal and akinetic hypertonic symptoms
d. Loss of spatial orientation.

After 2 or 3 years, dementia (memory loss) becomes well established and focal symptoms occur, such as aphasia (speech disorder), apraxia (inability to perform voluntary movements and agnosia (inability to recognize objects in spite of intact sensory modality). Similar features in the old age (over 65 years) are called senile dementia. Both the conditions are caused by degeneration of cholinergic nerve terminals in the cerebral cortex and hippocampus.

GAIT

A patient's gait is a coordinated action requiring integration of motor and sensory functions. It therefore often provides clues to a patient's underlying diagnosis and is a critical part of any neurological examination. The most common gaits are shown in Figure 11.75.

Hemiplegic Gait

The patient stands with unilateral weakness on the affected side, arm flexed, adducted and internally rotated. When walking, the patient will hold his or her arm to one side and drags his or her affected leg in a semicircle (circumduction) due to weakness of distal muscles (foot drop) and extensor hypertonia in lower limb. This is most commonly seen in stroke.

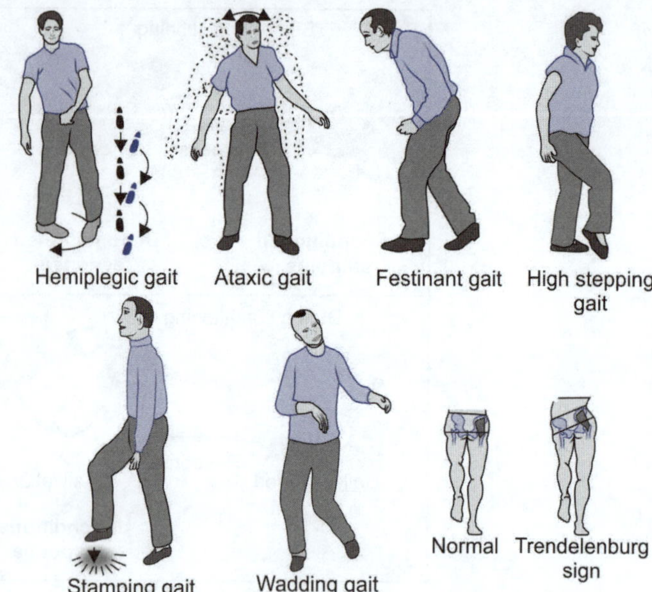

Fig. 11.75: Abnormal Gaits

High Stepping Gait

Seen in patients with foot drop (weakness of foot dorsiflexion), the cause of this gait is due to an attempt to lift the leg high enough during walking so that the foot does not drag on the floor. Causes include peroneal nerve palsy, other peripheral neuropathies including those associated with uncontrolled diabetes.

Waddling Gait

Hip girdle muscles are responsible for keeping the pelvis level when walking. If you have weakness on one side, this will lead to a drop in the pelvis on the contralateral side of the pelvis while walking (Trendelenburg sign). With bilateral weakness, you will have dropping of the pelvis on both sides during walking leading to waddling. Affected person walks like a duck. This gait is seen in patient with myopathies, such as muscular dystrophy.

Ataxic Gait (Cerebellar)

Most commonly seen in cerebellar disease, this gait is described as clumsy, staggering movements with a wide-based gait. Patients will not be able to walk in a straight line. The gait of acute alcohol intoxication will resemble the gait of cerebellar disease.

Parkinsonian Gait

In this gait, the patient will have rigidity and bradykinesia. He or she will be stooped with the head and neck forward, with flexion at the knees. The whole upper extremity is also in flexion with the fingers usually extended. The patient walks with slow little steps. The patient may show an involuntary inclination to take accelerating steps, known as festination. This gait is seen in Parkinson's disease or any other condition causing parkinsonism, such as side effects from drugs.

Sensory/Stamping Gait

As our feet touch the ground, we receive proprioceptive information to tell us their location. The sensory ataxic gait occurs when there is loss of this proprioceptive input. In an effort to know when the feet land and their location, the patient will slam the foot hard onto the ground in order to sense it. A key to this gait involves its exacerbation when patients cannot see their feet (i.e. in the dark). This gait is also sometimes referred to as a stamping gait since patients may lift their legs very high to hit the ground hard. This gait can be seen in disorders of the dorsal columns (B_{12} deficiency or tabes dorsalis) or in diseases affecting the peripheral nerves (uncontrolled diabetes).

CLINICAL QUESTIONS

1. **An elderly patient came with the complaints of inability to coordinate muscle movements and loss of balance. On examination, nystagmus and intention tremors were present, knee jerk was pendular.**
   a. Identify the condition.
   b. Give causes.
2. **A patient attending neurology clinic was having following findings:**
   - Loss of fine sensations and joint sense in lower extremities.
   - High steppage gait.
   - Romberg's sign was positive.

   Identify the condition and explain the above findings.
3. **A patient came to the clinic with complaints of weakness on left side of the body. On examination there was spasticity, exaggerated deep reflexes and positive Babinski's sign on left side.**
   a. Identify the condition.
   b. What is the cause of exaggerated reflexes and spasticity?
4. **A known hypertensive patient was brought to the clinic. He was unable to speak and do any movement on right side. On examination there was hypotonia in the muscles on right side. All reflexes were absent on right side.**
   a. Identify the condition with probable cause.
   b. What is the cause of aphasia?
5. **A patient was brought to the clinic 15 days after a road traffic accident with inability to move both his legs. On examination there was hypertonia, exaggerated ankle and knee jerk with positive Babinski's sign on both the sides.**
   a. What is the condition?
   b. Explain the clinical findings.
6. **An elderly patient came to the clinic with rigidity, resting tremors and akinesia.**
   a. Identify the condition.
   b. What is the cause of rigidity?
   c. Give the physiological basis of treatment.
7. **A person traveling in a bus developed vertigo, nausea and vomiting during the journey.**
   a. What is the probable condition?
   b. Explain the physiological basis.
8. **An elderly patient came to the clinic with jerky gait. On examination, he was having tremors at rest in fingers and there was lead pipe rigidity in upper and lower extremities.**
   a. Identify the condition.
   b. Explain the features.
   c. Give physiological basis of treatment.
9. **An elderly patient came to clinic with inability to balance himself. On examination there was hypotonia in all the muscles. Finger nose test showed in coordination with open and closed eyes and action tremors.**
   a. Identify the condition.
   b. Explain the features.

Answers for Clinical Questions are given in the Appendix

CHAPTER 12

Special Senses

VISION

Structure of Eye

The eye (Fig. 12.1) is a special organ of the sense of sight. In the adult human eyeball the A-P diameter is about 24 mm. The human eyeball has three principle layers:

a. Outer protective layer, sclera
b. Middle vascular layer, choroid (uveal tract)
c. Inner neural retina (lines the posterior 2/3rd of the choroid).

The light rays enters through the transparent cornea (sclera is modified anteriorly to form transparent cornea). The crystalline lens is a transparent structure held in place by suspensory ligament (zonule). The zonule is attached to thickened rim of smooth muscle, the ciliary body. The functions of the ciliary body are:

a. Formation of aqueous humor
b. Keeps lens in position.

The ciliary body contains circular and longitudinal muscle fibers that attach near the corneoscleral junction. In front of the lens, lies the pigmented and opaque iris (colored portion of the eye). Iris has two sets of smooth muscles:

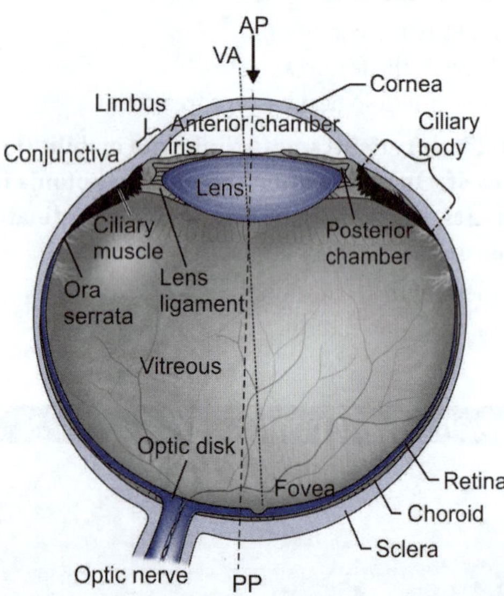

Fig. 12.1: Structure of eye

1. Sphincter pupillae (circular) constricts the pupil and is supplied by parasympathetic fibers through oculomotor nerve (nucleus is Edinger-Westphal).
2. Dilator pupillae (radial) is supplied by sympathetic fibers.

Retina

The retina extends from the margin of the optic disk to just behind the ciliary body where it ends abruptly as a dentated border known as ora serrata. It is organized in 10 layers and contains the rods and cones, which are the visual receptors (Fig. 12.2).

Retina has four types of neurons; bipolar cells, ganglion cells, horizontal cells and amacrine cells. The rods and cones which are next to the choroids, synapse with bipolar cells, and the bipolar cells synapse ganglion cells. The axons of ganglion cells converge and leave the eye as the optic nerve. Horizontal cells connect receptor cells to other receptor cells in the outer plexiform layer. Amacrine cells connect ganglion cells to one

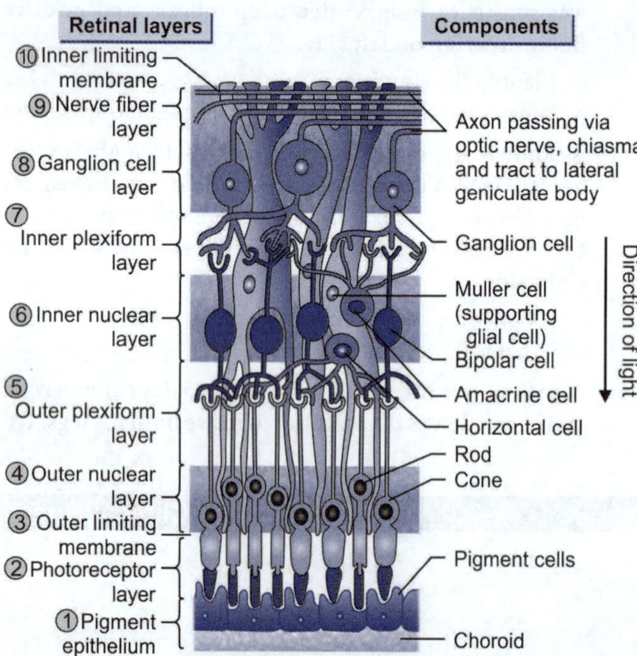

Fig. 12.2: Layers of retina

another in the inner plexiform layer via processes of varying length and patterns. The neural elements of retina are bound together by glial cells called Muller cells. The processes of these cells form an internal limiting membrane on the inner surface of the retina and an external limiting membrane in the receptor layer. Optic nerve leaves retina from optic disk which lies 3 mm medial to and slightly above posterior pole.

Fundus Oculi/Fundus

The posterior part of interior of the eyeball is called fundus oculi or fundus. The fundus can be examined by ophthalmoscope. The fundus has two important structures:

1. *Optic disc/blind spot:* It is situated near the center of the posterior wall of eyeball. Optic disc (1.5 mm in diameter) is formed by the convergence of axons from ganglion cells. It contains all the layers of retina except rods and cones. Therefore, it is insensitive to light (object is not seen if image falls on this area). Because of this, the optic disc is known as blind spot.
2. *Macula lutea/yellow spot:* Near the posterior pole of the eye is a yellowish pigmented spot called macula lutea (5.5 mm in diameter). The central 1.5 mm of the macula is termed as fovea, which has a small, central depression called *foveola.* The fovea is region of greatest acuity of vision as it contains:
   a. Only cones
   b. Each cones directly relay to a single cone
   c. Wide presentation in occipital primary visual area
   d. All layers of retina are shifted aside leaving cones to be hit directly by the cones.

Vitreous Humor

Space between lens and the retina is filled primarily with a clear gelatinous material called vitreous humor containing water, collagen fibrils, mucopolysaccharides and hyaluronic acid.

Functions

a. Prevents collapse of the eyeball.
b. Helps in maintaining normal intraocular pressure.
c. Keeps intraocular structures in position and thus helps in normal positioning of image on retina.

Aqueous Humor

Aqueous humor is a thin clear liquid that fills the space between the lens and cornea. It is produced in the ciliary body by ultrafiltration and active transport from the plasma at the rate of 2 mm^3/min. It flows through the pupil and fills the anterior chamber of the eye. It is normally reabsorbed through a network of trabaculae into the canal of Schlemm and uveoscleral outflow (venous channel at the junction between iris and cornea). Refractive index of aqueous humor is 1.336 and pH is 7.1–7.3. The space between the lens and cornea is divided into anterior and posterior chamber by iris. Space between iris and cornea is anterior chamber, space between iris and lens is posterior chamber. Both the chambers are filled with aqueous humor and they communicate with each other through the pupil.

Functions

a. Helps to maintain normal intraocular pressure.
b. It is the 2nd medium of refraction.
c. Provides nutrition to cornea and lens.
d. Takes the place of lymph that is absent in eye.

Contents

Protein, electrolytes (Na^+, K^+, HCO_3^-, Cl^-), non-electrolytes (glucose, urea and uric acid), organic acid (ascorbic acid, lactic acid and hyaluronic acid), dissolved O_2.

Mechanism of formation

Mainly ultrafiltration and some amount by active secretion.

Circulation of aqueous humor: Formed in posterior chamber by ciliary processes.

Posterior chamber → pupil → anterior chamber → canal of Schlemm (at the limbus) → episcleral venous plexus. Circulation is necessary for both metabolic process and to regulate the intraocular pressure.

Note: Any disturbance in this normal flow may increase the intraocular tension leading to glaucoma.

Glaucoma

It is a degenerative disease in which there is loss of retinal ganglia cells. Obstruction of canal of Schlemm leads to increased intraocular pressure. There are two types of glaucoma:

1. *Open angle glaucoma:* Here the cause of increased pressure is decreased permeability through the trabecular meshwork, through which aqueous humor is drained.
2. *Angle-closure glaucoma:* Here there is forward movement of iris, which obliterates the anterior chamber angle (angle between the iris and the cornea) thereby block the opening of trabecular meshwork at the angle.

Normal intraocular pressure is 10–21 mm Hg. Pressure in venous plexus is 10–15 mm Hg. This difference helps in continuous drainage of aqueous humor to venous plexus. The two important factors maintaining normal intraocular pressure are rate of formation and rate of reabsorption.

Visual Process

Receptors

The receptors (photoreceptors) of retina are rods and cones. Rods and cones communicate their message to bipolar cells. Bipolar cells, in turn, pass on the message to ganglion cells. The axon of ganglion cells forms the optic nerve which leaves the eye to reach the brain. Although there are approximately 100–120 million rods and cones, there are only about one million ganglion cells, indicating considerable convergence. That means there is no one-to-one relationship of photoreceptors with bipolar cells and ganglion cells (except at fovea).

The two photoreceptors differ from each other in several ways. Rods and cones differ in number, structure, retinal distribution, photochemical molecules, sensitivity, wavelength, color, synaptic connections and functions. There are total 100–120 million photoreceptors (rods and cones) in each eye, the ratio of rodes to cones being 20:1. Number of rods is about 90–100 millions and of cones is approximately is 3–46 millions.

Although the total number of rods is much more than cones, there is small area in the central retina which has more cones than rods. This area is called the macula lutea (macula). At the center of macula, there is a small area called as fovea centralis (fovea). The center of fovea, i.e. fovela contains only cones and no rods. The extremely high density of cones in the fovea and the one-to-one relationship with bipolar and ganglion cells (i.e. no convergence), endows this region with the capacity to mediate high visual acuity. As the cone density declines with eccentricity (periphery) and the degree of convergence onto retinal ganglion cells increases, acuity is markedly reduced. Visual pathway starts from receptors that respond to electromagnetic stimulation. Each rod and cone (Fig. 12.3) is divided into an outer segment, an inner segment that includes a nuclear region and a synaptic zone. The outer segments are modified cilia and are made up of regular stacks of flattened saccules or disks composed of membrane. These saccules and disks contain the photosensitive compounds that react to light, initiating action potentials in the visual pathways. The inner segments are rich in mitochondria. The rods are named for the thin, rod like appearance of their outer segments. Cones generally have thick inner segments and conical outer segments (Table 12.1).

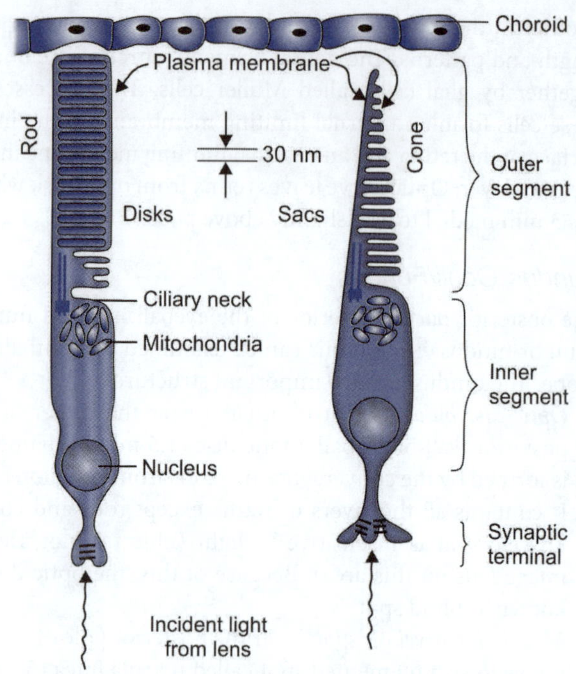

Fig. 12.3: Electron microscopic appearance of rods and cones

Table 12.1: Difference between rods and cones

Rods	Cones
Outer segment is rod shaped with regular stocks of membranes disks	Outer segment is cone shaped
Disks or saccules are separated from the cell membrane	Disks are infoldings of cell membrane
Has photo pigment called rhodopsin. It contains opsin (scotopsin) and vitamin C	Three types of cone pigments; erythrolabe (red), cyanolabe (blue), chlorolabe (green)
Except in fovea, rods predominates	Abundant in fovea
Helps in dim light vision	Helps in bright light vision, color vision, visual acuity
There are 120 million rods	There are 6 million cones

Photoreceptor Mechanism

Visual or phototransduction is the process by which light energy is converted into receptor potential in visual receptors. The potential changes that initiate action potentials in the retina are generated by the action of light on photosensitive compounds in rods and cones. The conformational change which happens when light falls on these substances triggers a sequence of events that initiate generation of action potential.

Ionic basis

In the dark Na^+ channels in the outer segments of the photoreceptors are kept open by cGMP, so there is a steady current flow from the inner to the outer segments of the rods. The steady current also flows in the synaptic ending of the photoreceptors. Light leads to increased conversion of cGMP to 5′-GMP, resulting in the closing of Na^+ channels (due to decrease in concentration of cGMP). This decreases current flow and resulting hyperpolarization generates local graded potentials (generator potential) in the synaptic terminal of the photoreceptor. In the dark, retinine1 in rhodopsin is present in 11 *cis* configuration (Figs 12.4 and 12.5).

Development of receptor potential or phototransduction (Fig. 12.6).

It is a local graded potential generated in the ganglion cells only. The sequence of events involved in phototransduction of rods and cones are:

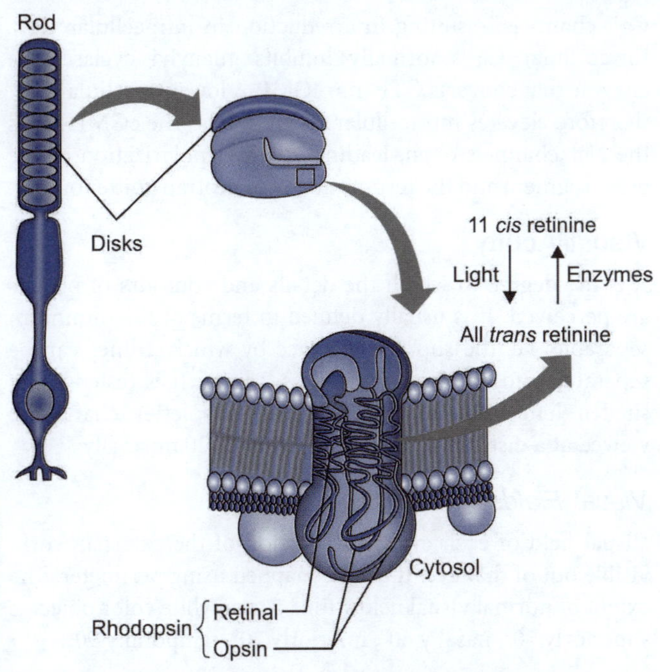

Fig. 12.4: Ionic basis of photoreceptor mechanism

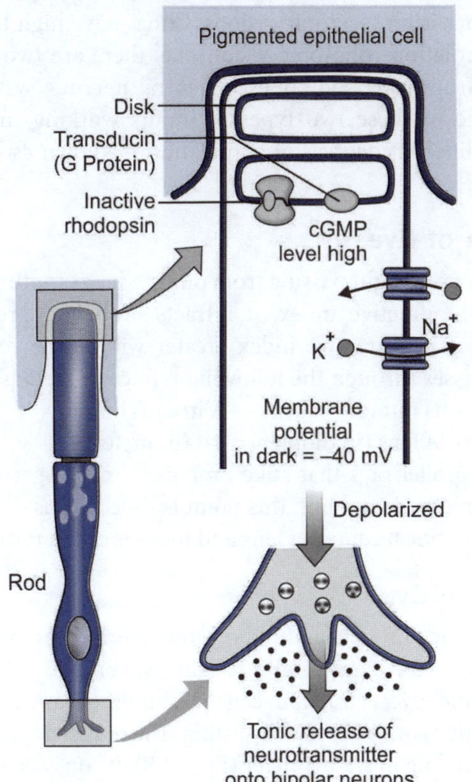

Fig. 12.5: Events involved in the depolarization step (in dark) of phototransduction in rods and cones

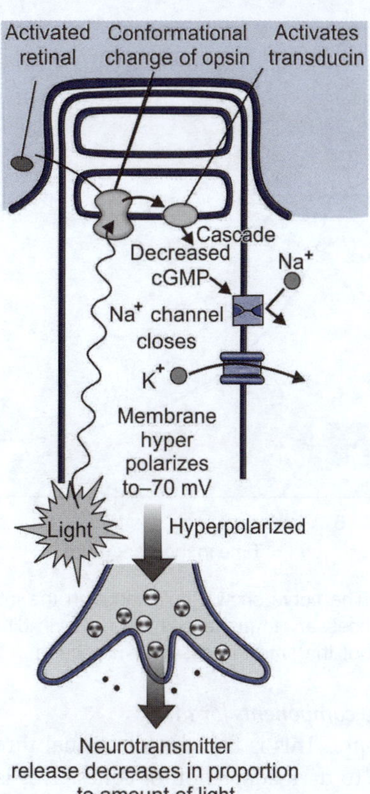

Fig. 12.6: Events involved in the hyperpolarization (activation) step of phototransduction in rods and cones

Light stimulus → structural changes in the retinine1 of rhodopsin (11 *cis* retinine → all transretinine) → conformational change of opsin → activation of tiransducin (G protein; Gt1 in rods and Gt 2 in cones) → α subunit separates from G protein → activation of phosphodiesterase converts cGMP → 5'GMP → decreased intracellular concentration of cGMP → closure of Na^+ channels → hyperpolarization of receptor → decreased release of synaptic transmitter (glutamate) cause disinhibition of bipolar cells and thus an action potential develops in ganglion cells.

Dark Adaptation

When a person enters a dark room from a brightly lit outdoor, at first he sees nothing but gradually gets adapted to the dark.

Reason

In bright light, vision was only due to cones. Cones have high threshold for stimulation. So when the person enter darkroom, the low intensity light that is available in the dark is unable to stimulate cones, but visual perception improves quickly at first and more slowly thereafter. This decrease in visual threshold and increase in sensitivity of eye to light is dark adaptation (Fig. 12.7)

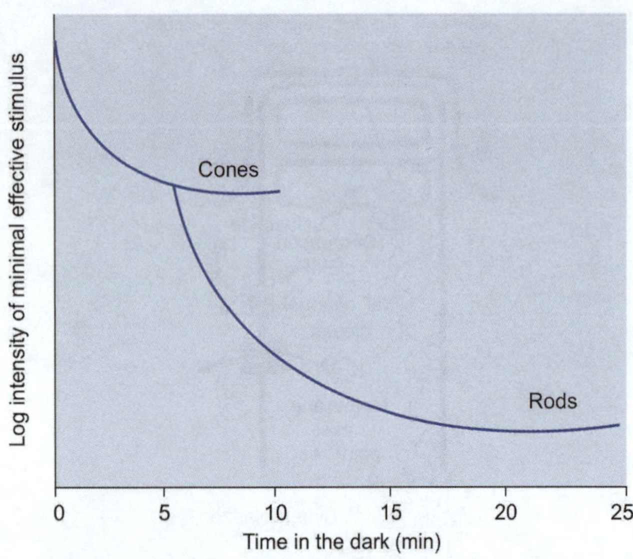

Fig. 12.7: The curve shows the change in the intensity of a stimulus necessary to just excite the retina in dim light as a function of the time the observer has been in the dark

There are two components for this:

1. *Fast response:* This is first drop in visual threshold and is rapid due to dark adaptation of cones. This is called paradoxical adaptation of cones. Its duration is 4–5 min.
2. *Slow response:* Further drop in visual threshold occurs over a period of 20–25 min due to dark adaptation of rods. Time for dark adaptation depends on time taken for resynthesis of rhodopsin.

Important Changes

a. Dilatation of pupil (mydriasis).
b. Change of photoreceptors from cones to rods.
c. Resynthesis of rhodopsin (occurs when the activated rhodopsin is inactivated by the enzyme rhodopsin kinase thereby a reversal of all reactions occurs).

Light Adaptation

When one passes suddenly from a dim to a brightly lit environment, the light seems intense until the eyes adapt to the increased illumination. This adaptation occurs over a period of about 5 minutes and is called light adaptation. Photoreceptors signal light by decreasing their neurotransmitter output. Intense light reduces their neurotransmitter output to zero so that no further decrease is possible. This renders rods useless for signaling bright light, but the neurotransmitter output of cones gradually increases again even in the continued presence of bright light. Ca^{2+} plays an important role in this recovery of conal sensitivity to bright light. When light falls on the cone, there is closure of Na^+ channels resulting in membrane hyperpolarization. The hyperpolarization causes closure of Ca^{2+} channels, resulting in a reduction in intracellular Ca^{2+}. Intracellular Ca^{2+} normally inhibits guanylyl cyclase; the enzyme that converts GTP into cGMP. A low intracellular Ca^{2+} therefore elevates intracellular cGMP levels. The cGMP keeps the Na^+ channels open, leading to the depolarization of the outer segment and the resumption of neurotransmitter output.

Visual Acuity

It is the degree to which the details and contours of objects are perceived. It is usually defined in terms of the minimum separable, i.e. the shortest distance by which 2 lines can be separated and still be perceived as 2 lines. It is tested using snellen letter charts. Normally, Snellens letter charts are viewed at a distance of 20 ft (6 m). It is 20/20 normally.

Visual Fields

Visual field of each eye is the portion of the external world visible out of that eye. It can be mapped using perimeter. The extent of normal visual field with a 5 mm white color object is superiorly 50°, nasally 60°, inferiorly 70°, temporally 90°.

Duplicity Theory

The rods are extremely sensitive to light and they are receptors for night vision (scotopic vision). Cones have high threshold for stimulation (photopic vision), i.e. there are two types of inputs from rods and cones to central nervous system. The existence of these two types of inputs working maximally under different degrees of stimulation is known as duplicity theory.

Optics of Eye

When a ray of light passing from one media to another having different refractive index, it refracts or bends; greater the difference in refractive index greater will be the refraction. Light passes through the following refractive medias: Cornea → Aqueous humor → Lens → Vitreous humor.

Power of lens (in diopter) = 1/f (in meter)

All parallel rays that stike on biconvex lens get refracted and converge to a point; this point is called focus. Difference between optical center of lens and focus is called focal length.

Reduced Eye

Due to the differences in the refractive indices of the eye structures, the refraction of light is complex. Therefore, compound eye refraction can be simplified as reduced or schematic eye as proposed by listing. The reduced eye of listing is 24 mm long in AP diameter (Fig. 12.8). It consists of a single refracting plane (resultant of all refractive media in the eye) situated 1.5 mm behind the anterior surface of cornea and a single nodal point N (nodal point-center of optical system). A ray passing through nodal point suffers no refraction. In

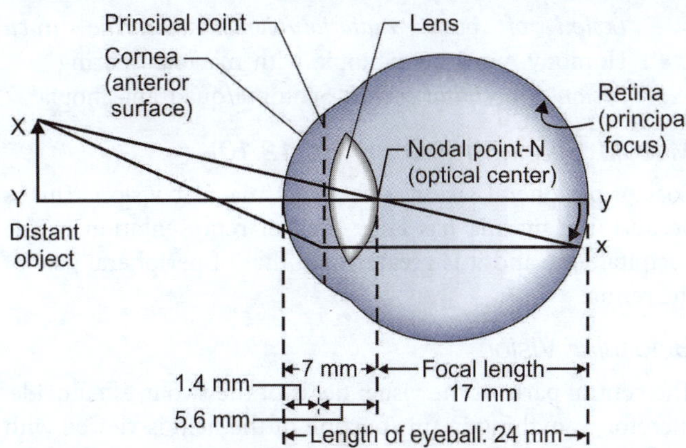

Fig. 12.8: Reduced/schematic eye

Listing's reduced eye, the nodal point is 17 mm anterior to retina (focal length of the optical system). Hence, power of the single lens of Listing's eye (equivalent to combined powers of all lenses of natural eye) is about 59 D (1000/17).

Visual Pathway

It is a three order neuronal pathway. The visual fibers arise in the layer of nerve cells (bipolar and ganglion cells) in the retina.

- *1st order neuron:* These are bipolar cells with which receptors synapse. It is of 3 types: rod bipolar cell with rods, flat bipolar cell with cones, midget bipolar cell. Bipolar cell synapse with ganglion cell.
- *2nd order neuron:* These are ganglion cells. Ganglion cells are of two types: Large magno and small parvo. Axons of ganglion cells emerge out of the eyeball as optic nerve. Optic nerve consists of two groups of fibers:
  - Fibers from the nasal half of retina which carry light sensation from temporal half of field of vision.
  - Fibers from temporal half of retina which carry light sensation from nasal half of field of vision.

  Partial crossing of optic nerve fibers occurs at optic chiasma and two optic tracts are thus formed. The optic tract ends in lateral geniculate body (LGB).
- *3rd order neurons:* These arise from LGB and ends in visual cortex. LGB has 6 layers, the layer 1 and 2 of LGB form magnocellular pathway and from layers 3–6 parvocellular pathway projects to visual cortex (Fig. 12.9).

Magnocellular pathway is concerned with detection of movement, depth, flicker. Parvocellular pathway is concerned with color of object, texture, shape and other fine details of object. Some fibers in intralaminar region of LGB ends in blobs in visual cortex and is concerned with color vision only.

Pathways ends in 1° visual area 17, visual association area 18 (concerned with depth perception, visual orientation, relay of information), area 19 (occipital eye field for conjugate movement of eye to opposite side) and area 8 (frontal eye field for visual reflexes).

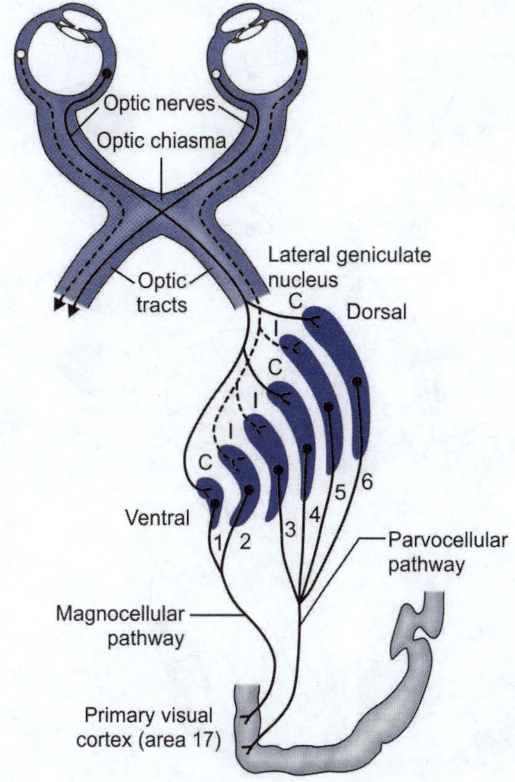

Fig. 12.9: Visual pathway

Some fibers from optic tract deviate from main tract and end in:

a. Midbrain (which mediate visual reflexes).
b. Suprachiasmatic nucleus (which mediate light and dark cycles).

Effects of Lesion of Optic Pathway

The effect of lesion of the visual pathways are described in term of field of vision. The following definitions will help to understand these defects.

- *Anopia:* Complete loss of visual field in an eye.
- *Hemianopia:* Blindness of ½ of visual field.
- *Quadrant anopia:* Loss of ¼ of visual field.
- *Homonymous hemianopia:* When same side (right/left) of visual field of both eyes are lost.
- *Heteronymous hemianopia:* When different sides of field of vision of both eyes are lost.
- *Scotoma:* Loss of vision in eye which is confined to center of visual field.
  - *Lesion of optic nerve (at A in Fig. 12.10):* Anopia of affected side.
  - *Lesion of optic chiasma (at B in Fig. 12.10):* Heteronymous hemianopia.
  - *Lesion of optic tract (at C in Fig. 12.10):* Homonymous hemianopia.
  - *Lesion of LGB:* Homonymous hemianopia.

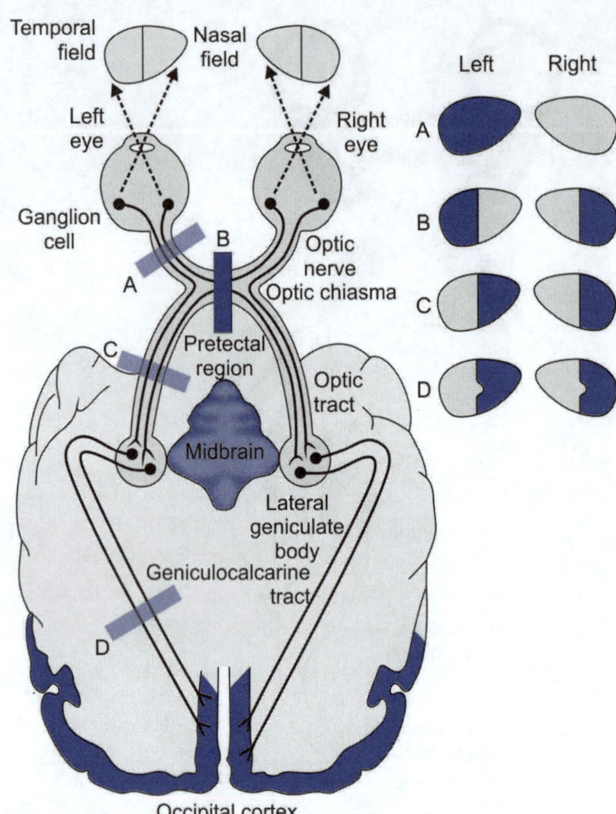

Fig. 12.10: Efffect of lesion on optic pathway

– *Lesion of optic radiation/Geniculocalcarine tract:* Homony-mous hemianopia with macular sparing.
– *Lesion of occipital cortex:* Scotoma/quadrant anopia

Macula Sparing (at D in Fig. 12.10)

Loss of peripheral vision with intact macular vision. This is because the macula has large area of representation in the occipital lobe and it is greater than that of peripheral part of the retina.

Binocular Vision

The central parts of the visual fields of the two eyes coincide, therefore, anything in this portion of the field is viewed with both eyes and is fused at the cortical level into a single image and is important in depth perception.

Visual Reflexes

Light Reflex (Direct, Indirect)

When light is directed to one of the eye, pupil of that eye constricts, it is called direct/pupillary light reflex. In addition it also results in the constriction of pupil of the opposite eye, called as indirect/consensual light reflex both sides it forms the basis of indirect light reflex.

Pathway of light reflex (Fig. 12.11)

Light sensation → optic nerve → optic chiasma → optic tract → enter midbrain via superior colliculus → pretectal nucleus of both sides → Edinger-westphal nucleus of 3rd cranial nerve

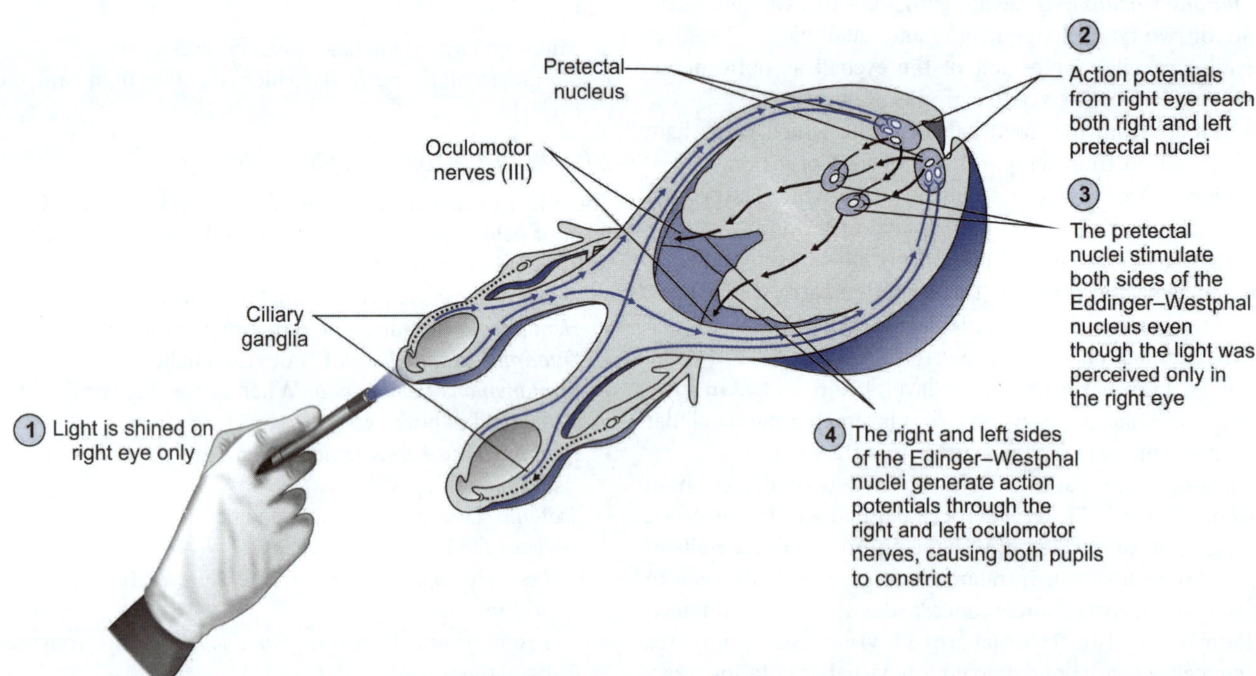

Fig. 12.11: Pathway of light reflex

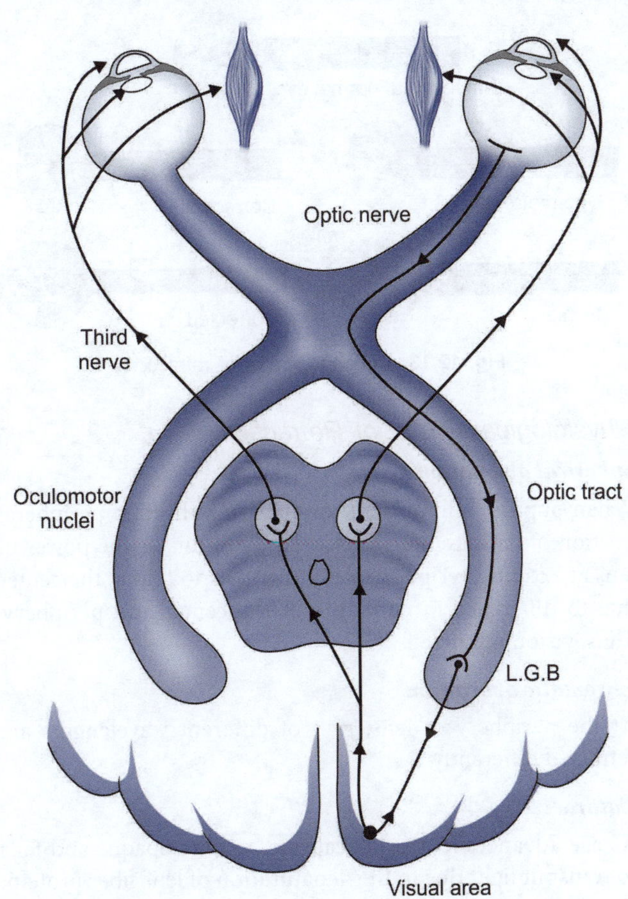

Fig. 12.12: Pathway of accommodation reflex

(parasympathetic) → ciliary ganglion → short ciliary nerve → sphincter pupillae of iris.

Effect is constriction of pupil of both sides.

Accommodation Reflex (Fig. 12.12)

Accommodation is defined as the ability of the eye to focus an object at varying distances. It is a reflex action. When a person changes his gaze from distant object to a near object, three adjustments are made in the eyeballs (Flowchart 12.1).

a. Convergence of eyeball due to the contraction of medial recti.
b. Constriction of the pupil due to contraction of constrictor pupillae of iris.
c. Increase in anterior curvature of lens due to contraction of ciliary muscle.

This is also called near response.

Afferent pathway

Visual impulse from retina pass through the optic nerve, optic chiasma, optic tract, LGB and optic radiation to visual cortex. From here, the association fibers carry the impulses to the frontal lobe.

Flowchart 12.1: Schematic diagram of accommodation reflex

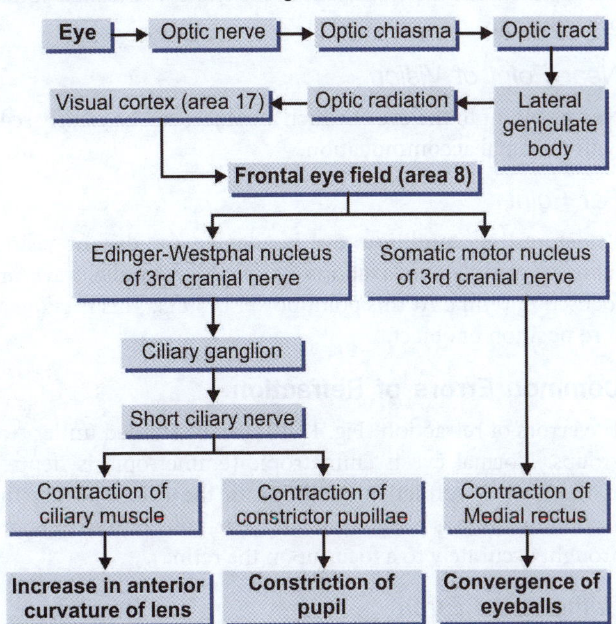

Center: Center for accommodation lies in the frontal eyefield, situated in the frontal lobe area 8.

Efferent pathway

a. *Efferent fibers to ciliary muscle and sphincter pupillae:* From area 8, the corticonuclear fibers pass via internal capsule to the Edinger-Westphal nucleus of 3rd cranial nerve on both sides. From here, the preganglionic fibers pass through the 3rd cranial nerve to ciliary ganglion. The postganglionic fibers from ciliary ganglion pass via the short ciliary nerves and supply the ciliary muscle and sphincter pupillae.
b. *Efferent fibers to medial rectus:* Some of the fibers from frontal eyefield terminate in the somatic motor nucleus of 3rd nerve. The fibers fro motor nucleus supply the medial rectus.

Applied Aspects

Argyll Robertson Pupil

In this condition pupillary constriction in response to a light stimulus is absent or decreased while the response to accommodation is present. Pupillary reflex pathway is dorsal to the pathway for near response. Cosequently, even if the light response is lost the response to accommodation still remains intact. Usually seen in midbrain lesion. The effects can be remembered like this (ARP—Accommodation reflex present, PRA—Pupillary reflex absent).

Strabismus or Squint

Normally visual axis of the two eyes are parellel to each other and this alignment is maintained in all positions of gaze. A misalignment of the visual axis of the two eyes is called squint or strabismus.

Near Point of Vision

Nearest point to the eye at which an object can be clearly seen with maximal accommodation.

Far Point

Under resting condition, eye is adapted for distant vision, there is complete relaxations of lens. So parallel rays are focused in retina. At this point power is 59 D. This is taken as zero position of object.

Common Errors of Refraction

The errors of refraction (Fig. 12.13) can be studied under two groups. Normal eye is emmetropic (emmetropia is defined as the normal refractive condition of the eye in which the accommodation is relaxed and all the parallel rays of light are brought accurately to a focus upon the retina).

Pathological Errors

Myopia /shortsightedness

Parallel rays are focused in front of retina. Person fails to see distant objects but near vision is normal.

Causes

i. Increased A-P diameter of eyeball.
ii. Changes in curvature of lens and cornea.

Correction: Using biconcave lens.

Hypermetropia/longsightedness

Parallel rays are focused behind the retina.

Causes

i. Smaller A-P diameter of eye.
ii. Abnormalities in curvature of lens and cornea.

Correction: Using biconvex lens.

Astigmatism

In some cornea, curvature varies from meridian to meridian. Refractive index of astigmatic cornea is different in different meridians, all the rays are not focused in retina and the image is blurred.

Correction: Using cylindrical lens.

Presbyopia

Clinical condition seen after 40 years due to the loss of accommodation.

Causes: Loss of elasticity of crystalline lens due to changes in lens protein. So lens become rigid and during accommodation, though the ciliary muscles are contracting, curvature of lens is not changed and person cannot see near objects when held at normal distance.

Correction: Use convex lens.

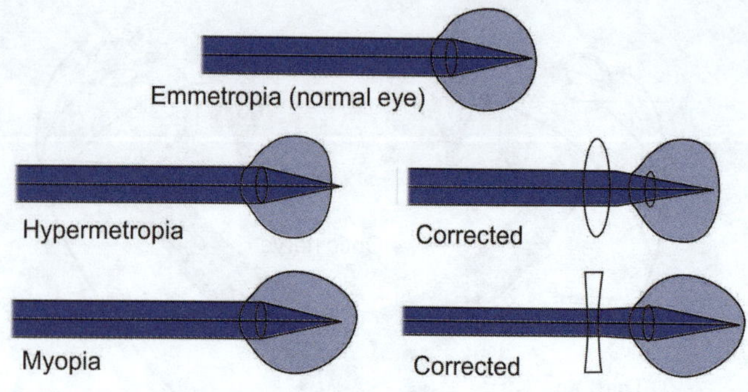

Fig. 12.13: Common errors of refraction

Physiological Errors of Refraction

Spherical aberration

When pupil is fully dilated, rays passing through peripheral portion of lens are not focused on the retina as the power of lens at extreme periphery is not identical to that at the center due to difference in curvature at the center and periphery. Thus, vision is blurred.

Chromatic aberration

At the periphery of lens, rays of different wavelengths are refracted differently.

Cataract

As age advances lens or its capsule become opaque and fails to transmit light due to the denaturation of lens fiber protein; elevated by exposure to strong sunlight and UV rays.

Correction: Surgical removal and artificial insertion of lens.

Aphakia

Condition where lens is absent. It may congenital or surgical.

Amplitude of accommodation: This is the difference in refractive power of the eye between the two states, complete relaxation and maximal accommodation.

Color Vision

The Young-Helmholtz Theory

The Trichromatic theory states that color vision is possible due to three types of cones: 1. Long (L) or red cones, 2. Medium (M) or green cones and 3. Short (S) or blue cones. It assumes that the signals generated in the three cone types, which are independent and have different spectral sensitivities (L for long wavelength sensitivity, M for medium wavelength sensitivity, and S for short wavelength sensitivity), are transmitted directly to the brain where '*color sensations*' are experienced that correlate in a simple and direct way to the three cone signals. The underlying premise of the theory is that it is possible to create all colors of the spectrum by mixing two primary colors.

Color Blindness

It is a clinical condition when people are unable to distinguish certain colors or have color weakness. It is an X-linked recessive disorder.

Types

There are following type of color blindness. Color blindness is tested using ishihara charts. When green cones are absent, the person is green blind. The condition is called deuteranope and the person is called deuteranope. When red cones are absent, the person is red blind. The condition is called protanopia and the person is called protanope.

These two are the two most common types of color blindness. Six percent of all men are green color blind (deuteranopes) and two percent of all men are red color blind (protanopes) making a total of about 8 percent who are red-green blind. These two types are grouped together and called red-green color blindness because these are the most common type of color blindness and as both are unable to differentiate between red and green colors. When blue cones are absent, the person is blue blind. The condition is called tritanopia and the person is called tritanope. This is a very rare condition. As all these patients can appreciate only two primary colors, this defect is called dichromatic color blindness.

Sometimes person does not have color blindness, but has color weakness for a particular color because color cones are not missing but they are under represented. The person can appreciate all three primary color but is defective for one or two of them, therefore called trichromatic color blindness. Three types of such anomalies are there: red color defective–protanomaly, green color defective—deuteranomaly, blue color defective—protanomaly.

Achromatopsia

Color blindness due to lesion of V8 (projection area for color vision).

Nyctalopia/night blindness

Prolonged deficiency of vitamin A leads to anatomic changes in the rods and cones followed by degeneration of neural layers of the retina causing visual abnormalities leading to nyctalopia.

As individual taking sildenafil (viagra), used for treating erectile dysfunction cause trasient color blindness as it inhibit the enzyme phosphodiesterase.

AUDITION

Structure of Ear

The ear consists of three parts namely external ear, middle ear and internal ear. The external ear is formed of two parts: auricle/pinna and the external auditory meatus (Fig. 12.14).

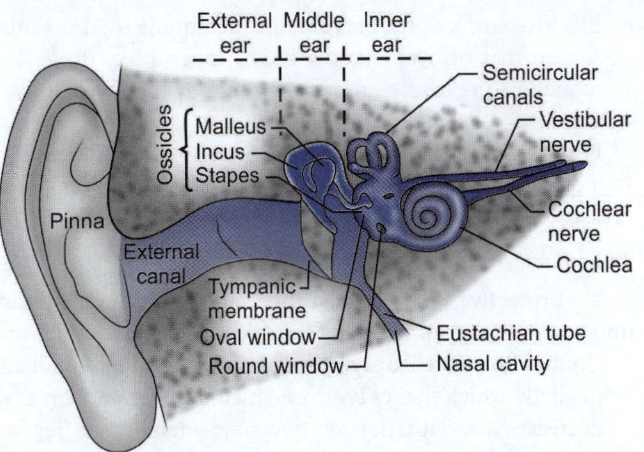

Fig. 12.14: Structure of ear

External Ear (24 mm Length)

External ear funnels sound waves to the external auditory meatus. From the meatus, the external auditory canal passes inward to the tympanic membrane.

Middle Ear

The middle ear is an air-filled cavity in the temporal bone that opens via the auditory (Eustachian) tube into the nasopharynx and through it to the exterior. The 3 auditory ossicles, the malleus, incus, and stapes are located in the middle ear. The ear ossicles are arranged in the form of a chain extending across the middle ear from the tympanic membrane to oval window. Function of ear ossicles is to magnify the intensity of sound waves to about 1.2–1.3 times.

Functions of middle ear

Tympanic membrane as resonator

It acts as a resonator, i.e. it starts vibrating (in and out movements) freely when the sound waves strike.

Impedance matching

The sound waves have to pass from the air to the liquid medium in the internal ear. So there will be resistance to the transmission of sound waves. This is overcome by increasing the pressure of sound waves at the level of oval window. The mechanisms are:

a. Ear ossicles move as a single unit. The size of handle of malleus is less than the size of incus, while size of stapes is less than the incus; moreover handle of malleus is longer than the long processes of the incus. The auditory ossicles thus function as a lever system that converts the resonant vibrations of the tympanic membrane into movements of the stapes against the perilymph-filled scala vestibuli of the cochlea. The lever action of the malleus and incus multiplies the intensity of sound waves to about 1.3 times.

b. Effective surface area of tympanic membrane is 50–54 mm sq and that of oval window is 3–4 mm sq, i.e. there is a reduction in surface area by 17 times at the level of oval window.

Both these mechanisms lead to corresponding increase in sound pressure at the oval window. So total increase in sound pressure is about 22 times (17 × 1.3).

Tympanic/acoustic/attenuation reflex

It is a protective reflex against the loud sound. Loud sound initiates a reflex contraction of the middle ear muscles.

a. Contraction of tensor tympani pulls the handle of malleus medially which makes tympanic membrane more taut and decreases the vibration of tympanic membrane. Tensor tympani is the muscle attached to neck of malleus. It is supplied by 5th CN.
b. Stapedius is attached to neck of stapes which is supplied by the 7th CN. Its contraction pulls footplate of stapes away from the oval window, thus, preventing transmission of sound waves to internal ear.

Both of these muscles contract reflexly in response to loud sound and thus excessive sound is prevented from going to oval window. This is known as tympanic/acoustic/attenuation reflex.

Equalization of pressure on either side of tympanic membrane

It equalizes the pressure on both sides of tympanic membrane with the help of eustachian tube. The eustachian tube is usually closed, but during swallowing, chewing and yawning it opens and equalizes the pressure on both sides of tympanic membrane.

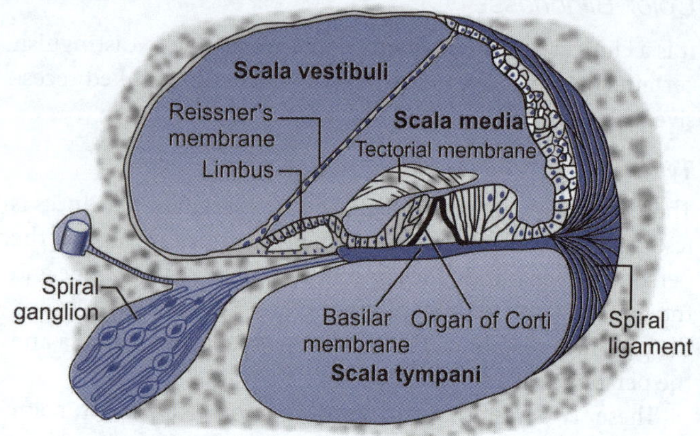

Fig. 12.15: Vertical section through cochlea

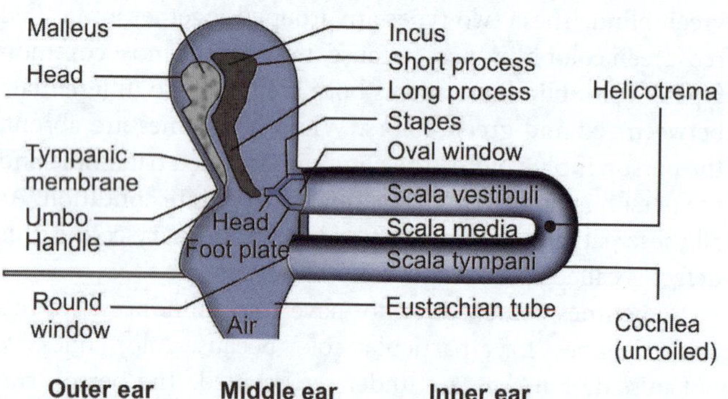

Fig. 12.16: Schematic diagram showing outer, middle and inner ear

Inner Ear

The inner ear (labyrinth) is made up of two parts; the bony labyrinth and the membranous labyrinth. The bony labyrinth is a series of channels in the petrous portion of temporal bone. The membranous labyrinth is present inside these channels and it is surrounded by a fluid called perilymph. This membranous labyrinth more or less duplicates the shape of bony channels and is filled with a fluid called endolymph. There is no communication between the spaces filled with endolymph and those filled with perilymph.

Internal ear is divided into 3 chambers; scala vestibuli, scala media and scala tympani by 2 membranes: Reissner's and Basilar membrane (Figs 12.15 and 12.16). Scala vestibuli and tympani are filled with perilymph and are continuous at the apex (helicotrema). Scala media is continuous with membranous labyrinth and is filled with endolymph.

Organ of Corti

It is located on the basilar membrane and it contains the hair cells. Hair cells are receptor cells that transduce sound energy into electrical energy. It extends from the apex to the base of the cochlea and has a spiral shape. There is one organ of Corti in each ear. The processes of hair cells pierce the tough, membrane-like reticular lamina that is supported by rods of Corti. The hair cells are arranged in 4 rows; 3 rows of outer hair cells lateral to the tunnel formed by rods of Corti and 1 row of inner hair cell medial to the tunnel (Fig. 12.17). There are 3500 inner hair cells which are important for fine sensory transduction. There are about 20,000 outer hair cells which is responsible for detecting the presence of sound.

Outer hair cells are capped with gelatinous material called tectorial membrane. Cell bodies of afferent neuron that surround the bases of hair cells are located in the spiral ganglion. About 90–95% fibers innervate inner hair cells and only 5–10% innervates outer hair cells. In each hair cell, there are about 30–50 hairs called stercocilia. It has actin and myosin. Very fine processes called tip links tie the tip of each stercocilia to the side of its higher neighbor. At the junction, there are cation channels which are mechanically sensitive. When hair cells move in one direction towards longer stercocilia, channels open and there is Ca^{2+} and K^{+} influx. If hair cells move in opposite direction the ion channel closes.

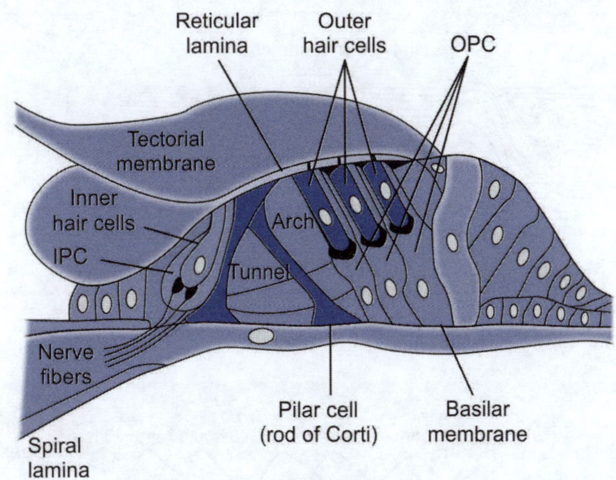

Fig. 12.17: Organ of corti

Supporting cells are:

- Inner phalangeal cells (for supporting inner hair cells).
- Outer phalangeal cells/dieter's cell (support outer hair cells).

The outer phalangeal cells are supported by Hansen's cells which is again supported by Claudius cells. The junctions between hair cells and other supporting cells are tight junctions to prevent mixing of endolymph and perilymph.

Sound Transduction

Sound waves which enter the cochlea gets transmitted along the scala vestibuli and spreads towards helicotrema. At the same time sound waves are also transmitted to fluid in other chambers. This will lead to vertical up and down movement of basilar membrane. This results in up and down and side to side movement of hair cells. The processes of hair cells project into the endolymph whereas the bases are bathed in perilymph.

Mechanism

When tip links pull stercocilia the ion channels open, there is K^+ influx → receptor potential in hair cells → Ca^{2+} influx causes depolarization → release of neurotransmitter (glutamate) into synaptic cleft between receptor cell and afferent sensory nerve → neurotransmitter binds with specific receptor on the sensory nerve → ligand gated ion channels open → action potential in cochlear division of 8th cranial nerve → auditory pathway.

Auditory Pathway

The afferent fibers in the auditory division of the 8th cranial nerve is the 1st order neuron and it ends in dorsal and ventral coclear nucleus (Fig. 12.18). There are three sets of fibers from this level:

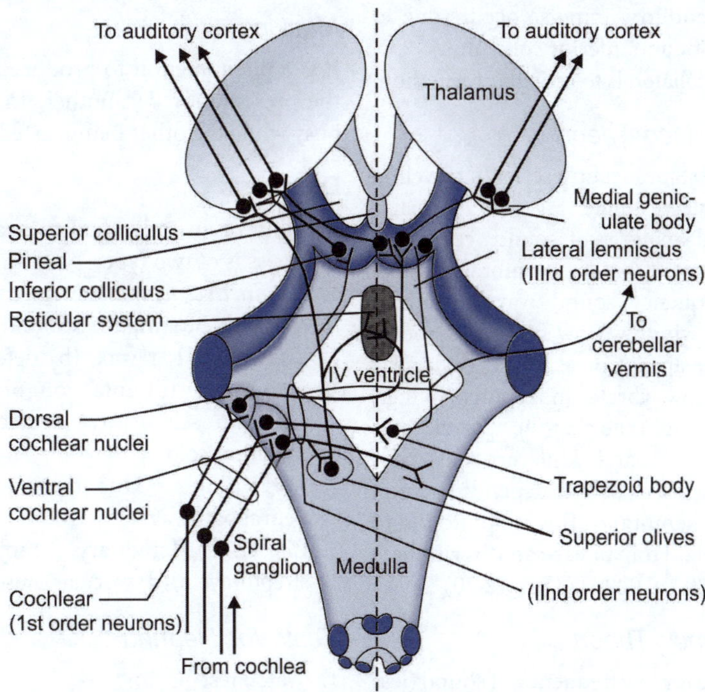

Fig. 12.18: Auditory pathway

1. Dorsal cochlear nucleus → 2nd order fibers cross to opposite side → ascend and end in inferior colliculus (many collaterals given to reticular formation) → 3rd order neurons arise → end in medial geniculate body of same and opposite → 4th order neurons arise → end in auditory cortex (primary auditory area 41, association area 20, 21, 22).
2. Ventral cochlear nucleus → 2nd order fibers cross to opposite side → end in trapezoid body → 3rd order neuron arises → end in inferior colliculus → 4th order neuron arises → medial geniculate body (no relay) → end in auditory cortex.
3. Ventral cochlear nucleus → 2nd order fibers end in superior olive → 3rd order fibers arise → ends in medial geniculate body (collaterals to inferior colliculus and reticular formation → 4th order neurons arise → ends in auditory cortex.

Efferent Pathway

Some fibers from cortex descend and ends in outer hair cells.

Neurotransmitter released is ACh, although these inhibitory fibers end in outer hair cells, they actually modify the activity of inner hair cells.

Salient features of the pathway

a. Bilateral representation due to extensive crossing of fibers.
b. There is a descending pathway.
c. Integration of visual and auditory impulse occurs due to connection between superior and inferior colliculus.
d. General arousal as it gives collaterals to reticular formation.

Traveling Wave Theory/Place Theory

The movement of foot plate of stapes set up a series of traveling waves in the perilymph of scala vestibule (Fig. 12.19). Basilar membrane is the mechanical analyzer of sound frequency. The basic pattern of movement of basilar membrane is like a traveling wave. High frequency sound waves produce maximum height at the oval window. Low frequency sound has maximum height near the apex. Correspondingly basilar membrane near the oval window vibrates in response to high frequency sound and basilar membrane near the apex vibrates in response to low frequency. That is different hair cells respond to different frequencies of sound depending upon their location on the basilar membrane. This is applicable to frequencies of 2000–20,000 Hz. Human ear can discriminate sound of frequency between 20–20,000 Hz (Fig. 12.20).

Volley's Principle/Frequency Theory

Volley's principle is applicable for low frequency of sound (less than 2000 Hz). There is a relation between frequency of sound and action potential developed in sensory nerve endings. For low frequency sound, frequency of action potential is less. If greater frequency, a volley of action potential is produced.

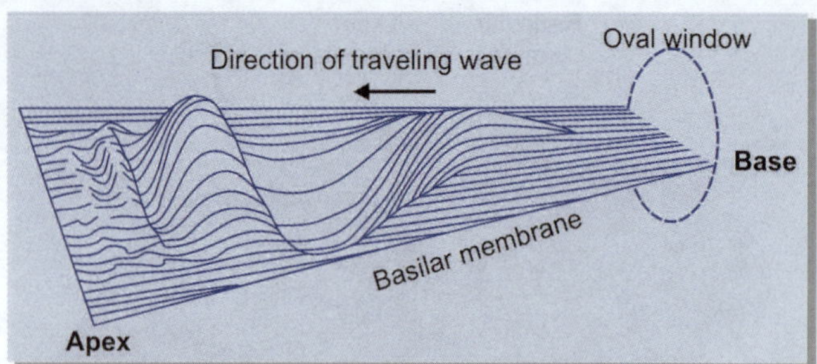

Fig. 12.19: Traveling wave theory

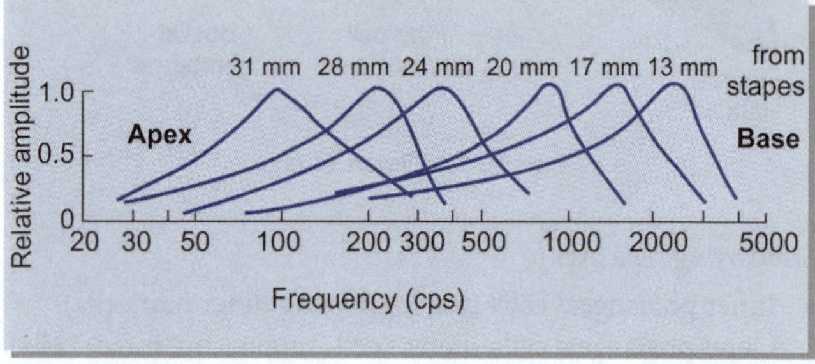

Fig. 12.20: Graphical representation of frequency of sound with the amplitude of vibrations in relation to distance from the stapes

Masking

It is a phenomenon to produce inaudibility of one sound by the presentation of another. In audiometry one ear is kept busy while the other being tested by a sound.

Deafness

Inability of an individual to hear either wholly or partially. Deafness is of two types:

1. *Conductive deafness:* Here the defect is in conduction of sound due to impaired sound transmission.
   Causes: (a) Ear wax, (b) defect in vibration of tympanic membrane, (c) infection of middle ear (otitis media), (d) auto sclerosis,(e) eustachian tube blocked due to common cold.
2. *Nerve deafness:* Due to damage to the hair cells or in the neural pathway.
   Causes: (a) Hereditary, (b) injury to 8th CN, (c) drugs like streptomycin, (d) vascular cause, (e) industrial noise pollution.

Tests for Hearing

1. Watch test
2. Tuning fork tests (Table 12.2)
3. Audiometry test

Table 12.2: Tests of hearing

Text	Method	Normal	Conductive deafness	Nerve deafness
Rinne test	Base of the vibrating tunning fork is placed on the mastoid process until subject no longer hears it (bone conduction), then it is held in the air, next to ear (air conduction)	Subject hears vibrations in air after bone conduction is over. Air conduction is better than bone conduction (Rinne's test positive)	Vibration in air not heard after bone conduction is over, that is bone conduction is better than air conduction (Rinne's test negative)	If partial nerve deafness. Rinne's test is positive. If complete nerve deafness, both air conducted and bone conducted sounds are not perceived
Weber test	Base of the vibrating tunning fork is placed on the vertex of skull in midline or over the mandible	Both the ears 'hear' the sound equally well	Sound is better heard in the affected ear	The 'deaf' ear remains deaf to bone conducted sound and sound is thus better heard and perceived by the normal ear, i.e. 'lateralized' to healthy ear
Schwabach test	Bone conduction of the subject is compared with that of the examiner's assuming that the latter is normal	Both the subject and examiner 'hear' the sound equally well	Subject's bone conduction is better than the examiner's	Subject's bone conduction is worse than the examiner's

Auditory acuity (sharpness of hearing) can be measured with the help of an audiometer. This test helps to assess the degree of deafness and the frequency range in which deafness is most affected. The device consists of the following parts:

a. Electronic oscillator
b. Intensity dial
c. Head phone

Vestibulo-ocular reflex: It is actually a reflex that maintains visual fixation on stationary points while the body rotates. When rotation starts, the eyes move slowly in a direction opposite to the direction of rotation, maintaining visual fixation.

Nystagmus: The regular and rhythmic to and fro involuntary oscillatory movements of the eyes. Meniere's disease/endolymphatic hydrops. It is a disorder of the inner ear where the endolymphatic system is distented with endolymph.

Endocochlear/Endolymphatic potential: An potential difference of about +80 millivolts exists all the time between endolymph and perilymph, with positivity inside the scala media and negativity outside. It is generated by continual secretion of K^+ ions into the scala media by the stria vascularis.

SENSATION OF TASTE

Taste buds are the sense organs for taste. Size of taste bud is about 50–70 μm and they are ovoid in shape with 40 mm diameter. Each taste bud is made of three types of cells (Fig. 12.21):

a. Taste/gustatory cells-type 3 cells.
b. Supporting/sustentacular cells-type 1 and 2 cells.
c. Basal cells: They differentiate into new receptor cells.

Chemoreceptors are present in taste buds on walls of papilla. There are four types of papillae.

1. *Fungiform:* They are rounded structures most numerous near the tip of the tongue. It contains five taste buds located on the tip of the papillae.

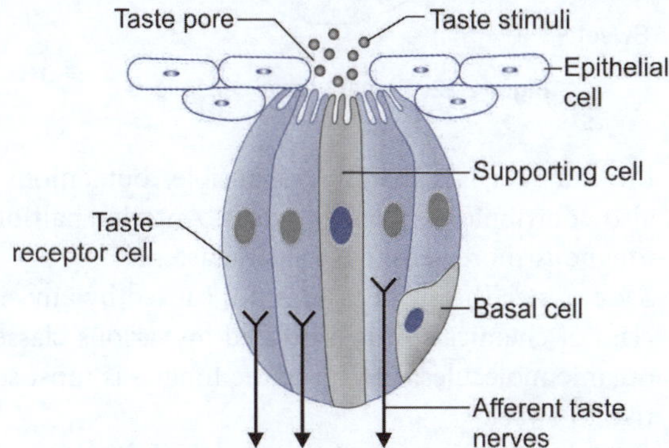

Fig. 12.21: Taste receptor (or taste bud)

2. *Filiform:* Small conical structures that cover the dorsum of the tongue. No taste buds are present on filiform papillae.
3. *Foliate:* These are found occasionally upon the posterolateral surfaces of tongue.
4. *Circumvallate:* They are prominent structures arranged in a V on the back of the tongue. They are 10–12 in number. Larger vallate papillae contains up to 100 taste buds located along the sides of the papillae.

Total number of taste buds is 10,000 and its number decreases with age. Taste bud is stimulated only at the tip as the necks of taste cells and sustentacular cells are connected to each other and to the surrounding epithelial cells by tight junctions so that only tip is exposed to oral fluids. At the base of taste bud, afferent nerve fibers are attached. Each taste bud is innervated by 50 nerve fibers.

All taste sensations result from various combinations of four basic tastes (primary taste sensations in Figure 12.22:

a. *Sour taste:* The sour taste is caused by acids, i.e. hydrogen ions. More acidic the food, more sour is the taste. The edges of tongue are more sensitive to sour.
b. *Salty taste:* The salty taste is elicited by ionized salts mainly by sodium ion concentration. The cation of

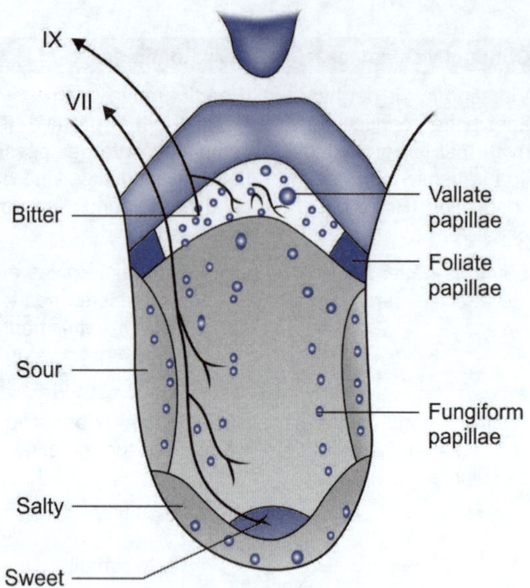

Fig. 12.22: Primary taste sensations

the salt (Na^+) is mainly responsible, but anions can also contribute, to a lesser extent. Anterior half of the tongue is more sensitive to salty taste.

c. *Sweet taste:* The sweet taste is not caused by any single class of chemicals. It is produced by various classes of organic molecules. The tip of the tongue is most sensitive to sweet.
d. *Bitter taste:* Bitter taste is produced by long-chain organic substances containing nitrogen and by alkaloids such as quinine and caffeine. The back of the tongue is particularly sensitive to bitter.

Taste Pathway

It is a three orders uncrossed pathway (Fig. 12.23). 1st order neurons are:

a. Chorda tympani branch of 7th CN, which carries sensation from anterior 2/3rd of tongue.
b. 9th CN, which carries sensation from posterior 1/3rd of tongue.
c. 10th CN, which carries sensation from areas other than tongue, i.e. epiglottis, pharynx and palate.

From taste cells in taste bud, 1st order neurons arise → reach nucleus tractus solitarius of medulla → 2nd order neurons ascend ipsilaterally in medial lemniscus → end in thalamus (ventral posteromedial nucleus) → 3rd order neurons arise → end in face area of somatosensory cortex in postcentral gyrus. Some fibers end on anterior part of insula.

The basic taste modalities are:

a. Sweet: Receptor is G protein activated gustducin.
b. Bitter: Receptor same as sweet.
c. Salt: Receptors are E NaCs (i.e. epithelium Na^+ channels).

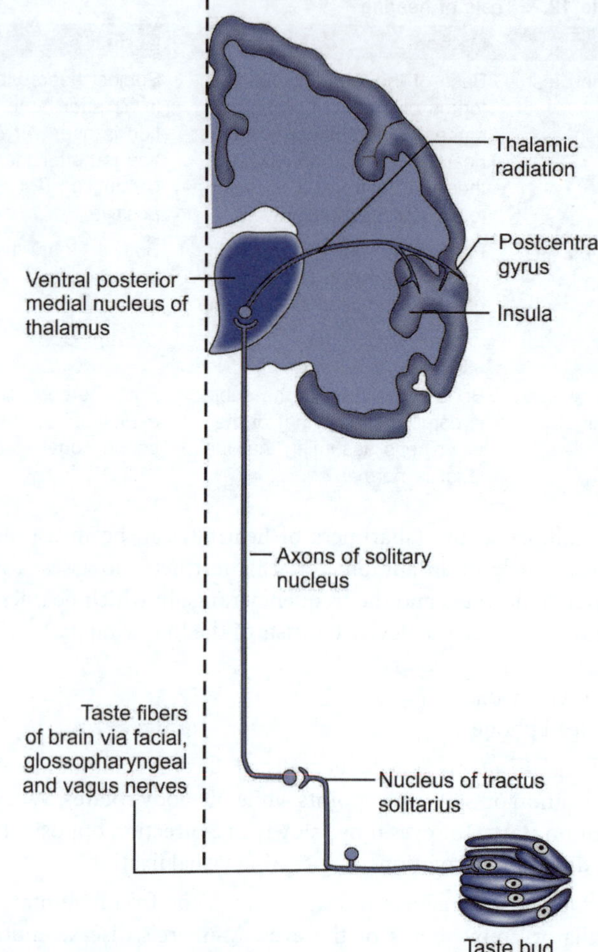

Fig. 12.23: Taste pathway

d. Sour: Receptors are E NaCs HCN (hyperpolarization activated cyclic nucleotide gated cation channels).
e. Umami (sweet pleasant taste evoked by monosodium glutamate): Receptor is mGluR4 receptor.

Note: Miraculin-taste modifier protein which when applied to tongue makes acid taste sweet.

Abnormalities

1. Ageusia: Absence of taste and it is commonly drug induced
2. Hypogeusia: Diminished taste sensitivity
3. Dysgeusia: Disturbed sense of taste.

OLFACTION

The olfactory receptor cells are located in a specialized portion of the nasal mucosa, the yellowish pigmented olfactory mucous membrane. Olfactory mucous membrane is constantly covered by mucous which is produced by Bowman's cells, present under the basal lamina of the membrane. Receptors are bipolar neurons with lifespan of 60 days. The olfactory receptors are unique in that the receptor cell itself is a neuron. In between the receptor cells, there are supporting cells and basal cells. Each neuron has a short and thick dendrite with expanded end called as olfactory rod, from these rods 10–20 cilia (unmyelinated process) project to the surface of the mucosa.

Odoriferous substances combine with receptors on surface of cilia. This will initiate G protein coupled reaction, finally leading to opening of Ca^{2+} channels. Ca^{2+} influx initiates receptor potential, then action potential develops which gets transmitted along olfactory nerve.

Olfactory Bulb

Olfactory bulb is the part of cerebral hemisphere located at the base of cerebral cortex, just below the frontal lobe.

In the olfactory bulb, the axons of the receptors enter olfactory bulb via cribriform plate and synapse with primary dendrites of the mitral cells and tufted cells to form the olfactory glomeruli. In addition to mitral and tufted cells, it also contains inhibitory interneurons, i.e. granular and periglomerular cells. Each glomerulus receives information from 26,000 receptors but there are only 24 mitral cells and 68 tufted cells (Figs 12.24A and B). So olfactory glomeruli is a special synaptic unit in olfactory bulb.

Olfactory Pathway

Olfactory nerve → pierce cribriform plate of ethmoid → reach olfactory bulb → synapse with mitral and tufted cell → axons of mitral and tufted cells form olfactory stria. The olfactory striae are 3 in number (Fig. 12.25) They are:

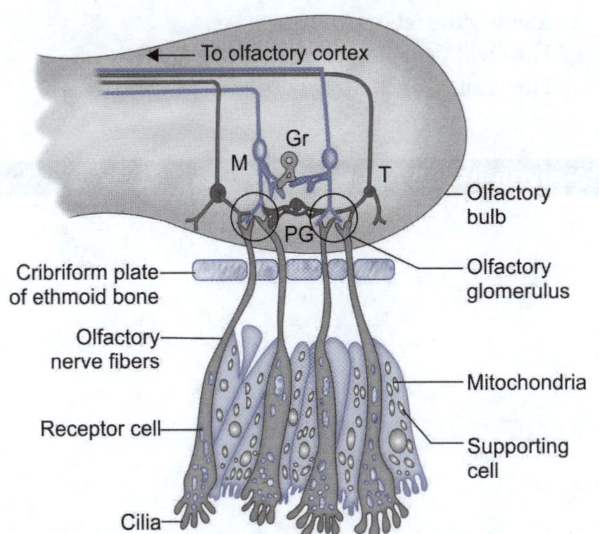

Fig. 12.24A: Olfactory receptor cells

a. Medial striae (formed by axons of tufted cells)-cross the midline in the anterior commissure to form synapses with granule cells in the opposite olfactory bulb.

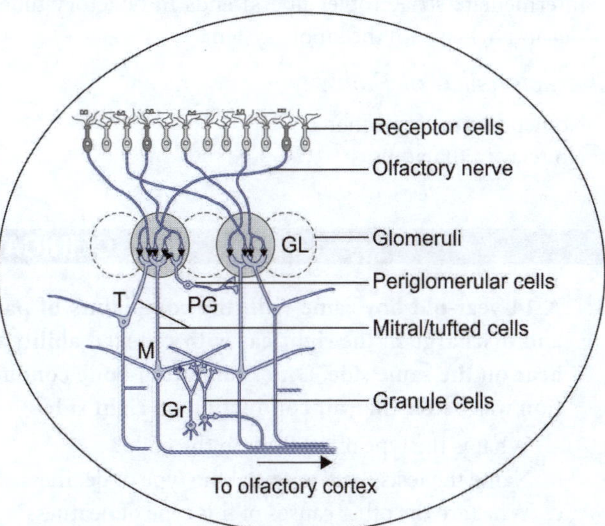

Fig. 12.24B: Magnified view of olfactory bulb, T = tufted cell, M = mitral cell, PG = periglomerular cell, Gr = granular cell

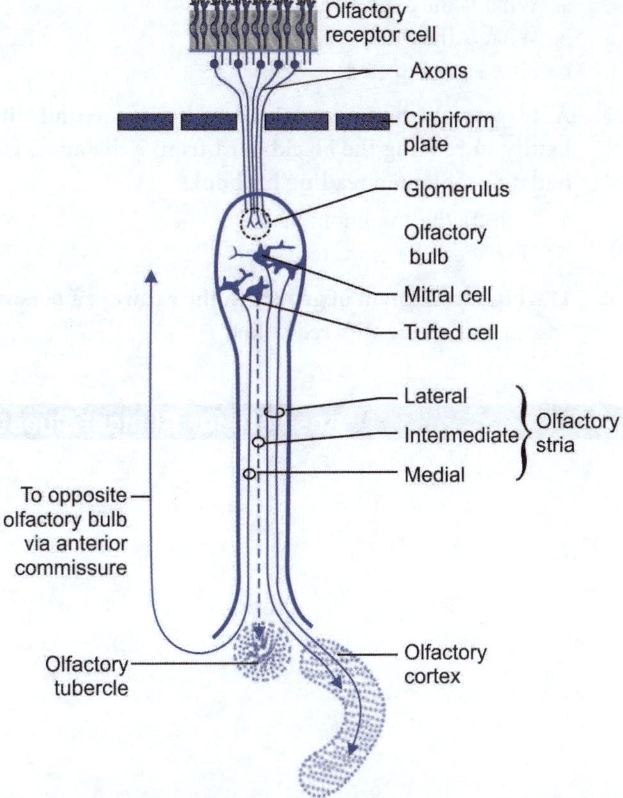

Fig. 12.25: Olfactory pathway

PHYSICON—The Reliable Icon in Physiology

b. Lateral striae (formed by axons of mitral cells)-runs to the olfactory cortex on the same side. Olfactory cortex includes the part of limbic system, i.e. the anterior olfactory nucleus, piriform cortex, olfactory tubercle, amygdala and entorhinal cortex.
c. Intermediate striae (other fibers)-ends in olfactory tubercle, and hence with the limbic system.

Characteristics of Pathway

a. No neocortical projections.
b. No relay in thalamus.
c. Receptors are directly in contact with atmosphere.
d. Receptors are tele and chemoreceptors.
e. Rapid and early adapting.

Abnormalities

- *Anosmia:* Complete absence of smell.
- *Parosmia:* Change in character of smell.
- *Hyposmia:* Diminished olfactory sensitivity.
- *Dysosmia:* Distorted sense of smell.

CLINICAL QUESTIONS

1. **A 14-year-old boy came with the complaints of pain and discharge in the right ear with reduced ability to hear on the same side. On examination bone conduction was better than air conduction on right side.**
   a. What is the type of deafness in the child?
   b. Name the tests done to reveal the type of deafness.
   c. What are the other causes of this type of deafness?
2. **An elderly gentleman complained of difficulty in reading the newspaper but could read it by holding at a distance.**
   a. What is the condition?
   b. What is the cause?
   c. How is it corrected?
3. **A 15-year-old boy complained of headache and difficulty in reading the blackboard from a distance. He had no problem in reading his books.**
   a. Identify the condition.
   b. How it can be corrected?
4. **During recruitment of guards in the railways a person was unable to identify red color.**
   a. What is the disorder he is suffering from?
   b. Which tests are used to detect this condition?
   c. What is the genetic basis?
5. **A person with high myopia complains of excruciating pain in right eye with watering while seeing a movie in theater. On examination anterior chamber was shallow, intraocular pressure was 40 mm of Hg.**
   a. Identify the condition.
   b. What is the cause?
   c. What is the physiological basis of treatment?
6. **An elderly diabetic came with complaints of diminished vision. On examination opacity was seen in both the eyes.**
   a. Identify the condition.
   b. What is the cause?
   c. Give the treatment.
7. **A young patient's visual acuity for both right and left eye is 6/24 on Snellen's chart and he was able to read the smallest print on Jaeger's chart.**
   a. Identify the refractive error.
   b. How will you interpret the finding 6/24?
   c. How is it corrected?

Answers for Clinical Questions are given in the Appendix

Section 2

PRACTICALS

CHAPTER

13

Hematology

DETERMINATION OF ERYTHROCYTE SEDIMENTATION RATE

Apparatus

Westergren's pipette, blood sample, Westergren's stand and 3.8% sodium citrate solution. Westergren's pipette is a narrow cylindrical glass tube of 300 mm length with a uniform bore of 2.5 mm. It is open at both ends and is graduated from 0 to 200 above downwards. The anticoagulant used is 3.8% sodium citrate solution in the ratio 4:1, i.e. 4 parts blood and 1 part anticoagulant.

Principle

When a column of blood taken in narrow tube is kept vertically undisturbed, the red blood cells (RBC's) settle down due to higher specific gravity than plasma. Erythrocyte sedimentation rate (ESR) is the number of millimeters of clear plasma seen above the cell layer, and is expressed in millimeters at the end of 1st hour.

Mechanism of ESR

Sedimentation occurs in three stages:

Stage 1 (10 to 15 minutes): Rouleaux formation (piling of RBC's) and aggregation occurs.

Stage 2 (40 to 45 minutes): Sinking of aggregates at constant speed.

Stage 3 (10 to 12 minutes): Aggregated cells pack at the bottom of the tube.

Normal Values (Westergren's Method)

Adult male: 1 to 3 mm at the end of 1 hour

Adult female: 3 to 7 mm at the end of 1 hour

Infants: 0 to 0.5 mm at the end of 1 hour.

Note

Wintrobe's method can also be used for determination of ESR. However, it is used for determination of PCV. Value will be higher than that in Westergren's method.

Adult male: 0 to 9 mm at the end of 1 hour

Adult female: 0 to 20 mm at the end of 1 hour.

Viva Questions

1. Why do the red cells settle down in a sample of anticoagulated blood?
   Since, the blood is not moving, the red cells settle down because they are heavier (sp. gr. = 1.095) than the plasma (sp. gr. = 1.032) in which they are suspended.
2. What is rouleaux formation?
   Rouleaux formation is the piling of RBC one on top of each other like a stack of coins (Fig. 13.1). Fibrinogen neutralizes the negative charges imparted by sialic acid moieties on the cell membrane and thereby makes the RBCs sticky so that they tend to adhere to each other and form larger rouleaux.
3. Mention the factors responsible for rouleaux formation.
   - Concentration of fibrinogen, albumin and globulin.
   - Bacterial proteins and toxins, products of inflammation and tissue destruction released into the blood neutralize the surface charges of red cells.
   - Concentration of glycoprotein in plasma.
   - Biconcave shape of red cells favors rouleaux formation.
   - Number of red cells.
4. What are the factors influencing ESR?
   - Rouleaux formation favors sedimentation.
   - Increase in concentration of fibrinogen in plasma increases the rouleaux formation and hence increases ESR.

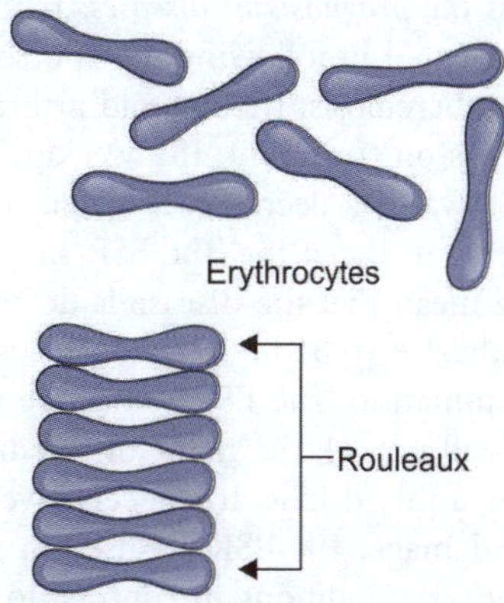

Fig. 13.1: Rouleaux formation

- Concentration of α and β globulins increases ESR.
- Albumin decreases ESR.
- The biconcave disk shape of RBCs help in rouleaux for-mation. Variation in size of RBCs or anisocytosis and variations in shape of RBCs or poikilocytosis interferes with rouleaux formation and hence decreases ESR.
- *RBC count:* When the RBC count increases ESR decreases.
- ESR is influenced by viscosity of blood, specific gravity, acid-base balance, temperature, age of the blood since withdrawal and the anticoagulant used. Excess oxalate will slow sedimentation.
- *Position of the tube:* Slanting position of the tube increases ESR.

5. Name the physiological and pathological variations of ESR.
   - *Physiological*
     a. ESR is low in newborn.
     b. ESR is high in pregnancy, lactation and old age.
     c. ESR is more in females and less in males.
   - *Pathological*
     ESR is increased in:
     - Chronic infections like tuberculosis.
     - Rheumatic fever.
     - Collagen diseases.
     - Malignancies like leukemias and multiple myeloma.
     - Acute infections.
     - Anemias except sickle cell anemia.

     ESR is reduced in:
     - Allergic conditions.
     - Sickle cell anemia.
     - Afibrogenemia.
     - Polycythemia.
6. What is the clinical significance of ESR?
   - *To assess the prognosis of diseases:* ESR is a valuable prognostic tool in following the course of a disease, such as tuberculosis, rheumatoid arthritis, etc. while a patient is on treatment. If a weekly ESR shows a trend towards a decrease, it would indicate an improvement. But if the The ESR shows an increase, it would mean that the disease is deteriorating.
   - As an indicator of bodily reaction to tissue injury and inflammation. The ESR values are not diagnostic, i.e. they will not tell the name of the disease that is causing a raised ESR. It is a sensitive indicator of tissue damage. The ESR is raised in all organic (pathological) conditions in contrast to functional disorders (anxiety neurosis, hypochondria).
7. Can you use oxalate mixture in Westergren method and citrate in Wintrobe method?
   No. The anticoagulants employed for each method have been standardized and cannot be interchanged.
   Sodium citrate cannot be used in Wintrobe method because the blood will be too much diluted as compared to the height of the tube; and this will give high false values for ESR.
8. What are the disadvantages of Wintrobe method?
   The disadvantage is that, this method is less sensitive because the column of blood is not as high as is desirable for good results and the chances of errors are high, especially when the ESR is increased, say to over 50 mm.

PACKED CELL VOLUME (HEMATOCRIT)

Apparatus

Wintrobe's tube, copper sulfate solution and double oxalate mixture. Double oxalate mixture consists of potassium and calcium oxalate. Here, the anticoagulant is used in the ratio 3:2, i.e. 3 parts blood mixed with 2 parts of anticoagulant.

Wintrobe's hematocrit tube is a cylindrical tube with a uniform bore and opens at the top. It is 11 cm long and is graduated from 0-10 cm from above downwards on one side and 10-0 cm on the other side. The diameter of the tube is 2.5 mm.

Principle

When tube containing the blood sample is subjected to centrifugal forces, heavier RBCs settle at the bottom and the lighter elements remain above the RBC layer. RBC layer denotes the packed cell volume (PCV)/hematocrit.

Observations

The tube shows:

- An uppermost layer of clear plasma, it is straw colored.
- A whitish and thin layer of platelets above and leukocytes below just below the plasma layer. This is called buffy coat and is 0.5 -1 mm thick (Fig. 13.2).
- A tall bottom layer of packed red cells. This red cell layer is separated from the buffy coat by the black line. This line is due to the presence of reduced Hb, present in the red cells lying adjacent to the white cells. This line marks the upper limit of red cell layer. Height of the red cell column varies from 4.2–4.7 cm. The packed cell volume percentage is obtained by multiplying the reading obtained by 10.

Normal Value

Adult male: 46 ± 5%
Adult female: 42 ± 5%.

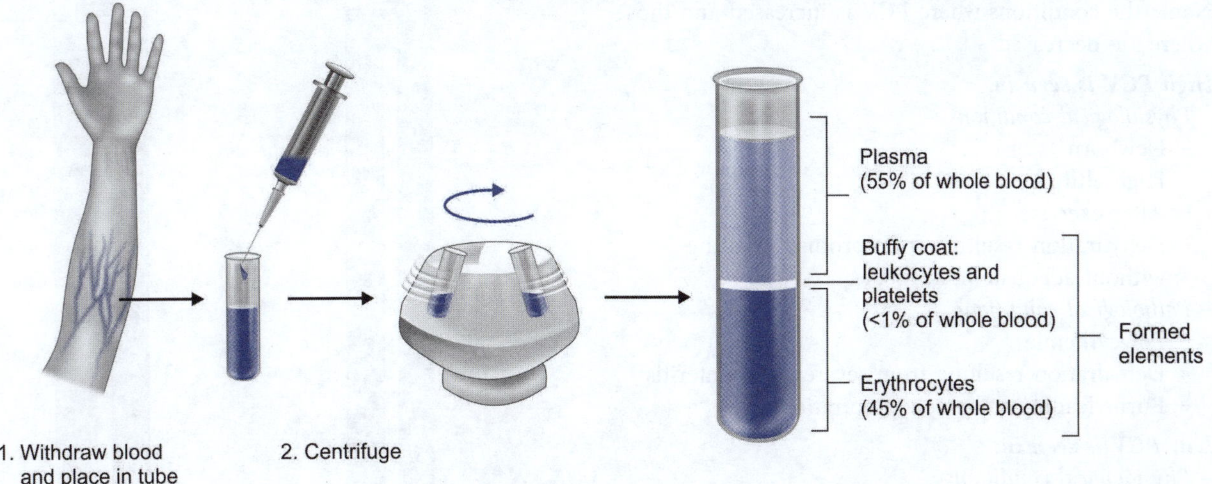

Fig. 13.2: Packed cell volume

Note

- Hematocrit value of blood in microcirculation vessels (meta arterioles, arterioles, capillaries) is lower than that of actual blood. In these small vessels, the red cells tend to move in the center of the bloodstream (axial flow). As a result, the blood along the sides of the vessels has a low hematocrit, and branches leaving at right angles may receive cell–poor blood. In capillaries, the effect is marked because the RBCs move in a single file in the middle of the stream. This phenomenon called plasma skimming, may be responsible for the capillary blood hematocrit being about 25% lower than the whole body hematocrit.
- The PCV of venous blood is slightly higher (3%) than that of arterial blood (refer page 59).

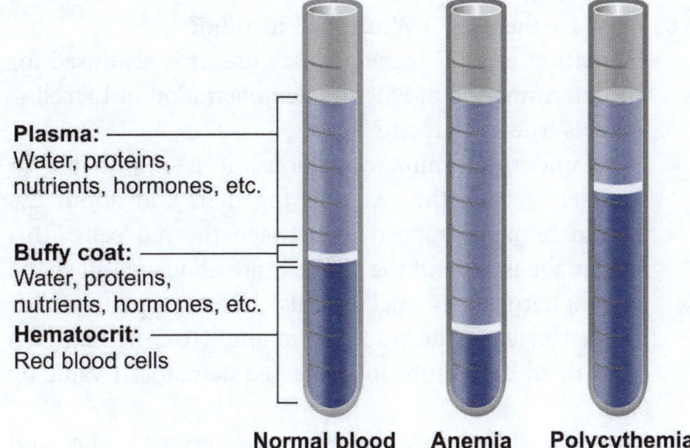

Fig. 13.3: PCV in anemia and polycythemia

Viva Questions

1. What is PCV?
   It is the volume of cellular elements per unit volume of whole blood. In a normal adult it is approximately 45%.
2. What do you mean by hematocrit value ?
   It is the volume percentage of the packed RBC only (not all the formed elements) with respect to the whole blood. In a normal person, PCV and hematocrit are almost the same. But in conditions where there is abnormal proliferation of WBC (as in leukemia) the values can be different.
3. What is the importance of determining hematocrit?
   It is simple, but accurate method for determining the presence of anemia or polycythemia (Fig. 13.3). It is also used for the screening of anemia.
4. What cells make up the buffy layer? Mention its clinical significance.
   The buffy layer consists of packed platelets and leukocytes. A rough estimate of WBC count may be made from the thickness of the buffy coat. A thickness of 1 mm corresponds to 10,000 WBC. The thickness increases in cases of leukemia, severe leukocytosis and primary thrombocytosis. Smears from buffy coat are useful when WBC count is very low and may be of use in detecting the LE cells in systemic lupus erythematosus, blast cells in aleukemic leukemia and plasma cells in multiple myeloma.
5. Briefly mention about the plasma column.
   It is normally straw colored. It is red in hemolysis, pale in anemia, yellow in jaundice, milky and opaque in lipemia.
6. What is the effect of a high hematocrit?
   Increase in hematocrit increases the viscosity of blood which leads to an increase in peripheral resistance, and thus the blood pressure.

7. Name the conditions where PCV is increased and those where it is decreased.

   High PCV is seen in:
   – *Physiological conditions*
     - Newborn
     - High altitude
     - After exercise
     - Dehydration resulting from profuse sweating without adequate fluid intake.
   – *Pathological conditions*
     - Polycythemia
     - Dehydration resulting from severe gastroenteritis.
     - Burns leading to hemoconcentration.

   Low PCV is seen in:
   – *Physiological conditions*
     - During pregnancy due to hemodilution
     - In females.
   – *Pathological conditions:* In various types of anemias.
8. What are the uses of Wintrobe's method?
   Estimation of PCV is the primary use. It is also used for the determination of ESR and demonstration of LE cells.
9. What is true hematocrit?
   Even under optimum conditions, it is impossible to completely pack the red cells together, and about 2% plasma remains trapped in between the red cells. This percentage is more if the red cells are abnormal in shape (e.g. spherocytosis, sickle cells). To compensate for trapped plasma, the true cell volume (true hematocrit) is obtained by multiplying observed hematocrit value by 0.98.
10. How to differentiate between Westergren tube and Wintrobe?

Table 13.1: Difference between Westergren tube and Wintrobe tube (Fig. 13.4)

Westergren tube	Wintrobe tube
It is a long tube	It is a short tube
Total length 300 mm	Total length 110 mm
Diameter 2.5 mm	Diameter 3 mm
Both ends are open	Lower end is closed
Marking from top of the tube to the bottom, i.e. Upper reading = 0 mm Lower reading = 200 mm	Marking from top of the tube to the bottom and vice versa. Left side lower reading = 10 cm
	Right side Upper reading = 10 cm Lower reading = 0 cm
For ESR only	For both ESR and PCV

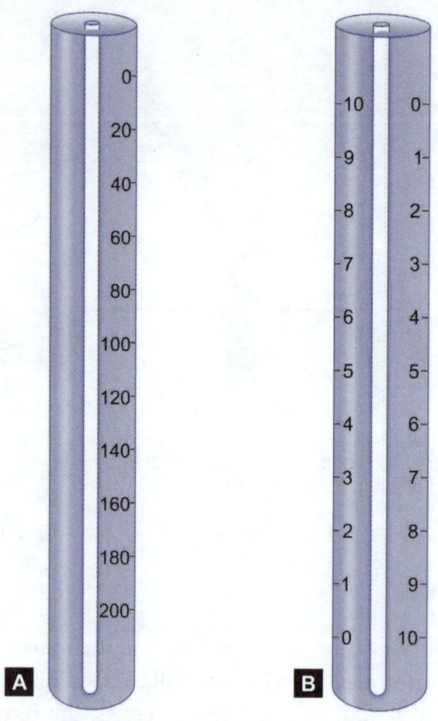

Figs 13.4A and B: A. Westergren tube; **B.** Wintrobe tube

ESTIMATION OF HEMOGLOBIN (SAHLI'S METHOD)

Apparatus

Sahli's hemoglobinometer, N/10 HCl.

Principle

Hemoglobin is converted to acid hematin. Then it is estimated by matching the color with a standard plate of the same derivative after diluting it with distilled water.

Preparation of the standard. The standard color in Sahli's hemoglobinometer is prepared by treating blood containing 14.4 gm of Hb with N/10 HCl and diluting the same with distilled water 100 times.

Normal Values

Adult male: 14-8 gm%
Adult female: 12-16 gm%
Newborn: 18-23 gm%

The high value in the newborn is due to the increased RBC count. The newborn has been living in state of relative hypoxia, which is a very potent stimulus for the secretion of erythropoietin. The value decreases gradually and reaches the adult value by 16–18 months.

Viva Questions

1. Can strong acids (such as nitric, sulfuric acid, concentrated HCl) or alkalies be used in place of decinormal HCl?
The strong acids, which are very strong oxidizing agents and alkalies will cause disruption of Hb and thus cannot be used. Only N/10 HCl is used because standardization has been done for acid hematin.
2. Can tap water be used for diluting and color matching?
No, it cannot be used because its soil may cause turbidity which will interfere with color matching.
3. Can N/10 HCl be used instead of distilled water for diluting and color matching?
Yes, it can be used because it being transparent, it cannot further deepen the color once all the Hb has been converted into acid hematin.
4. What will happen if quantity of N/10 HCl is changed?
The minimum quantity should be present so as to form complete acid hematin.
5. What are the disadvantages of Sahli's method?
   – The method estimates only oxy Hb and reduced Hb, other forms such as carboxyHb and met Hb are not estimated.
   – In the long-term use, the standard coloration on the hemoglobinometer may fade and become lighter. This will lead to wrong result.
6. What are the other methods of Hb estimation?
   – Spectrophotometric methods
     - Cyanmethemoglobin method
     - Oxyhemoglobin method
     - Haldane's carboxyHb method
     - Wu's alkaline hematin method.
   – Tallqvist method
   – Copper sulfate falling drop method
7. Name some derivatives of hemoglobin.
   – Oxyhemoglobin
   – Reduced hemoglobin (deoxygenated Hb)
   – Carbaminohemoglobin
   – Carboxyhemoglobin
   – Methemoglobin
   – Sulfhemoglobin
   – Cyanmethemoglobin (hemoglobincyanide).
8. Why is it required to allow the solution to stand for 10 minutes before dilution?
This time is required for complete hemolysis of RBCs and maximum conversion of hemoglobin in blood to form acid hematin.
9. What are the functions of hemoglobin?
   – Carriage of O_2
   – Carriage of CO_2
   – Homeostasis of pH (buffer action of Hb)
   – It preserves iron in the body.
10. How is heme synthesized from the body?
Heme portion of Hb is synthesized from glycine and succinyl CoA. Heme is synthesized by cells of erythroid series in red bone marrow.
11. Name the physiological and pathological variations of Hb content in RBC.
   – *Physiological*
     - *Age:* Hb% is more in newborn.
     - *Sex:* Higher in males.
     - *At high altitudes:* Hb% is increased at high altitudes as hypoxia stimulates erythropoiesis which in turn increases Hb count.
     - *Exercise:* Hb content is increased after exercise.
   – *Pathological:* Hb content is increased in polycythemia and decreased in all types of anemias.

12 What would happen if Hb were present freely in the plasma instead of in the red cells?
Normally, only a very small amount is present in the plasma (about 3 mg/dL), most of it being confined to red cells. If it were present in the plasma, it would increase the viscosity (thus raising BP), and the osmotic pressure of blood (thus affecting fluid exchanges). It would also be excreted in the urine, besides being taken up and rapidly destroyed by the reticuloendothelial system.

13. Calculate the oxygen carrying capacity of blood.
Normal oxygen carrying capacity of blood per gram of Hb is 1.34 ml. For 15.79 gm/dL of Hb, the oxygen carrying capacity becomes $15.79 \times 1.34 = 20.2$ ml/dL of blood.
14. Discuss the differences between adult Hb and fetal Hb. (Table 13.2).
15. What is anemia and how it is graded to Hb concentration?
Refer Page no. 28.
16. What are the normal variants of hemoglobin ?
Refer Page no. 21.
17. What is the fate of Hb?
Refer Page no. 22.

Table 13.2: Adult and fetal Hb compared

Adult hemoglobin	Fetal hemoglobin
1. Contains 4 polypeptide chains (2 alpha and 2 beta)	1. The 2 beta chains replaced by gamma chains
2. Appears in red cells of the fetus in 5th month. At birth 20% of total Hb is Hb A	2. HbF at birth makes up 80% of total Hb disappear by 5th month after birth
3. Lifespan long—120 days	3. Lifespan short—about 2 weeks
4. It has the usual affinity for oxygen	4. It has greater affinity for oxygen as it binds 2,3 DPG less avidly
5. Percentage saturation at pO_2 of 20 mm Hg = 30–35%	5. Percentage saturation at pO_2 of 20 mm Hg = 70%

18. What is the structure of Hb, where is it synthesized?
Refer Page no. 21.

RBC COUNT

Apparatus

Improved Neubauer's counting chamber (Fig. 13.5), RBC pipette, RBC diluting fluid (Hayem's fluid).

Composition of Hayem's Fluid

- *Sodium sulfate:* To prevent rouleaux formation.
- *Sodium chloride:* To maintain isotonicity of fluid (RBC remains suspended in solution).
- *Mercuric chloride:* Act as preservative (antifungal and antibacterial).
- *Distilled water:* As a solvent.

Normal Values

Males: 4.5–6.5 million/mm^3

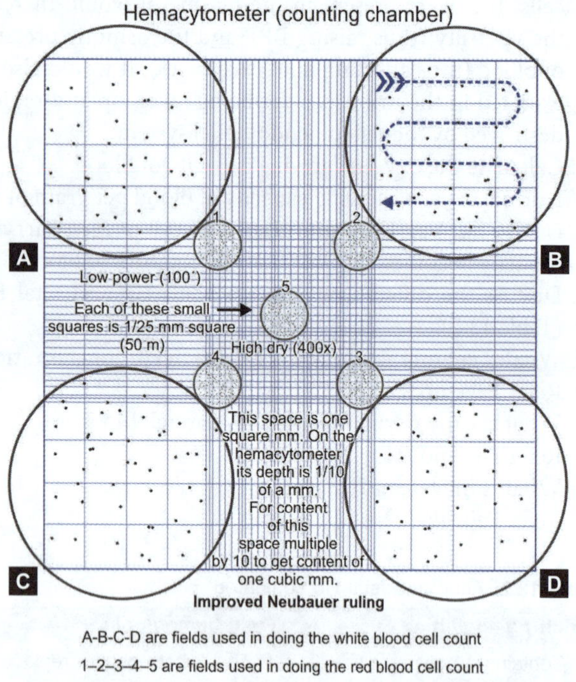

Fig. 13.5: Improved Neubauer's counting chamber

> The hemacytometer is divided into sections. WBCs are counted in the outer four sections (each section contains a 4 × 4 grid with 16 total squares in each section). To determine the number of leukocytes per cubic millimeter, use the following formula:
> Total WBCs in all four sections × 50 = Total WBCs/mm^3
> The center section of the hemacytometer contains a 5 × 5 grid. RBCs are counted in the four corner squares and the central square (each square contains a 4 × 4 grid, also). To get the total number of RBCs per cubic millimeter (or microliter), use the following formula:
> Total RBCs in all five squares × 10,000 = Total RBCs/mm^3 (see Fig. 13.5)

Females: 3.9–5.6 million/mm^3
Newborn: 6–7 million/mm^3

Viva Questions

1. How is diluting factor calculated?
   0.5 part of blood is mixed 100.5 part of Hayem's fluid in pipette. Blood mixes with diluting fluid only in the bulb. So, 1 part diluting fluid that remains in the stem does not mix with the blood, i.e. 0.5 part blood and 99.5 part diluting fluid in blood, to form 100 part of solution.
   $$\text{Dilution factor} = \frac{\text{Final volume}}{\text{Original volume}} = \frac{100}{0.5} = 200$$
2. What is the function of bead in the bulb?
   - Bead act as stirrers.
   - Free rotation of bead in the bulb signifies pipette is dry
   - Beads are distinguishing feature - Red bead for RBC pipette, white bead for WBC pipette.
3. Would not the bead decrease the dilution due to its own volume?
   The volume of bead is taken into consideration during manufacture of the pipette.
4. Why the fluid in the stem is discarded?
   The fluid from the stem portion of the pipette is discarded because the actual mixing is taking place only in the bulb and stem contains only the diluting fluid.
5. Since, the mature red cells do not contain 'nuclei, are they dead cells?
   The RBCs, though without nuclei, are not dead in the usual sense. Since there are no mitochondria (and other organelles), energy is not available from oxidative phosphorylation (Kreb's cycle). However, they contain a number of enzymes which control important functions. The cells contain all enzymes necessary for energy supply from anaerobic glucose metabolism via the Embden-Meyerhof pathway (hexose monophosphate shunt). (Glucose enters RBCs by an active process which is insulin-independent).
6. What are the uses of Neubauer's chamber?
   It helps in finding out: RBC count, WBC count, platelet count and also cells in CSF, peritoneal, pleural fluids, etc.
7. What are the physiological and pathological variations in RBC count?
   Increase in RBC Count
   - Physiological-males, high altitude, high temperature, low O_2 tension, after exercise, infants.
   - Pathological-polycythemia vera, hyperthyroidism, Cushing's syndrome, dehydration, chronic lung disease, congenital cyanotic heart disease.

   Decrease in RBC Count
   Seen in all types of anemia.

8. What is the site of RBC formation during fetal life and after birth?
   Refer Page no. 26
9. What is the lifespan and fate of red cells?
   Refer Page no. 25
10. What is erythropoiesis and what are the stages of differentiation and maturation of red cells?
    Refer Page no. 26, 27
11. How is erythropoiesis regulated?
    Refer Page no. 27
12. Mention the sites of erythropoietin formation.
    Refer Page no. 27
13. What is polycythemia?
    Refer Page no. 30

WBC COUNT

Apparatus

Improved Neubauer's counting chamber, WBC diluting fluid (Turk's fluid).

Composition of Turk's Fluid

- Glacial acetic acid-lyses membrane of RBC, platelets and causes swelling of nucleus of WBC.
- Gentian violet-stains nucleus of WBC.
- Distilled water-as a solvent.

Calculation of Dilution Factor

$$\text{Dilution factor} = \frac{\text{Final volume}}{\text{Original volume}} = \frac{10}{0.5} = 20$$

Normal Values

Adults: 4000–11000/mm^3
Newborn: 10000–25000/mm^3
Children up to 4 years: 18000 cells/mm^3 (count decreases after 4 years).

Viva Questions

1. What are the other uses of WBC pipette?
   The WBC pipette can be used for diluting the blood much less for counting RBCs in cases of severe anemia, or for counting platelets. It can also be used for counting sperms and bacteria.
2. Why are the red cells not seen when counting the leukocytes?
   The red cells are not seen because they are hemolyzed by glacial acetic acid in the WBC diluting fluid, i.e. Turk's fluid. The remnants of red cells membranes are faintly visible, the so called ghost cells.
3. How you differentiate a WBC pipette from a RBC pipette (Table 13.3).

Table 13.3: RBC and WBC pipette compared (Fig. 13.6)

RBC pipette	*WBC pipette*
Calibrations are 0.5 and 1.0 below the bulb, and 101 above the bulb	Calibrations are 0.5 and 1.0 below the bulb, and 11 above it
The capillary bore is narrow, thus it is a slow speed pipette	The capillary bore is wider, hence it is a fast speed pipette
Bulb is larger and has a red bead	Bulb is smaller and has a white bead
The volume of the bulb is 100 times the volume contained in stem	The volume of the bulb is 10 times the volume contained in stem
The dilution can be 1 in 100 or 1 in 200	The dilution can be 1 in 10 or 1 in 20

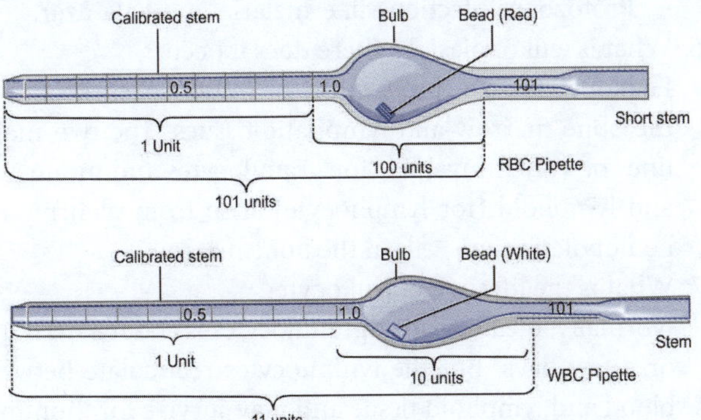

Fig. 13.6: RBC and WBC pipette compaired

4. Are WBCs also lyzed while doing WBC count ?
   Yes. WBCs are also lyzed, this is to destroy the plasma membrane to expose the nucleus for staining. So while counting we actually count the nucleus of WBC and not WBC as a whole.
5. What are the physiological and pathological variations in WBC count?
   Increase in leukocyte count > 11000/mm^3 is called leukocytosis. It generally refers to an increase in neutrophils and hence it is synonymous with neutrophilia.

   Increase in TLC

   a. *Physiologically*
      - *Diurnal variations:* The count is lowest in the morning and rises during miday. It is the highest in the evening. Count is lowest after rest.
      - *After exercise:* Count is increased after strenuous muscular exercise. It is probably due to redistribution of cells and it becomes normal within 1 hour.
      - Count is higher in newborns and infants.
      - Count is increased in pregnancy and is highest during labor. It is also increased in menstruation.

b. *Pathologically*
   - Leukocytosis is seen in acute bacterial infections like boils, abscesses, pneumonia, etc.
   - It is increased in allergic conditions like asthma, hay fever, etc.
   - Hemorrhage, burns and malignant disease also show leukocytosis.

Decrease in TLC

Leukopenia is the reduction in leukocyte count below normal. It is pathological and occurs in:
- Certain bacterial infections like typhoid and paratyphoid.
- Viral infections like influenza, measles and smallpox.
- Protozoan infections like malaria and kala-azar.

6. What is leukopoiesis? Where does it occur?
   Leukopoiesis, i.e. production of WBCs occurs both in the bone marrow and lymphatic tissues. The two major lines of WBCs myeloid (for granulocytes and monocyte) and lymphoid (for lymphocyte) arise from pleuripotent hemopoietic stem cells in the bone marrow.
7. What is the lifespan of leukocyte?
   Normally, the lifespan of granulocytes is about 8-10 hours or a few days. But the lymphocytes recirculate between blood and lymphoid tissue and may survive for months.
8. What is meant by the term agranulocytosis, leukocytosis, leukopenia and leukemia?

Agranulocytois: Decrease in the number of granulocytes.

Leukocytosis: Increase in the number of WBC beyond 11,000/mm^3 irrespective of the type of cells (granulocytes, monocytes, leukocytes).

Leukopenia: Decrease in the number of white cells below 4000/mm^3.

Leukemia: It is a group of malignant neoplasms of WBC forming organs–bone marrow and lymphoid tissue. The TLC is generally above 40,000 - 50,000/mm^3 or even a few lakhs.

DLC

Apparatus

Glass slide, Leishman's stain, Cedar wood oil.

Composition of Leishman's Stain

Eosin: Acidic dye, stains positively charged particles. For example, nuclei of RBC's, granules of eosinophils.

Methylene blue: Basic dye, stains negatively charged particles. For example, nuclei of WBC's, granules of basophils.

Acetone free methyl alchohol: Fixative and preserves cells. The methyl alcohol should be acetone free to prevent shrinkage, crenation and lysis of cells.

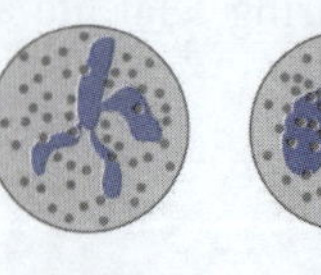

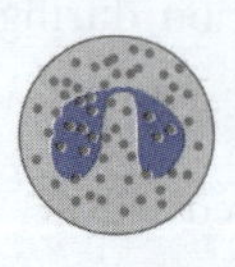

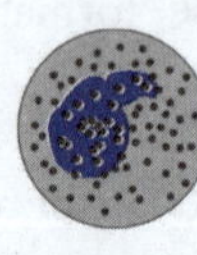

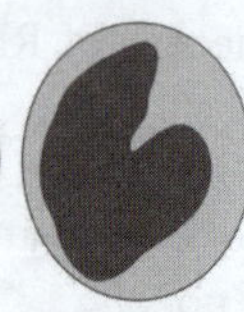

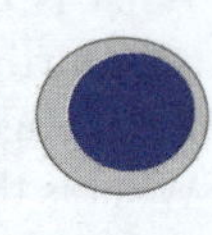

Fig. 13.7: White blood cells

Points of Identification

- *Neutrophil (Fig. 13.7)*
  - Multilobed nucleus
  - Fine pink granules
- *Eosinophil*
  - Bilobed spectacle shaped nucleus
  - Coarse brick red granules
- *Basophil*
  - Roughly S-shaped nucleus
  - Coarse bluish black granules which may even mask the nucleus
- *Monocyte*
  - Large kidney-shaped nucleus
  - Cytoplasm more
- *Lymphocyte*
  - Unlobed nucleus (sometimes it may be indented)
  - Thin rim of cytoplasm.

Comparison with RBC Size

- Neutrophil, eosinophil, basophil, large lymphocyte: Double the size of RBC.
- *Monocyte:* Double/triple the size of RBC.

Viva Questions

1. Discuss the significance of DLC.
   The differential count is done to find if there is an increase or decrease of a particular type of WBC. Knowing the TLC, the absolute number of each type can be calculated. This information is important in detecting infection or inflammation, allergic and parasitic infections, and effects of chemotherapy and radiation therapy.
2. Why is Leishman's stain diluted after 1–2 minutes? What happens to the blood film during this period?
   During the fixation period of 1–2 minutes, the pure absolute alcohol serves two purposes:
   a. It precipitates the plasma proteins, which act as glue and attach (fix) the blood cells on to the glass slide.
   b. It preserves the shape and chemistry of cells to as, near the living state as possible.

   The cells are not stained during this time, because the stain particles cannot enter the cells in their unionized state. Their ionization occurs only when water is added to the salts in the undiluted stain. (If diluted stain were added to start with, the blood smear itself would be washed away. Diluted Leishman's stain can be used if the blood film is first fixed in absolute alcohol).

3. Mention the absolute count, percentage and size (diameter) of various leukocytes?
   Neutrophil: 2000–7500/mm^3, 40–75%, 10–14 m.
   Eosinophils: 4–440/mm^3, 1–6%, 10–14 m
   Basophil: 0–100/mm^3, 0–1%, 10–14 m
   Monocyte: 500–800/mm^3, 2–10%, 10–18 m
   Lymphocytes: 1300–3500/mm^3, 20–45%, 10–14 m (large), 7–10 m (small).
4. What are the functions of various leukocytes?
   Refer Page no. 30, 31
5. Enumerate the conditions that cause neutrophilia and neutropenia, eosinophilia and eosinopenia, basophilia and basopenia, monocytosis and monocytopenia, lymphocytosis and lymphocytopenia.
   Refer Page no. 30, 31
6. Mention the steps of phagocytosis.
   Refer Page no. 32
7. What is Arneth count ?
   Refer Page no. 32

DETERMINATION OF BLOOD GROUP

Apparatus

Antisera A, B and D (Rh), 0.9% NaCl/3.8% sodium citrate solution, capillary dropper.

Principle

Surfaces of red cell membrane contain genetically determined antigens-agglutinogens while plasma contains antibodies Red cells allowed to react with commercially available antisera with agglutinins. Clumping/hemolysis as a result of antigen-antibody reaction (Fig. 13.8).

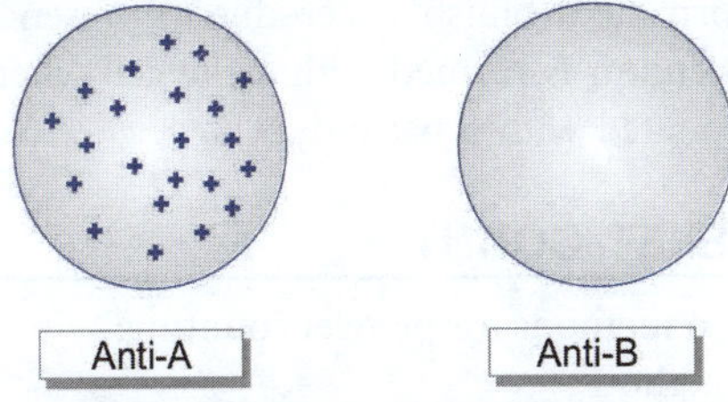

Fig. 13.8: Blood group estimation

Anti-A serum has been added to the blood in the left well causing agglutination, which gives the mixture 'beaded' appearance. When anti-B serum was added to the right well, agglutination did not occur. For this particular sample of blood, this test indicates that the A antigen is present and the B antigen is not present; therefore this individual has type A blood.

Viva Questions

1. What is agglutination?
   Clumping and hemolysis of red cells during antigen - antibody interaction.
2. What are the different blood group systems?
   Different blood group systems include ABO, Rh, M and N, Kell and Duffy, MNS, Lutheran, etc.
3. How will you differentiate agglutination from rouleaux formation?
   Dilution with saline disperses rouleaux, but agglutinated cells are not dispersed.
4. What is Bombay blood group?
   This blood type is a rare phenomenon in which the H antigen is absent. Since there is no H antigen, there is no antigen A or antigen B on the red cells. However, the plasma contains anti-A, anti-B and anti-H antibodies. As a result, such a person can receive blood only from a person having Bombay blood type.
5. What is reverse blood typing?
   The blood grouping (typing) procedure in which the red cells of a person (whose blood type is to be determined) are tested against anti-A and anti-B sera, is called 'blood typing' or 'forward blood typing'.
   In another but related procedure called 'reverse blood typing' (also called 'serum typing' or 'backward blood typing') the serum of the would-be recipient is tested against red cells containing known antigens, i.e. red cells from persons with blood types A, B, AB, and O. It agglutination occurs with A and AB red cells, the blood type is B; if agglutination occurs with B and AB red cells, the blood type is A; if agglutination occurs with A, B, and AB red cells, the blood type is O and if there is no agglutination in any RBCs the blood type is AB. [In AB blood type there are no antibodies in the plasma (serum).
6. What are cold and warm antibodies?
   Refer Page no. 42
7. What is Landsteiner's law?
   Refer Page no. 37
8. What is cross matching?
   Refer Page no. 37
9. What is Rh factor and what is its clinical significance?
   Refer Page no. 37
10. How can HDN be prevented? What is its treatment?
    Refer Page no. 38
11. What are the indications of blood transfusion?
    Refer Page no. 38
12. What are the hazards of blood transfusion?
    Refer Page no. 38
13. How is donated blood stored?
    Refer Page no. 38

RETICULOCYTE COUNT

Apparatus

Microscope, Petri dish, blotting paper, reticulocyte stains (supravital stains).

Reticulocyte Stains

- *Brilliant cresyl blue:* 1g of this dye is dissolved in 100 ml of citrated saline (1 volume of 3.8% sodium citrate and 4 volumes of normal saline).

  Uses
  - Brilliant cresyl blue stains the RNA of reticulocytes.
  - Citrate prevents the clotting of blood.
  - Normal saline provides tonicity.
- *New methylene blue:* It stains the reticulum of reticulocytes unlike brilliant cresyl blue. It is chemically different and stains more deeply and uniformly. One gram of this dye is dissolved in 100 ml of citrated saline.

Theory of Reticulocyte Staining

The basophilic remnants of RNA and ribosomes in the cytoplasm of reticulocytes is stained by brilliant cresyl blue. The dye enters the cells and stains the basophilic material to form bluish precipitates of dots, short strands and filaments. This reaction can occur only in supravitally (vitally) stained cells, i.e. in 'unfixed' and 'living' cells. The more the immature cells, greater is the amount of precipitable material present in them.

Points of Identification of Reticulocytes

Reticulocytes are non-nucleated cells and are slightly larger (diameter-8 μm) than RBCs (7.5 μm). They also stain lighter than the red cells, and contain dots, strands and filaments of bluish-stained material.

Normal Values

Newborn: 30–40% (no: decreases to 1–2% during 1st week of life).
Infants: 2–6%
Children and adults: 0.2–1%

Viva Questions

1. What is a reticulocyte?
   Reticulocytes are the non-nucleated immediate precursors of red cells that develop in the red marrow from the PHSCs. They contain large amounts of remnants of RNA and ribosomes. They are present in large numbers in bone marrow and small numbers in blood.
2. What are the indications of doing reticulocyte count?
   - Assessment of erythroid activity of bone marrow.
   - It can also help in assessing the effectiveness of a drug used in the treatment of anemia.
3. What is the importance of reticulocytes count?
   An increase in the reticulocyte count is indicative of regeneration of red cells.
4. How do you differentiate between a reticulocyte and RBC?
   - Size of reticulocyte: 8 μm^3 and size of erythrocyte is 6.7-7.7 μm^3 (reticulocyte is bit larger than RBC).
   - DNA: Reticulocyte has central core of RNA have takes up basic stains. RBC's do not have a central core of RNA.
   - Cytoplasm of reticulocyte is coarse and appears to contain granules (ribosomes) while that of RBC does not.
5. What is reticulocytosis? Name the conditions in which it occurs.
   Increase in the number of reticulocytes in blood is referred to as reticulocytosis. The conditions in which reticulocytes count is high are:
   - Recovery from anemia.
   - After acute hemorrhage.
   - Proliferation of bone marrow.
     Physiologic conditions: In newborn; hypoxic conditions (high altitude); menstruation.
     Pathological conditions: Hemolytic anemia, sickle cell anemia; polycythemia.
6. What is vital and supravital staining?
   The term 'vital' suggests that this method has to do with living cells. Vital staining is a special method of staining employed for unfixed, 'living cells' (or as nearly living as possible), including tissue cultures. There are two types of vital staining:
   Supravital staining: It is *in vitro* method where the living cells are stained by immersing them in a dye solution.
   Intravital staining: It is *in vivo* method where a dye is injected into a living organism for selective staining.
7. What are the characteristics of reticulocyte?
   - Size is 7.2 μm^3.
   - Uniform light-bluish violet–due to presence of RNA
   - A reticulum is formed within the cell when RNA is precipitated with a basic dye.

PLATELET COUNT

There are two methods for platelet counting:
1. Direct method
2. Indirect method

Direct Method

Apparatus

Microscope, RBC pipette, counting chamber with cover slip, Rees-Ecker diluting fluid or freshly prepared 1% ammonium oxalate solution. Ammonium oxalate destroys red cells but preserves platelets; it also acts as an anticoagulant.

- Rees-Ecker diluting fluid contains the following:
- Brilliant cresyl blue (0.1 g) – Stains platelets
- Sodium citrate (3.8 g) – Prevents clotting and makes the fluid isotonic.
- Formalin – Prevents fungal growth and lyses RBCs.

Calculation of Platelet Count

With the knowledge of platelet count, and the RBC count, the actual number of platelets per mm^3 blood can now be calculated. Normal platelet count is 2,50,000–5, 00,000/mm^3.

Automated Method

It is a very accurate method. It is carried out on an Eleccell counter. The red cells and platelets in the diluted blood sample pass through an aperture. The particles between 2 and 10 µm^3 are counted as platelets.

Viva Questions

1. What are the physiological variations of platelet count?
   Minor variations in platelet count occurs in the following conditions:
   - Increased counts may be seen after severe exercise, and sometimes at high altitudes.
   - Decreased counts, near the lower side of the normal, may be seen in the newborns and in females, during menstruation.
2. What are the different types of granules present in the platelets?
   Alpha-granules, dense granules and glycogen granules.
3. What are megakaryocytes ?
   Platelets are produced from the giant cells which are called megakaryocytes in the bone marrow. Diameter is about 100 µm.
4. What is meant by the terms thrombocytopenia and thrombocytosis?
   Thrombocytopenia: The term refers to a decreased count 'of platelets. It may be due to decreased production or increased destruction.
   Thrombocytosis: The term refers to an increase in platelet count above 4,50,000/mm^3 of blood.
5. Mention the causes of thrombocytopenia.
   - Deficient production, hypoplastic and aplastic anemia, various drugs and antibiotics.
   - Thrombocytopenic purpura.
   - Pernicious anemia.
6. Mention the causes of thrombocytosis.
   - Following hemorrhage, severe injury or any major surgical operation.
   - Removal of spleen.
   - Chronic myeloid leukemia.
   - Polycythemia vera.
7. How is hemostais brought about by platelets?
   - Increased tendency to aggregation
   - Vasoconstriction by serotonin and norepinephrine causing closure of ruptured blood vessels.
8. What is the normal platelet count? Describe their site of formation, lifespan and functions.
   Refer Page no. 32
9. How does aspirin act as an antiplatelet agglutinating agent and what is its clinical value?
   Refer Page no. 33

BLEEDING TIME AND CLOTTING TIME

Bleeding Time

It is the time taken from the puncture of the blood vessels to the stoppage of bleeding. It can be found by two methods - Duke's method and Ivy's method. Normal time: 2–6 minutes (according to the Duke's method).

Clotting Time

It is the time taken from the puncture of blood vessels to the formation of the fibrin thread (Fig. 13.9). It can be found by two methods. Capillary glass tube method and Lee and White method. Normal values: 3–8 minutes at 37°C.

Viva Questions

1. What is the clinical importance of doing bleeding time (BT) and clotting time (CT)?
   BT and CT are important in the following situations:
   - History of frequent and persistent bleeding from minor injuries, or spontaneous bleeding into tissues.

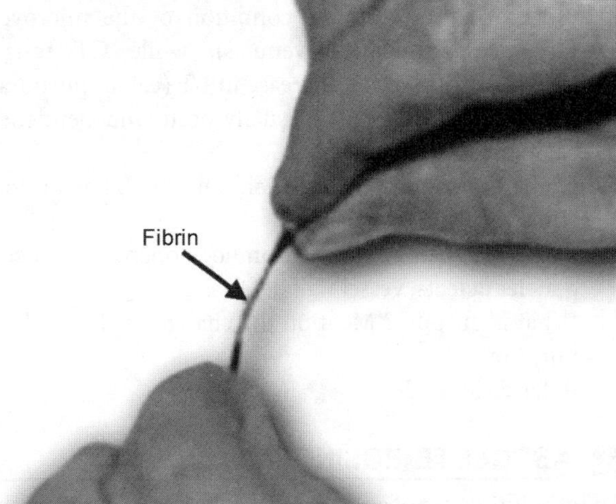

Fig. 13.9: Breaking the capillary tube to view insoluble fibrin strands

- Before every minor and major surgery (tooth extraction, etc).
- Before taking biopsy, especially from bone marrow, liver, kidney, etc.
- Before and during anticoagulant therapy.
- Family history of bleeding disorders.

2. What are the factors on which BT and CT depend?
   Bleeding time depends on: Breadth and depth of the wound, degree of hyperemia of the skin puncture site, number of platelets and their functional status, functional status of the blood vessels, temperature (in cold weather, low temperature promotes vasoconstriction and thus shorten BT).
   Clotting time depends on: Nature of contact surface (glass in this case: siliconized surface would prolong the CT, presence or absence of clotting factors, temperature (low temperature may prolong the CT).
3. Name the conditions in which BT is prolonged?
   Deficiency of vitamin C, thrombocytopenic purpura.
4. Name the conditions in which CT is prolonged.
   Hemophilia (due to lack of factor VIII), liver disease, lack of Christmas factor (factor IX), vitamin K deficiency.
5. What is hemophilia? Mention the changes of BT and CT in hemophilia.
   Hemophilia is a disorder in which clotting time is prolonged. In 85% of cases, it is due to deficiency of factor VIII and in about 15% patients it is due to deficiency of factor IX. BT is normal in hemophilic person; only CT is prolonged.
6. How does BT differ from CT? What is the interrelation between them, and which aspects of hemostasis are tested by them?
   Both BT and CT are done together in all disorders of hemostasis. They are interrelated in the sense that platelets are involved in both tests. The BT tests the platelet plug formation and the condition of the microvessels (arterioles, capillaries, venules), while CT tests the formation of the clot. Increase in BT (e.g. in purpura), or CT (e.g. in hemophilia) usually occur independently of each other.
7. Name the conditions in which only the BT is prolonged while the CT is normal.
   Low platelet count (thrombocytopenia), functional platelet defects, vessel wall defects.
8. What is purpura? Mention the changes of BT and CT in purpura.
   Refer Page no. 36

ABSOLUTE EOSINOPHIL COUNT

The absolute count of eosinophils can be done by two methods:

1. *Direct method:* The cells are counted directly by employing hemocytometry.
2. *Indirect method:* Here the percentage of eosinophils is determined from a blood smear counting of leukocytes. From the TLC value, the absolute eosinophil count can be calculated. For example, If TLC = 8000/mm^3 and eosinophils are 2% in DLC, then the absolute count = $2/100 \times 8000 = 160/\text{mm}^3$ of undiluted blood.
   In this experiment, the direct method of hemocytometry will be used.

Principle: Blood is diluted 10 times in a WBC pipette using Pilot's diluting fluid that lyses RBCs and leukocytes other than eosinophils. The stained cells are then counted in a counting chamber.

Apparatus

Microscope, counting chamber, WBC pipette, Pilot's diluting fluid (for eosinophil counting).

Composition

Stock Solutions

- Propylene glycol
- *Phloxine:* 1% solution in water (0.5% eosin may be used but phloxine is superior)
- *Sodium bicarbonate:* 10% solution in water

Working solution: It is made by mixing and filtering the following:

- Propylene glycol = 50 ml
- Phloxine (1%) = 10 ml
- Sodium bicarbonate (10%) = 1 ml
- Heparin = 100 units
- Distilled water = 40 ml

Note: The diluting fluid is freshly prepared from stock solution when required. Propylene lyses the red cells, phloxine stains the eosinophil granules and sodium carbonate solution lyses all leukocytes except eosinophils.

Normal absolute eosinophil count: 10-400/mm^3 (Eosinophil count of capillary blood is usually 10–15% higher).

Viva Questions

1. What is the clinical significance of absolute eosinophil count?
   Formerly, eosinophil count was considered as an index of ACTH activity in the blood. When ACTH is injected into a person with normal adrenocortical function, there is a drastic reduction in the absolute eosinophil count. This test, called 'Thorn's test' used to be employed to assess adrenocortical function. However, with better hormone assay tests, this test is no longer employed. However, the absolute count helps in diagnosing various allergic and parasitic conditions.

CHAPTER

14

Amphibian Experiments

GASTROCNEMIUS MUSCLE AND SCIATIC NERVE PREPARATION OF FROG

Composition of Amphibian Ringer Solution

- 0.65% NaCl: Isotonic with the amphibian plasma.
- 0.14% KCl: Maintaining membrane potential.
- 0.012% $CaCl_2$: Maintaining membrane potential.

The amphibian Ringer's solution stimulates ATPase activity. The optimal pH is about 0.02% $NaHCO_3$.

Note

- The tissues used to demonstrate the properties of skeletal muscles are sciatic nerve, gastrocnemius muscle of frog.
- Stimulus is defined as a sudden change in external or internal environment of a tissue due to which a response is obtained.
- The different types of stimuli used to stimulate a tissue are electrical, mechanical, chemical and thermal.
- Of these different stimuli, electrical stimuli is preferred because we can adjust the strength of current, also the duration and frequency of the stimulus can be varied. Current does not damage the tissue.

RECORDING OF A SIMPLE MUSCLE CURVE

Simple muscle curve is recording of simple muscle twitch. Total muscle twitch of frog's gastrocnemius muscle is 0.1 second.

Simple Muscle Twitch

Simple muscle twitch (Fig. 14.1) is the contraction and relaxation of muscle following a single stimulus.

The different phases of simple muscle curve are described as follows.

Latent Period (LP)

It is the period between the point of stimulus and the onset of contraction. *Normal duration:* 0.01–0.012 second.

Causes for LP

- Time taken for the generation of impulse.
- Time taken for the transmission of impulse along the nerve fiber.
- Neuromuscular delay.

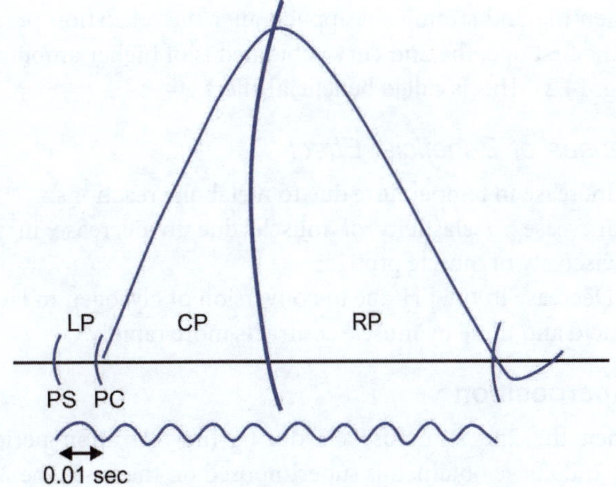

Fig. 14.1: Simple muscle twitch

- Time taken for release of Ca^{2+} in muscle fiber (excitation contraction coupling time).
- Inertia of lever.

Factors influencing LP

- Stimulating near the vertebral end increases the LP and if at the muscle end the LP decreases.
- *Temperature:* High temperature decreases LP.
- Fatigue increases LP.
- Increase in pH increases the LP.

Contraction Period (CP)

It is the period between the point of contraction and to point of maximum contraction. *Normal duration:* 0.04 second.

Factors influencing CP

- *Temperature:* Increase in temperature increases speed of contraction, therefore decreases CP and vice versa.
- *Fatigue:* When muscle is at fatigue, CP increases.

Relaxation Period (RP)

It is the period between the point of maximum contraction to the point of relaxation of muscle. *Normal duration:* 0.05–0.06 second.

Factors influencing RP

- *Temperature:* As temperature increases, RP also increases.
- *Fatigue:* As fatigue increases, RP also increases.

EFFECT OF TWO SUCCESSIVE STIMULI ON SKELETAL MUSCLE

This experiment is meant to study the refractoriness of skeletal muscle. Skeletal muscle is refractive only during LP.

Beneficial Effect

When the 2nd stimulus is applied after the relaxation period of the first one, the 2nd curve obtained is of higher amplitude (Fig. 14.2). This is called beneficial effect.

Causes of Beneficial Effect

- Increase in temperature due to metabolic reactions.
- Increase in elasticity of muscle due to decrease in the viscosity of muscle protein.
- Decrease in the pH due to conversion of glycogen to lactic acid and there by muscle contracts more rapidly.

Superposition

When the 2nd stimulus falls during the relaxation period, the 2nd curve obtained is superimposed on the first. The 2nd contraction will be of higher amplitude (Fig.14.3).

Summation

This results when the 2nd stimulus falls during the contraction period of the first one. Here the effects of the two stimuli are fused together and leads to a forceful contraction. The curve has higher amplitude and a broader base than the normal curve and also it has two points of stimulation (Fig. 14.4).

There are two types of summation:

1. *Wave/temporal summation:* The stimuli are of same strength, but the frequency of stimuli are increased and the contractions are fused.
2. *Multifiber/quantal summation:* The strength is increased, so that the number of motor units contracting is increased.

Refractory Period

Refractory period is the period after the application of the 1st stimulus during which a 2nd stimulus of adequate strength fails to produce a response. In skeletal muscle the refractory period is less than 0.005 second and is represented by the early part of LP in the simple muscle twitch.

It has two phases:

1. *Absolute refractory period:* It is the period during which a 2nd stimulus will not produce a response, whatever be the intensity of the stimulus.

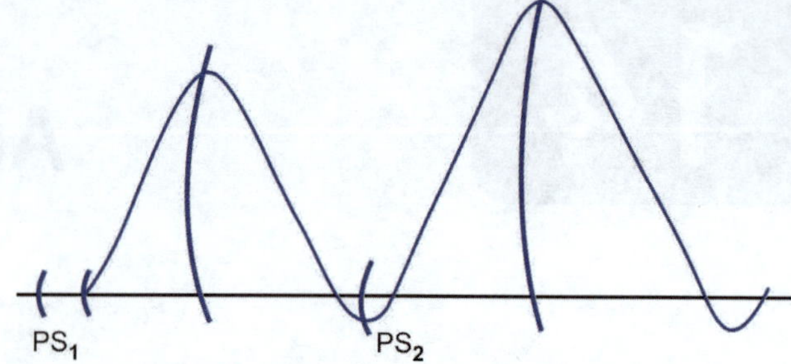

Fig. 14.2: Effect of second stimulus after relaxation period on muscle contraction

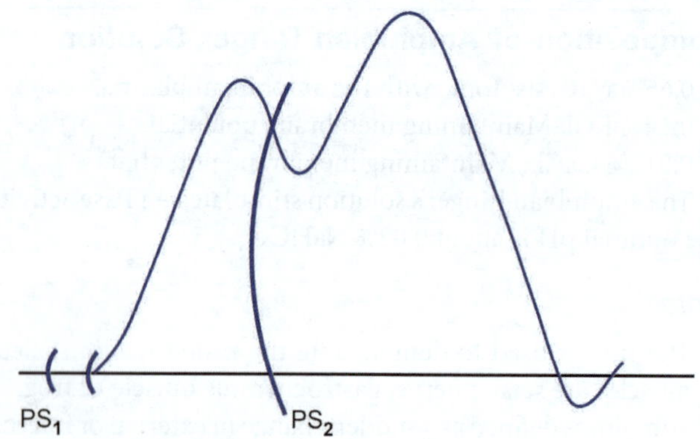

Fig. 14.3: Effect of second stimulus during relaxation period on muscle contraction

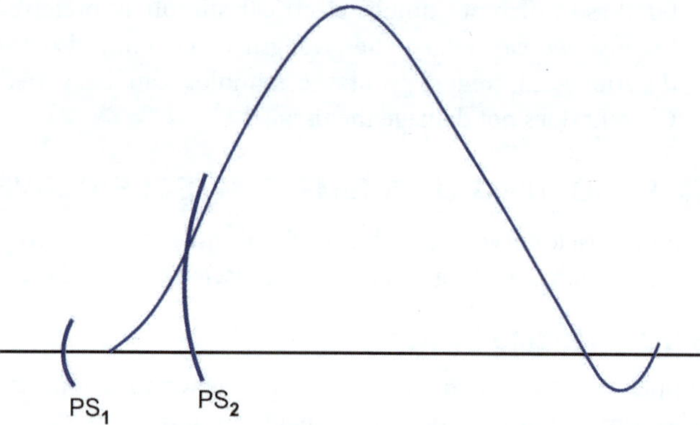

Fig. 14.4: Effect of second stimulus during contraction period on muscle contraction

2. *Relative refractory period:* It is the period during which a second stimulus of stronger intensity can produce a response.

Inference

In skeletal muscle, the 2nd stimulus is effective during relaxation period and contraction period, but ineffective during latent period (Fig. 14.5).

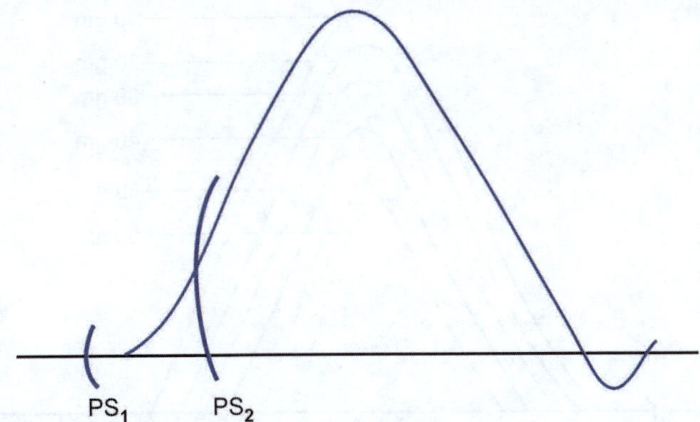

Fig. 14.5: Graph showing the importance of refractory period on muscle contraction

EFFECT OF TEMPERATURE ON SIMPLE MUSCLE TWITCH

Effects of Warm Ringer's Solution (Figs 14.6A and B)

- Decrease in LP.
- Decrease in CP and RP.
- Increase in amplitude or strength of muscle contraction.

Causes for These Changes

- Increase in enzymatic and metabolic processes.
- Increase in velocity of nerve conduction and transmission.
- Decrease in viscosity of muscle protein.

Heat Rigor

At temperature above 42°C, the muscle proteins coagulate causing a condition known as heat rigor, which is an irreversible process.

Effects of Cold Ringer's Solution (Figs 14.6A and B)

- Increase in LP.
- Increase in contraction and relaxation period.
- Decrease in amplitude or strength of muscle contraction.

Causes for These Changes

- Decrease in enzymatic and metabolic processes.
- Decrease in velocity of nerve conduction and transmission.
- Increase in viscosity of muscle protein.

Cold Rigor

With very low temperature the muscle fails to contract and there will be no response to stimulus, which is a reversible process.

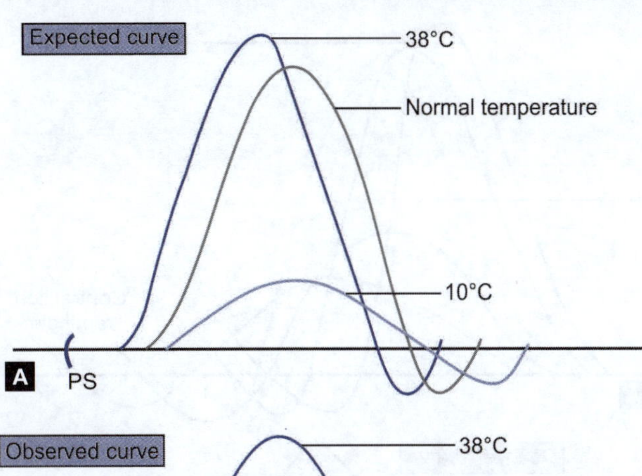

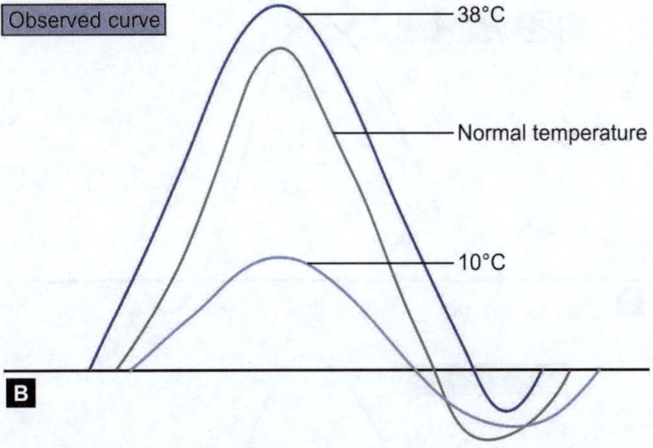

Figs 14.6A and B: **A.** Expected curve of effect of temperature on muscle contraction; **B.** Observed curve of effect of temperature on muscle contraction

GENESIS OF FATIGUE

Fatigue

Fatigue is defined as the inability of muscle to respond to a stimulus following repeated stimulation. Neuromuscular junction is the site of fatigue in muscle nerve preparation.

When a muscle is repeatedly stimulated the first few contractions increase in amplitude due to beneficial effect. When further stimulated, amplitude decreases and there is incomplete relaxation, ultimately the muscle does not respond to any stimulation (Fig. 14.7A).

Causes of Fatigue

- Anoxia.
- Accumulation of metabolic waste products like lactic acid. Small amounts of lactic acid increases excitability, but high concentration decreases it.
- Depletion of acetylcholine.
- Shortage of energy producing substances like glycogen, creatine phosphate.
- Failure to reestablish the electrical potential due to repeated stimulation.

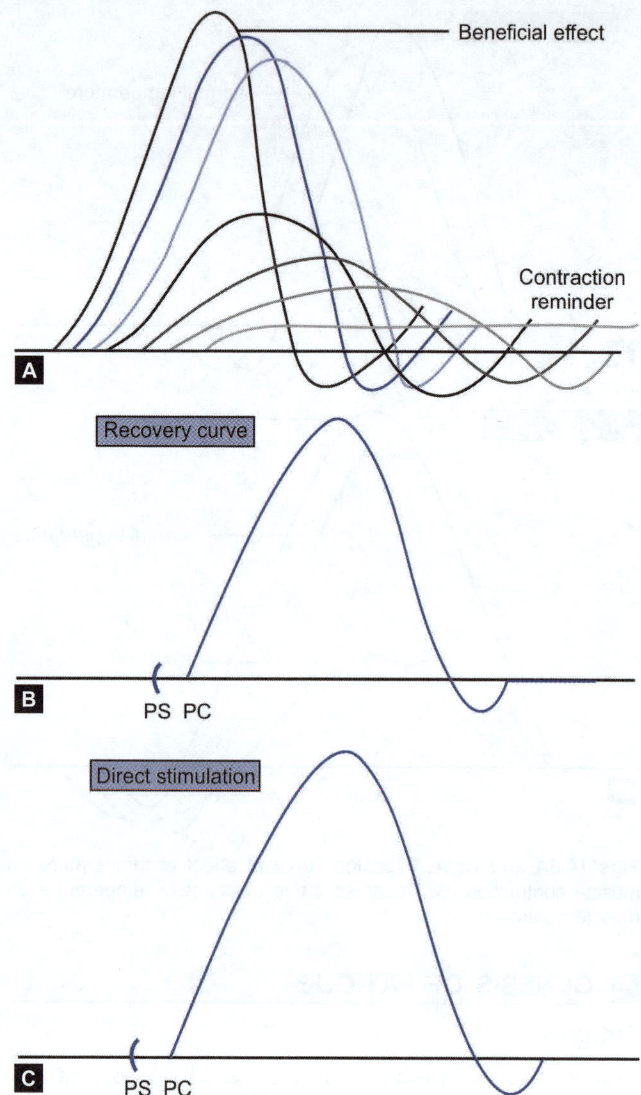

Figs 14.7A to C: **A.** Phenomenon of fatigue; **B.** Recovery curve; **C.** Effect of direct stimulation on muscle contraction

Synapse is the site of fatigue in an intact animal. Neuromuscular junction is the site of fatigue in an isolated preparation. Fatigue is reversible which is proved by the recovery curve (Fig. 14.7B).

Factors Affecting Fatigue

- Fatigue is enhanced by:
  - Increasing the frequency of stimulation.
  - By application of load.
  - Increase in temperature.
  - Lack of O_2.
- Factors favoring recovery:
  - Giving rest
  - Giving O_2

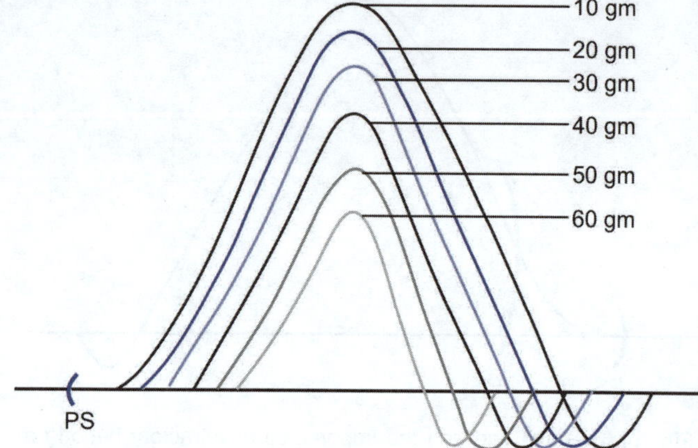

Fig. 14.8: Effect of afterload on muscle contraction

Inference

Repeated stimulation causes fatigue of muscle. Site of fatigue is the neuromuscular junction in an isolated gastrocnemius sciatic preparation (Fig. 14.7C). Fatigue is a reversible process.

EFFECT OF AFTERLOAD AND FREE-LOAD ON MUSCLE CONTRACTION

Afterload

It is the load acting on the muscle after it starts contracting. It has no effect on the muscle before it contracts and so there is no initial stretching of the muscle fiber (Fig. 14.8).

Free-load

It is the load acting on the muscle even before it starts contracting. It will stretch the muscle fiber before it contracts.

Observation

With increase in load, the amplitude decreases. In free-load, the contraction obtained for a given weight is of higher amplitude than that obtained for the same weight in afterload. This is because in free-load, the initial length of the muscle is increased. So there is increase in force of contraction. This proves Starling's law. This law is also applicable to cardiac muscle. When venous return to the heart is increased. So there is an increase in the initial length of the muscle fiber and force of contraction is increased.

For example for free-load: Throwing the ball in shot put.

For example for afterload: Lifting a weight from the ground.

Calculation of work done

Force applied to move an object through a given distance is called work done.

$$W = F \times h$$

From the Figure 14.9, $h = \dfrac{H \times I}{L}$

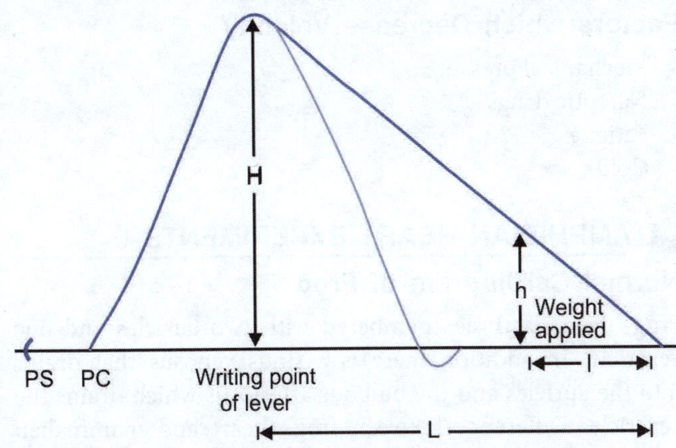

Fig. 14.9: Schematic diagram for the calculation of work done

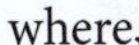

where,
W = Work done
F = Force applied
H = Apparent height of contraction for each weight applied
h = Actual height to which weight is lifted
l = Distance between fulcrum of lever and weight applied
L = Distance from the fulcrum and the writing point of the lever.

GENESIS OF TETANUS

It is incomplete tetanus where subsequent stimuli fall during relaxation period of the previous one. So the curves obtained will have a wavy appearance. This occurs at a frequency of 20 vib/sec, there is partial fusion of individual contractions which is due to incomplete relaxation and curves do not touch baseline. This is called clonus.

Tetanus

It is a smooth sustained contraction due to mechanical fusion of curves. Here subsequent stimuli fall during contraction period of previous one, but electrical properties are separate.

The minimum frequency at which tetanus occurs is called ***critical fusion frequency***. In frog it is 25 vib/sec. The critical fusion frequency depends on duration of contraction period. It is inversely proportional to the contraction period of the muscle. Conditions which increase the contraction period such as cold, fatigue, etc. will decrease the critical fusion frequency.

At a frequency of 30 vib/sec complete fusion of contractions take place, thereby producing a smooth sustained contraction called tetanus (Figs 14.10A to F).

Tetany

It is a clinical condition where there is a spasm of muscle due to hypocalcemia, alkalosis.

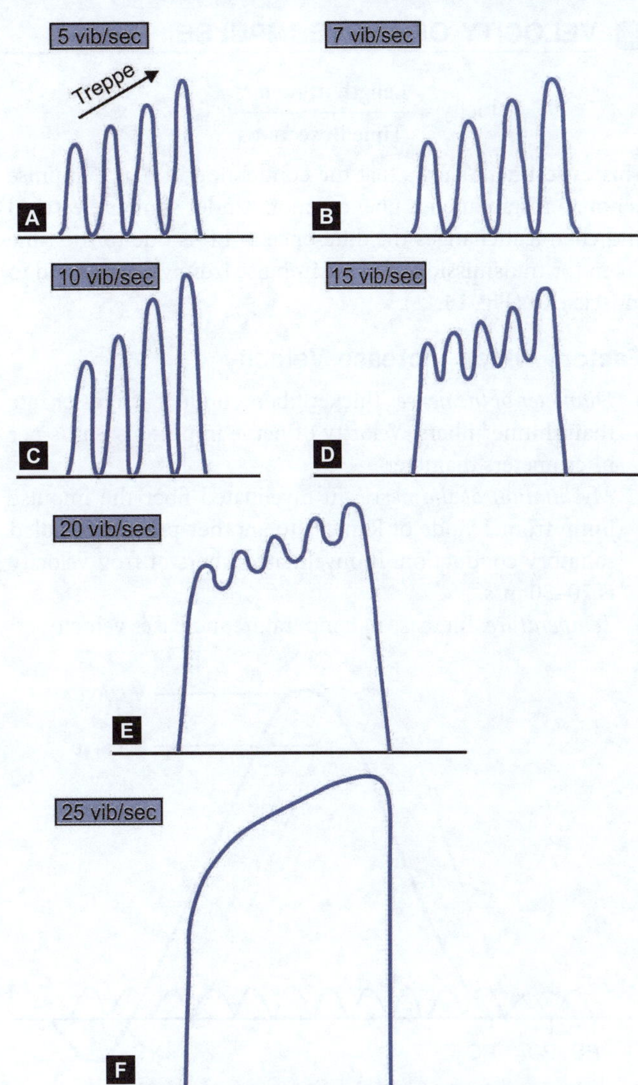

Figs 14.10A to F: Genesis of tetanus. The approximate rate of stimulation is indicated above each set of recording

Factors affecting the genesis of tetanus

- *Type of muscle:* In fast white muscle, tetanizing/critical fusion frequency is small compared to slow red muscle.
- *Temperature:* When temperature decreases, tetanus occurs at lower frequency of stimuli.
- *Fatigue:* A fatigued muscle undergoes tetanus with low frequency of stimulus.
- *Refractory period:* In skeletal muscle, refractory period is very short therefore they can undergo tetanus very easily. Cardiac muscle cannot be tetanized because of its long refractory period.

Note: The duration of one simple muscle twitch is 0.1 second so we do not get fusion of frequency up to a frequency of 10 vib/second.

VELOCITY OF NERVE IMPULSE

$$\text{Velocity} = \frac{\text{Length in meters}}{\text{Time in seconds}}$$

This experiment shows that the conduction of nerve impulse is not an instantaneous phenomenon. Under similar electrical and chemical changes the difference in LP is due to the time taken for transmission of nerve impulse from vertebral end to muscle end (Fig. 14.11).

Factors which Increase Velocity

- *Diameter of the nerve:* Thicker fibers conduct at a faster rate than thinner fibers. Velocity of nerve impulse is 5 m/s per micrometers diameter.
- *Myelination of the nerve:* In myelinated fiber the impulse jump from 1 node of Ranvier to another process is called saltatory conduction. In myelinated fibers of frog velocity is 20–30 m/s.
- *Temperature:* Increase in temperature increases velocity.

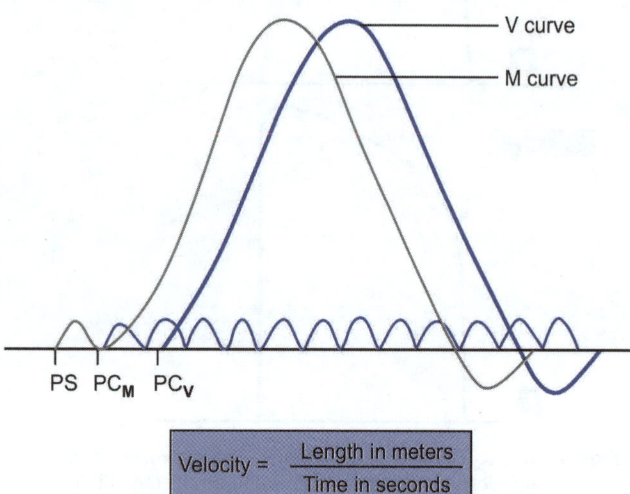

Fig. 14.11: Velocity of transmission of nerve impulse when stimulated from vertebral end and muscle end

Factors which Decrease Velocity

- Mechanical pressure
- Narcotic drugs
- Fatigue
- Cold.

AMPHIBIAN HEART EXPERIMENTS

Normal Cardiogram of Frog

Frog's heart is three chambered with two auricles and one ventricle. In addition there is a sinus venosus that drains into the auricles and the bulbous arteriosus which drains the ventricle. Difference between frog's heart and mammalian heart is given in Table 14.1.

Composition

Ringer's Solution

NaCl : 0.65 g%, it maintains rhythmicity
KCl : 0.014 g%, necessary for relaxation
$CaCl_2$: 0.012 g%, necessary for relaxation
$NaHCO_3$: 0.02 g%, it acts as a buffer
Distilled water : 100 mL

Ringer Locke's Solution

NaCl : 0.9 g%
KCl : 0.042 g%
$CaCl_2$: 0.02 g%
$NaHCO_3$: 0.02 g%
Glucose : 0.1 g%

Note: When normal cardiogram (NCG) is recorded using a simple lever (Figs 14.12A and B), the upstroke indicates systole and the downstroke indicates diastole.

There are three waves in the systole S, A, V as shown in Figures 14.12A and B. 'S' wave is due to contraction of sinus venosus. 'A' wave is due to contraction of atria and 'V' wave is due to contraction of ventricle. The contraction of ventricle is followed by relaxation. These are the sequences of events

Table 14.1: Differences between frog's heart and mammalian heart

Frog's heart	Mammalian heart
Three chambered	Four chambered
Sinus venosus is the pacemaker of heart	SA node is the pacemaker
Nutrition of heart is from the surrounding tissue fluid	Nutrition is from the coronary blood vessels which supply the heart
Chamber perfusion	Coronary perfusion
Specialized conducting system is absent	Specialized conducting system is present
Ringer's solution is used in the experiment	Ringer's lock solution is used
Oxygen, pressure and temperature need not be maintained	Oxygen, temperature and pressure have to be maintained

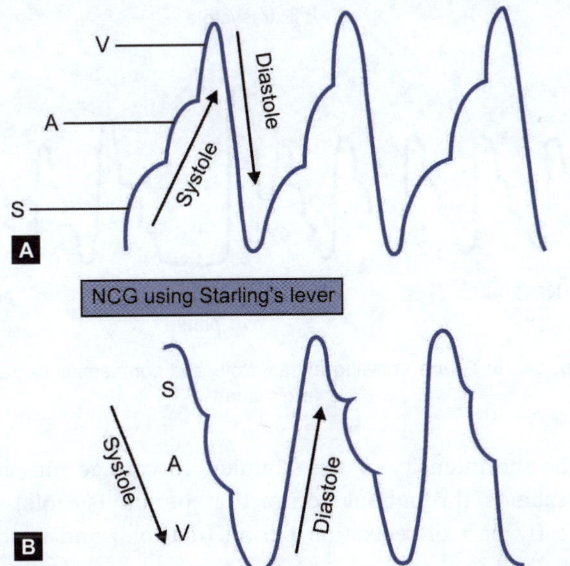

Figs 14.12A and B: A. Record of normal cardiogram of frog using simple lever; **B.** Record of normal cardiogram of frog using Starling's lever

occurring in the heart and it indicates the rhythmicity if the heart. It also helps to determine the heart rate with the help of time tracing below the NCG.

Bulbus Arteriosus

On the ventral aspect of the frog's heart there is an initial dilated portion of the aorta called as bulbus arteriosus.

White crescentic lie on the dorsal aspect of the frog's heart. The auricles and the sinus venosus are separated by white crescentic line which represents the parasympathetic nerve ganglion.

Effect of Temperature on Frog's Heart

The effect of temperature (heat and cold) on frog's heart can be studied separately in two parts:

Effect on Sinus Venosus

Effect of heat on sinus venosus (SV) (Fig. 14.13A)

Two effects are as follows:

1. *Increase in heart rate (1° effect):* Sinus venosus is the pacemaker in the frog's heart. Application of warm saline increases the rate at which impulse is generated. Therefore the heart rate is increased.
2. *Force of contraction of heart decreases (2° effect):* This is because increase in the heart rate will decrease the diastolic pause. Therefore ventricular filling decreases. So end-diastolic volume (EDV) decreases, so there is decreased stretching of ventricular muscle fibers, so force of contraction decreases (Frank-Starling law).

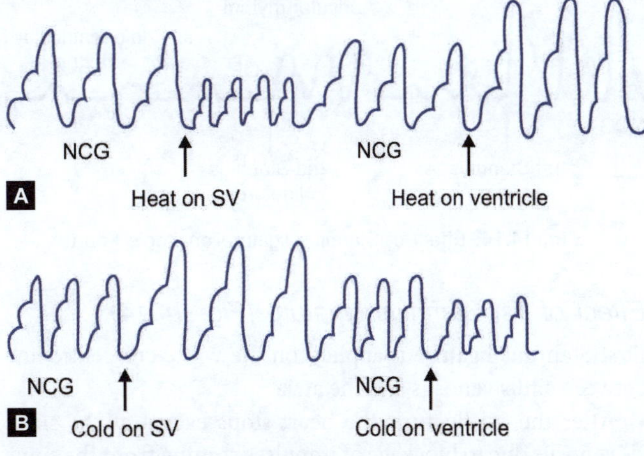

Figs 14.13A and B: A. Effect of heat on sinus venosus and ventricles of frog's heart; **B.** Effect of cold on sinus venosus and ventricles of frog's heart

Effect of cold on sinus venosus (Fig. 14.13B)

Two effects are as follows:

1. *Decrease in heart rate (1° effect):* This is due to decrease in the rate of impulse generation at sinus venosus.
2. *Force of contraction of heart increases (2° effect):* When cold saline is applied on sinus venosus the heart rate decreases, but the diastolic pause increases. Therefore, there will be increased diastolic filling, which increases the EDV. Hence, there will be increased stretching of ventricular muscle fibers, thereby increasing the force of contraction (according to Frank-Starling law of cardiac muscle).

Effect on Ventricles

Effect of heat on ventricles (Fig. 14.13A)

1. No change in heart rate
2. Force of contraction of heart increases.

There is no change in heart rate as ventricle is not the pacemaker of the frog's heart. Further the force of contraction increases because of increase in metabolism of the ventricle and also there is decrease in the viscosity of muscle protein.

Effect of cold on ventricles (Fig. 14.13B)

1. No change in heart rate
2. Force of contraction of heart decreases.

There is no change in heart rate as ventricle is not the pacemaker of the frog's heart. The force of contraction decreases because of decrease in metabolism of the ventricle and also there is increase in the viscosity of muscle protein.

Effect of Stannius Ligature on Frog's Heart

Application of ligature is an attempt to block the transmission of cardiac impulse from sinus venosus to auricles in the 1st ligature and from atria to ventricles in the 2nd ligature.

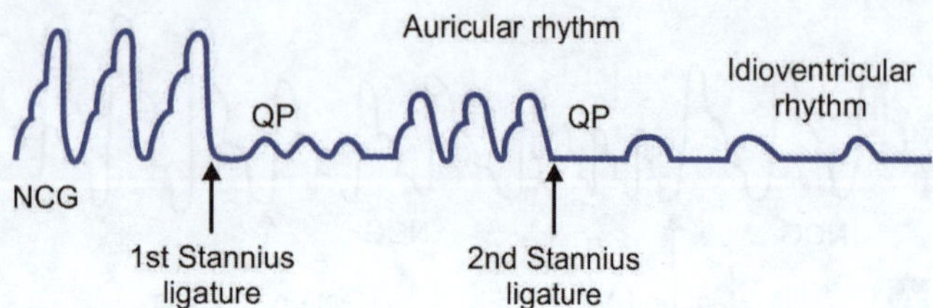

Fig. 14.14: Effect of Stannius ligature on frog's heart

Effect of 1st Stannius Ligature (Fig. 14.14)

First Stannius ligature is applied on the white crescentic line between sinus venosus and the atria.

- After the 1st ligature, the heart stops except at the sinus venosus due to blockage of impulses coming from the sinus venosus. Therefore sinus venosus will continue to beat on its own because it is the pacemaker of the heart. This is called ***sinus rhythm.***
- The atria and ventricle stop beating in diastole. But after sometime the atria initiate their own impulse and start beating on their own at a slower rate independent of the sinus rhythm. This is called ***auricular rhythm.*** The impulse from the atria reach the ventricle and they also start beating.

Effect of 2nd Stannius Ligature (Fig. 14.14)

Second Stannius ligature is applied on the atrioventricular groove between two atria and the ventricle in the frog's heart.

When the 2nd Stannius ligature is applied, the auricles stop contracting whereas the ventricles continue to contract at its own rhythm. This is the ***idioventricular rhythm.***

- Average rate of impulse production (human heart)
  SA node = 72/min
  AV node = 50/min
  Ventricle = 30/min
- Velocity of conduction (human heart)
  SA node = 0.05 m/s
  AV node = 0.05 m/s
  Atrial and ventricular musculature=1 m/s
  Bundle of His = 1 m/s
  Purkinje fibers = 4 m/s
  In frog's heart
  Heart rate = 50–60/min
  Auricular rhythm = 20–30/min
  Idioventricular rhythm = <10/min

Refractory Period and Extrasystole in Frog's Heart

Refractory period is a brief period during which cardiac muscle does not respond to restimulation. It has two phases:

1. *Absolute refractory period:* It is the period during which a 2nd stimulus will not produce any response whatever be the intensity of the stimulus. In cardiac muscle, it extends throughout contraction period (systole) and early part of relaxation period (diastole) and is about 0.25–0.3 sec.
2. *Relative refractory period:* It is the period during which a 2nd stimulus of stronger intensity can produce a response. The rest of diastole is in the relative refractory period and is about 0.05 second.

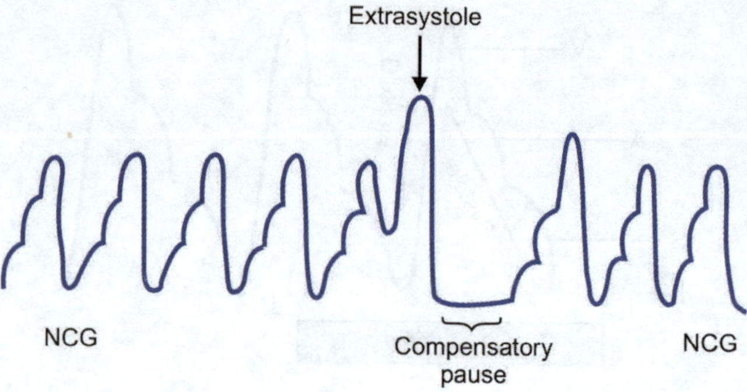

Fig. 14.15: Graph showing extrasystole and compensatory pause in frog's heart

Note: Summation and tetanus are not possible in cardiac muscle because whole of contraction is in absolute refractory period. A long refractory period is due to prolonged repolarization in cardiac muscle.

Functional Significance of Long Refractory Period

- It maintains the normal rhythm of heart.
- Summation and tetanus are not possible in heart muscle.
- Under normal condition it would not produce any extra-systole.
- If extrasystole occurs the compensatory pause helps to regain the normal rhythm.

Normally the impulse passes from atria to ventricle in an orderly sequence. When the ventricle is stimulated in the later part of diastole, an extrasystole is produced because the heart is in the relative refractory period. During this time a normal impulse from SA node reaches the ventricle but it fails to produce a contraction because the heart is in the absolute refractory period of extrasystole. This missing of 1 beat produces the compensatory pause. Only when the next normal impulse from SA node reaches the ventricle it will respond. So the total duration of extrasystole, preceding contraction and compensatory pause equals to two normal cardiac cycle.

Extrasystole (Fig. 14.15)

It is the response of myocardium to a stimulus other than one from the normal pacemaker. It can be auricular, nodal or ventricular in man.

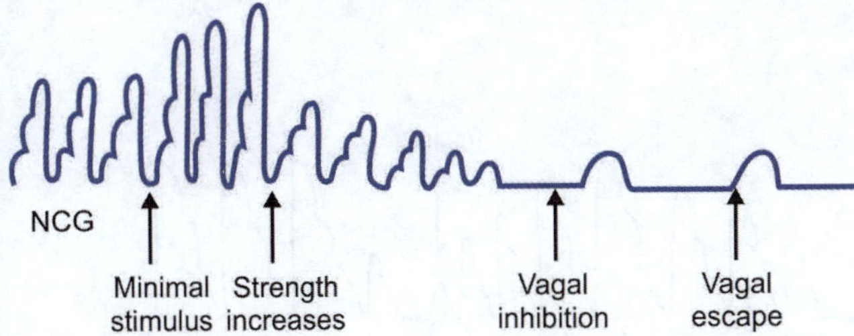

Fig. 14.16: Effect of vagal stimulation on frog's heart

Causes of extrasystole

- Physiological
  - Excessive consumption of alcohol, coffee and smoking
  - Occasionally in pregnancy.
- Pathological
  - Digitalis toxicity
  - Ischemic heart disease
  - Rheumatic carditis
  - Thyrotoxicosis.

Effect of Vagal Stimulation on Frog's Heart

With weak stimuli, the heart may beat faster and more forcefully due to the excitation of sympathetic fibers present in the vagal trunk. With increase in the strength of stimuli the heart beat becomes slower and weaker. Finally the heart stops in diastole. This is called ***vagal inhibition.*** With continued stimulation of the vagus (do not increase the strength of current), the heart starts beating at a slower rate inspite of the stimulation which is the idioventricular rhythm. This phenomenon is called the ***vagal escape*** **(Fig. 14.16).** Then when the stimulus is stopped the heart beats normally.

Vagal Escape

It is the escape of the heart from the inhibitory effect of vagus.

Cause of vagal escape

- Depletion of acetylcholine due to continuous stimulation.
- Idioventricular rhythm: The lower 2/3rd of the ventricle is not supplied by the vagus. So it starts contracting on its own even while the vagus is being stimulated.
- Stimulation of sympathetic fibers present in the vagal nerve.

Effect of Adrenaline, Acetylcholine on Frog's Heart

Adrenaline

Adrenaline is stimulatory to frog's heart.

Actions of adrenaline

It increases:

- *Rate of contraction:* Positive chronotropic effect
- *Force of contraction:* Positive inotropic effect

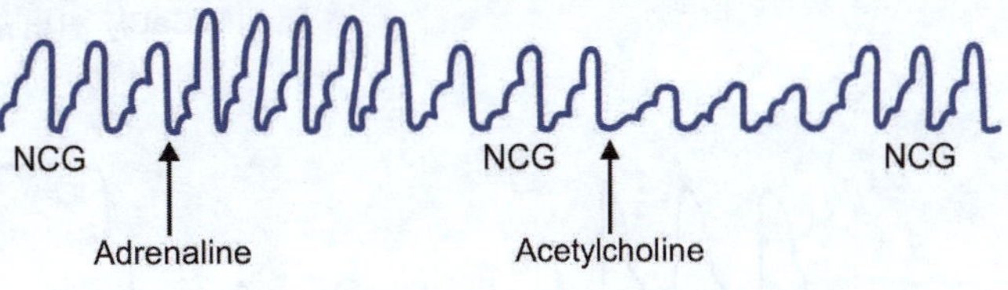

Fig. 14.17: Effect of adrenaline, acetylcholine on frog's heart

- *Velocity of contraction:* Positive dromotropic effect
- *Irritability:* Positive bathmotropic effect.

Explanation

Adrenaline increases the heart rate due to its effect on sinus venosus (Fig. 14.17). Increase in the force of contraction is due to its direct effect on ventricular contraction. Action of adrenaline in heart is mediated through β-receptors.

Acetylcholine

It is inhibitory to frog's heart.

Actions of acetylcholine

It decreases:

- *Rate of contraction:* Negative chronotropic effect
- *Force of contraction:* Negative inotropic effect
- *Velocity of contraction:* Negative dromotropic effect.

Perfusion of Frog's Heart and Effect of Ions on it

Frog's Heart is Perfused with Ringer's Solution

- *Solution I:* Contains 0.65% NaCl. The heart beats rhythmically but becomes weaker and weaker and finally stops in diastole. Solution I is removed and solution II is added (Fig. 14.18).
- *Solution II:* Contains 0.012% $CaCl_2$ in addition to NaCl. The heart regains rhythmicity but contractions become slow and sustained. Relaxation becomes less and less. Now when 1 drop of 1% $CaCl_2$ is added the heart stops in systole. This is called *calcium rigor.* Solution II is removed and solution III is added.
- *Solution III:* Contains 0.014% KCl in addition to the above ions. The heart relaxes quickly and gradually begins to beat normally, but after sometime the amplitude falls. Now when 1 drop of 1% KCl is added heart stops in diastole. This is called *K^+ inhibition.* Now when the solution is removed and Ringer's solution is added, heart regains its normal amplitude and rhythm.

Discussion

- **Action of NaCl**—Na^+ ions are essential for:
  - Excitation of heart
  - Maintaining rhythmicity.

PHYSICON—The Reliable Icon in Physiology

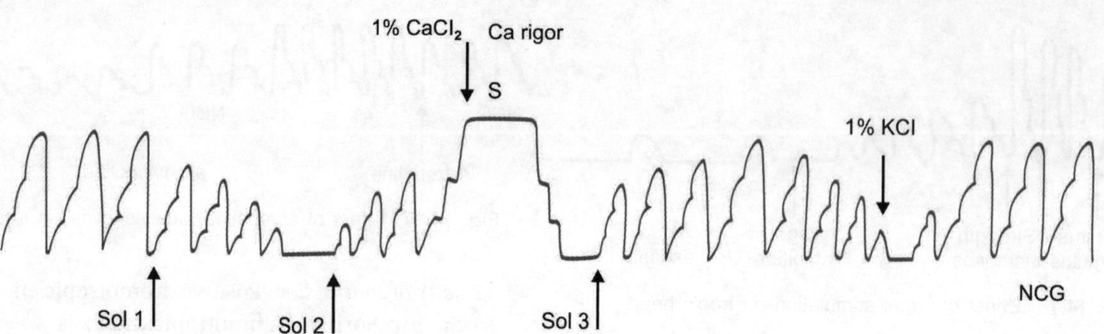

Fig. 14.18: Effect of perfusion of frog's heart and effect of ions on it

- **Action of Ca^{2+}**
  - Maintain contractibility
  - For sliding action of actin and myosin Ca^{2+} is necessary.

Causes of calcium rigor

When contraction increases more ATP is utilized and complete loss of ATP occurs. Relaxation depends on ATP, which when lost relaxation is ultimately inhibited. Excess of Ca^{2+} causes heart to go into spastic contractions and the heart stops in systole.

- **Action of K^+**—Necessary for relaxation
  - *K^+ inhibition:* When excess of K^+ is present in ECF, it causes heart to become extremely dilated and flaccid. The heart is slowed and stops in diastole.

CHAPTER

15

Clinical Examinations

CLINICAL EXAMINATION PROFORMA

Name :
Age :
Sex :
Occupation :
Address :

General Examination

Built and nourishment : Moderately built and adequately nourished
Height :
Weight :
Pallor : No pallor
Jaundice/Icterus : Not jaundiced
Cyanosis : Not cyanosed
Clubbing : No clubbing of fingers or toes
Lymphadenopathy : No significant lymph node enlargement
Edema : No edema
Skin and hair : Skin and hair healthy
Pulse (Figs 15.1 and 15.2): 72/min regular, normal in volume, character and tension, no thickening of vessel walls, all peripheral pulsations are felt equally and normally on both sides and there is no brachiofemoral delay

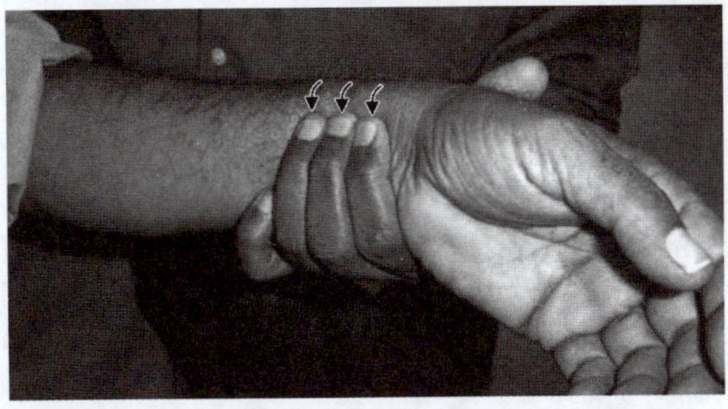

Fig. 15.1: Examination of radial pulse: The radial pulse is felt with the tips of the fingers (preferably three: index, middle, and ring) compressing the vessel against the head of the radius, with the patient's forearm slightly pronated and the wrist slightly flexed

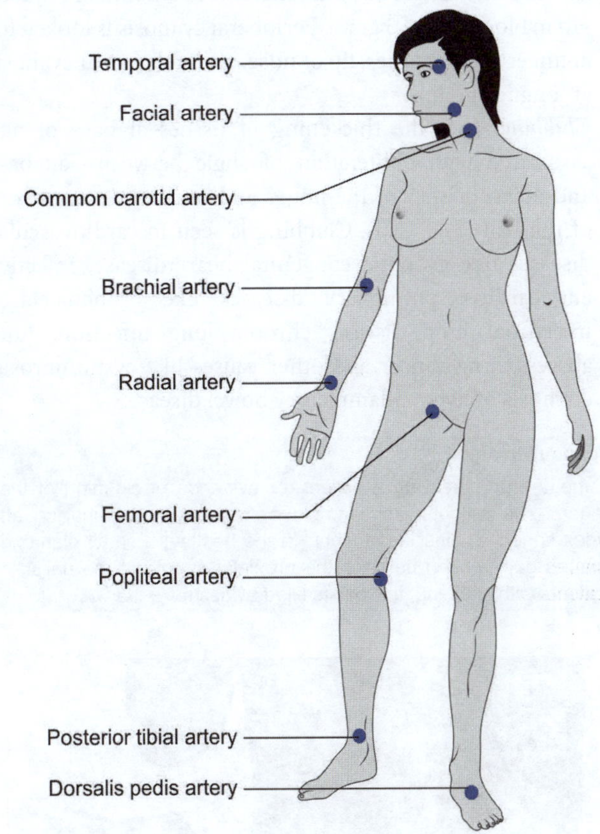

Fig. 15.2: Sites to look for pulse

Blood pressure : 120/80 mm Hg in the right upper limb in supine position.
JVP : Not raised
Respiratory rate : 14/min, regular
Body temperature : 37 °C

Impression

On general examination, the subject appears to be normal.

Note

- *Pallor:* It gives a rough assessment of degree of anemia of the patient. It is looked for by retracting the lower eyelids and observing the color of palpebral conjunctiva. It is normally red in color. Pallor is also noted by color of skin, especially of palms, nail bed, mucosa of tongue and oral cavity.

- *Jaundice/Icterus:* It is the yellowish discoloration of skin, sclera and mucous membrane due to deposition of bilirubin in tissues. Clinically obvious when serum bilirubin exceeds 2 mg/dL. Jaundice is looked for in upper sclera by asking the patient to lower his eyeballs.
- *Cyanosis:* It is the bluish discoloration of the skin and mucous membrane due to an increase in amount of reduced Hb in blood above 5 gm%. Peripheral cyanosis is looked for at fingertips, ear lobes, tip of nose, etc. and central cyanosis at tongue and lips.
- *Clubbing:* It is the thickening of tissues at base of nail associated with obliteration of angle between nail base and adjacent skin of the finger and increase in convexity of the nail (Fig. 15.3). Clubbing is seen in cardiovascular diseases like cyanotic congenital heart disease, infective endocarditis; pulmonary diseases like bronchiectasis, interstitial lung disease, chronic lung infection, lung abscess, lung cancer and other causes like cystic fibrosis, cirrhosis of liver, inflammatory bowel disease.

Schamroth sign

A method of assessing a patient for evidence of clubbing of the fingers. The patient is asked to place the nails of the right and left index fingers against each other. In the healthy, a small diamond shaped gap is seen between the proximal margin of the nails. In patients with clubbing, this gap is filled by tissue.

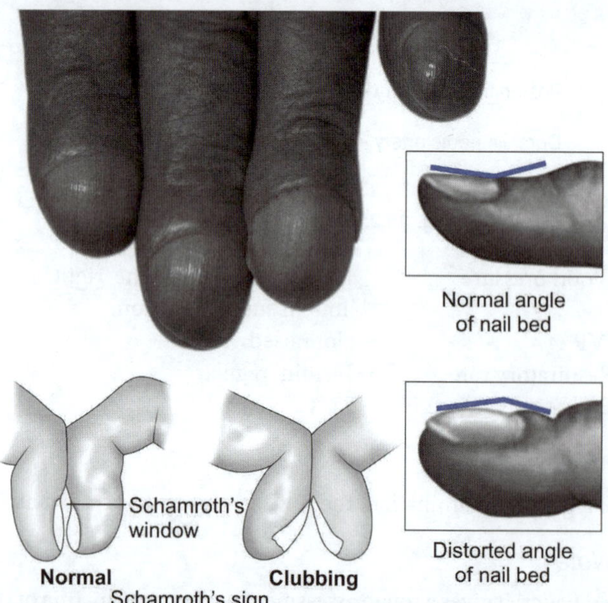

Fig. 15.3: Clubbing nails

- *Lymphadenopathy:* The lymph nodes in the drainage area of any organ are prone to be affected in diseases of that organ. There may be enlargement or tenderness or both. Generalized lymphadenopathy is seen in conditions like leukemia and Hodgkin's disease. Local lymphadenitis is seen in inflamations affecting drainage area. Different groups of lymph nodes are palpated, e.g. cervical, axillary, inguinal, etc.
- *Edema:* Edema is an abnormal accumulation of fluid in the intercellular spaces of body. Edema may be detected from the glossy appearance of the skin. It is seen in congestive heart failure, renal failure, hepatic failure, venous insufficiency etc. Presence of dependent edema in ambulant persons is usually detected by applying sustained firm pressure with the thumb against medial malleolus or shaft of tibia (for about 30 sec) and see for pitting or depression at pressure point.

HUMAN ARTERIAL BLOOD PRESSURE

In clinical medicine, blood pressure is the lateral pressure exerted by the flowing blood in the systemic arteries.

Apparatus

Sphygmomanometer and stethoscope

Sphygmomanometer has three important parts:

1. A mercury manometer
2. A rubber bag with linen cuff
3. An air pump.

Definitions

- *Systolic blood pressure (SBP):* It is the highest BP recorded during systole of cardiac cycle.
- *Diastolic blood pressure (DBP):* It is the lowest BP recorded during diastole of cardiac cycle.
- Pulse pressure (PP) = SBP–DBP
- Mean arterial BP is the weighted mean pressure of blood. Mean arterial BP = DBP + 1/3PP

Procedure

Measurement is done by two methods:

Palpatory Method

Here the radial pulse is palpated. Pressure in the cuff is elevated until the pulse disappears. The cuff is then slowly deflated. Reading at which the pulse reappears corresponds to the systolic BP.

Auscultatory Method

Here brachial artery is auscultated during the measurement. Cuff is inflated 20–30 mm Hg above the systolic BP got by palpatory method. Slowly deflate the cuff and observe the manometer reading when a first tapping sound is heard. This corresponds to systolic BP. Now the cuff is slowly deflated listening to serial changes in the sound. The manometer reading when the sound completely disappears corresponds to diastolic BP. Series of sound heard during deflation are called Korotkoff sound and they are divided into five phases:

- *Phase I:* Sudden reappearance of a clear tapping sound. It becomes louder during 10–15 mm Hg fall of pressure.
- *Phase II:* Sound becomes soft and murmuring in the next 10–15 mm Hg fall of pressure.
- *Phase III:* Murmuring character continues but becomes louder and clear in the next 5–7 mm Hg fall of pressure.
- *Phase IV:* Sound becomes soft and muffled.
- *Phase V:* Sound completely disappears.

Basis of Korotkoff's sounds

Normal blood flow is laminar and streamlined and is always silent. Flow through a partially occluded vessels produces turbulence, hence a sound is produced. There is no sound in a completely occluded vessel. When the vessel is partially occluded by the pressure cuff there is turbulence. These sounds of vibration are transmitted and heard by auscultation. Appearance and disappearance of sounds are observed which corresponds to systolic and diastolic BP respectively (Fig. 15.4).

Auscultatory gap and its significance

In some patients of hypertension, there may be a gap in the Korotkoff sound. As the Hg is lowered, a few faint sounds are heard which soon disappear only to reappear once again at a lower pressure. This brief interruption, which may range from 40–60 mm Hg is called the 'auscultatory' or 'silent' gap. If the Hg column is raised to this gap and then the pressure lowered, one may miss the first appearance of sounds, which indicate systolic pressure, and thus record a false low systolic pressure.

To avoid this mistake, the BP should always be recorded by the palpatory method first. Then during auscultatory method, the Hg column must be raised 30–40 mm Hg above the level found by palpatory method. If we record BP only by auscultatory method, systolic BP may be underestimated due to the presence of auscultatory gap (particularly in HT individuals). But, during palpatory method this gap is not seen so there will be an idea of actual BP so, palpatory method is done before auscultatory method to get an approx value of systolic BP.

Normal Values

Systolic BP: 100–140 mm Hg.

Diastolic BP: 60–90 mm Hg.

Results

BP by palpatory method (systolic BP)

BP by auscultatory method

- Sitting :
- Standing :
- Recumbent :
- After exercise :

EXAMINATION OF RESPIRATORY SYSTEM

Name :

Age :

Sex :

Occupation :

Address :

General Examination

Built and nourishment : Moderately built and adequately nourished

Height :

Weight :

Pallor : No pallor

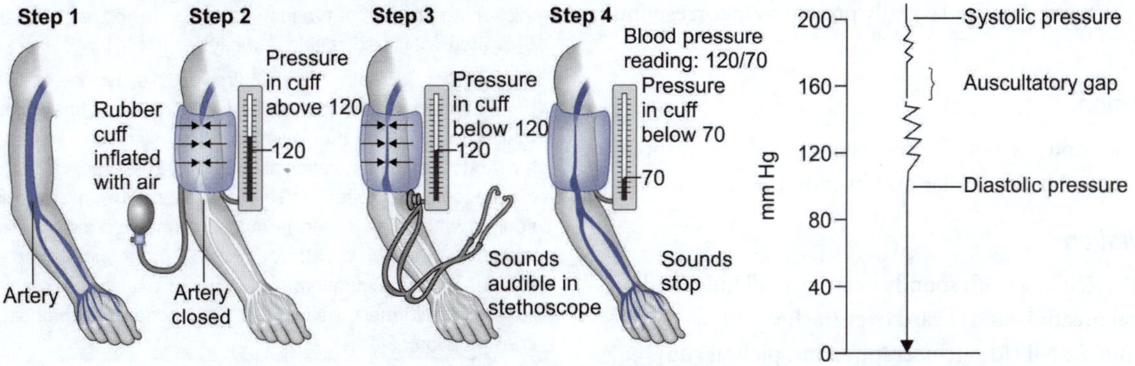

Fig. 15.4: Measurement of BP

Jaundice/Icterus : Not jaundiced
Cyanosis : Not cyanosed
Clubbing : No clubbing of fingers or toes
Lymphadenopathy : No significant lymph node enlargement
Edema : No edema
Skin and hair : Skin and hair healthy
Pulse : 72/min regular, normal in volume, character and tension, no thickening of vessel walls, all peripheral pulsations are felt equally and normally on both sides and there is no brachiofemoral delay
Blood pressure : 120/80 mm Hg in the right upper limb in supine position
JVP : Not raised
Respiratory rate : 14/min, regular
Body temperature : 37 °C

Systemic Examination

Inspection

Nostrils and throat normal
Trachea-central
Shape of the chest normal bilaterally symmetrical
Apex beat visible below and medial to the nipple
Respiratory movements: Equal on both sides
Respiratory rate: .... /min. Rhythm: Regular/irregular.
Type: Abdomino thoracic or thoracoabdominal
No dilated veins or visible pulsations over the chest
No localized prominence/depression/intercostal edema

Palpation

Trachea-central
Apex beat-palpable (note the site also)/not palpable.
Respiratory movements equal over corresponding areas.
Chest expansion—cms
Vocal fremitus normal and equally present over corresponding areas.

Percussion

Percussion note is equally resonant overall corresponding areas except over the cardiac and liver dullness.

Auscultation

Normal vesicular breath sounds heard overall lung fields
Bronchial breath sounds heard over trachea
Added sounds: Nil (Rhonchi, crepitations, pleural rub)

Vocal resonance is normal and equal overall corresponding areas.

Impression

The respiratory system of the given subject appears to be normal.

Note: For the purpose of physical examination and description of findings, the chest wall is divided into different areas bilaterally, i.e.

Front

- Supraclavicular area
- Clavicular area
- Infraclavicular area
- Mammary area.

Sides

- Axillary area
- Infra-axillary area.

Behind

- Suprascapular area
- Scapular area
- Interscapular area
- Infrascapular area.

Inspection: Undue prominence of sternocledomastoid muscle on either side indicates tracheal shift (Trail's sign). Scoliosis (lateral bending of vertebral column), kyphosis (forward bending of vertebral column), pigeon chest (sternum projects forwards; seen in rickets). In chronic airway obstruction, transverse diameter becomes more than the anteroposterior diameter. In females it is thoracoabdominal and in males it is abdominothoracic.

Palpation: In fibrosis of lung, the trachea is shifted to the same side of lesion and to opposite side in pleural effusion. Shift in position of apex beat can occur in conditions like pleural effusion and pneumothorax. In dextrocardia, it is felt on the right side. Normal chest expansion is 2–5 cms. Vocal fremitus is decreased in pleural thickening, fibrosis of the lung, pleural effusion, etc. It is increased over areas of consolidation and cavities in the lung.

Auscultation: Breath sounds are of two types—vesicular and bronchial breath sounds. Normal vesicular breath sounds have a rustling quality and are louder during inspiration and usually only the first third of expiration is audible. There is no gap between inspiration and expiration. This is in contrast with bronchial breath sounds where the sound is much harsher (sounding like blowing through a hollow tube), there is a pronounced gap between inspiration and expiration, and you can usually hear the whole of expiration. Normally heard over the trachea and pathologically in consolidation of lung.

EXAMINATION OF CARDIOVASCULAR SYSTEM

Name :
Age :
Occupation :
Address :

General Examination

Built and nourishment : Moderately built and adequately nourished
Height :
Weight :
Pallor : No pallor
Jaundice/Icterus : Not jaundiced
Cyanosis : Not cyanosed
Clubbing : No clubbing of fingers or toes
Lymphadenopathy : No significant lymphnode enlargement
Edema : No edema
Skin and hair : Skin and hair healthy
Pulse : 72/min regular, normal in volume, character and tension, no thickening of vessel walls, all peripheral pulsations are felt equally and normally on both sides and there is no brachiofemoral delay.
Blood pressure : 120/80 mm Hg in the right upper limb in supine position
JVP (Figs 15.5A and B): Not raised
Respiratory rate : 14/min, regular
Body temperature : 37 °C

Systemic Examination

Inspection

Shape of precordium: Normal, no bulging/deformity
Apex beat: Visible below and medial to the left nipple
Jugular venous pulse: Just visible/not visible
Other visible pulsations: Suprasternal, carotid and epigastric pulsation not visible

Palpation

Apex beat is felt in the 5th left intercostal space 1 cm medial to the midclavicular line.
Thrills: No thrills
Left parasternal heave: No LPH.

Percussion

The upper border of the liver percussed out in the 5th space in the midclavicular line, 7th space in the midaxillary line and 9th space in the scapular line on the right side. The right border of the heart corresponds with in the right border of the sternum and left border corresponds with the apex beat.

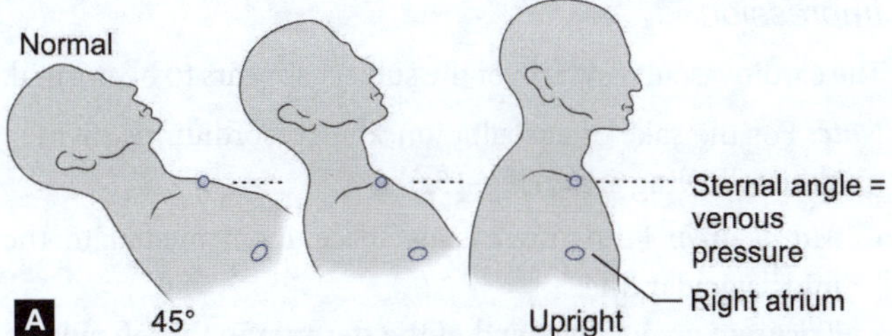

The distance between the sternal angle and center of the RA remains relatively constant regardless of the position of the thorax

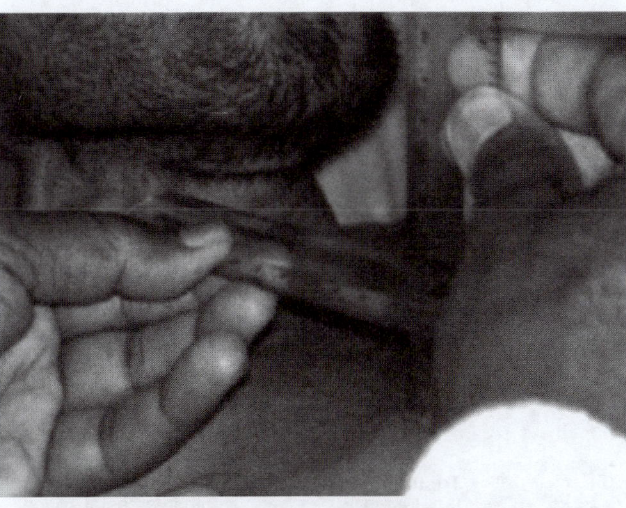

Measurement of JV pressure by two scale method—A horizontal scale at the top of the oscillating venous column in IJV cuts the vertical scale at the sternal angle. The vertical distance from the sternal angle gives the RA pressure in cm.

Figs 15.5A and B: Measurement of JVP

Auscultation

Mitral area : S1 and S2 sounds heard-normal intensity (S1 louder)
No additional sounds
No murmur/click/pericardial rub

Tricuspid area : S1 and S2 sounds heard-normal intensity (S1 louder)
No additional sounds
No murmur

Pulmonary area : S1 and S2 sounds heard-normal intensity (S2 louder)
No additional sounds
No murmur

Aortic area : S1 and S2 sounds heard-normal intensity (S2 louder)
No additional sounds
No murmur

Impression

The cardiovascular system of the subject appears to be normal.

Note: For the sake of auscultation, the precordium is divided into the following areas (Fig. 15.6):

- *Mitral area:* Fifth intercostals space 1 cm medial to the midclavicular line.
- *Tricuspid area:* Lower end of the sternum to the left side.
- *Aortic area:* Second right intercostal space close to the sternum.
- *Pulmonary area:* Second left intercostal space close to the sternum.

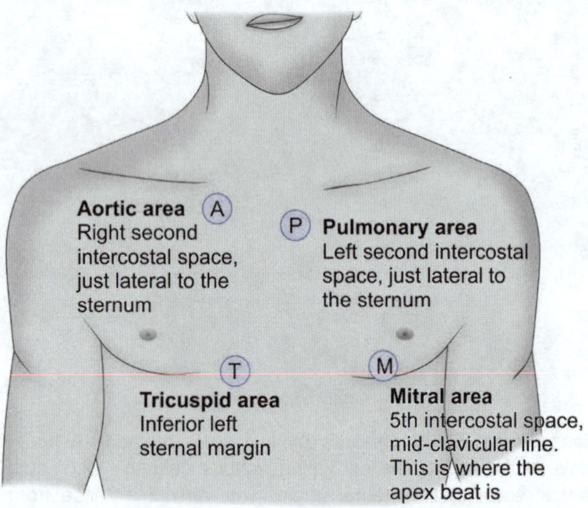

Fig. 15.6: Cardiac auscultatory areas

Inspection: Bulging or prominence of the precordium is seen in mediastinal tumours, pericardial effusion, left sided pleural effusion, etc. Engorged veins over the precordium is present in superior or inferior vena caval obstructions. Apex beat is defined as the lowermost and outermost point of definite cardiac impulses that can be best seen or felt. It is invisible in persons with thick chest wall, pericardial effusion or when located behind a rib. Suprasternal pulsations are visible in persons with aneurysms of arch of aorta. Carotid pulsations are prominent in hypertension. Epigastric pulsations is seen in aneurysm of abdominal aorta.

Palpation: Thrill is a palpable murmur. It is associated with very loud murmurs and can be felt over the precordium or over major vessels in diseases. Left parasternal heave is sign present in right ventricular hypertrophy.

Auscultation: In mitral and tricuspid areas both the 1st and 2nd heart sounds are heard, but the 1st heart sound is better heard. In aortic and pulmonary areas both the 1st and 2nd heart sounds are heard, but the 2nd heart sound is better heard. Murmur is the vibration produced by the turbulence of flow in the heart. Similar sound produced at the level of blood vessels outside the precordium is called bruit. Opening snap and clicks are produced in valvular diseases. Any split in the 1st or 2nd heart sound should be also observed.

EXAMINATION OF HIGHER FUNCTIONS AND SENSORY SYSTEM

Name :
Age :
Occupation :
Address :

General Examination

Built and nourishment	:	Moderately built and adequately nourished
Height	:	
Weight	:	
Pallor	:	No pallor
Jaundice/Icterus	:	Not jaundiced
Cyanosis	:	Not cyanosed
Clubbing	:	No clubbing of fingers or toes
Lymphadenopathy	:	No significant lymph node enlargement
Edema	:	No edema
Skin and hair	:	Skin and hair healthy
Pulse	:	72/min regular, normal in volume, character and tension, no thickening of vessel walls, all peripheral pulsations are felt equally and normally on both sides and there is no brachiofemoral delay
Blood pressure	:	120/80 mm Hg in the right upper limb in supine position
JVP	:	Not raised
Respiratory rate	:	14/min, regular
Body temperature	:	37 °C

Higher Functions

General appearance and behavior	:	Normal
Level of consciousness	:	Conscious
Mental and emotional state	:	Cooperative
Delusions and hallucinations	:	No hallucinations or delusions
Orientation in place and time	:	Well-oriented in time, place and person
Memory	:	Normal
Intelligence	:	Normal
Sleep	:	Normal
Gait	:	Normal
Speech	:	Normal

Sensory System

Stereognosis :

Sense of position :

Joint Sense :

Touch, pain, temperature, tactile localization, two point discrimination, vibration sense (Table 15.1).

Sensory inattention :

Any abnormal sensations (pins and needles, numbness, tingling sensations, crawling of insects).

Impression: The higher functions and sensory system of the subject appears to be normal.

Stereognosis is the ability to recognize an object purely from the feel of its shape, size, texture, weight and form. Sensations could be lost in lesions of sensory pathways at any level. Cortical sensations like tactile localization, two point discrimination, stereognosis as well as joint position sense and vibration sense are lost in lessions of parietal lobe, where as the sensations like crude touch, pain and temperature probably appreciated at the thalamic level are preserved. In sensory inattention, he fails to appreciate the stimulus on one side of the body. This is seen in parietal lobe lesion, on the opposite side of body.

EXAMINATION OF MOTOR SYSTEM

Name :

Age :

Sex :

Occupation :

Address :

General Examination

Built and nourishment : Moderately built and adequately nourished

Height :

Weight :

Pallor : No pallor

Jaundice/Icterus : Not jaundiced

Cyanosis : Not cyanosed

Clubbing : No clubbing of fingers or toes

Lymphadenopathy : No significant lymph node enlargement

Edema : No edema

Skin and hair : Skin and hair healthy

Pulse : 72/min regular, normal in volume, character and tension, no thickening of vessel walls, all peripheral pulsations are felt equally and normally on both sides and there is no brachiofemoral delay

Blood pressure : 120/80 mm Hg in the right upper limb in supine position

JVP : Not raised

Respiratory rate : 14/min, regular

Body temperature : 37 °C

Higher Functions

General appearance and behavior :

Emotional state :

Delusions and hallucinations :

Sleep :

Orientation in place and time :

Table 15.1: Examination of sensory system

Sensation		Trunk				Limbs				Face	
		Front		Back		Upper		Lower		Rt	Lt
		Rt	Lt	Rt	Lt	Rt	Lt	Rt	Lt		
Touch											
Fine touch											
Crude touch											
Tactile localization											
Two point discrimination											
Vibration sense											
Pain											
Superficial pain											
Pressure pain											
Temperature	Heat										
	Cold										

Level of consciousness :
Memory :
Intelligence :
Gait :
Speech :

Motor System (Examine both Upper Limb and Lower Limb)

- Bulk of the muscle :
- Tone of the muscle :
- Strength (Power) of the muscle :

Muscles of upper limb (Fig. 15.7)

- Abductor pollicis brevis :
- Opponens brevis :
- Dorsal interossei :
- Interossei and lubricals :
- Flexors of the fingers :
- Flexors of the wrist :
- Extensors of the wrist :
- Brachioradialis :
- Biceps, triceps, supraspinatus
- Deltoid, infraspinatus :
- Pectoralis :
- Serratus anterior :
- Latissimus dorsi :

Muscles of the trunk

- Muscles of the abdomen :
- Erector spinae and muscles of back :
- Trapezius :
- Diaphragm :

Muscle of the lower limb (Fig. 15.8)

- Intrinsic muscles of foot :
- Flexors and extensors of toes and foot :
- Flexors of the knee :
- Extensors of the knee :
- Extensors of thigh :
- Flexors of thigh :

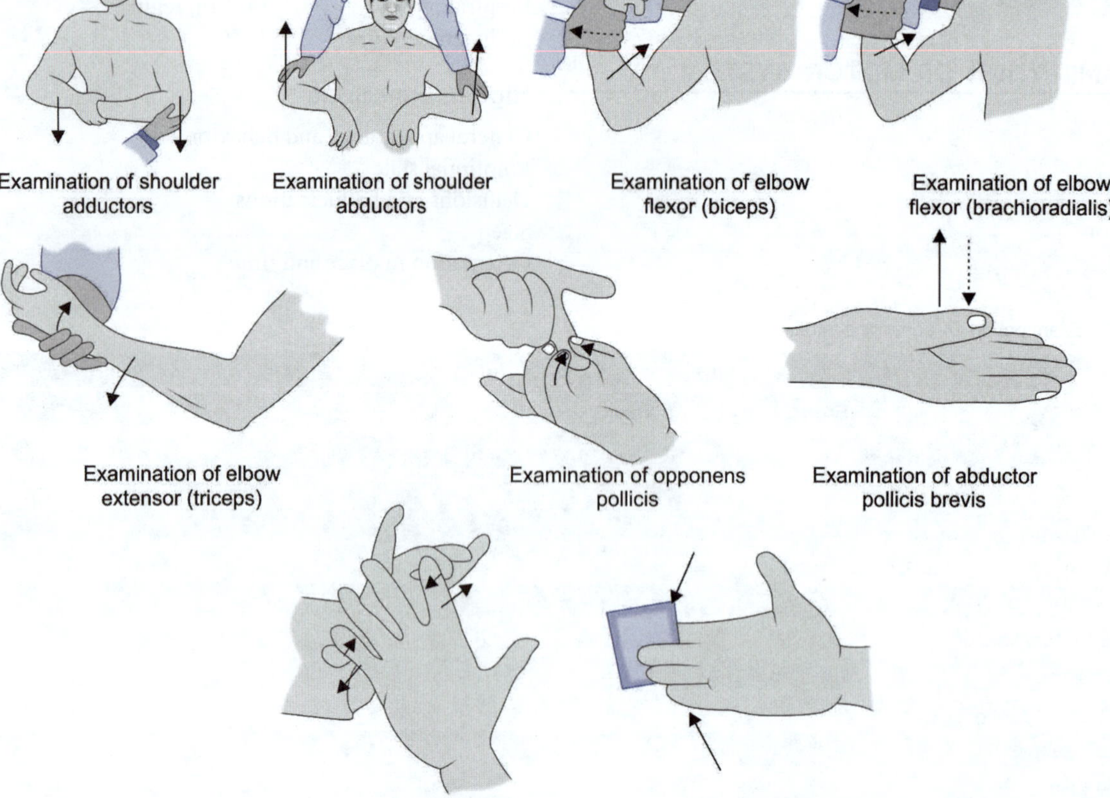

Fig. 15.7: Examination of power in upper limb

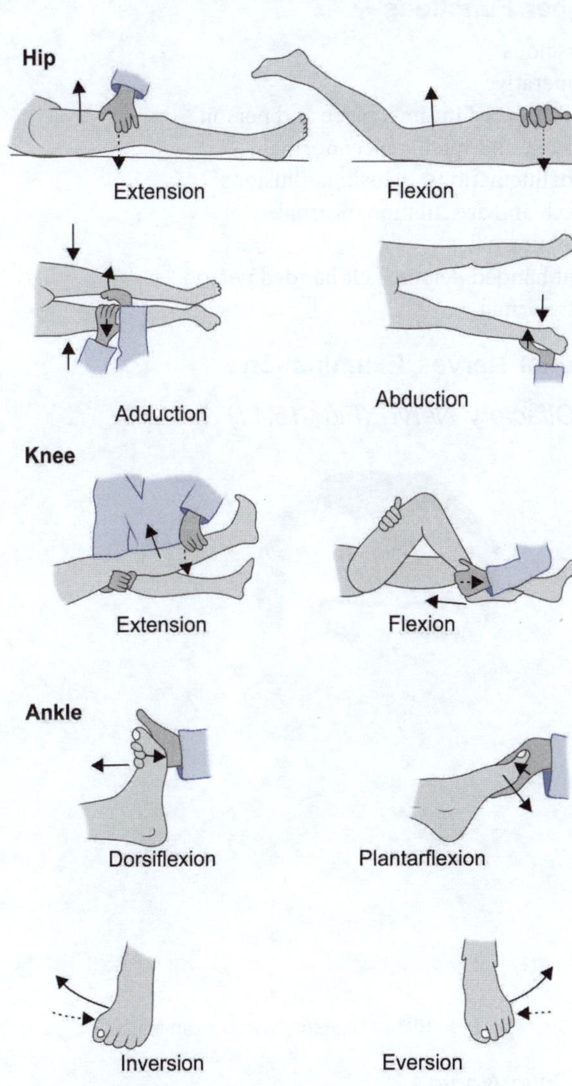

Fig. 15.8: Examination of power in lower limb

- Adductors of thigh :
- Abductors of thigh :
- Rotators of the thigh :

Coordination of Movements (Fig. 15.9)

Upper limb

- Finger-nose test
- Finger-to-finger test
- Rapid alternation movement (Dysdiadochokinesis)

Lower limb

- Straight line test
- Heel-knee test
- Romberg's test (Fig. 15.10)

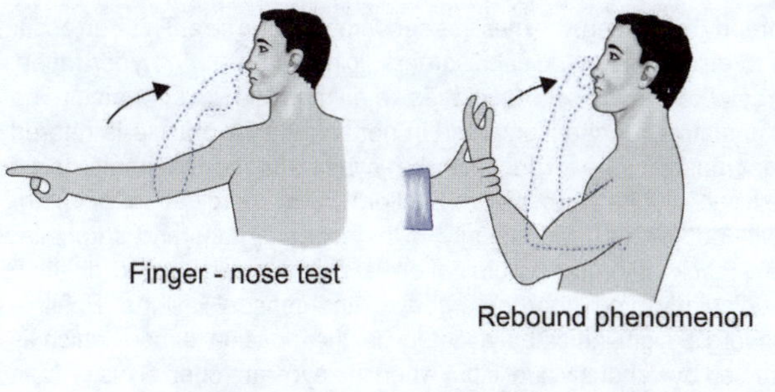

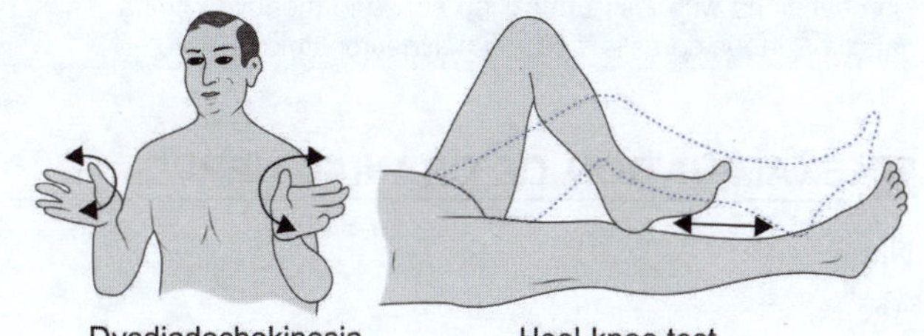

Fig. 15.9: Examination of coordination

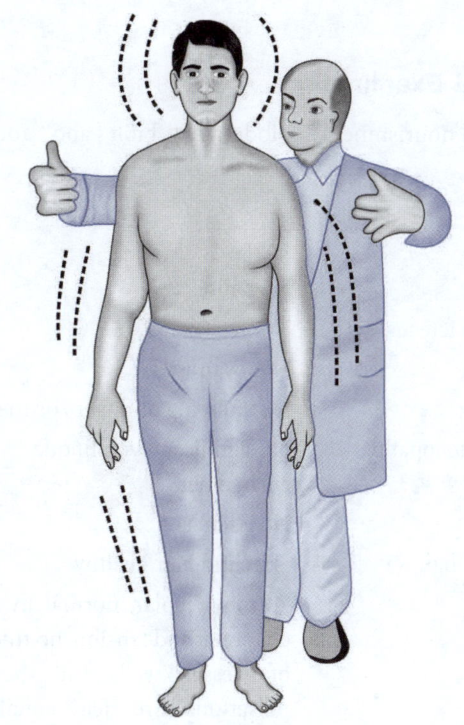

Fig. 15.10: Romberg's test

- Gait (spastic, drunken/ataxic festinant, high stepping, waddling, staming) :
- Motor cranial nerves :
- Involuntary movements (tremor, chorea, athetoses) :

Impression: The motor system of the subject appears to be normal.

PHYSICON—The Reliable Icon in Physiology

In atrophy or wasting, the muscles becomes small in size. This can occur due to disuse, neurological disorders, joint diseases. In hypertrophy, the bulk of the muscle increases, e.g. muscular dystrophies. The partial state of contraction found in normal healthy muscle is refered to as muscle tone. Tone can be hypertonia or hypotonia (read spasticity, rigidity from theory section). The coordination of motor activity depends on the integrity of the sensory paths and cerebellar tracts. Lack of proper coordination is called ataxia. Incoordination is particularly prominent in cerebellar and sensory lesions. Positive Romberg's sign indicates a defect in the position sense which is corrected by various visual input when the eyes are open. This is seen in conditions with loss of position sense in the lower limbs (sensory ataxia) - tabes dorsalis, sensory polyneuropathies.

EXAMINATION OF CRANIAL NERVE

Name :
Age :
Sex :
Occupation :
Address :

General Examination

Built and nourishment	: Moderately built and adequately nourished
Height	:
Weight	:
Pallor	: No pallor
Jaundice/Icterus	: Not jaundiced
Cyanosis	: Not cyanosed
Clubbing	: No clubbing of fingers or toes.
Lymphadenopathy	: No significant lymphnode enlargement
Edema	: No edema
Skin and hair	: Skin and hair healthy
Pulse	: 72/min regular, normal in volume, character and tension, no thickening of vessel walls, all peripheral pulsations are felt equally and normally on both sides and there is no brachiofemoral delay.
Blood pressure	: 120/80 mm Hg in the right upper limb in supine position.
JVP	: Not raised
Respiratory rate	: 14/min, regular
Body temperature	: 37 °C

Higher Functions

Conscious
Cooperative
Well-oriented in time, place and person
Memory and intelligence: normal
No hallucinations, delusions/illusions
Speech and articulation: normal
Sleep: normal
Right handed person/Left handed person
Gait: normal

Cranial Nerves Examination

1. Olfactory Nerve (Fig. 15.11)

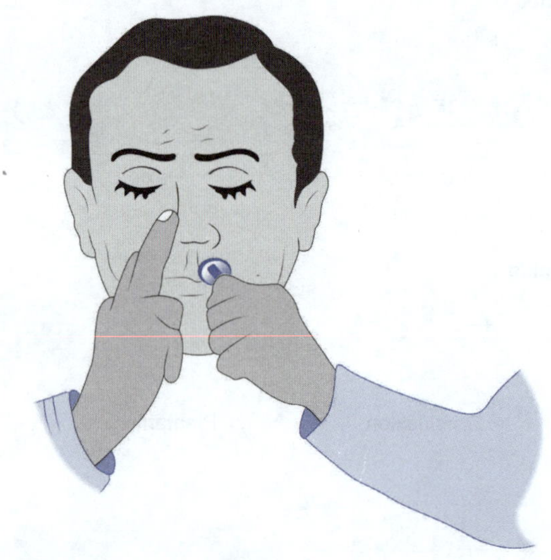

Fig. 15.11: Olfactory nerve examination

2. Optic Nerve

- Visual acuity
  - Distant vision (using Snellen's chart)
  - Near vision (using Jager's chart)
- Field of vision [Confrontation test (Fig. 15.12)]
- Color vision (using Ishihara chart)

3. Occulomotor (Fig. 15.13) 4. Trochlear 6. Abducent Nerves

- Presence of squint, nystagmus and ptosis
- Size and shape of pupil
- Ocular movements
- Light reflex
  - Direct
  - Indirect (consensual)
- Accomodation reflex

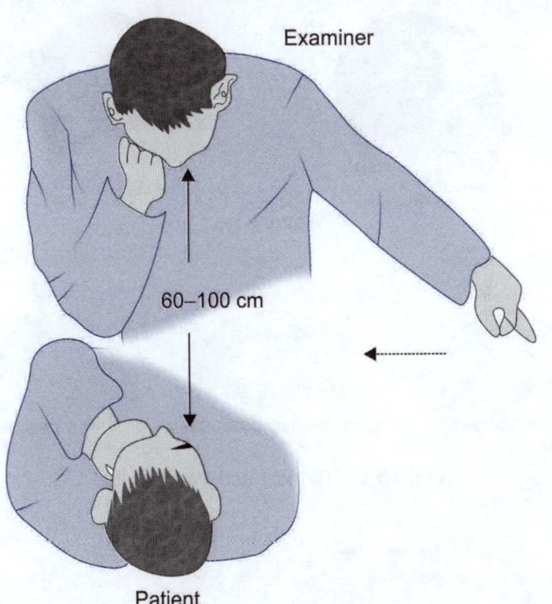

Fig. 15.12: Confrontation test

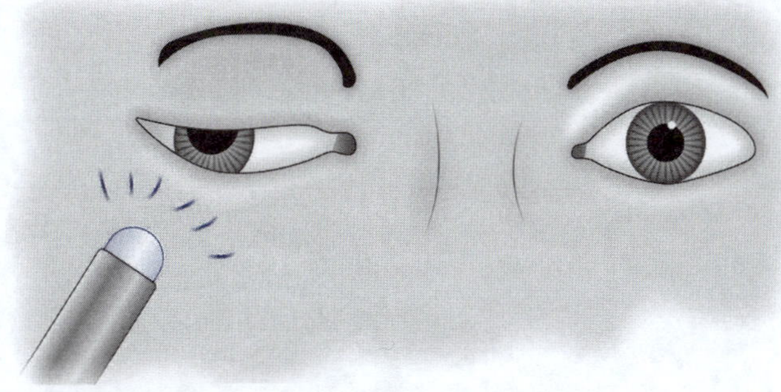

Fig. 15.13: 3rd nerve lesion, See ptosis, dilated and fixed pupil

Note: Both light reflex and accommodation reflex are included under pupillary reflexes.

5. Trigeminal (Fig. 15.14)

Test for sensory functions

- Sensations over face
- Corneal reflex
- Conjunctival reflex
- Jaw jerk

Test for motor functions

- Ask the patient to clench his teeth
- Ask the patient to open his mouth

7. Facial Nerve

Test for sensory functions (Fig. 15.15)

- Taste sensation over anterior two-third of tongue

Motor
Temporalis - with jaws clenched
Masseter - with jaws clenched
Pterygoids - with open mouth and fixed

1
2
3

Sensory
Test sensation of face both sides and each division

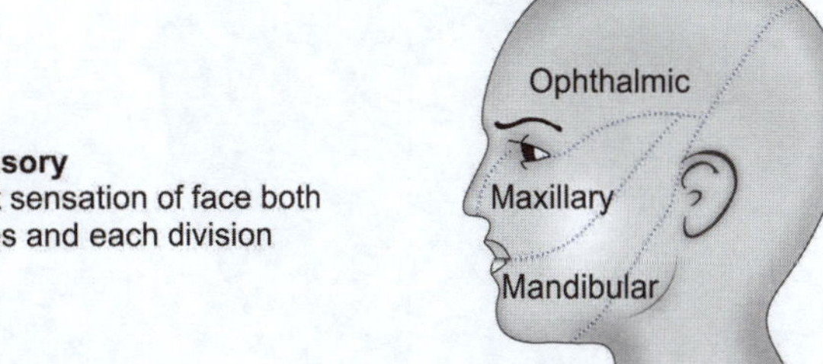

Reflex

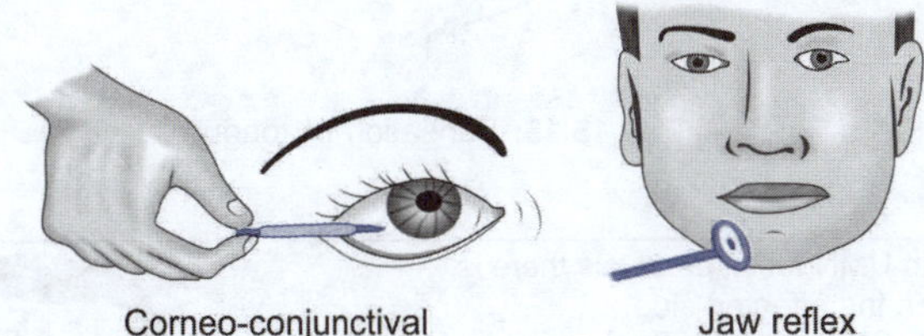

Fig. 15.14: 5th nerve examination

Test for motor functions (Fig. 15.16)

- Look for wrinkle over forehead
- Ask subject to close his eyes tightly and then tell him to open it against resistance
- Look for nasolabial folds on both sides
- Ask the subject to smile
- Ask the subject to inflate both cheeks (inflation test)
- Ask the subject to whistle

8. Vestibulocochlear Nerve (Fig. 15.17)

- Watch test
- Rinne's test
- Weber's test

9. Glossopharyngeal Nerve

Test for sensory functions

- Taste sensation over posterior 1/3rd of tongue
- Sensations in mucous membrane of soft palate and palate

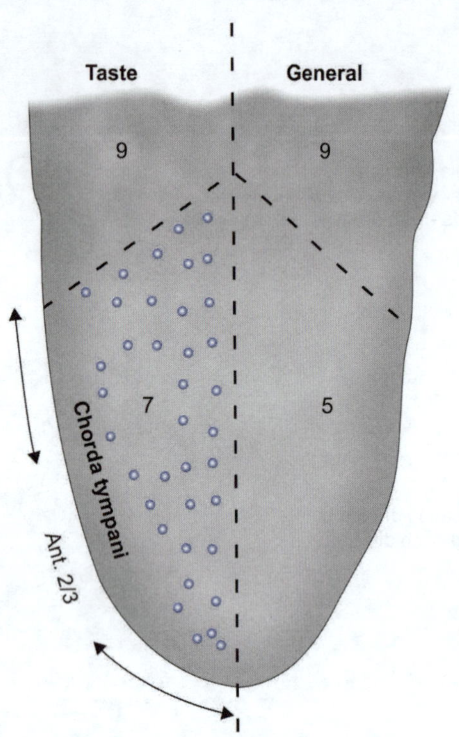

Fig. 15.15: Sensation of tongue

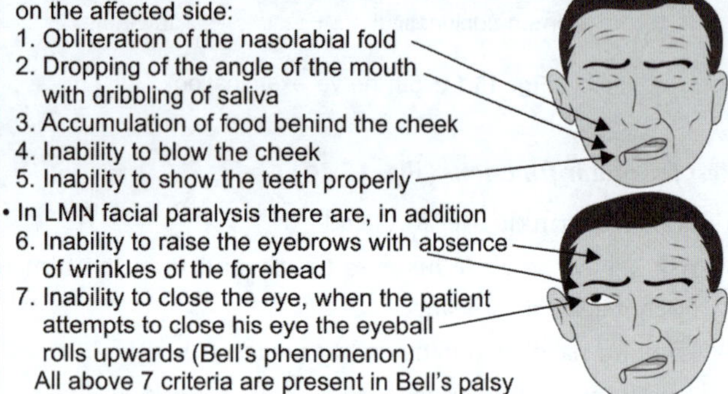

Fig. 15.16: Facial palsy

Test for motor functions

- Pharyngeal reflex (Gag reflex)
- Palatal reflex
- Nasal twang
- Nasal regurgitation
- Dysphagia and dysphonia

10. Vagus Nerve (Fig. 15.18)

- Nasal twang
- Nasal regurgitation

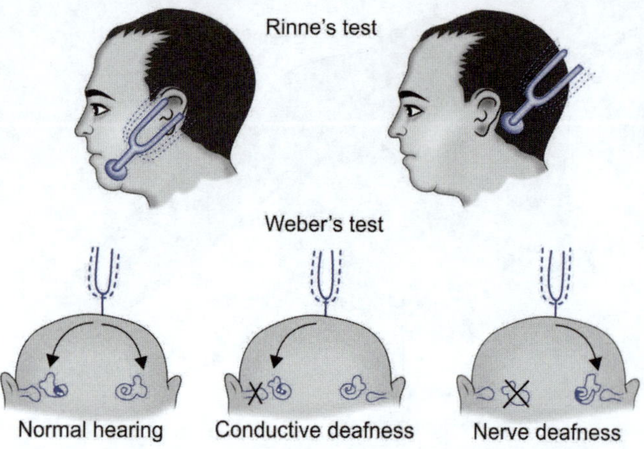

Fig. 15.17: Rinne's and Weber's test

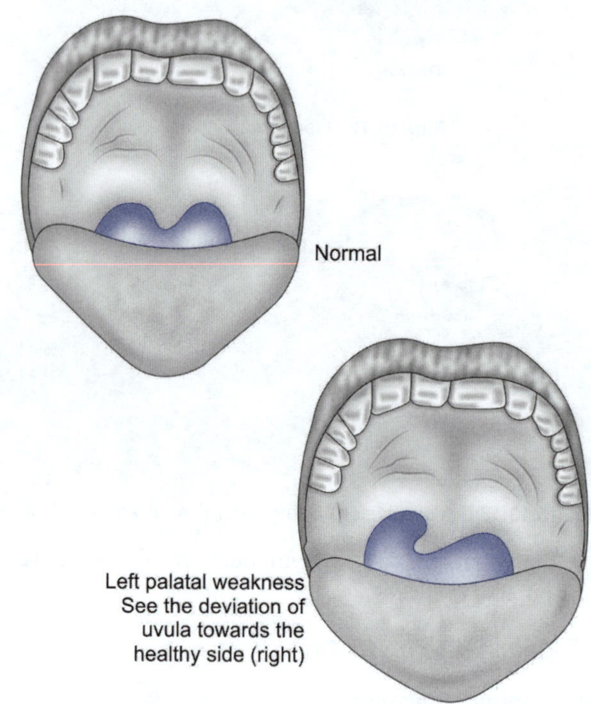

Fig. 15.18: Glossopharyngeal and vagus nerves

- Test palatal arch during phonation (by saying 'Ah')
- Deviation of uvula
- Pharyngeal reflex (Gag reflex)
- Palatal reflex

11. Accessory Nerve (Spinal) (Fig. 15.19)

- Ask the subject to shrug his shoulders against resistance
- Ask the subject to turn his head against resistance with a hand on side of face.

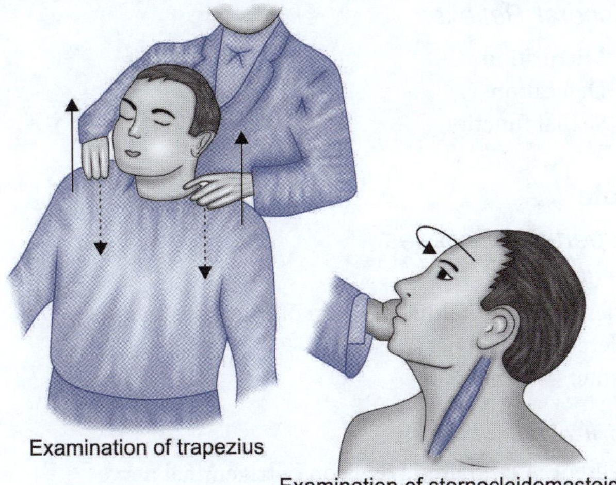

Fig. 15.19: Examination of 11th nerve

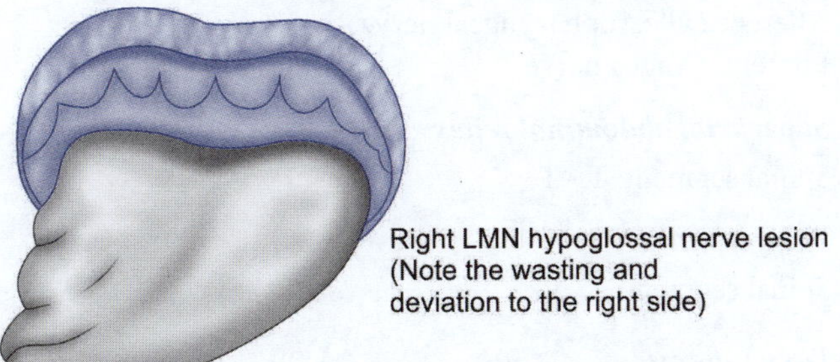

Fig. 15.20: Right hypoglossal nerve lesion

12. Hypoglossal Nerve (Fig. 15.20)

- Look for any deviation on protrusion of tongue
- Movements of the tongue
- Look for any fasciculation, wasting and tremors of tongue
- Look for protrusion of cheek on pushing with tongue

Impression: The cranial nerves of the subject appears to be normal.

Loss of sense of smell is called anosmia, which occurs as a result of common cold, frontal lobe tumors, head injury, etc. Parosmia is peverted sense of smell (e.g. pleasant smell may be felt as offensive smell). Read defects in field of vision, color vision from theory section. Squint (strabismus) is a condition in which the visual axis do not meet at the point of fixation. Nystagmus is involuntary conjugate, often rhythmical oscillations of the eyes, which may be horizontal, vertical or rotatory. Ptosis is drooping of the upper eyelid, usually due to paralysis of levator palpebrae superioris. Trigeminal nerve carries both motor and sensory fibers. Facial nerve consists of two parts. The larger motor part supplies all the muscles of facial expression. The smaller part comprises of special sensory component which carries taste fibers from the anterior two-third of the tongue and parasympathetic efferents to the salivary glands. Read UMN vs LMN facial palsy (see Figure 15.16). Eighth cranial nerve comprises of two components - auditory fibers which arise from the cochlea and subserve hearing, the vestibular fibers which arise from the saccule, utricle and semicircular canals and subserve equilibrium, balance and positional sense. In conduction deafness, bone conduction is better than air conduction (Rinne's test is negative). While doing Webers's test, in lesions of the inner ear of one side (sensory neural deafness) the sensation will be less on that side than on the normal side, i.e. the patient lateralizes or hears better in the healthy ear. In unilateral conductive deafness (disease of outer or middle ear) the sound is better heard in the abnormal ear because the conduction defect excludes background noise due to air conduction (sound is better heard in the abnormal affected side). IXth nerve has sensory and motor functions. The motor part of this nerve innervates middle pharyngeal sphincter and stylopharyngeus muscle. The sensory component carries taste fibers from posterior one-third of the tongue, soft palate and pharynx. Vagus nerve is a mixed nerve. The motor part of this nerve supplies the muscles of the soft palate, pharynx and larynx. The sensory fibers convey impulses from part of external auditory meatus and the pharynx. The vagus also carries parasympathetic fibers to heart, lungs and gut. Hypoglossal nerve is purely motor, supplying the tongue and the depressors of the hyoid bone.

EXAMINATION OF REFLEXES

Name :
Age :
Sex :
Occupation :
Address :

General Examination

Built and nourishment	: Moderately built and adequately nourished
Height	:
Weight	:
Pallor	: No pallor
Jaundice/Icterus	: Not jaundiced
Cyanosis	: Not cyanosed
Clubbing	: No clubbing of fingers or toes
Lymphadenopathy	: No significant lymphnode enlargement
Edema	: No edema
Skin and hair	: Skin and hair healthy
Pulse	: 72/min regular, normal in volume, character and tension, no thickening of vessel walls, all peripheral pulsations are felt equally and normally on both sides and there is no brachiofemoral delay.
Blood pressure	: 120/80 mm Hg in the right upper limb in supine position.

JVP : Not raised
Respiratory rate : 14/min, regular
Body temperature : 37 °C

Examination of Reflexes (Fig. 15.21)

Superficial Reflexes

Conjunctival

- Corneal
- Palatal
- Pharyngeal
- Abdominal
- Cremasteric
- Plantar

Deep Tendon Reflexes

- Jaw Jerk
- Biceps Jerk
- Triceps Jerk
- Supinator Jerk
- Knee Jerk
- Ankle Jerk

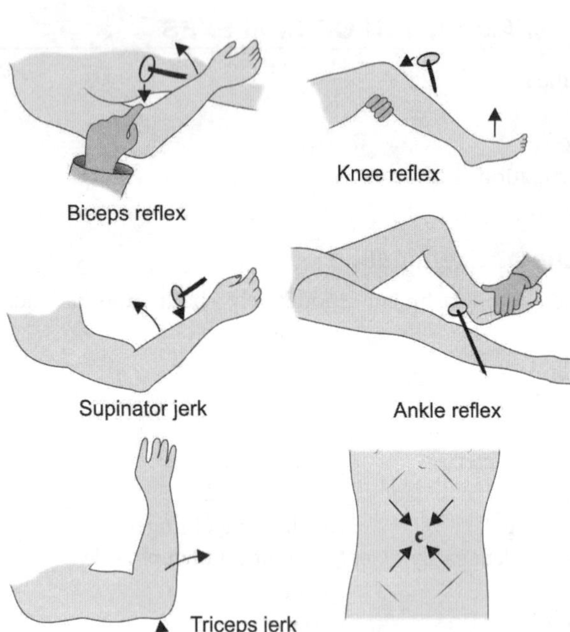

Fig. 15.21: Examination of reflexes

Visceral Reflexes

- Micturition
- Defecation
- Sexual function

Note

Superficial Reflexes

Conjunctival reflex

Afferent : Ophthalmic division of trigeminal nerve
Efferent : Facial nerve
Center : Pons

Corneal reflex

Afferent : Ophthalmic division of trigeminal nerve
Efferent : Facial nerve

Palatal reflex

Afferent : Glossopharyngeal nerve
Efferent : Vagus nerve

Superficial abdominal reflex

Spinal segment: T_7–T_{12}

Plantar reflex

Spinal segment: L_5, S_1

Deep reflexes

Knee jerk : L_2–L_4
Ankle jerk : S_1, S_2
Triceps jerk : C_6, C_7
Biceps jerk : C_5, C_6
Supinator jerk : C_5, C_6

Alterations in Tendon Reflexes

Absent or decreased in lesions affecting any part of the spinal reflex arc:

- ***Tabes dorsalis:*** Posterior root is affected
- ***Poliomyelitis:*** Anterior horn cells are affected
- ***Peripheral neuropathies:*** Sensory or motor neuron is affected

Hyper Reflexia

Exaggerated tendon reflexes are present in UMN lession (hemiplegia). Hyperreflexia may also occur in anxiety, nervousness and thyrotoxicosis, but usually bilateral in these cases.

Section 3

EXTRA MILE

CHAPTER 16

Multiple Choice Questions

GENERAL PHYSIOLOGY

1. **Glucose is transported into the cell by:**
   a. Simple diffusion b. Primary active transport
   c. Facilitated diffusion d. Endocytosis
2. **Resting membrane potential develops mainly due to:**
   a. K^+ efflux b. Cl^- influx
   c. Ca^{2+} influx d. Na^+ efflux
3. **Part of action potential that coincides with absolute refractory period is:**
   a. Depolarization
   b. Hyperpolarization
   c. Depolarization and 1/3 of repolarization
   d. After repolarization
4. **Decrease in colloidal osmotic pressure leads to:**
   a. Dehydration
   b. Edema
   c. No change in the body fluid
   d. Acidosis
5. **One of the following is not a second messenger:**
   a. NO b. cGMP
   c. IP3 d. cAMP
6. **Na-K pump contribution to RMP in excitable tissue is:**
   a. 4 mV b. 15 mV
   c. 60 mV d. 10 mV
7. **Depolarization in an excitable tissue may be due to the following factors except:**
   a. Na^+ influx
   b. Ca^{2+} influx
   c. Associated with increased membrane permeability to Na^+ in nerves and striated muscle
   d. K^+ influx
8. **Gap junctions are present in one of the following tissues:**
   a. Skeletal muscles b. Neurons
   c. Cardiac muscle d. Epithelial tissue
9. **Isotonic fluids should contain:**
   a. 300 mOsm/L b. 350 mOsm/L
   c. 10 mOsm/L d. 400 mOsm/L
10. **Minimum strength of stimulus required to elicit an impulse when applied for long duration is:**
    a. Chronaxie b. Rheobase
    c. Utilization time d. Threshold stimulus
11. **Cell shape and motility are provided by:**
    a. Microfilament b. Microtubules
    c. Golgi apparatus d. Both a and b
12. **A unique characteristics of smooth muscle is that:**
    a. It can sustain a contraction for prolonged periods
    b. Calcium is not required for contraction
    c. Repetitive contractions are not possible
    d. Myosin filaments are not required
13. **The ionic channels in excitable membrane are lined by:**
    a. Cephalins b. Proteins
    c. Lipids d. Carbohydrates
14. **ECF volume is measured by using:**
    a. Insulin b. Inulin
    c. Evans blue d. D_2O
15. **Cyclic AMP acts a second messenger in the secretion of all except:**
    a. FSH b. Estrogen
    c. Glucagon d. Epinephrine
16. **The most important buffer in the extracellular fluid is:**
    a. Hemoglobin b. Protein
    c. Phosphate d. H_2CO_3: HCO_3^-
17. **The substance essential for the transfer of fatty acids across mitochondrial membrane:**
    a. Creatine b. Creatinine
    c. Carnitine d. Coenzyme A
18. **Which of the following does not act intracellularly to produce physiological effects:**
    a. Triiodothyronine
    b. Inositol triphosphate
    c. Aldosterone
    d. Cyclic AMP
    e. Dopamine

19. **Ca^{2+} binding proteins are involved in excitation-contraction coupling in:**
a. Skeletal muscle b. Smooth muscle
c. Both d. Neither

20. **Aquaporin channels transport mainly:**
a. H_2O b. Na^+
c. Ca^{2+} d. Glucose

21. **Exocytosis requires**
a. Na^+ b. K^+
c. Ca^{2+} d. Mg^{2+}

22. **Microfilaments are made up of:**
a. Calmodulin b. Myosin
c. Actin d. Titin

23. **Gated ion channels open or close by:**
a. Alteration in membrane potential
b. Binding to an internal ligand
c. Binding to an external ligand
d. Depending upon lipid solubility of an ion

CIRCULATING BODY FLUIDS

1. **Hemophilia B (Christmas disease) is produced by deficiency of coagulating factor:**
a. VII b. V
c. IX d. X

2. **Which of the plasma protein is not synthesized primarily in the liver:**
a. Angiotensinogen b. Fibrinogen
c. Gamma globulin d. Prothrombin

3. **Normal lifespan of RBC:**
a. 1 hour b. 1 day
c. 1 week d. 120 days

4. **Colloidal osmotic pressure contributed mainly by:**
a. Albumin b. Fibrinogen
c. Thrombin d. Prothrombin

5. **Humoral antibody formation response is shown by:**
a. Neutrophil b. T lymphocytes
c. B lymphocytes d. Monocytes

6. **The following are present in circulating blood except:**
a. Fibrinogen b. Prothrombin
c. Thrombin d. Albumin

7. **Erythropoietin is secreted by:**
a. Stomach
b. Adrenal cortex
c. Kidney
d. Bone marrow

8. **Adult hemoglobin has:**
a. 2 alpha and 2 delta chains
b. 2 alpha and 2 beta chains
c. 4 alpha chains
d. 2 alpha chains

9. **The conversion of fibrinogen to fibrin is caused by:**
a. Prothrombin b. Thrombin
c. Plateletes d. Fibrin stabilizing factor

10. **Plasma osmolality in a normal adult (in mOsm/L) is:**
a. 250 b. 310
c. 280 d. 320

11. **Cyanosis occurs when the reduced Hb level in the blood is:**
a. More than 5 g/100 ml b. Less than 5 mg/100 ml
c. Less than 5 g/100 ml d. More than 5 mg/100 ml

12. **Conversion of prothrombin to thrombin requires:**
a. Factor X
b. Factor VII, X, V, Ca^{2+}
c. Factor V
d. Ca^{2+}, Va, phospholipid and factor Xa

13. **This is not a vitamin K dependent blood clotting factor:**
a. Factor I b. Factor II
c. Factor VII d. Factor X

14. **Kernicterus is a condition characterized by:**
a. Bilirubin deposition in basal ganglia
b. Excessive greed to eat meat
c. Severe anemia
d. Mild anemia

15. **Megaloblastic anemia is not a feature of the:**
a. Vitamin B_{12} (cyanocobalamine)
b. Folic acid
c. Iron
d. Gastric juice secretion

16. **With regard to blood transfusion:**
a. Transfusion cannot be done with one's own blood
b. ABO group antigens are present in the cytoplasm of the RBCs
c. ABO antigens are not present in any other tissue of the body
d. Cross matching is necessary before transfusion

17. **The total blood protein in 100 ml of blood is about:**
a. 7.3 g b. 23 g
c. 45 g d. 23 mg

18. **Megaloblastic anemia is due to the deficiency of:**
a. Vitamin C b. Iron
c. Vitamin E d. Vitamin B_{12}

19. **The biggest cell in the bone marrow is:**
    a. Reticulocytes
    b. Megakaryocytes
    c. Erythrocytes
    d. Metamyelocytes

20. **Which of the following is true about stored blood:**
    a. Decrease in intracellular Na
    b. Increase in intracellular Na
    c. Decrease in plasma K
    d. None of the above

21. **Microcytic hypochromic RBCs are seen in:**
    a. Hemorrhagic anemia
    b. Folic acid deficiency anemia
    c. Pernicious anemia
    d. Iron deficiency anemia

22. **Normal reticulocyte count in adult is ________ % of normal RBC count:**
    a. 0.1–0.2 b. 1–2
    c. 5–10 d. 10–12

23. **Decreased MCHC is found in:**
    a. Microcytic hypochromic anemia
    b. After acute hemorrhage
    c. Vitamin B_{12} deficiency
    d. Aplastic anemia

24. **von Willebrand factor has role in:**
    a. Platelet adhesion against injured vascular surface
    b. Activation of clotting factor
    c. Clot lysis
    d. Vasoconstriction

25. **Dicoumarol therapy inhibits synthesis of all the following factors except:**
    a. Factor IX b. Factor II
    c. Factor VII d. Factor I

26. **The fragility of RBC is decreased in all the following except:**
    a. Thalassemia
    b. Sickle cell anemia
    c. Spherocytic anemia
    d. Microcytic hypochromic anemia

27. **Macrophages are involved in the function of:**
    a. Destroying senescent red cells and catabolism of hemoglobin
    b. Phagocytosis of the organisms
    c. Releasing chemicals which are toxic to the larvae of the parasites
    d. Production of antibodies

28. **Lymphatics:**
    a. Collects and transports proteins and lipids from the intestinal spaces
    b. Exhibits bidirectional flow due to absence of valves
    c. Do not have any role to play in the defense of the body
    d. Drains directly into the arterial system

29. **Interleukins are secreted mainly by the:**
    a. RBCs b. Macrophages
    c. Hepatic cells d. Platelets

30. **Blood group of father being AA and mother BO, the child can belong to:**
    a. A and B b. B and AB
    c. O and A d. A and AB

31. **Citrate is useful anticoagulant because of its ability to:**
    a. Bind vitamin K b. Chelate calcium
    c. Bind factor XII d. Both a and b

32. **Increased erythrocyte production will occur in persons who:**
    a. Live at high altitude
    b. Have chronic pulmonary disease
    c. Experience hemorrhage
    d. All

33. **The integral membrane glycoprotein of human RBC is:**
    a. Porrin b. Ankyrin
    c. Spectrin d. Glycophorin

34. **Blood group antigens are:**
    a. Attached to plasma proteins
    b. Attached to hemoglobin molecule
    c. Found in saliva of all persons
    d. None

35. **Thromboxane A2 is released mainly by the:**
    a. Platelets b. Vascular endothelium
    c. Liver d. Muscles

36. **Reticulocytes are stained with:**
    a. Brilliant cresyl blue b. Sudan black
    c. Indigo carmine d. None

37. **Arneth count is:**
    a. Counting the lymphocytes
    b. Counting the lobes in the neutrophil
    c. Counting the granules in the eosinophil
    d. WBC counting in the bone marrow

38. **Iron is stored in the body in the following except:**
    a. RE system b. Spleen
    c. Gallbladder d. Bone marrow

39. What prevents blood loss after rupture of small blood vessels:

a. Vasoconstriction
b. Formation of fibrin threads
c. Formation of platelet plug
d. Production of hematoma to increase perivascular pressure
e. All of the above

40. Neutropenia is seen in all except:

a. Pernicious anemia
b. Bone marrow depression
c. Trauma
d. Megaloblastic anemia

41. The best screening test for hemophilia is:

a. BT b. PT (prothrombin time)
c. CT d. CRT

42. Hemoglobin is a buffer because of its:

a. Histidine residue b. Glycoprotein nature
c. Weak acidic nature d. Iron molecule

43. Mean life of RBC in transfused blood is (in days):

a. 120 b. 100
c. 60 d. 90

44. Lifespan of neonatal RBC is:

a. 120 days b. 100 days
c. 6 months d. 1 year

45. Heparin, an anticoagulant, is manufactured by:

a. Plasma cells b. Mast cells
c. Lymphocytes d. Blood platelets

46. When infection occurs in tissue, what type of WBC is first attracted from the blood into the tissue by the process of chemotaxis:

a. Neutrophils b. Monocytes
c. Eosinophils d. Basophils
e. Plasma cells

47. Which of the following reflects glycemic control in diabetics:

a. HbA b. HbA2
c. HbA1C d. HbC

48. For what aspect of blood cell production is vitamin-B_{12} essential:

a. Formation of hemoglobin
b. Extrusion of the nucleus from the normoblasts
c. Formation of DNA
d. Activation of erythropoietin
e. Promotion of iron absorption from the intestinal tract

49. Blood group antigens are:

a. Unconjugated proteins b. Glycoproteins
c. Amino acid derivatives d. Steroidal hormones

50. The cell membrane of human erythrocyte is more permeable to:

a. Cl^- than K^+
b. K^+ than Na^+
c. K^+ than urea

51. Aggregation of platelet is inhibited by:

a. Ca^{2+} b. ADP
c. Thrombin d. Prostacyclin

52. Neutrophil count tends to fall in all except:

a. Bacterial infection
b. Pernicious anemia
c. Drugs depressing bone marrow

53. Intrinsic factor is secreted by:

a. Liver
b. Chief cells of stomach
c. Parietal cells of stomach
d. Beta cells of pancreas

54. Stuart prower factor is factor:

a. VIII b. IX
c. X d. XII

55. Lymphocyte is how much % of white cell count:

a. 1–2% b. 80%
c. 20–40% d. 10%

56. Total blood volume is _____ % of body weight:

a. 8 b. 20
c. 40 d. 80

57. Human cell membrane is composed of:

a. Protein molecules
b. Carbohydrate and phospholipid
c. Lipoprotein mainly
d. Amino acid residues

58. Patients with anemia tend to have:

a. Decrease in cardiac output
b. Low oxygen tension in the arterial blood
c. Pallor of the mucous membrane

59. Iron deficiency anemia is:

a. More common in male than female
b. Caused by large pale erythrocytes
c. Followed by chronic blood loss from the body

60. Factor used in the extrinsic pathway of blood coagulation is:

a. V b. VIII
c. Tissue factor d. X

61. **Hemostasis is normally accomplished by or associated with:**
a. Polymerization of plasma fibrinogen molecule
b. Blood coagulation
c. Vascular spasm
d. Formaton of platelet plug
e. All of the above

62. **Anticoagulants that prevent coagulation when placed in a blood sample outside the body include all except:**
a. Citrate
b. Oxalate
c. Heparin
d. Coumarins

63. **Increased amounts of erythropoietin might be released from the kidneys in all cases except when the:**
a. Arterial pO_2 is normal and arterial O_2 content is reduced
b. Arterial pO_2 and arterial O_2 content are reduced
c. Arterial pO_2 is low and the saturation of hemoglobin with O_2 is much reduced
d. Tissue pO_2 and renal blood flow are both increased

64. **Which of the plasma protein has got the highest molecular weight:**
a. Fibrinogen
b. Albumin
c. Globulin

65. **What is the most important event in trival injury:**
a. Blood coagulation
b. Formation of platelet plug
c. Vascular spasm
d. Formation of thromboplastin
e. Formation of prothrombin activator

66. **Which is true about serum albumin:**
a. Contributes maximally to plasma oncotic pressure
b. It is anionic
c. Freely filterable in renal filter
d. Not synthesized in liver

67. **Decreased MCHC is found in:**
a. Microcytic hypochromic
b. Megloblastic anemia
c. Sideroblastic anemia
d. Vitamin B_{12} deficiency

68. **Blood clotting can be prevented by the use of potassium oxalate. It is due to:**
a. Checking of conversion of fibrinogen into fibrin
b. Inactivation of all factors for blood coagulation
c. Neutralization of acidic medium
d. Removal of free Ca^{2+} ion

69. **Histocompatibility complexes are the:**
a. Groups of proteins set to recognize antigen, by specific genes
b. Nonspecific antigen
c. Agglutination product of antibody-antigen reaction
d. Colonies of B and tumor cells

70. **Which one of the following is related to vasoconstriction produced by blood platelets during hemorrhage:**
a. 5HT b. Histamine
c. Thrombothenin d. Bradykinin

71. **After hemorrhage, restoration of blood volume is due to:**
a. Arterial constriction
b. Shift of intracellular fluid to extracellular space
c. Increased venous return
d. Intravenous infusion

72. **Structure of Hb is normal but decreased in amount in:**
a. Chronic blood loss c. Sickle cell anemia
c. Hemolytic anemia d. Thalessemia

73. **T lymphocyte differentiate into all except:**
a. Helper cells b. Plasma cells
c. Cytotoxic cells d. Suppressor cells

74. **Abnormality of hereditary spherocytosis lies in:**
a. Spectrin molecule b. CD4 Cells
c. Amino acid d. Hb

RESPIRATORY SYSTEM

1. **Compared with the apex of the lung, the base of the lung has:**
a. Same V/P ratio
b. A higher pulmonary capillary pO_2
c. A lower V/P ratio
d. A higher pulmonary capillary pCO_2

2. **Normal value of functional residual capacity is:**
a. 250 cc. b. 500 cc.
c. 1200 cc. d. 2200 cc.

3. **CO_2 is carried in venous blood mostly in the form of:**
a. Carbonic acid b. Bicarbonate
c. Dissolved CO_2 d. Carbamino Hb

4. **Most potent respiratory stimulant is:**
a. Oxygen b. CO_2
c. K^+ d. H^+

5. **Type II pulmonary epithelial cells secrete:**
a. Mucus b. Polypeptide
c. Serotonin d. Surfactant

6. **Which of the following change does not occur in high altitude acclimatization:**
   a. Reticulocytosis
   b. Increased serum cortisol
   c. Increased rate of respiration
   d. Decreased serum erythropoietin.

7. **Compliance of lungs is decreased in all conditions except:**
   a. Fibrosis of lungs b. Pulmonary edema
   c. Emphysema d. IRDS

8. **Alveolar ventilation is increased in:**
   a. In rapid shallow breathing
   b. In slow deep breathing
   c. While breathing under the sea with SCUBA apparatus.
   d. Immediately after hyperventilation

9. **The difference of amount of oxygen present in 100 ml of arterial blood and 100 ml of venous blood at rest is equal to:**
   a. 20 ml b. 5 ml
   c. 19.4 ml d. 14.4 ml

10. **The lung volume which cannot be measured by using spirometer is:**
   a. Residual volume
   b. Vital capacity
   c. Inspiratory reserve volume
   d. Tidal volume

11. **Oxygen content of saturated arterial blood is:**
   a. 11.2 ml/100 ml b. 25 ml/100 ml
   c. 19 ml/100 ml d. 14.5 ml/100 ml

12. **CA is found in:**
   a. Leukocytes b. Erythrocytes
   c. Plasma d. Lymphocytes

13. **The pO_2 of alveolar air is:**
   a. 40 mm Hg
   b. 158 mm Hg
   c. 104 mm Hg

14. **The respiratory center:**
   a. Is located in hypothalamus
   b. Is activated during swallowing
   c. Sends out regular rhythmic impulses to the respiratory muscle at rest

15. **Under normal respiratory conditions greatest resistance to air flow occurs in:**
   a. Alveolar duct
   b. Nose
   c. Large bronchi
   d. Terminal bronchiole

16. **In stagnant (ischaemic) hypoxia and histotoxic hypoxia, which of the following is abnormal:**
   a. Arterial pO_2
   b. Arterial O_2 content
   c. Arterial %-O_2 saturation of Hb
   d. A-V pO_2 difference

17. **Which of these are not lung capacities:**
   a. Inspiratory capacity b. TLC
   c. MVV d. FRC

18. **In restrictive type of lung diseases, VC:**
   a. Increases b. Decreases
   c. Normal d. May increase or decrease

19. **Which of the following shifts oxy-Hb dissociation curve to the left:**
   a. Increase in body temperature
   b. Increase in pH
   c. Increase in CO_2
   d. Increased 2,3 DPG

20. **The type of adrenergic receptor present in the smooth muscle of bronchi is:**
   a. Beta 1 b. Beta 2
   c. Alpha 1 d. Alpha 2

21. **Oxygen:**
   a. Carriage by fetal and adult hemoglobin does not differ in their capacity
   b. Transport increases if administered at high pressure
   c. Molecular combination with hemoglobin occurs with the same ease
   d. Is indicated for therapy in histotoxic hypoxia

22. **What is the primary function of pneumotaxic center located in the pons:**
   a. To limit the duration of inspiration
   b. Inhibition by vagal afferents
   c. To initiate basic rhythm of respiration

23. **Which of the following statement about pulmonary blood flow during exercise is true:**
   a. It increases by the same amount as systemic blood flow
   b. It increases less than systemic blood flow
   c. It decreases
   d. It does not change

24. **The dead space is what percent of the tidal volume:**
   a. 10% b. 1%
   c. 30% d. 50%

25. **Volume of air inspired and expired in each breath in normal respiration is called:**
   a. Total lung capacity b. Tidal volume
   c. Residual volume d. Inspiratory capacity

26. Inherent rhtymicity of respiration is controlled by neurons located in the:

a. Carotid body
b. Lungs
c. Reticular formation in the medulla
d. Pneumotaxic center

27. O_2 therapy is not effective in:

a. Histotoxic hypoxia b. Ischemic hypoxia
c. Anemic hypoxia d. Hypoxic hypoxia

28. Respiratory quotient of fat, protein and carbohydrate are respectively:

a. 0.7, 0.8, 1 b. 0.8, 0.7, 1
c. 0.8, 1, 0.7 d. 1, 0.8, 0.7

29. During starvation, the nonprotein RQ value is close to:

a. 1 b. 0.5
c. 0.25 d. 0.75
e. 0

30. Bohr effect is:

a. Effect of Zn on carbonic anhydrase activity
b. Effect of pCO_2 on oxyhemoglobin dissociation
c. HCO_3^- leaving the RBC in exchange of Cl
d. H^+ leaving RBC for each CO_2 that inters

31. Haldane effect is:

a. Binding of O_2 to Hb-favors exalation of CO_2
b. Binding of CO_2 to Hb-favors release of O_2
c. Important mechanism of O_2 trasport in body
d. All of the above

32. J receptors are situated in:

a. Heart b. Blood vessels
c. Alveolar interstitium d. Carotid body

33. Stimulation of baroreceptor leads to:

a. Increase in BP and heart rate
b. Decrease in BP and rise in heart
c. Increased intracranial tension
d. Decreased intracranial tension

34. Respiratory acidosis can cause:

a. Decreased pCO_2 and decreased pH
b. Increased pCO_2 and decreased pH
c. Increased pCO_2 and increased pH
d. Decreased pCO_2 and increased pH

35. The most important factor in transport of CO_2 as bicarbonate is:

a. Affinity to Hb
b. Basic nature of HCO_3
c. Increased solubility of CO_2
d. Carbonic anhydrase in RBC

36. Normal value of FEV1 % in an adult male is:

a. 80% b. 95%
c. 65% d. 50%

37. Sympathetic vasoconstrictor tone is diminished in response to increased activity of:

a. Carotid body chemoreceptors
b. Carotid sinus pressor receptors
c. Pain receptors
d. Medullary chemoreceptors.

38. Structures through which O_2 must diffuse in passing from alveolar lumen to hemoglobin:

a. Surfactant containing liquid
b. Alveolar membrane, basement membrane
c. Capillary endothelium, plasma and RBC membrane
d. All of the above

39. An increase in ventilation occurs in all situations except:

a. Fall in plasma bicarbonate
b. Sleep
c. Fall in pH of CSF
d. Rise in blood adrenalin level

40. During the initial part of inspiration which of the following does not occur:

a. Intrapulmonary pressure falls
b. Intrathoracic pressure rises
c. Intra-abdominal pressure rises
d. The partial pressure of O_2 in dead space rises

41. When the atmospheric pressure is halved which of the following is not likely to develop:

a. An increase in pulmonary ventilation
b. A fall in arterial pO_2
c. A fall in arterial pH
d. A rise in cerebral blood flow

42. The most important substance controlling alveolar ventilation is:

a. O_2 b. CO_2
c. H_2O d. None of the above

43. The diffusing capacity for CO_2 compared to that for oxygen is:

a. 20 times b. 10 times
c. 5 times d. 2 times

44. Total vital capacity is decreased but timed vital capacity is normal in:

a. Bronchial asthma
b. Scoliosis
c. Chronic bronchitis
d. All of the above

45. Compliance of lung is decreased in all conditions except:
a. Fibrosis of lung b. Emphysema
c. Pulmonary oedema d. Kyphosis

46. Arterial pO_2 is reduced in:
a. Anemia
b. KCN poisoning
c. Pulmonary hypoventilation
d. CO poisoning

47. Maximum voluntary ventilation is:
a. 20–50 L/min b. 50–75 L/min
c. 75–125 L/min d. 125–170 L/min

48. In cigarette smoking, surfactant is:
a. Increased
b. Decreased
c. Increased following decrease
d. Unaltered

49. CO_2 affects respiratory center via:
a. CSF H^+ concentration
b. Carotid body
c. Inflation and deflation receptors
d. Aortic body

50. Hyperbaric oxygenation is useful in all except:
a. Congenital heart disease
b. Gas gangrene
c. CO poisoning
d. Nitrogen toxicity

51. Chemoreceptor mechanism is not triggered in:
a. Anemic hypoxia b. Hypoxic hypoxia
c. Stagnant hypoxia d. Histotoxic hypoxia

52. Which of the following statements is correct:
a. Breathing and respiration are the same
b. Breathing results in intake of O_2 and removal of CO_2 from lungs
c. Breathing provides energy to the body

53. Exchange of gases between blood and alveolar air in the lungs occur by:
a. Simple diffusion b. Osmosis
c. Active transport d. All of these

54. In a normal adult, the ratio of physiological and anatomical dead space is:
a. 2 : 1 b. 1 : 3
c. 3 : 1 d. 1 : 1

55. O_2 transported from lung to tissues is:
a. 70% b. 86%
c. 91% d. 97%

56. When CO_2 is removed from the lungs which of the following also occur:
a. Efflux of HCO^-_3 from RBC
b. Efflux of Cl^- from RBC
c. Efflux of O_2 and influx of CO_2

57. When CO_2 in inspired air increases beyond 10% at atmospheric pressure it causes:
a. Decreased ventilation
b. Depression of CNS
c. Diminished sensory acuity
d. All of the above

58. Destruction of pneumotaxic center in pons causes:
a. Apnea
b. Forceful respiration
c. Apneustic respiration
d. Accelerated respiration

59. When under certain conditions the P50 value of hemoglobin rises, the affinity of the pigment for combining with O_2 will:
a. Remain the same b. Fall
c. Rise d. First rise, then fall

60. If under certain conditions the P50 value of hemoglobin rises to 100 mm Hg, a person will die of O_2 deficiency because the pigment:
a. Is not loading enough oxygen in the lungs
b. Can load enough oxygen in the lungs but cannot unload it in tissues
c. Can neither load or unload oxygen
d. Suffers degradation and cannot function normally

61. Work during normal respiration is mainly done for overcoming:
a. Lung elasticity
b. Respiratory air passages
c. Alveolar air spaces
d. Creating negative pleural pressure

62. Hypoxia may be characterized by:
a. Low arterial pO_2
b. Intense chemoreceptor response
c. Favorable response to 100% oxygen
d. All of the above

63. Oxygen therapy has significant value in all of the following types of hypoxia except:
a. Atmospheric hypoxia
b. Hypoventilation hypoxia
c. Hypoxia due to pulmonary edema
d. Hypoxia due to decreased hemoglobin in the blood
e. Histotoxic hypoxia due to cyanide poisoning.

64. Combination of hemoglobin with O_2 in the lungs can be promoted by:

a. Decreasing O_2 concentration in blood
b. Increasing O_2 concentration in blood O_2
c. Increasing CO_2 concentration in blood
d. Introducing CO_2 into the blood

65. Alveolar hyperventilation causes:

a. Respiratory acidosis b. Respiratory alkalosis
c. Metabolic acidosis d. Metabolic alkalosis

66. The partial pressure of oxygen in the arterial blood is normally lower than that of alveolar gas primarily because:

a. Lungs use oxygen
b. Blood moves through the lungs too fast
c. Oxygen requires a pressure gradient to diffuse into blood
d. Some portions of the lungs are ventilated but not perfused
e. Some portion of the lungs are perfused but not ventilated

67. Contraction of which of the following muscles is most important for causing forceful expiration:

a. Internal intercostal
b. Diaphragm and abdominal muscles
c. External intercostal
d. Sternocleidomastoid

68. For cyanosis to be manifested the amount of reduced hemoglobin in blood should be:

a. 1 g% b. 3 g%
c. 5 g% d. 7 g%

69. Respiratory movements are under control of:

a. Cerebral hemispheres
b. Cerebellum
c. Crura cerebri
d. Medulla oblongata

70. Which of the following can be measured by using the helium dilution method:

a. Functional residual capacity
b. Tidal volume
c. Dead space
d. Total lung volume

71. O_2 is transported from alveoli into blood in the pulmonary capillaries by:

a. Filtration
b. Secondary active transport
c. Facilitated diffusion
d. Passive diffusion

72. During quiet breathing which of the following discharge spontaneously:

a. Inspiratory neurons
b. Neurons in apneustic center
c. Expiratory neurons
d. Stretch receptors in the lungs

73. O_2 therapy is not effective in:

a. Hypoxic hypoxia b. Anemic hypoxia
c. Ischemic hypoxia d. Histotoxic hypoxia

74. Normal anatomical dead space is:

a. 250 ml b. 150 ml
c. 175 ml d. 200 ml

75. Respiration during exercise is regulated by:

a. Cerebral cortex b. Hypoxia at muscles
c. Joint proprioceptors d. All the above

76. The normal intrapleural pressure:

a. Is less negative during inspiration
b. Helps lung expansion
c. Reduces venous return to heart
d. Both a and b are correct

77. O_2 therapy is of significance in:

a. Pulmonary fibrosis
b. Cyanide poisoning
c. Sever anemia
d. Right to left shunt in heart

78. Pulmonary fibrosis would be expected to produce:

a. Histotoxic hypoxia
b. Stagnant hypoxia
c. Decreased vital capacity
d. Cyanosis
e. Emphysema

79. Airway resistance:

a. Is increased if the lungs are removed and inflated with saline
b. Does not affect the work of breathing
c. Is increased in paraplegic patients
d. Makes up 80% of work of breathing

80. Surfactant deficiency is the primary cause for:

a. Acute respiratory distress syndrome
b. Emphysema
c. Chronic bronchitis
d. Bronchial asthma

81. p50 is decreased by:

a. Fever
b. Increase in blood pH
c. Exercise
d. Acclimatization to high altitude

CARDIOVASCULAR SYSTEM

1. **T wave of ECG occurs:**
   a. At the beginning of atrial contraction
   b. After atrial contraction
   c. At the beginning of ventricular contraction
   d. At the end of ventricular contraction

2. **The QRS complex of ECG represents:**
   a. Atrial depolarization
   b. Atrial repolarization
   c. Ventricular depolarization
   d. Ventricular repolarization

3. **Cardiac index is cardiac output:**
   a. Per unit body weight b. Per unit surface area
   c. Per unit body volume d. Per unit time

4. **The most important cardiac and vasomotor center are located in:**
   a. Pons b. Medulla
   c. Hypothalamus d. Cerebellum

5. **The region of heart having the lowest inherent rhythmicity is:**
   a. SA node b. AV node
   c. Atrial muscle d. Ventricular muscle

6. **Parasympathetic stimulation:**
   a. Increases heart rate b. Decreases heart rate
   c. No effect on heart rate d. Initiates heart rate

7. **If all the nerves to the heart are cut, then heart will:**
   a. Beat rhythmically b. Stop
   c. Beat arrythmically d. Shrink

8. **In a healthy adult male, the diastolic pressure is:**
   a. 120 mm Hg b. 100 mm Hg
   c. 90 mm Hg d. 80 mm Hg

9. **The increase in vascular permeability responsible for 'wheal' formation in triple response is due to:**
   a. Serotonin b. Acetyl choline
   c. Histamine d. Adrenaline

10. **Closure of semilunar valves occurs at the onset of which phase of cardiac cycle:**
    a. Isovolumetric contraction
    b. Isovolumetric relaxation
    c. Rapid ejection
    d. Rapid filling

11. **A heart attack occurs when blockage takes place in artery carrying blood to:**
    a. Lungs b. Kidneys
    c. Heart d. Brain

12. **Maximum peripheral resistance is offered by:**
    a. Blood capillaries b. Arteries
    c. Arterioles d. Venules

13. **Negative bathmotrophic effect can be produced by:**
    a. Stimulation of vagus
    b. Section of vagus
    c. Stimulation of sympathetic chain
    d. Increasing the temperature

14. **Maximum blood flow in the left coronary artery occurs during:**
    a. Early ventricular systole
    b. Late ventricular systole
    c. Early ventricular diastole
    d. Late ventricular diastole

15. **ECG:**
    a. Helps in the diagnosis of serum K^+ abnormalities
    b. Is the direct recording of the ventricular muscle action potentials
    c. Is the recording of the SA nodal pace maker potentials
    d. Mean electrical axis is >110 degree in left axis deviation

16. **Cardiac output:**
    a. Can be measured by using echocardiography
    b. Is dependent on the length of the muscle fiber
    c. Decreases after adrenaline infusion
    d. Is not altered in digitalis administration

17. **When pulse rate is 100 per minute, R-R interval in ECG will be:**
    a. 0.8 sec b. 0.8 minutes
    c. 0.6 sec d. 1 sec

18. **During ventricular diastole blood pressure in the blood capillary is:**
    a. About 80 mm Hg
    b. About 120 mm Hg
    c. About 30 mm Hg
    d. About 100 mm Hg

19. **Thrombus means:**
    a. Increase in thrombocyte count
    b. Blood clot in a test tube
    c. Decreased thrombocyte count
    d. Blood clot inside a blood vessel

20. **Capacitance vessels are:**
    a. Aorta b. Large veins
    c. Capillaries d. Arterioles

21. **Normal coronary blood flow is:**
    a. 70 mL/min b. 250mL /min
    c. 5000 mL /min d. 1250 mL /min

22. The Jugular venous:

a. Pulse can not be seen in the people with normal heart
b. Pressure is typically raised in right ventricular failure
c. Pulse is not exaggerated in patients suffering from tricuspid incompetence

23. First HS occurs with:

a. Closure of aortic and pulmonary valves
b. Rapid ventricular filling
c. Closure of AV valves

24. Which of the following is NOT a property of cardiac muscle:

a. Excitability
b. Rhythmicity
c. Short refractory period

25. When the HR is 100 beats/min, the cardiac cycle time is:

a. 0.8 sec b. 0.8 min
c. 0.6 sec d. 1 sec

26. The EDV of ventricle increases when:

a. The person is upright
b. There is increase in venous tone
c. There is increase in intrapericardial pressure
d. There is decrease in ventricular compliance

27. Incisura in the aortic pressure curve is:

a. Because of increased aortic pressure
b. Associated with third HS
c. Rapid peripheral emptying
d. Backward flow of blood from aorta to ventricle

28. Fast response action potential is seen in:

a. SA node b. AV node
c. Ventricular muscle d. All the above

29. In which of the following, the blood flow is least during exercise:

a. Brain b. Heart
c. Skeletal muscle d. GIT

30. ST segment elevation in the ECG indicates:

a. 1° heart block b. 2° heart block
c. 3° heart block d. Acute MI

31. Tall T waves of ECG are associated with:

a. Hypernatremia b. Hypokalemia
c. Hyperkalemia d. Hyponatremia

32. The catecholamine useful for increasing the systolic pressure while treating circulatory shock is:

a. Dopamine b. Noradrenaline
c. Adrenaline d. Glutamine

33. Hypertension is a common complication of all of the following conditions except:

a. Anaphylaxis
b. Pregnancy
c. Cushing's syndrome
d. Posterior pituitary fossa tumor
e. Pyelonephritis

34. PR interval in an electrocardiogram is measured by finding the interval between the:

a. Beginning of the P wave and the beginning of the R wave
b. Beginning of the P wave and the beginning of QRS complex
c. End of P wave and end of QRS complex
d. End of P wave and beginning of the QRS complex

35. Stroke volume is increased by:

a. Digitalis in failing heart
b. Sympathetic stimulation
c. Stretched cardiac muscle fibers
d. Decreased systemic blood pressure

36. PR segment in the ECG corresponds to:

a. Time interval between onset of atrial contraction and onset of ventricular contraction
b. Time delay in the AV node
c. SA nodal conduction time
d. Ventricular depolarization

37. The first reactive change to occur after hemorrhage is:

a. Vasoconstriction
b. Tachycardia
c. Raised cortisol
d. Raised epinephrine

38. Blood flow through left coronary artery is:

a. Regulated by sympathetic vasodilator nerves
b. Increased when myocardial hypoxia is present
c. Greater during early systole
d. Decreased in reflex response to fall in blood pressure

39. Dicrotic notch in aortic pressure curve is:

a. Magnified by aortic regurgitation
b. Absent in arterioscle: rosis
c. Of no diagnostic value
d. Coincident with 2nd heart sound

40. What is not true of jugular venous pulse:

a. Pressure typically raised in right ventricular failure
b. Pressure typically raised in partial obstruction of SVC
c. Commonly visible in normal persons
d. Pulsations exaggerated in tricuspid incompetence

41. Capacitance is least in the following vascular segment:

a. Pulmonary artery b. Systemic artery
c. Systemic vein d. Pulmonary vein

42. What prevents blood loss after rupture of a very small blood vessel:

a. Vasoconstriction
b. Formation of fibrin threads
c. Formation of platelet plug
d. All of the above

43. Work performed by the left ventricle is greater than that performed by the right ventricle due to differences in:

a. Blood velocity b. Stroke volume
c. Arterial pressure d. Atrial pressure

44. The arterial pulse pressure in the femoral artery is normally:

a. Slightly less than the pulse pressure in the upper aorta
b. Greater than the pulse pressure in the upper aorta
c. Equal to the peak pressure in the upper aorta
d. One of the above

45. The Purkinje fibers:

a. Are myelinated axons
b. Do not have a very high conduction velocity
c. Have action potentials which has a long duration
d. All of the above

46. In athletes bradycardia is because of:

a. Decreased sympathetic tone
b. Increased vagal tone
c. Cardiac output
d. Low venous return

47. Velocity of transmission is fastest through following part of the heart:

a. AV node b. Bundle of His
c. Atria d. Purkinje fibers

48. Plateau phase of action potential curve of cardiac tissue is due to:

a. Opening of sodium channels
b. Opening of potassium channels
c. Opening of slow calcium channels
d. Closing of sodium channels

49. Tachycardia at the onset of exercise is due to stimulation of

a. Chemoreceptors b. Baroreceptors
c. Stretch receptors d. Joint proprioceptors

50. Left ventricular systole corresponds to:

a. Auricular diastole b. Auricular systole
c. ST wave of ECG d. P wave of ECG

51. During exercise, blood flow does not decrease in:

a. Cutaneous circulation
b. Hepatosplanchnic circulation
c. Coronary circulation
d. Renal circulation

52. Difference of pulmonary microcirculation from systemic is:

a. Resistance low; pulsatile flow
b. Resistance low; capillary pressure low
c. Capillary pressure high; pulsatile flow
d. None of the above

53. Heart rate is under the control of:

a. Vagus nerve
b. Autonomic nervous system
c. Both
d. None

54. Tricuspid valve is present between:

a. Right atrium and right ventricle
b. Two atria
c. Two ventricles
d. Left atrium and ventricle

55. When sympathetic nerve supply to heart is cut off, the heart rate will:

a. Increase b. Decrease
c. Show no change d. None

56. If heart is stimulated through its vagus supply, heart rate will:

a. Decrease b. Increase
c. Show no change d. None

57. The dicrotic notch on the aortic pressure curve is caused by:

a. Closure of aortic valve
b. Closure of tricuspid valve
c. Closure of pulmonary valve
d. Closure of mitral valve

58. PR interval is said to be prolonged if it exceeds:

a. 0.2 sec b. 0.25 sec
c. 0.30 sec d. 0.35 sec

59. Total blood volume is ______% of body weight:

a. 8 b. 20
c. 40 d. 80

60. Blood volume is greater in:

a. Aorta
b. Capillaries
c. Arteries and arterioles
d. Venules and veins

61. Blood brain barrier is made up of:

a. Astrocytes b. Oligodendrocytes
c. Oligodendroglia d. Microglia

62. Cerebrospinal fluid:

a. Has a pressure which is slightly lower than venous pressure in the recumbent position (5 cm H_2O)
b. Has the main function of protecting the brain from injury when the head is struck
c. Is an ultrafiltrate of plasma
d. Both a and b

63. Shock always involves:

a. External hemorrhage
b. Internal hemorrhage
c. Central nervous system
d. Decreased tissue perfusion

64. Plateau phase of plateau type of action potential is mainly caused by:

a. Sustained K^+ efflux b. Ca^{2+} influx
c. Na^+ influx d. Na^+-K^+ pump

65. Mean blood pressure is:

a. Systolic blood pressure + diastolic blood pressure/2
b. Systolic blood pressure–diastolic blood pressure
c. Systolic blood pressure + 1/3 pulse pressure
d. Diastolic blood pressure + 1/3 pulse pressure

66. Normal adult lumbar CSF pressure in mm CSF is:

a. 5–100 b. 70–180
c. 100–200 d. 200–280

GASTROINTESTINAL SYSTEM

1. Vitamin B_{12} is absorbed primarily in:

a. Stomach b. Duodenum
c. Jejunum d. Ileum

2. Following statement about colon is incorrect:

a. Movement include segmentation contraction
b. Mass peristalsis present
c. Net absorption of K^+ occurs
d. Net secretion of HCO^-_3 occurs

3. The following are some of the gastrointestinal hormones except:

a. Secretin b. VIP
c. Trypsin d. Villikinin

4. Which one of the following statement is correct:

a. Salivary secretion per day is about 1500 ml
b. Gastric secretion per day is about 2500 ml
c. Bile secretion per day is about 500 ml
d. All the above are correct

5. Which of the following is not an enzyme of digestive system:

a. Enterokinase b. Amylase
c. Trypsin d. Streptokinase

6. Intrinsic factor is secreted in:

a. Intestine b. Pancreas
c. Stomach d. Liver

7. Chymotrypsin acts upon:

a. Starch in duodenum
b. Proteins in stomach
c. Proteins in duodenum in alkaline medium
d. Proteins in duodenum in acidic medium

8. Gallbladder is stimulated by:

a. Enterogastrone b. Secretin
c. CCK d. Enterokinase

9. Dysphagia means:

a. Loss of speech
b. Inhibition of breathing
c. Difficulty in breathing
d. Difficulty in swallowing

10. The major mediator for gastric acid HCl secretion during cephalic phase is:

a. Histamine b. Gastrin
c. Somatostatin d. ACh

11. Vomiting is NOT associated with the following event:

a. Contraction of the lower esophageal sphincter
b. Deep breath
c. Closure of glottis
d. Elevation of the soft palate

12. All are pancreatic enzymes except:

a. Chymotrypsinogen b. Trypsinogen
c. Amylase d. Insulin

13. The inhibition of gastric juice secretion is brought about by:

a. Food b. Cholecytokinin
c. Acetylcholine d. Gastrin

14. Parietal cell is stimulated by all the following except:

a. Insulin
b. Gastrin
c. Stretch of stomach wall
d. Histamine

15. This is the main function of large intestine:

a. Absorption of proteins
b. Digestion of proteins
c. Absorption of water and electrolytes
d. Digestion and absorption of fats

16. **Which salivary gland contributes to maximum quantity of saliva secreted:**
    a. Parotid
    b. Submandibular
    c. Sublingual
17. **The potent choleretic agent is:**
    a. Gastrin b. Secretin
    c. Bile salts d. Glucagon
18. **Submandibular glands are:**
    a. Serous gland
    b. Mucous gland
    c. Mixed gland
    d. Predominating mucous gland
19. **Liver bile and gallbladder bile have the respective pH as:**
    a. 6.4–7.2 and 8.6–9.4 b. 8.2–9.0 and 4.2–6
    c. 6–7 and 8-9 d. 7.8–8.6 and 7.0–7.4
20. **In which of the following jaundice do we see biphasic reaction to Van Den Bergh test:**
    a. Prehepatic jaundice b. Hemolytic jaundice
    c. Hepatic jaundice d. Posthepatic jaundice
21. **Urinary bilirubin is absent in which type of jaundice:**
    a. Hepatic jaundice b. Hemolytic jaundice
    c. Obstructive jaundice d. Prehepatic jaundice
22. **Stimulation of the parasympathetic nerve to the salivary glands cause:**
    a. Profuse secretion of watery saliva
    b. Xerostomia
    c. Profuse secretion of mucinous saliva
    d. Produces no change
23. **Potent stimulus for bile secretion:**
    a. Bilirubin b. Biliverdin
    c. Secretin d. Bile salts
24. **Which of the following is seen in obstructive jaundice:**
    a. Excess of urobilinogen
    b. Excess of unconjugated serum bilirubin
    c. Excess of bile salts in the urine
    d. All of the above
25. **The enzyme primarily responsible for protein degradation in stomach is:**
    a. Trypsin
    b. Pepsin
    c. Chymotrypsin
26. **Antiperistalsis may sometimes be seen in:**
    a. Stomach b. Ileum
    c. Colon d. None
27. **Glycogenolysis in muscle does not raise blood sugar level due to lack of:**
    a. Lactate dehydrogenase
    b. Pyruvate kinase
    c. G-6-phosphatase
    d. Argininosuccinase
28. **Infant's gastric juice pH is:**
    a. Generally high
    b. Generally low
29. **The rate of absorption of sugars by small intestine is highest for:**
    a. Disaccharides b. Polysaccharides
    c. Hexoses d. Pentose
30. **Which of the following is not secreted by the pancreas:**
    a. Procarboxypeptidases b. Trypsinogen
    c. Phospholipase A d. Pepsinogen
31. **Which of the following is found in conjunction with bile acids:**
    a. Cholic acid b. Pregnenolone
    c. Glycine d. Cholylacetyl CoA
32. **Alpha amylase acts on which bond**
    a. Alpha 1- 4 bond b. Alpha 1- 6
    c. Beta 1- 4 d. Beta 1- 6
33. **The gastric phase of gastric secretion is brought about by:**
    a. Neural factors
    b. Hormonal factors
    c. Gastric distension
    d. Presence of proteins in the stomach
    e. All of the above
34. **Gastric secretion is stimulated by all of the following except:**
    a. Secretin b. Gastric distension
    c. Gastrin d. Vagal stimulus
35. **Most potent stimulus for secretion of secretin is:**
    a. Dilatation of intestine b. Acid chyme
    c. Protein d. Fat
36. **Gastric emptying is decreased, by all except:**
    a. Fatty meal
    b. Hyperosmolarity in duodenum
    c. Distension of the duodenum
    d. Vagal stimulation
37. **Vagal stimulation following intake of food does not affect secretion of:**
    a. Stomach b. Pancreas
    c. Parotid gland d. Gallbladder

38. **Brunner's glands are located in:**
a. Mucosa of duodenum
b. Stomach
c. Pancreas

39. **Small intestinal peristalsis is controlled by:**
a. Myenteric plexus b. Meissner's plexus
c. Vagus nerve d. Parasympathetic system
e. Both a and b

40. **Fat is maximally absorbed in:**
a. Ileum b. Colon
c. Stomach d. Jejunum

41. **The enzyme that acts on milk is:**
a. Rennin b. Renin
c. Lipase d. Amylase

42. **Which of the following is not produced from intestine:**
a. Gastrin b. Enterogastrone
c. Secretin d. Pancreozymin

43. **Emulsification of fat by bile occurs in:**
a. Liver b. Pancreas
c. Duodenum d. Stomach

44. **Digestion of fats, proteins and carbohydrates is completed in:**
a. Liver b. Large intestine
c. Stomach d. Small intestine

45. **Fat splitting enzyme is not present in:**
a. Saliva b. Pancreatic juice
c. Succus entericus d. Gastric

46. **Which cells of gastric mucosa secrete pepsinogen:**
a. Parietal cells b. Argentaffin cells
c. Goblet cells d. Zymogen (chief) cells

47. **A large greasy smelly stool usually indicates failure of digestion of:**
a. Carbohydrates b. Fats
c. Proteins d. Peptones

48. **Pancreatic juice takes part in digestion of:**
a. Proteins, carbohydrates
b. Proteins and fats, carbohydrates
c. Proteins and fats
d. Proteins only

49. **Trypsin differs from pepsin in that:**
a. It digests proteins in alkaline medium and not in acid medium
b. It digests proteins in acidic medium and not in alkaline medium
c. Both of these
d. None of these

50. **Stored fat is usually transported from one part of the body to another in the form of:**
a. Triglyceride b. Free fatty acids
c. Glycerol d. Neutral fat
e. Cholesterol

51. **Emulsification of fats is brought about by:**
a. Bile pigments b. Bile salts
c. Vitamin B_{12} d. HCI

52. **Removal of entire colon would be expected to cause:**
a. Malnutrition b. Megaloblastic anemia
c. Jaundice d. None.

53. **Vomiting center is situated in the:**
a. Hypothalamus b. Amygdala
c. Pons d. Medulla

54. **Which is essential for absorption of glucose from complex carbohydrates:**
a. Salivary amylase b. Enterokinase
c. Na^+- K^+ ATPase d. Secretin

55. **Wharton's ducts are associated with:**
a. Parotid glands
b. Submaxillary gland
c. Sublingual glands

56. **Paneth cells are found in:**
a. Crypts of Lieberkuhn b. Peyer's patches
c. Organ of Corti d. Islet of Langerhans

57. **Conversion of starch into maltose is brought about by:**
a. Invertase b. Diastase
c. Zymase d. Lipase

58. **Obstructive jaundice is caused by:**
a. Defective pancreas
b. Impacted-gallstone in common bile duct
c. Liver deficiency
d. When bile is not removed from the blood

59. **Fatty acids can be absorbed only in the presence of:**
a. Glycerol b. Lipase
c. Bile salts d. Bile pigments

60. **Products of digestion that enter the lacteals of villi of small intestine are poured into:**
a. Jugular vein b. Left jugular vein
c. Lymphatic vessels d. Hepatic portal vein

61. **Products of digestion that enter the capillaries of villi of small intestine are carried to the liver via:**
a. Jugular vein
b. Left jugular vein
c. Lymphatic vessels
d. Hepatic portal vein

62. Glycerol is one of the digestive products of:
a. Carbohydrates b. Fats
c. Proteins d. Nucleic acids

63. The inactive trypsin is converted to active trypsin by:
a. HCl b. Enterokinase
c. a and b d. None of these

64. Peristaltic waves are integrated by:
a. Meisner's plexus
b. Auerbach's plexus
c. Circular muscle fraction is
d. Longitudinal muscle fibers

65. Pancreozymin stimulates increase of:
a. Pancreatic juice rich in bicarbonate
b. Pancreatic juice rich in enzymes
c. Gastric juice
d. Bile from liver

66. The primary contractile pattern of small intestine during digestive period is:
a. Segmentation b. Peristalsis
c. Retropulsion d. Pendular movements

67. Gallbladder function does not include:
a. Storage of bile b. Acidification of bile
c. Concentration of bile d. Secretion of bile

68. The GIT secretion without hormonal regulation is:
a. Bile
b. Saliva
c. Small intestinal juice
d. Gastric hydrochloric acid

69. Mass peristalisis is seen in:
a. Stomach b. Rectum
c. Colon d. Small intestine

RENAL PHYSIOLOGY

1. Sodium reabsorption from distal tubule will be increased if there is an increase in:
a. Plasma potassium concentration
b. Plasma volume
c. Mean arterial pressure
d. Urine flow rate

2. Glomerular filtration rate is decreased by the following:
a. An increase in glomerular capillary pressure
b. A decrease in plasma oncotic pressure
c. A decrease in intrarenal pressure
d. An increase in plasma protein concentration

3. Renal plasma flow is:
a. 125 ml/min b. 700 ml/min
c. 500 ml/min d. 1250 ml/min

4. Assuming GFR is 125 ml/min and plasma glucose level is 100 mg%, the amount of glucose filtered by glomerular membrane in 10 min would be:
a. 125 mg b. 1.25 g
c. 2 g d. 2.5 g

5. Which of the following statements about the PCT is false?
a. About 60% of water is reabsorbed here
b. Glucose is completely reabsorbed here
c. Hydrogen ions are secreted here
d. The fluid leaving the PCT is hypotonic

6. More than two-third of the salt and water from the glomerular filtrate in the kidney is absorbed from:
a. PCT b. Loop of Henle
c. DCT d. Collecting duct

7. When dialysis is done in a patient with renal failure, the dialyzing fluid will contain:
a. Creatinine b. Urea
c. No creatinine or urea d. RBCs

8. Which of the following is not an example for osmotic diuretic:
a. Urea b. Glucose
c. Chlorthiazide d. Mannitol

9. The normal inulin clearance is about:
a. 126 ml/min b. 80 ml/min
c. 650 ml/min d. 1.5 liters

10. ADH acts on:
a. PCT b. Urinary bladder
c. Collecting ducts d. Loop of Henle

11. Renal threshold for glucose is:
a. 160 mg/100 ml of blood b. 120 mg/100 ml of blood
c. 180 mg/100 ml of blood d. 375 mg/100 ml of blood

12. Net filtration pressure in kidney:
a. 20 mm Hg b. 10 mm Hg
c. 30 mm Hg d. 15 mm Hg

13. Severe diarrhea leads to:
a. A decreased K^+ contents of the body fluid
b. Alkalosis
c. Increased Na^+ contents of the body

14. The substance used to measure GFR should be:
a. Freely filtered b. Should be reabsorbed
c. Should be secreted d. Both a and c are correct

15. **The normal RBF is:**
a. 1400 ml/min b. 1273 ml/min
c. 1500 ml/min d. 1000 ml/min

16. **Inulin is used to measure:**
a. RBF b. RPF
c. Urinary volume d. GFR

17. **ADH secretion is induced by all the following except:**
a. Stress b. Dehydration
c. Hypovolemia d. Hyponatremia

18. **Which one of the following is not suitable for the substance used in measuring GFR:**
a. Will be stored in kidney
b. It should not be toxic and biologically inert
c. It should not have an effect on filtration rate
d. It should not be metabolized in the body

19. **TmG in male is:**
a. 375 mg/min b. 200 mg/min
c. 180 mg/100 ml of blood d. 400 mg/min

20. **Which is the loop diuretic among the following:**
a. Spironolactone b. Furosemide
c. Chlorothiazide d. Ethanol

21. **Renin is released from the juxtaglomerular apparatus when afferent arteriolar:**
a. Hydrostatic pressure increases
b. Hydrostatic pressure decreases
c. Oncotic pressure increases
d. Oncotic pressure decreases

22. **Glucose transport in the PCT of kidney takes place by:**
a. Active transport
b. Passive transport
c. Bulk flow
d. Secondary active transport

23. **Which of the following causes the greatest increase in the amount of K^+ excreted in the urine:**
a. Mannitol b. Calcium chloride
c. Aldactone d. Furosemide
e. Ethanol

24. **GFR is increased when:**
a. Plasma oncotic pressure is increased
b. Glomerular hydrostatic pressure is increased
c. Tubular hydrostatic pressure is increased
d. Renal blood flow is increassed

25. **Where is active Na^+-K^+-$2Cl^-$ pump located:**
a. Proximal tubule
b. Thick ascending limb of loop of Henle
c. Distal convoluted tubule

26. **In renal glycosuria, the renal thresold for glucose is:**
a. Low b. High
c. Same d. Greatly increased

27. **Major portion of glomerular filtrate is reabsorbed in:**
a. Loop of Henle b. Distal convoluted tubule
c. Collecting duct d. Proximal segment

28. **Regarding potassium reabsorption in kidneys all are true except:**
a. Partly in PCT and loop of Henle
b. Under the influence of ADH
c. Coupled with sodium loss
d. Only in PCT.

29. **Ammonia in the kidney tubules is excreted in exchange for**
a. HCO_3^- b. Na^+
c. Cl^- d. PO_4^{3-}

30. **Two substances that can be used to determine filtration fraction are:**
a. Insulin and mannitol b. Urea and diodrast
c. PAH and phenol red d. Diodrast and PAH

31. **Diuresis is caused by:**
a. Mannitol b. Glycerol
c. Urea d. All of the above

32. **Where in the kidney does active reabsorption of sodium ions occur:**
a. Collecting duct
b. Distal tubule
c. Ascending limb of loop of Henle
d. All of the above
e. Both b and c

33. **One of the following does not form filtration barrier in nephrons:**
a. Mesangium
b. Podocytes
c. Endothelial cells
d. Parietal layer of Bowman's capsule

34. **Blood flows in glomerular capillaries with a pressure of about:**
a. 30 mm Hg b. 60 mm Hg
c. 15 mm Hg d. 18 mm Hg

35. **What is the normal urea clearance (nearest correct value):**
a. 4.4 ml/min
b. 88 ml/min
c. 440 ml/min
d. 44 ml/min
e. 22 ml/min

36. Automatic bladder is seen in:

a. Spinal shock
b. Cauda equina lesion
c. Filum terminale lesion
d. Superior sagittal sinus thrombosis

37. The major source of NH_3 produced by the kidney is:

a. Glycine b. Alanine
c. Glutamine d. Uric acid

38. If the renal plasma flow is 600 ml /min and the hematocrit is 40%, what is the renal blood flow in ml/min (nearest value):

a. 1,500 b. 1,000
c. 960 d. 1,800

39. The glomerular filtration rate is regulated primarily by:

a. Glomerular capillary pressure
b. Glomerular capillary blood flow
c. Plasma-colloid osmotic pressure
d. All

40. Hydrostatic pressure in glomerular capillary (mm Hg) is

a. About 45 b. About 10
c. About 5 d. 60

41. Which of the following changes would tend to decrease glomerular filtration rate:

a. Increased afferent arteriolar resistance
b. Increased glomerular capillary filtration coefficient
c. Decreased hydrostatic pressure in Bowman's capsule
d. Decreased plasma colloid osmotic pressure.

42. The maximum amount of each substance that can be transported in one minute by the kidney tubules is called:

a. Transport maximum b. Tubular maximum
c. Secretion maximum d. Diodrast clearance

43. Action of renal nerves on urine formation is limited to their effect on:

a. Release of angiotensin
b. Pressure and flow of renal blood
c. Reabsorption of glucose
d. Reabsorption of sodium by the tubules

44. The glomerular:

a. Efferent arteriole is smaller in diameter
b. Capillaries are more permeable than are most other capillaries in the body
c. Capillary blood is separated from glomerular filtrate by the capillary membrane only
d. Capillary ressure is normally 15–35 mm Hg.

45. Normal filtration fraction is:

a. 0.12–0.16 b. 0.16–0.20
c. 0.20–0.25 d. 0.25–0.30

46. Hyperosmolar coma is seen in all except:

a. Hyperglycemia
b. Uremia
c. Increased concentration of plasma proteins
d. Increase in plasma Na^+ concentration

47. Glucose reabsorption occurs in:

a. PCT
b. LH
c. Distal tubule
d. Cortical collecting tubule
e. Medullary collecting tubule

48. H^+ secretion in renal tubule is affected by

a. Increase in pCO_2
b. Minerelocorticoids
c. Decreased K^+ level
d. Carbonic anhydrase inhibitor

REPRODUCTIVE SYSTEM

1. Normal average sperm count in semen is:

a. 5 million/m^3
b. 50 million/ml
c. 100 million/m^3
d. 100 million/ml

2. Mechanism of action of IUCD is by:

a. Preventing LH surge
b. Making the vaginal mucosa hostile for sperms
c. Preventing the implantation of fertilized ovum
d. Preventing fertilization

3. Testosterone is secreted by:

a. Sertoli cells
b. Leydig cell
c. Epididymis
d. Seminiferous tubules

4. The precursor of testosterone is:

a. Aldosterone b. Estradiol
c. Androsterone d. Pregnenolone

5. The number of chromosomes in human sperm is:

a. 42 b. 23
c. 21 d. 46

6. Ovarian follicle growth is influenced by:

a. FSH
b. ACTH
c. TSH
d. Progesterone

7. **Postmenopausal women:**
   a. Have decreased libido
   b. Have no circulating estrogen in the blood
   c. Sexual activity persists in them due to release of estrogen by adrenals
   d. Are less prone for fractures due to decreased estrogen level.

8. **Estrogen:**
   a. Is secreted by theca interna cells of grafian follicle
   b. Has no effect on epiphyseal closure
   c. Has plasma cholesterol lowering activity
   d. Both a and c are correct

9. **Capacitation of the sperms:**
   a. Occurs mainly in the testis
   b. Involves very gross morphological changes of the sperm
   c. Is not required for the fertilization function of the sperm
   d. Is an important physiological event for fertilization

10. **Uterine endometrium is thinnest:**
    a. At the end of bleeding phase
    b. On the 14th day of menstrual cycle
    c. On the 25th day of menstrual cycle
    d. Before the start of menstruation

11. **Oral contraceptive pills contain:**
    a. Testosterone
    b. Human chorionic gonadotropin
    c. Relaxin
    d. Estrogen

12. **Cryptorchidism means:**
    a. A method of family planning
    b. Disturbances in menstrual cycle
    c. Delayed puberty
    d. Undescended testis

13. **The hormone responsible for conversion of Wolffian: duct into vas deferens in male fetus is:**
    a. Estrogen
    b. Progesterone
    c. Testosterone
    d. Cortisone

14. **Thermogenesis shown during ovulation is because of:**
    a. Estrogen b. Progesterone
    c. FSH d. LH

15. **Sertoli cell secrete all the following except:**
    a. Inhibin b. ABP
    c. cytokines d. Testosterone

16. **Menopause means:**
    a. Excessive bleeding
    b. Intermittent bleeding
    c. Absence of menstrual cycle
    d. Stoppage of menstrual cycle

17. **Entire period of spermatogenesis:**
    a. 8 days b. 74 days
    c. 700 days d. None of the above

18. **Lactation:**
    a. Is inhibited by estrogen and progesterone
    b. Is initiated due to lactogenic effect of prolactin within 1 to 7 days after the birth of baby
    c. Is controlled by hypothalamus
    d. All the above

19. **Fertilization of the ovum normally occurs in:**
    a. Uterus b. Cervix of uterus
    c. Fallopian tube d. None of the above

20. **Basis of pregnancy immunologic test is:**
    a. Excretion of hCG in urine
    b. Presence of progesterone in urine
    c. Excretion of estrogen in urine
    d. None of the above

21. **Blood testis barrier is chiefly produced by:**
    a. Sertoli cells b. Leydig cells
    c. Both the cells d. Mesangial cells

22. **Life span of corpus luteum in absence of fertilization:**
    a. 7 days b. 28 days
    c. 4 days d. 14 days

23. **All are true regarding vasectomy, except:**
    a. It is easily reversible
    b. It is a surgical method
    c. It is a permanent method
    d. It is done in males

24. **Sperms have:**
    a. 22 autosomes + Y chromosome
    b. 22 autosomes + X chromosome
    c. 23 pairs of chromosomes
    d. 22 autosomes + either X or Y chromosome

25. **Which of the following contraceptive method has high failure rate:**
    a. IUCD b. Oral pills
    c. Tubectomy d. Rhythm method

26. **Human chorionic gonadotropin is secreted from:**
    a. Ovary b. Pituitary gland
    c. Placenta d. Corpus luteum

27. **Spermatozoa matures in the following organs:**
    a. Prostate gland b. Epididymis
    c. Vas deferens d. Rete testis
28. **The role of progesterone is:**
    a. To thicken myometrium
    b. To increase blood supply to uterine wall
    c. To build up fat and glycogen in uterine wall
    d. All of the above
29. **A decrease in blood levels of estrogen and progesterone causes:**
    a. Loss of endometrium
    b. Release of ova from ovaries
    c. Growth and dilatation of myometrium
    d. Constriction of uterine blood vessels leading to sloughing of uterine epithelium
30. **Uterine contractility is increased by the hormone:**
    a. Vasopressin b. LH
    c. FSH d. Oxytocin
31. **Which one is not found in semen:**
    a. Testosterone b. Fructose
    c. Citric acid d. Ascorbic acid
    e. Acid phosphatase
32. **Ejection of milk from the breast or let down:**
    a. Frequently occurs in both breasts even though the baby is nursing at only one breast
    b. Can be stimulated by mechanical stimulation of the breast
    c. Can be stimulated by the sight or sound of the baby
    d. Is caused by oxytocin-induced contraction of the myoepithelial cells
33. **Important effects of testosterone include all of the following except:**
    a. Formation of fetal penis
    b. Descent of testis into the scortum
    c. Increased muscle development
    d. Initiation of ejaculation
    e. Increased thickness of the skin
34. **Which of the following statements regarding capacitation of spermatozoa is true:**
    a. It occurs in epididymis
    b. It is stimulated by testosterone
    c. It is accompanied by release of acrosomal enzymes
35. **Which of the following hormones is responsible for the development of ovarian follicles prior to ovulation:**
    a. Follicle-stimulating hormone (FSH)
    b. Human chorionic gonadotropin (hCG)
    c. Estradiol
    d. Leutenising hormone (LH)
36. **Functions of the Sertoli cells in the seminiferous tubules include:**
    a. Synthesis of estrogen after puberty
    b. Synthesis of androgen-binding protein
    c. Secretion of testosterone into the tubular lumen
37. **Progesterone has the ability to:**
    a. Inhibit ferning of cervical mucus
    b. Antagonize the effect of aldosterone
    c. Give rise to secretory endometrium
    d. Prevent ovulation if given in sufficient doses
38. **The site of spermatogenesis is:**
    a. Seminiferous tubules
    b. Leydig's cells
    c. Gram cells
39. **Testis does not produce:**
    a. Estradiol b. Testosterone
    c. Fructose d. Inhibin
40. **Levels of which of the following hormones are increased in postmenopausal women:**
    a. Estrogen b. FSH
    c. Progesterone d. Cortisone
41. **The viability of the spermatozoa within the female genital tract is up to hours:**
    a. 6 b. 12
    c. 24 d. 48
42. **Function of leutenizing hormone is:**
    a. Follicle maturation and ovulation
    b. Milk secretion
    c. Progesterone secretion during ovulation
    d. To maintain placenta
43. **Precursor of testosterone is:**
    a. Pregnenolone b. Methyltestosterone
    c. Aldosterone d. Cortisone
44. **Estrogen receptors are in:**
    a. Nucleus b. Mitochondrion
    c. Cell membrane d. Cytoplasmic receptor
45. **Which is not caused by estrogen:**
    a. Decreased folate levels b. Decreased HDL
    c. Increased blood sugar d. None
46. **Menopausal hot flushes are due to:**
    a. Decreased estrogen b. Decreased progesterone
    c. LH surge d. FSH surge
47. **Spermatozoa mature in which of the following organs:**
    a. Epididymis b. Vas deferens
    c. Rete testis d. Prostate

48. If a lady presents with a very regular 29 day menstrual cycle, ovulation should occur on day:

a. 14 b. 15
c. 17 d. 19

49. Maturation of graffian follicle occurs under the influence:

a. FSH b. ACTH
c. LH d. Cortisol

50. The nourishment to the development of spermatozoa is provided by:

a. Seminiferous tubules b. Leydig's cells
c. Sertoli's cells d. Any of the above

51. The seminiferous tubules require the following for full development:

a. LH b. Oxytocin
c. FSH d. Androgen and FSH

52. Testosterone, the male sex hormone, is synthesized in:

a. Interstitial cells b. Seminiferous tubules
c. Prostate gland d. Vas deferens

53. Mature sperms are stored in:

a. Interstitial cells b. Seminiferous tubules
c. Prostate gland d. Epididymis

54. Alkaline component of the semen is secreted by:

a. Seminal vesicles b. The prostate gland
c. Bulbourethral glands d. Testis

55. Sertoli cell secretes:

a. Testosterone b. Progesterone
c. Androstenedione d. Inhibin

56. Testosterone:

a. Causes salt and water retention
b. Has protein catabolic effect
c. Inhibits erythropoiesis
d. None of the above

57. Genetic make up in Klinefelter's syndrome is:

a. XO b. XX
c. XXY d. XXYY

58. Corpus luteum is maintained by:

a. Progesterone b. Estrogen
c. LH d. FSH

ENDOCRINOLOGY

1. Effect of epinephrine includes:

a. Hyperglycemia
b. Decrease in metabolic state
c. Lipid synthesis and promotion
d. Inhibition of phosphorylase

2. Hyperglycemia is induced by all of the following hormones except:

a. Cortisol b. Aldosterone
c. Thyroxin d. Glucagon

3. The supraoptic nucleus of hypothalamus controls the secretion of:

a. Prolactin b. FSH
c. Vasopressin d. TSH

4. Thyroid hormones act on the target cells via:

a. Receptors in cytoplasm
b. Receptors in plasma membrane
c. Cyclic AMP second messenger system
d. Receptors in the nucleus

5. Myxoedema is due to:

a. Hypothyroidism b. Hypopituitarism
c. Hyperthyroidism d. Hyperpituitarism

6. The organ not directly involved in the control of Ca^{2+} level in blood is:

a. Skin b. Bone
c. Kidney d. GIT

7. Insulin is not involved in the glucose transport to the following cell:

a. Adipose tissue b. Liver
c. Alveolar epithelial cells d. Muscle

8. All are true regarding adrenocorticotropic hormone except:

a. It causes pigmentation
b. Its concentration increases during Cushing's syndrome
c. Its secretion increases during stress
d. It is a polypeptide

9. Acromegaly is due to:

a. Hyposecretion of ACTH
b. Hyposecretion of growth hormone in children
c. Hypersecretion of growth hormone in adults
d. Hypersecretion of thyroxin in adults

10. Glucagon secretion is decreased by all except:

a. Hyperglycemia b. Starvation
c. Somatostatin d. Insulin

11. Insulin increases glucose entry into:

a. Skeletal muscle b. Intestine
c. Renal tubular cells d. Cortical neuron

12. Glucocorticoids can induce:

a. Neutropenia
b. Eosinopenia
c. Anemia
d. Thrombocytosis

13. Growth hormone:
a. Enhances utilization of glucose by cells
b. Favors utilization of amino acids for energy
c. Favors utilization of fatty acids for energy
d. Promotes deposition of fat in adipose tissue
e. All are true

14. In Addison's disease:
a. There is decreased volume of ECF
b. Pigmentation of skin
c. Extreme muscle weakness
d. All the above

15. Cortisol release increases:
a. In trauma
b. When ACTH level in blood increases
c. In mental stress
d. All the above

16. Parathyroid hormone:
a. Is a polypeptide
b. Increases Ca excretion in urine
c. Reduces blood Ca level
d. Causes reduced excretion of phosphate in urine

17. Milk secretion by mammary gland occurs due to:
a. Estrogen b. Prolactin
c. Oxytocin d. Progesterone

18. All the statements are true regarding cortisol except:
a. It increases blood sugar level
b. Hyposecretion of it produces Cushing's syndrome
c. Increases blood volume
d. It shows anti-inflammatory action

19. All are steroid hormones except:
a. Relaxin b. Estrogen
c. Testosterone d. Progesterone

20. All are true regarding Diabetes Insipidus, except:
a. It is caused due to the lesion of hypothalamus
b. Increased water reabsorption at renal tubule
c. Polyuria
d. Polydipsia

21. The active form of Vitamin D is:
a. Cholecalciferol b. Calcitonin
c. 1,25 DHCC d. Parathyroid hormone

22. Normal body temperature can be raised by:
a. Estrogen b. Progesterone
c. Gonadotropins d. Androgens

23. Beta cells of pancreas secrete:
a. Glucagon b. Insulin
c. Gastrin d. Somatostatin

24. Oxytocin causes all except:
a. Milk ejection
b. Contraction of uterine muscle
c. Lactogenesis
d. Myoepithelial cell contraction

25. Hyperglycemia is induced by all of the following hormones except:
a. ACTH b. Aldosterone
c. Thyroxine d. Epinephrine
e. Glucagon

26. Thyroid gland function is best monitored by which of the following:
a. BMR
b. Total thyroxine and triiodothyronine uptake
c. Level of protein bound iodine
d. Level of thyroid stimulating hormone

27. Which of the following statements about the action of the somatomedins is not true:
a. Inhibit protein synthesis
b. Promote growth of the bone and cartilage
c. Stimulate the secretion of hormones by pancreatic islet cells

28. A true statement about calmodulin is that it is:
a. A plasma binding protein for calcium
b. An intracellular calcium binding protein
c. Involved in intestinal absorption of calcium

29. Thyroxine and triiodothyronine are transported in plasma bound to several different proteins which do not include:
a. Thyroglobulin
b. Thyroxine binding globulin (TBG)
c. Albumin
d. Thyroxine binding prealbumin

30. Glucocorticoids decrease the number of circulating:
a. Eosinophils
b. Platelets
c. Leukocytes

31. Somatostatin is produced in the:
a. Hypothalamus b. Anterior pituitary
c. Delta cells of pancreas d. Both a and c

32. Panhypopituitarism causes all except:
a. Pigmentation
b. Infertility
c. Loss of secondary sexual character
d. Cold tolerance
e. Both a and d

33. In Addison's disease, the following is seen:

a. Hyperkalemia b. Hypernatremia
c. Hyperglycemia d. High blood pressure

34. Calcium necessary for blood coagulation and muscle contraction is:

a. Bound, nonionized calcium
b. Free, ionized calcium
c. Both

35. Increased fetal cortisol just before birth results in:

a. Uterine contraction
b. Release of oxytocin
c. Placental steroid biogenesis
d. Fetal lung maturation

36. The 'diuretic' activity of the anterior pituitary can be explained in terms of the actions of:

a. ACTH
b. TSH
c. Growth hormone
d. All of the above

37. Which is false regarding insulin:

a. Secreted by beta cells
b. Glycopeptide in nature
c. Causes lipogenesis
d. Promotes glycogenesis

38. A patient with hypothyroidism is likely to have all except:

a. Subnormal mouth temperature
b. Tendency to fall asleep frequently
c. Decreased body hair
d. Moist hands and feet

39. Cortisol:

a. Secretion increases following gross injury
b. Favors protein synthesis
c. Enhance effects of antigen-antibody reactions
d. Tends to lower blood pressure

40. Adrenal insufficiency causes:

a. A rise in plasma sodium/potassium ratio
b. Low blood pressure
c. A fall in extracellular fluid volume
d. Both b and c

41. In Cushing's syndrome the following features are found except:

a. Rapidly increasing adiposity
b. Polycythemia
c. Hypotension
d. Impotence with atrophy of testes

42. Regarding myxoedema the following are true except:

a. Swollen, Edematous look of the face
b. Amenorrhea
c. BMR increased by 30-45%
d. Dullness, loss of memory

43. Polypeptide hormone includes all except:

a. Insulin b. Angiotensin
c. Growth hormone d. Progesterone

44. If piluitary is surgically removed, blood level of sodium falls and that of potassium rises because of:

a. Atrophy of adrenal cortex
b. Atrophy of adrenal medulla
c. The fact that LTH from pituitary is no longer available
d. The fact that oxytocin from pituitary is no longer available

45. The hormone secretin is produced in:

a. Pancreas and influences conversion of glycogen into glucose
b. Adrenal glands and accelerates heart beat
c. Testis and produces male secondary sexual charecteristics
d. Small intestine and stimulate pancreas

46. Renal calculi is seen in:

a. Hyperthyroidism b. Hyperparathyroidism
c. Cushing's disease d. Addison's disease

47. The excretion of estrogen and progesterone are through:

a. Bile b. Sweat
c. Urine d. Feces

48. Cortisol increases the blood glucose concentration either directly or indirectly by:

a. Decreasing glucose uptake by the cells
b. Decreasing the rate of gluconeogenesis
c. Increasing the rate of glucose utilization by the cells
d. Inhibiting hormone sensitive lipase

49. All of the following hormones mediate their major effects without actually entering the target cell except:

a. Cortisol b. Insulin
c. Growth hormone d. Glucagon
e. Parathyroid hormone

50. Growth hormone increases all of the following except:

a. Blood glucose concentration
b. Blood free fatty acid concentration
c. Protein synthesis
d. Storage of proteins in cells
e. Metabolism of carbohydrates
f. All

51. **Thyroid stimulating hormone stimulates thyroid function in many ways but it does not increase:**
   a. Synthesis of thyroxine-binding globulin
   b. Rate of synthesis of thyroglobulin
   c. Iodine uptake from the blood
   d. Iodination of tyrosine
   e. Size of the thyroid gland

52. **Which of the following is true about adrenalin:**
   a. Converted to norepinephrine by methylation
   b. Increases glygogen breakdown in liver and muscle
   c. Is a polypeptide
   d. Increases triglyceride deposition in adipose tissue

53. **The coupling of MIT and DIT and iodination of thyroglobulin is blocked by:**
   a. TSH b. TRH
   c. Propylthiouracil d. Monovalent anions

54. **Steroid hormone has:**
   a. Receptors in cytoplasm or nucleus of the target cell
   b. Receptor in the plasma membrane of the target cell
   c. Both

55. **Anti-inflammatory action of glucocorticoid is due to:**
   a. Stabilization of lysosomal membrane
   b. Decreased capillary permeability
   c. Inhibition of WBC migration
   d. All of the above

56. **Cyclic AMP mediate the action of all except:**
   a. Glucagon b. FSH
   c. LH d. Estrogen

57. **Hormone that is a derivative of a single amino acid is:**
   a. Estrogen b. Epinephrine
   c. Thyroxine d. Progesterone

58. **True about insulin action is:**
   a. Causes gluconeogenesis
   b. Not useful for growth and development
   c. Required for transport of glucose, amino acid, K^+
   d. Catabolic hormone

59. **Cushing's syndrome is characterized by:**
   a. Eosinophilia b. Hypericalemia
   c. Nitrogen retention d. Poor wound healing

60. **Action of epinephrine in liver is:**
   a. Glycogenolysis b. Gluconeogenesis
   c. Glycolysis d. Lipolysis

61. **Acidophil cells of pituitary secrete:**
   a. ACTH b. Prolactin
   c. Growth hormone d. TSH
   e. Both b and c

62. **Neurotransmitter which controls secretion of prolactin is:**
   a. Serotonin b. GABA
   c. Somatostatin d. Dopamine

63. **Parathyroid hormones are responsible for all EXCEPT:**
   a. Increases the absorption of phosphorus from the renal tubule
   b. Increases the formation of 1, 25 dihydroxycholecalciferol
   c. Mobilizes calcium from bone
   d. Increases intestinal absorption of calcium

64. **The testes does not produce:**
   a. Estradiol b. Testosterone
   c. Fructose d. Inhibin

65. **The chemical nature of hormones of adrenal cortex is:**
   a. Amino acids b. Steroids
   c. Eicosanoids d. Glycoproteins

NERVE MUSCLE PHYSIOLOGY

1. **During isotonic contraction:**
   a. I band remains constant
   b. A band changes in length
   c. Z line approach each other
   d. H zone remains constant

2. **Troponin C binds with:**
   a. Actin b. ATP
   c. Tropomyosin d. Calcium

3. **At neuromuscular junction, the receptor present are:**
   a. Adrenergic b. Nicotinic
   c. Muscarinic d. Dopaminergic

4. **Which of the ion is responsible for release of transmitters by exocytosis at nerve endings:**
   a. Mg^{2+} b. Ca^{2+}
   c. Na^+ d. K^+

5. **The nerve fiber easily blocked by local anesthetics is:**
   a. C type b. A beta
   c. A alpha d. A gamma

6. **Depolarizing type of neuromuscular blocking agent is:**
   a. Neostigmine b. Physostigmine
   c. Succinyl choline d. Tubocurarine

7. **The fastest conducting nerve fiber is:**
   a. B fiber b. C fiber
   c. δ fiber d. A α fiber

8. **Glial cell responsible for the formation of BBB is:**
   a. Microglia b. Astrocyte
   c. Ependymal cells d. Oligodendrocytes

9. **The part of sarcomere that disappears on muscle contraction:**
a. M line b. H zone
c. I band d. A band

10. **Phagocytosis in CNS is done by:**
a. Astrocytes b. Schwann cells
c. Microglia d. Oligocytes

11. **Chronaxie is minimum in:**
a. Large myelinated nerve fiber
b. Skeletal muscle fiber
c. Unmyelinated nerve fiber
d. Cardiac muscle

12. **Glycogen content is lowest in:**
a. Slow oxidative fibers b. Fast glycolytic fibers
c. Fast oxidative fibers d. All the above

13. **Ryanodine receptor control:**
a. K^+ efflux from the sarcoplasmic reticulum
b. Na^+ influx from the sarcoplasmic reticulum
c. Ca^{2+} efflux from the sarcoplasmic reticulum
d. Cl^- influx from the sarcoplasmic reticulum

14. **Myasthenia gravis is due to:**
a. Old age
b. Non-production of ACh
c. Excess destruction of ACh
d. Destruction of ACh receptors

15. **Force of contraction of following muscle does not depend on the extracellular calcium ion concentration:**
a. Skeletal muscle
b. Sphincter muscle
c. Smooth muscle
d. Cardiac muscle

16. **Energy for muscle contraction is:**
a. Actin-tropomyosin b. ATP
c. Lactic acid d. Nicotinamide

17. **The nuclear bag portion of the muscle spindle is innervated by:**
a. Type I fiber b. Type II fiber
c. Both d. None

18. **The band which disappears on muscular contraction is:**
a. H b. I
c. A d. Z

19. **A decrease in extracellular calcium causes:**
a. Decreased membrane permeability
b. Hyperpolarization
c. Increased excitability
d. All of the above

20. **Myosin found in muscle cell is:**
a. Myosin I b. Myosin II
c. Both d. None

21. **The value of resting membrane potential in a nerve fiber is:**
a. –50 mV b. –70 mV
c. –110 mV d. –130 mV

22. **All are steps in contraction of skeletal muscle except:**
a. Discharge of motor neuron
b. Ca^{2+} release from sarcoplasmic reticulum
c. Binding of Ca^{2+} to troponin C
d. Release of Ca^{2+} from troponin C

23. **Which of the following is an excitatory neurotransmitter:**
a. GABA
b. Glycine
c. Melatonin
d. Glutamate

24. **The strength of contraction of an entire skeletal muscle is dependent on the:**
a. Number of muscle fibers that contract simultaneously
b. Frequency of contraction of each muscle fiber
c. Number of active cross-bridges in each muscle fiber
d. Degree of plasticity of the muscle

25. **Which of the following statements about release of acetylcholine at the neuromuscular junction is not correct?**
a. Produces an endplate potential
b. Increases sodium movement into the muscle cell
c. Always causes the muscle fiber to contract
d. Is followed by rapid destruction of acetylcholine
e. Both c and d

26. **The repolarization of an action potential is associated with all of the following except:**
a. Loss of positive charges from inside the cell
b. Outward diffusion of K^+
c. Return of the membrane potential toward its resting value
d. Closure of sodium channels in the cell membrane
e. Decreased potassium permeability of cell membrane

27. **Resting membrane potential of a cell is established by or maintained by all of the following except:**
a. Sodium and potassium pump
b. Outward movement of sodium ions
c. Inward movement of potassium ions
d. A net inward movement of positive ions
e. Adenosine triphosphate

28. **Enzyme involved in acetylcholine synthesis is:**
    a. Choline acetyl transferase
    b. Choline esterase
    c. Pseudocholinesterase
    d. Glycine

29. **Which of the following statements is true:**
    a. The transmitter secreted at the endings of sympathetic preganglionic neurons is norepinephrine
    b. The transmitter secreted at the endings of the preganglionic neurons of the parasympathetic neuron is epinephrine
    c. The transmitter secreted at the postganglionic neuron ending of the parasympathetic neurons is atropine
    d. The transmitter secreted at most postganglionic neuron endings of sympathetic nervous system is norepineiphrine

30. **When energy is derived from creatine phosphate to cause muscle contraction, what is the first step in the transfer of energy:**
    a. Creatine phosphate transfers the energy to the cross-bridges to cause them to become locked
    b. Creatine phosphate causes the power stroke of the cross-bridges
    c. Creatine phosphate transfers its energy to the myosin filament
    d. The energy of creatine phosphate is used to convert ADP into ATP

31. **End plate potential is characterized by:**
    a. Hyperpolarization
    b. Normal polarity
    c. Depolarization
    d. None of the above

32. **The type of nerve fiber that has a conduction velocity of approximately 1 meter per second:**
    a. Type A alpha b. Type A beta
    c. Type A delta d. Type A gamma
    e. Type C

33. **Which of the following transmitter substances always or almost always tend to inhibit the postsynaptic neuron?**
    a. GABA
    b. Dopamine
    c. Norepinephrine

34. **The motor unit is:**
    a. Muscle fiber and neuron supplying it
    b. Afferent fiber-center-efferent fiber
    c. Motor neuron and muscle fibers supplied by it
    d. Single muscle fiber with its nerve

35. **At a given load, the velocity of muscle contraction is maximal at:**
    a. The resting length b. Twice the resting length
    c. Half the resting length d. The equilibrium length

36. **Neurotransmitter in nigrostrial pathway is:**
    a. Dopamine b. Epinephrine
    c. Norepinephrine d. Acetylcholine

37. **Myosin light chain kinase plays an important role in the contraction of:**
    a. Skeletal muscle b. Smooth muscle
    c. Cardiac muscle

38. **Smooth muscle has the following characteristic:**
    a. Threshold is higher
    b. RMP is greater
    c. Action potential is greater
    d. Chronaxie is longer

39. **Which of the following is caused by acetylcholine through nicotinic receptors?**
    a. Contraction of skeletal muscle
    b. Decrease of heart rate
    c. Secretion of saliva
    d. Contraction of pupils

40. **A patient complains of muscle weakness; on administration of neostigmine it disappears. Its mechanism of action is:**
    a. It blocks action of acetylcholine
    b. It interferes with the action of amino-oxidase
    c. It interferes with the action of carbonic anhydrase
    d. It interferes with the action of acetylchlorine esterase

41. **Actin combines with myosin to form actomyosin in the presence of:**
    a. Ca^{2+} and Mg^{2+}
    b. Mg^{2+} and ATP
    c. Ca^{2+} and ATP
    d. Ca^{2+} and K^{+}

42. **Repetitive stimulation of the muscle results in:**
    a. Tetany
    b. Tetanus
    c. Summation
    d. None of the above

43. **The action potential of skeletal muscle:**
    a. Has a prolonged plateau phase
    b. Spreads inward to all parts of the muscle via T tubules
    c. Causes immediate uptake of Ca^{2+} into the lateral sacs of the sarcoplasmic reticulum
    d. Is longer than the action potential of cardiac muscle
    e. Is not essential for contraction

44. The function of tropomyosin in skeletal muscle is:

a. Sliding on actin to produce shortening
b. Releasing Ca^{2+} after initiation of contraction
c. Binding to myosin during contraction
d. To act as a relaxing protein at rest by covering up the sites where myosin binds to actin

45. The cross-bridges in skeletal muscle are made up of:

a. Actin b. Myosin
c. Troponin d. Tropomyosin
e. Myelin

46. Denervation of skeletal muscle leads to all except:

a. Atrophy b. Flaccid paralysis
c. Spastic paralysis d. Fibrillations

47. Gap junctions:

a. Not present in cardiac muscle
b. Are present, but of little functional importance in case of cardiac muscle
c. Are present and are important in initiation of pathway for rapid spread of excitation from one cardiac muscle fiber to another
d. Are not present in smooth muscle

48. The I-bands of a sarcomere contains molecules of:

a. Mainly actin b. Mainly myosin
c. Mainly troponin d. Mainly tropomyosin

49. When the muscle is at rest, the myosin-binding sites on the actin molecule are blocked by:

a. Troponin b. Tropomyosin
c. Collagen

50. Group A fibers are most susceptible to:

a. Pressure b. Hypoxia
c. Local anesthetics d. Temperature

51. All or none response in a nerve is applicable to:

a. A mixed nerve b. A sensory nerve
c. A motor nerve d. A single nerve fiber

52. Tropomyosin:

a. Helps in the fusion of action and myosin
b. Slides over myosin
c. Covers myosin and prevent attachment of actin and myosin
d. Causes calcium release

53. d-tubocurarine in therapeutic doses:

a. Competes with acetylcholine for same nicotinic receptors on motor end plate
b. Prevents propagation of action potential in skeletal muscle
c. Enhances the action of catecholamines
d. Enhances the action of cholineesterase

CENTRAL NERVOUS SYSTEM

1. Normal blood flow to the brain in ml/min:

a. 150 b. 500
c. 750 d. 1000

2. The following is not related to stretch reflex:

a. Response is shortening of the same muscle
b. It is a monosynaptic reflex
c. It is a polysynaptic reflex
d. Voluntary movement
e. Involuntary movement

3. Pain is carried by:

a. A delta fibers b. A beta fibers
c. C fibers d. Both a and c

4. Nucleus Gracilis and Nucleus Cuneatus are the first synapse for:

a. Dorsal column tract
b. Dorsolateral tract
c. Lateral spinothalamic tract
d. Ventral spinothalamic tract

5. In the spinal cord:

a. Dorsal roots are motor and ventral roots are sensory
b. Dorsal roots are sensory and ventral roots are motor
c. There is no relay of sensory nerves
d. There is no crossing of nerve fibers

6. Primary visual area is located in the:

a. Limbic system b. Parietal lobe
c. Occipital lobe d. Frontal lobe

7. The area responsible for short term memory is located in:

a. Cerebellum b. Hypothalamus
c. Thalamus d. Hippocampus

8. Lateral spinothalamic tract carries the following sensation:

a. Vibration b. Proprioception
c. Pain d. Fine touch

9. Which of the following is the part of limbic system:

a. Red nucleus
b. Corpus striatum
c. Prefrontal lobe
d. Cingulate cortex

10. Nerve supply to the sweat glands is by:

a. Parasympathetic cholinergic
b. Sympathetic cholinergic
c. Sympathetic adrenergic
d. None of the above

11. **Dominant hemisphere:**
   a. Is located on the right side in most of the people
   b. Is also known as representational hemisphere
   c. Is concerned with language functions
   d. Concept does not apply to deaf mute
12. **The motor cortex (area 4):**
   a. Is in the precentral gyrus of the parietal lobe
   b. Receives inputs from a variety of sources, including cortical association fibers, the cerebellum, and the basal ganglia
   c. Has the muscles of the feet and legs represented laterally near the sylvian sissure
   d. Is the only area involved in motor function
13. **Stereognosis means:**
   a. Detecting pressure
   b. Detecting vibration
   c. Identifying an object by touch
   d. Sense of smell
14. **All are symptoms of Parkinsonism except:**
   a. Memory loss b. Mask like face
   c. Resting tremor d. Hypokinesia
15. **If a patient has involuntary athetoid movement probably he may have lesion in:**
   a. Thalamus b. Basal ganglia
   c. Cerebellum d. Limbic system
16. **Satiety center is located in:**
   a. Parietal lobe b. Thalamus
   c. Hypothalamus d. Medulla
17. **Satiety center is located in the following hypothalamic nucleus:**
   a. Supraoptic b. Ventromedial
   c. Lateral d. Dorsomedial
18. **Which of the following is an inhibitory neurotransmitter:**
   a. ACh b. Glutamate
   c. GABA d. Norepinephrine
19. **Limbic system is mainly concerned with:**
   a. Control of emotion
   b. Speech execution
   c. Voluntary movement
   d. Involuntary movement
20. **All are true regarding receptor potential except:**
   a. Is a graded response
   b. Generates action potential in the nerve fiber attached to receptor
   c. Can be propagated
   d. Does not obey all or none law
21. **All the following reflexes are multisynaptic except:**
   a. Cord righting reflex b. Withdrawal reflex
   c. Stretch reflex d. Golgi tendon reflex
22. **Parkinson's disease is due to damage to:**
   a. Putamen
   b. Globus pallidus
   c. Dopaminergic cells of substantia nigra
   d. All the above
23. **Wernicke's area:**
   a. Is present in parietal cortex
   b. Lies near auditory area of temporal lobe
   c. Is located in occipital cortex
   d. Is a motor area
24. **δ waves in EEG:**
   a. Occur in deep sleep
   b. Occur at a rate below 3 to 5 cycles/second
   c. Strictly occur in the cortex independent of activities of lower regions of brain
   d. All the above
25. **Dorsal column-medial lemniscus pathway:**
   a. Carries sense of temperature to the cortex
   b. Carries sense of crude touch and pain to the cortex
   c. Carries sensation of fine touch, vibration and propriocetion
   d. Does not help in detecting movt of different parts
26. **Muscle spindles:**
   a. Are stretch receptors
   b. Lie with their long axis parallel to extrafusal fibers
   c. Are present in more number in antigravity muscles
   d. All the above
27. **Brown-Sequard syndrome results:**
   a. On spinal transection
   b. On hemisection of spinalcord
   c. On sectioning brain stem at midcollicular level
   d. None of the above
28. **The primary function of basal ganglia is:**
   a. Sensory integration
   b. Planning motor movements
   c. Short-term memory
   d. REM sleep
29. **The following are considered as mechano receptors except:**
   a. Pacinian corpuscle b. Krause's end bulb
   c. Ruffini's end organ d. Bare nerve endings
30. **In Brown Sequard syndrome, all the sensations except one is lost on the same side:**
   a. Proprioception b. Stereognosis
   c. Vibration d. Pain

31. Spastic gait is seen in:
a. LMN lesion b. Thalamic syndrome
c. UMN lesion d. Cerebellar lesion

32. Crossed extensor reflex is a:
a. Monosynaptic reflex b. Postural reflex
c. Sympathetic reflex d. Withdrawal reflex

33. All are ascending tracts except:
a. Tract of Goll
b. Tract of Burdach
c. Rubrospinal tract
d. Lateral spinothalamic tract

34. Sensory area for speech is situated at:
a. Broca's area b. Temporal lobe
c. Occipital lobe d. Frontal lobe

35. The wave in EEG with highest frequency is:
a. Delta wave b. Beta wave
c. Theta wave d. Gamma wave

36. When environmental temperature is above body temperature, heat is lost from the body by:
a. Conduction b. Evaporation
c. Radiation d. Convection

37. Sensation of fine touch is carried by:
a. Pyramidal tract
b. Posterior column tract
c. Lateral spinothalamic tract
d. Ventral spinothalamic tract

38. Flocculonodular lobe of cerebellum is concerned with:
a. Coordination b. Chemoreception
c. Equilibrium d. Taste sensation

39. Center for body temperature regulation is located in:
a. Pons b. Medulla
c. Hypothalamus d. Thalamus

40. Neurotransmitter at the postganglionic sympathetic fiber is:
a. ACh b. Norepinephrine
c. Epinephrine d. Dopamine

41. Parkinsonism is due to the lesion of:
a. Corticostriate fibers
b. Thalamocortical fibers
c. Nigrostriatal fibers
d. Rubrothalamocortical fibers

42. Delta waves seen in:
a. REM sleep
b. Awake with eye closed
c. Deep sleep
d. Awake with eye open

43. Which one is a superficial reflex?
a. Knee b. Plantar
c. Ankle d. Jaw

44. The frequency of alpha waves in EEG is:
a. 8–12 cycles/sec b. 15–25 cycles/sec
c. 2–5 cycles/sec d. None of the above

45. Lesions in—lead to sensory ataxia:
a. Posterior column of cerebellum
b. Vermis of cerebellum
c. Flocculonodular lobe of cerebellum
d. Vestibular apparatus

46. Basal ganglia include all except:
a. Caudate nucleus
b. Putamen
c. Globus pallidus
d. Substantia gelatinosa of Rolando

47. The end plate potential is characterized by:
a. Propagation b. All or none loss
c. Depolarization d. Hyperpolarization

48. Vomiting center is situated in the:
a. Hypothalamus b. Amygdala
c. Pons d. Medulla

49. Swallowing center is situated in:
a. Midbrain b. Pons
c. Medulla d. Cerebellum

50. The intensity of sensory stimuli is determined by:
a. Frequency of action potential
b. Duration of latent period
c. Amplitude of action potential
d. Amplitude of generation potential

51. Which sensation is not lost on the side of lesion in Brown-Sequard syndrome:
a. Touch b. Vibration sense
c. Muscle sense d. Temperature

52. Conduction in which type of nerve is blocked maximally by pressure:
a. C-fibers b. A-alpha fibers
c. A-beta d. A-gamma

54. Broca's area is present in:
a. Superior temporal gyrus
b. Precentral gyrus
c. Postcentral gyrus
d. Inferior frontal gyrus

55. Following are seen in REM sleep except:
a. Bruxism b. Hypotonia
c. Tachycardia d. Dreams

56. In cerebellar disease all the statements are correct except:

a. The Romberg's sign is positive
b. There is adiadokokinesia
c. There is pendular knee jerk
d. There is static tremor

57. The cerebellum:

a. Has a totally inhibitory output from its cortex
b. Has only excitatory signal output from its deep nuclear layers
c. Has a conscious interpretation of motor activity
d. Has inhibitory influence on muscle tone in human.

58. The condition known as REM sleep is:

a. That point at which the individual becomes aware and alert
b. Referred to as paradoxical sleep
c. Characterized by total lack of all muscular activity
d. Characterized by slow high voltage regular EEG activity

59. True visceral pain arises in normal persons from:

a. Distension b. Mechanical irritation
c. Excessive heat d. Compression
e. Chemical stimulation

60. Interneurons are:

a. Essential part of stretch reflex
b. Essential part of all reflexes
c. Always excitatory
d. Always inhibitory
e. None of the above

61. What is true regarding the gamma efferent neuron:

a. An 'A' group motor neuron with a smaller diameter than that of alpha efferent neurons
b. Innervates intrafusal fibers
c. Innervates muscle fibers that stretch annulospiral endings
d. All of the above

62. A unilateral upper motor neuron lesion in the internal capsule is best characterized by:

a. Diminished use of contralateral limbs below the lesion
b. Muscle fasciculations
c. Ipsilateral hypotonicity
d. Flexion of the leg

63. Which of the following reflexes disappear in the absence of functional connections between the spinal cord and the brain:

a. Swallowing reflex b. Seating reflex
c. Withdrawal reflex d. Erection of penis
e. All of the above

64. Hyperkinetic syndromes such as chorea and athetosis are usually associated with pathological changes in:

a. Motor areas of cerebral cortex
b. Anterior hypothalamus
c. Pathways for recurrent collateral inhibition in the spinal cord
d. Basal ganglia complex

65. Muscle spindle is:

a. Receptor for a variety of multisynaptic reflexes
b. Receptor for myotatic or stretch reflex
c. Occurs only in antigravity extensor muscles
d. Excited by both stretch and contraction of the muscles in which it is located

66. The reticular formation is a diffuse collection of:

a. Sensory neurons only
b. Motor neurons only
c. Autonomic centers only
d. All the above

67. Classical decerebrate animal results from the following experimental procedure:

a. Removal of the cerebrum
b. Transection at the upper border of midbrain

68. The nerve fiber carrying which of the following sensations is the thickest in human:

a. Touch b. Pain
c. Temperature d. Proprioception

69. What percentage of pyramidal fibers are unmyelinated:

a. 20 b. 35
c. 50 d. 75

70. Gag reflex is mediated by cranial nerve:

a. VII b. IX
c. X d. XII

71. Flocculonodular lobe of cerebellum is concerned with:

a. Equilibrium b. Coordination
c. Baroreception d. Chemoreception

72. Vestibular fibers relay in:

a. Vermis
b. Lateral geniculate body
c. Flocculonodular lobe of cerebellum
d. Auditory cortex

73. Destruction of lateral nucleus of thalamus lead to:

a. Aphagia b. Hyperphagia
c. Satiety d. Somnolence

74. Chemical transmission of nerve impulses from one neuron to another or from a neuron to a muscle is by:

a. Cholesterol b. Acetylcholine
c. CCK d. ATP

75. Which part of the mammalian brain controls the voluntary muscular coordination:

a. Cerebellum b. Cerebrum
c. Corpus callosum d. Medulla

76. Parasympathetic nervous system increases the activity of:

a. Gut, iris, urinary bladder
b. Heart, adrenal and sweat glands
c. Heart, lacrimal glands, pancreas
d. Lacrimal glands, sweat glands, arrector pilli

77. Cerebellum of brain is concerned with all except:

a. Balance
b. Initiation of muscular contraction
c. Regulation of body posture and equilibrium
d. Coordination of muscular movements

78. Which of these is an example of conditioned reflex:

a. Withdrawal of hand on touching a hot plate
b. Watering of mouth at the smell of food
c. Flowing of tears while peeling and cutting onion
d. Cycling
e. Both b and d

79. During conduction of an impulse electric potential on inside of axolemma changes from:

a. Negative to positive and remains positive
b. Positive to negative and again positive
c. Negative to positive and again negative
d. Positive to negative and remains negative

80. The sensory ganglia concerned with spinal reflexes are located in:

a. Cutaneous sense organs
b. Gray matter of.spinal cord
c. Dorsal root ganglion of spinal nerves
d. Ventral root of spinal nerves

81. Commonest neurotransmitter in the synapse outside brain is:

a. Acetylcholine
b. Secretin
c. CCK
d. Acetylcholinesterase

82. 'All or none law' is applicable in the following events:

a. IPSP
b. EPSP
c. Nerve action potential

83. Pacinian corpuscles are:

a. Temperature receptor
b. A-beta nerve fibers
c. Touch - pressure receptor

84. Which of the following is a characteristic of chemical synapses:

a. One-way conduction b. Synaptic delay
c. Susceptible to drugs d. All the above

85. Stimulation of which of the following might be expected to produce itching:

a. Dorsal root C fibers
b. Touch receptors
c. A-beta fibers in peripheral nerves

86. Primary auditory cortex is located in the:

a. Limbic system
b. Occipital lobe
c. Parietal lobe
d. Superior part of temporal lobe

87. The extrapyramidal system is not directly concerned with:

a. Stretch reflexes b. Sensation from viscera
c. Spasticity d. All the above

88. Lesions of which of the following hypothalamic nuclei cause loss of the circadian rhythm in plasma cortisol secretion:

a. Ventromedial nuclei
b. Dorsomedial nuclei
c. Suprachiasmatic nuclei
d. Supraoptic and paraventricular nuclei

89. Lesions of which of the hypothalamic nuclei cause diabetes insipidus:

a. Supraoptic nuclei b. Ventromedial nuclei
c. Dorsomedial nuclei d. Medial preoptic nuclei

90. Which of the following are part of the limbic system:

a. Red nuclei
b. Amygdaloid nuclei
c. Posterior commissure
d. Cingulate cortex

91. The functions of the limbic system include all except:

a. Regulation of sexual behavior
b. Influencing rage and fear
c. Temperature regulation
d. Olfaction

92. A reflex action:

a. May be carried out by skeletal, smooth and cardiac muscles as well as by glands
b. Pathway is: efferent → spinal cord → brain → afferent
c. Pathway is: spinal cord → brain → afferent → efferent → target tissue
d. Pathway is: receptor → spinal cord → brain → efferent

93. **The ascending reticular formation:**
a. Is located in cerebral hemisphere
b. Has increased activity during sleep
c. Is located in brain stem
d. All the above

94. **Increased tendon reflexes are likely to be present a patient suffering from long-standing damage to:**
a. Anterior horn cells (poliomyelitis)
b. Primary sensory neurons (tabes dorsalis)
c. Internal capsule

95. **All are features of cerebellar dysfunction except:**
a. Ataxia b. Scanning speech
c. Dysmetria d. Resting tremor

96. **Which neurotransmitter is involved in sleep pattern:**
a. Serotonin b. Acetylcholine
c. Noradrenaline d. Dopamine

97. **Diseases of basal ganglia can produce:**
a. Athetosis b. Paralysis agitans
c. Chorea d. All

98. **Which of the following is the inhibitory neurotransmitter:**
a. Acetylcholine b. Serotonin
c. GABA d. Dopamine

99. **The output of cerebellum is:**
a. Mostly inhibitory
b. Mostly excitatory
c. Sometimes inhibitory and sometimes excitatory

100. **Granular cells of cerebral cortex have:**
a. Nutritive role b. Motor activity
c. Sensory action d. All

101. **The neurotransmitter released into synapse between neurons and muscle cells is:**
a. Epinephrine
b. Norepinephrine
c. Acetylcholine
d. Gamma-aminobutyric acid

102. **Broca's area:**
a. Is for planning and making decisions
b. Contains primary visual cortex
c. Contains somatic sensory area
d. Coordinates muscles used in speech production.

103. **Parietal lobe:**
a. Is for planning and making decision
b. Contains primary visual cortex
c. Contains somatic sensory area
d. Coordinates muscles used in speech production

104. **Neurotransmitter synthesized from tryptophan and responsible for production and regulation of sleep is:**
a. Acetylcholine b. Serotonin
c. Dopamine d. Adrenaline

105. **Occipital lobe:**
a. Is for planning and making decision
b. Contains primary visual cortex
c. Contains somatic sensory area
d. Coordinates muscles used in speech production

106. **Frontal lobe:**
a. Is for planning and making decisions
b. Contains primary visual cortex
c. Contains somatic sensory area
d. Coordinates muscles used in speech production

107. **The reticular formation is mainly responsible for:**
a. Homeostasis and control of emotional responses
b. Control of rate of breathing
c. Regulating brain alertness
d. Conveying visual information to the cortex

108. **Pacinian corpuscles are:**
a. Rapid touch receptors
b. Slow touch receptors
c. Temperature receptors
d. Innevated by a delta nerve fibers

109. **The primary auditory cortex is located in the:**
a. Limbic system
b. Superior part of temporal lobe
c. Posterior part of parietal lobe
d. Posterior part of occipital lobe

110. **Sleep is produced due to the stimulation of which of the following brain areas:**
a. Occipital cortex
b. Posterior hypothalamus
c. Cuneate nucleus
d. Gracile nucleus

111. **Thirst is produced when:**
a. Plasma osmolality is increased and plasma volume decreased
b. Plasma osmolality and volume are increased
c. Plasma osmolality and volume are decreased
d. Plasma osmolality is decreased and plasma volume is increased

112. **Which of the following is not the result of parasympathetic stimulation:**
a. Increased stomach activity
b. Increased saliva formation
c. Constriction of bronchi
d. Dilatation of the pupil

113. Stimulation of parasympathetic fibers not contained in cranial nerve can lead to:

a. Contraction of the bladder
b. Constriction of the pupil
c. Increased salivation
d. Simulation of gallbladder activity

114. The white matter of spinal cord consists mainly of:

a. Cell bodies b. Dendrites
c. Axons d. Synapses

115. Diencephalon contains:

a. Cerebral cortex b. Hypothalamus
c. Olfactory bulbs d. Basal ganglia

116. Crude touch sensations are carried by:

a. Lateral spinothalamic tract
b. Ventral spinothalamic tract
c. Posterior columntract
d. Spinocerebellar tract

117. The main excitatory neurotransmitter in the central nervous system is:

a. Glycine b. Acetylcholine
c. Aspartate d. Glutamate

118. Pain transmission is inhibited by all EXCEPT:

a. Morphine b. Enkephalin
c. Substance P d. Beta-endorphin

119. Receptor for vision are:

a. Telereceptor b. Exteroceptors
c. Interoceptors d. Chemoreceptors

120. Phagocytosis in the CNS is done by:

a. Astrocytes b. Schwann cells
c. Microglia d. Oligodendrogliocytes

121. Modality that is lost on the ipsilateral side in Brown sequard syndrome is:

a. Pain b. Temperature
c. Crude touch d. Proprioception

122. REM sleep is:

a. That point at which the individual become aware and alert
b. Referred to as paradoxical sleep
c. Characterized by loss of alt muscular activity
d. Characterized by slow high voltage regular EEG activity

123. Flocculonodular lobe has direct connection with:

a. Red nucleus
b. Inferior olivary nucleus
c. Vestibular nucleus
d. Dentate nucleus

124. Circadian rhythem is controlled by:

a. Suprachiasmatic nucleus of hypothalamus
b. Postero ventral nucleus of thalamus
c. Dentate nucleus of cerebellum
d. Pineal gland

125. Crossed extensor response is a:

a. Withdrawal reflex
b. Postural reflex
c. Monosynaptic reflex
d. Sympathetic reflex
e. Exaggerated in UMN lesion

SPECIAL SENSES

1. On comparing with perilymph, endolymph has:

a. Higher sodium concentration
b. Higher potassium concentration
c. Same sodium concentration
d. Same potassium concentration

2. Near response include all the following except:

a. Increase in anterior curvature of lens
b. Constriction of pupil
c. Dialatation of pupil
d. Convergence of eyeball

3. Refractive power of the lens is measured in:

a. Decibels
b. Diopters
c. Centimeters
d. Millimeters

4. Lateral geniculate body (LGB) is concerned with:

a. Hearing b. Smell
c. Taste d. Vision

5. Flavor of food is due to:

a. Taste sensation
b. Olfactory sensation
c. Warmth in the tongue
d. A combination of taste, smell and warmth sensations from the food

6. When light strikes the outer segment of the photoreceptor, the following reactions occur except:

a. Formation of hyperpolarizing receptor potential
b. Closure of the Na^+ channel
c. Activated phosphodiesterase hydrolyses cGMP
d. Opening of the Na^+ channel

7. Bitter taste is produced by:

a. Acids b. Alkaloids
c. Organic salts d. Alcohols

8. **Protonopia means:**
   a. Person cannot see green b. Cannot see blue
   c. Cannot see red d. No color sense

9. **Myopia can be corrected by using ________ lens.**
   a. Biconvex b. Cylindrical
   c. Biconcave d. Plain

10. **Dioptric power of the human eye in diopter is:**
    a. 50 b. 60
    c. 70 d. 80

11. **Cavity of middle ear contains:**
    a. Perilymph b. Endolymph
    c. Air d. ECF

12. **Which of the following is test for inner ear deafness:**
    a. Finger nose test b. Weber's test
    c. Rinne's test d. Barany's test

13. **Medial geniculate body receives:**
    a. Auditory fibers b. Visual fibers
    c. Proprioceptive fibers d. None of the above

14. **If light source in front of the eye suddenly becomes bright:**
    a. Focus of lens will change
    b. Retinal blood supply will be cut off
    c. Intraocular pressure will rise
    d. Pupils will constrict

15. **Which one of the following procedures is most likely to increase intraocular pressure of glaucoma patient:**
    a. Use of atropine
    b. Decreased pressure in jugular vein
    c. High doses of vitamin C
    d. Exposure to brilliant sunlit environment

16. **The Helmholtz theory of color vision states that**
    a. There are three kinds of cones in the retina responding to the three primary colors
    b. There are two kinds of cones called dominators and modulators
    c. There is only one kind of cone and the color is recognized only in area 17
    d. There are seven types of cones responding to the seven colors of the spectrum

17. **Which structure in the eye is pain-sensitive?**
    a. Iris
    b. Choroid
    c. All of the above

18. **Red color blindness is called:**
    a. Deuteranopia b. Protanopia
    c. Protanomaly d. Deuteranomaly

19. **Medial geniculate body is concerned with:**
    a. Hearing b. Vision
    c. Smell d. Taste

20. **Smell receptors are seen in:**
    a. Lower 1/3 of nasal mucosa
    b. Upper 1/3 of nasal mucosa
    c. Amygdaloid body
    d. Cribriform plate

21. **Intraocular fluid:**
    a. Is produced at the canal of Schlemm
    b. Is reabsorbed by ciliary process
    c. Helps to maintain the curve of cornea
    d. None of the above

22. **Most of the refraction in the eye occurs at the:**
    a. Anterior surface of cornea
    b. Posterior surface of cornea
    c. Anterior surface of lens
    d. Posterior surface of lens

23. **The medium with highest refractive index in the eye is:**
    a. Cornea b. Nucleus of the lens
    c. Cortex of the lens d. Aqueous humor

24. **The optical power of the eye is:**
    a. 25 diopters b. 50 diopters
    c. 59 diopters d. 75 diopters

25. **The portion of the ear involved in balancing is:**
    a. Sacculus
    b. Cochlea
    c. Three semicircular canals with ampullae
    d. Utriculus

26. **Impulses generated by the olfactory receptors in the nasal mucous membrane:**
    a. Relay through the thalamus
    b. Relay through the internal capsule
    c. Relay through the hypothalamus
    d. Pass through mitral cells and from there directly to olfactory cortex

27. **Impulses generated in the taste buds of the tongue reach the cerebral cortex via:**
    a. Thalamus b. Internal capsule
    c. Trochlear nerve d. Hypoglossal nerve

28. **Olfactory sensory cells:**
    a. Relay in the thalamus
    b. Are of little importance in appreciating the flavor of food after it enters the mouth
    c. Show adaptation
    d. All of above

29. **The cones in the eye:**
 a. Are responsible for dim light vision
 b. Are much more sensitive to light than the rods
 c. Have higher visual acuity than rods
 d. Have impaired function in the absence of vitamin A

30. **The rods in the retina:**
 a. Contain visual pigment which is more sensitive to dim light than cone pigments
 b. Are relatively more numerous in night shift workers
 c. Comprise one-fifth of the receptors cells in the fovea

31. **The stapes rests on:**
 a. Round window b. Oval window
 c. Tympanic membrane d. Semicircular canal

32. **In nerve deafness:**
 a. Air conducted sounds are perceived well
 b. Bone conducted sounds are perceived well
 c. Both air and bone conducted sounds are not perceived well

33. **Argyll Robertson pupil is a condition in which the pupillary constriction in response to light stimulus:**
 a. Is absent b. Is delayed
 c. Is not affected d. Is present only in one eye

34. **Myopia (shortsightedness) is a defect in human eyes where image is formed:**
 a. In front of retina and can be corrected by using concave lens
 b. In front of retina and can be corrected by using convex lens
 c. Behind retina and can be corrected by using concave lens
 d. Behind retina and can be corrected by using convex lens

35. **Function of iris is to:**
 a. Move the lens forwards and backwards
 b. Alter the diameter of pupil
 c. Close the eyelids
 d. Secrete aqueous humor

36. **Blind spot in an eye is located:**
 a. In fovea centralis
 b. In the middle of the lens
 c. Where optic nerve leaves the retina
 d. In the center of the pupil

37. **Area of the most acute vision in eyes which contains only cone and where sharp and bright images are formed is:**
 a. Blind spot b. Yellow spot (macula lutea)
 c. Pupil d. Lens
 e. Fovea centralis

38. **The low intensity light during night is detected by:**
 a. Cones b. Rods
 c. Both d. Crystalline lens

39. **Ear ossicles are arranged in the following order from eardrum:**
 a. Malleus, stapes, incus b. Malleus, incus, stapes
 c. Incus, malleus, stapes d. Stapes, malleus, incus

40. **Vitreous humor lies:**
 a. Behind the lens
 b. In front of the lens
 c. Between the choroid and retina
 d. Between sclera and choroid

41. **Chief function of semicircular canals of the internal ear is:**
 a. To perceive sound of high or low frequencies
 b. To transmit sound to the auditory nerves
 c. To maintain dynamic equilibrium of moving body
 d. To perceive changes in orientation of body in relation to gravity

42. **Internal ear is responsible for:**
 a. Fixation of gaze
 b. Sensing changes in atmospheric pressure
 c. Maintaining rotational balance of body at rest
 d. Maintaining gravitational balance of body at rest

43. **Organ of Corti is found in:**
 a. Middle ear b. Utriculus
 c. Sacculus d. Cochlea
 e. External ear

44. **Otoconia are suspended in:**
 a. Synovial fluid b. Endolymph
 c. Perilymph d. Hemolymph

45. **Membranous labyrinth is called statoacoustic organ because it is concerned with:**
 a. Hearing b. Balancing
 c. Both d. Sound production

46. **Taste and smell receptors are:**
 a. Mechanoreceptors
 b. Chemoreceptors
 c. Thermoreceptors
 d. Electromagnetic receptors

47. **The sensory cell for smell is a:**
 a. Receptor cell b. Sensory neuron
 c. Motor neuron d. Photoreceptor

48. **The part of the eye which transduces blue, green and red light is:**
 a. Cornea b. Fovea
 c. Periphery of retina d. Optic nerve

49. The part of eye which bends light and protects inner eye is the:
a. Cornea
b. Fovea
c. Pupil
d. Ciliary muscle

50. Transduction of light is responsible for functioning of:
a. Rods and cones in the retina
b. Opsin and retinal rhodopsin
c. Rods and retinal
d. Opsin and cones

51. The part of the ear where sound is transduced is:
a. Outer ear
b. Tympanic membrane
c. Semicircular canals
d. Cochlea

52. Impulses of the taste buds of the tongue come from cerebral cortex through:
a. Internal capsule
b. Thalamus
c. Trochlear nerve
d. Hypoglossal nerve

53. Visual accommodation involves:
a. Contractions of ciliary muscles
b. Increased intraocular pressure
c. Decrease in the curvature of lens
d. Increased tension on the lens ligaments

54. The fovea centralis of the eye:
a. Contains only rods
b. Is the region of highest visual acuity
c. Has lowest light threshold

55. To correct myopic vision one should use:
a. Concave lens
b. Convex lens
c. Plane glass plates
d. Convex glass plates

56. Bitter taste is mediated by the action of:
a. Guanylate cyclase
b. G protein
c. Tyrosine kinase
d. Epithelial Na channels

ANSWERS

GENERAL PHYSIOLOGY

1. c 2. a 3. c 4. b 5. a 6. a
7. d 8. c 9. a 10. b 11. d 12. a
13. b 14. c 15. b 16. d 17. c 18. e
19. a 20. a 21. c 22. c 23. a

CIRCULATING BODY FLUIDS

1. c 2. c 3. d 4. a 5. c 6. c
7. c 8. b 9. b 10. c 11. a 12. d
13. a 14. a 15. c 16. d 17. a 18. d
19. b 20. b 21. d 22. b 23. a 24. a
25. d 26. c 27. b 28. a 29. b 30. d
31. d 32. d 33. c, d 34. d 35. a 36. a
37. b 38. c 39. a 40. c 41. b 42. c
43. c 44. b 45. b 46. a 47. c 48. c
49. b 50. b 51. d 52. a 53. c 54. c
55. c 56. a 57. c 58. c 59. c 60. a, c
61. e 62. c 63. a 64. a 65. b 66. a
67. a 68. d 69. a 70. a 71. b 72. a
73. b 74. a

RESPIRATORY SYSTEM

1. c 2. d 3. b 4. b 5. d 6. d
7. c 8. b 9. b 10. a 11. c 12. b
13. c 14. c 15. c 16. d 17. c 18. b
19. b 20. b 21. b 22. a 23. a 24. c
25. b 26. c 27. a 28. a 29. d 30. b
31. a 32. c 33. b 34. b 35. d 36. a
37. b 38. d 39. b 40. b 41. c 42. b
43. a 44. b 45. b 46. c 47. d 48. b
49. a,b,d 50. a 51. d 52. b 53. a 54. d
55. d 56. b 57. d 58. c 59. b 60. a
61. a 62. d 63. e 64. a 65. b 66. e
67. b 68. c 69. d 70. a 71. d 72. a
73. d 74. b 75. d 76. d 77. a 78. d
79. d 80. a 81. b

CARDIOVASCULAR SYSTEM

1. d 2. c 3. b 4. b 5. d 6. b
7. a 8. d 9. c 10. b 11. c 12. a
13. a 14. c 15. a 16. b 17. c 18. a
19. d 20. b 21. b 22. b 23. c 24. c
25. c 26. b 27. d 28. c 29. d 30. d
31. c 32. a 33. a 34. b 35. c 36. b
37. a 38. b 39. b 40. c 41. b 42. a
43. c 44. c 45. c 46. b 47. d 48. c
49. d 50. a 51. c 52. b 53. c 54. a
55. b 56. a 57. a 58. a 59. a 60. d
61. a 62. d 63. d 64. b 65. d 66. b

GASTROINTESTINAL SYSTEM

1. d	2. a	3. c	4. d	5. d	6. c
7. c	8. c	9. d	10. d	11. a	12. d
13. b	14. a	15. c	16. a	17. c	18. c
19. d	20. c	21. c	22. a	23. d	24. c
25. b	26. c	27. c	28. a	29. c	30. d
31. c	32. a	33. e	34. a	35. b	36. d
37. c	38. a	39. e	40. d	41. a	42. a
43. c	44. d	45. d	46. d	47. b	48. b
49. a	50. b	51. b	52. d	53. d	54. c
55. b	56. a	57. b	58. b	59. c	60. d
61. d	62. b	63. b	64. b	65. b	66. a
67. d	68. b	69. c			

RENAL PHYSIOLOGY

1. a	2. d	3. b	4. b	5. d	6. a
7. b	8. c	9. a	10. c	11. c	12. d
13. a	14. b	15. b	16. a,d	17. d	18. a
19. a	20. b	21. b	22. d	23. d	24. b,d
25. b	26. a	27. d	28. d	29. b	30. d
31. d	32. e	33. d	34. b	35. b	36. a
37. c	38. b	39. d	40. d	41. a	42. b
43. a,b	44. a	45. b	46. c	47. a	48. d

REPRODUCTIVE SYSTEM

1. d	2. c	3. b	4. c	5. b	6. a
7. c	8. d	9. d	10. a	11. d	12. d
13. c	14. b	15. c	16. d	17. b	18. d
19. c	20. a	21. a	22. a	23. a	24. d
25. d	26. c	27. b	28. d	29. d	30. d
31. a	32. c	33. d	34. c	35. a	36. b
37. a	38. a	39. c	40. a	41. c	42. a
43. a	44. a	45. c	46. a	47. a	48. b
49. a	50. c	51. d	52. a	53. d	54. b
55. d	56. a	57. c	58. a		

ENDOCRINOLOGY

1. a	2. b	3. c	4. d	5. a	6. a
7. c	8. c	9. c	10. b	11. a	12. b
13. e	14. d	15. d	16. a	17. b	18. b
19. a	20. b	21. c	22. b	23. b	24. c
25. b	26. d	27. c	28. b	29. a	30. a
31. d	32. e	33. a	34. b	35. d	36. d
37. b	38. d	39. a	40. d	41. c	42. c
43. d	44. a	45. d	46. b	47. c	48. a
49. a	50. d	51. a	52. b	53. c	54. a
55. d	56. d	57. b	58. c	59. d	60. a
61. e	62. d	63. a	64. c	65. b	

NERVE MUSCLE PHYSIOLOGY

1. c	2. d	3. b	4. b	5. a	6. c
7. d	8. b	9. b	10. c	11. a	12. a
13. c	14. d	15. a	16. b	17. a	18. a
19. c	20. b	21. b	22. d	23. d	24. c
25. e	26. e	27. d	28. a	29. d	30. d
31. c	32. e	33. a	34. c	35. a	36. a
37. b	38. d	39. a	40. d	41. a	42. a
43. c	44. d	45. b	46. c	47. c	48. a
49. b	50. a	51. d	52. c	53. a	

CENTRAL NERVOUS SYSTEM

1. c	2. c	3. d	4. a	5. b	6. c
7. d	8. c	9. d	10. b	11. c	12. a
13. c	14. a	15. b	16. c	17. b	18. c
19. a	20. c	21. c	22. d	23. b	24. a
25. c	26. d	27. b	28. b	29. d	30. d
31. c	32. d	33. c	34. b	35. d	36. b
37. b	38. c	39. c	40. b,c	41. c	42. c
43. b	44. a	45. a	46. d	47. c	48. d
49. c	50. a	51. d	52. c	53. d	54. d
55. a	56. d	57. a	58. b,c	59. a	60. a
61. d	62. a	63. a	64. d	65. b	66. d
67. c	68. d	69. c	70. b	71. a	72. c
73. b	74. b	75. a	76. a	77. b	78. e
79. c	80. c	81. a	82. c	83. c	84. d
85. a	86. d	87. a,b	88. c	89. a	90. b,d
91. c	92. a	93. c	94. c	95. d	96. a,c
97. d	98. c	99. c	100. b	101. c	102. d
103. c	104. b	105. b	106. a	107. c	108. a
109. b	110. b	111. a	112. d	113. a	114. c
115. b,c	116. c	117. b	118. d	119. a	120. c
121. d	122. b	123. c	124. d	125. a	

SPECIAL SENSES

1. b	2. c	3. b	4. d	5. d	6. d
7. b	8. c	9. c	10. b	11. c	12. b,c
13. a	14. d	15. a	16. a	17. c	18. b
19. b	20. b	21. c	22. a	23. b	24. c
25. c	26. d	27. a	28. c	29. b	30. a
31. b	32. c	33. a	34. a	35. b	36. c
37. b	38. b	39. b	40. a	41. c	42. a,d
43. d	44. b	45. c	46. b	47. a	48. b
49. a	50. b	51. d	52. b	53. a	54. b
55. a	56. b				

CHAPTER

17

Reasoning Type Questions

CIRCULATING BODY FLUIDS

1. Blood does not clot *in vivo* (Page no. 35; anticlotting mechanism, velocity of blood flow)
2. Reverse anemia occurs after gastrectomy (Page no. 30)
3. Opsonization aids phagocytosis (Page no. 32)
4. Aspirin is given in MI (Page no. 33)
5. Dicumarol cannot be used as an *in vitro* anticoagulant (Page no. 35; In a collected blood sample, i.e. *in vitro*, the clotting factors are already present, so dicumarol (vitamin K antagonist) has practically no effect
6. Bleeding disorders in vitamin K deficiency or in liver diseases clotting time is prolonged (Page no. 35)
7. In thrombocytopenic purpuras BT is prolonged but CT remains normal (Page no. 36)
8. Reticulocyte count increases after vitamin B_{12} therapy (Page no. 28; reticulocyte response-due to proliferation of bone marrow and numerous young RBCs pass into circulation)
9. Parentral administration of vitamin B_{12} in pernicious anemia (Page no. 28)
10. Hematocrit value of capillary blood is lower than that of actual blood (Page no. 337)
11. Edema develops in hypoalbunemia (Page no. 44)
12. Bleeding tendency in obstructive jaundice (in obstructive jaundice, there is no release of bile from liver into the intestine, so no absorption of fat soluble vitamin, i.e. Vitamin K, thereby vitamin K deficiency so bleeding tendancy is there)
13. Bleeding occurs in chronic liver diseases (Page no. 35)
14. PCV of venous blood is greater than that of arterial blood (Page no. 59)
15. Calcium deficiency does not lead to bleeding disorders (Page no. 35)
16. Clot does not spread in the injured vessel after blood coagulation (Page no. 35)
17. In a Rh-negative mother carrying an Rh-positive fetus, the first child is usually normal (Page no. 37)
18. Stored blood is not suitable for transfusing WBCs and platelet to a recipient (blood stored for longer than 24 hours contains virtually no viable WBCs and platelets)
19. In case of extreme emergency, 'O' Rh negative blood should be transfused (As 'O' Rh negative blood contains no antigens and therefore no antigen - antibody reaction)
20. ABO incompatibilities rarely produce hemolytic disease of newborn (Page no. 38).

RESPIRATORY SYSTEM

1. Intrapleural pressure is always negative/subatmospheric (Page no. 49)
2. Alveoli are always kept dry (Page no. 53)
3. Pulmonary TB affects apex of lung first (Page no. 56)
4. Expiratory phase is longer than inspiratory phase of respiratory cycle (during expiration bronchial constriction occurs thereby resistance to air flow increases, more work has to be done)
5. Bronchial asthma is a disease of expiratory obstruction (during inspiration expansion of bronchioles take place but on expiration there is constriction of already constricted bronchioles)
6. High ventilation/perfusion (V/P) ratio in the apices of lungs (Page no. 56; At the apex intrapleural pressure more negative, so alveoli expand more → greater alveolar ventilation, perfusion also less at apex relative to base)
7. Compliance of lungs alone is greater than the combined compliance (Inside thorax, some energy is required to expand the thorax also)
8. Lung compliance increases in old age (due to some modification in the knitting arrangement of the elastic tissues)
9. Arterial PO_2 is less than alveolar PO_2 (blood leaving the pulmonary capillaries is joined by venous blood from bronchial circulation and from anterior cardiac and the basian veins)
10. Sigmoid shape of oxygen-hemoglobin dissociation curve (Page no. 57)
11. Myoglobin acts as a temporary O_2 storehouse (Page no. 58)
12. Blood is an ideal vehicle for O_2 transport (it can give off more O_2 to tissues at lower PO_2)

13. Central chemoreceptors respond only to abrupt changes in PCO_2 (H^+ penetrates blood brain barrier slowly, CO_2 penetrate rapidly thereby leading to increased H^+ concentration in brain interstitial fluid stimulating central chemoreceptors)
14. Respiratory chemoreceptors are not stimulated in anemia or CO poisoning (Page no. 65)
15. Mild-to-moderate hypoxia stimulates the respiration but severe hypoxia depresses it (severe hypoxia causes direct inhibition of respiratory center)
16. Pulmonary ventilation is not much affected until PO_2 of inspired air falls below 60 mm Hg (Hypoxia increase the amount of reduced Hb (weaker acid), bind with H^+ reducing H^+ concentration tending to inhibit respiration)
17. CO_2 increases pulmonary ventilation primarily by stimulating central chemoreceptors. (CO_2 is a potent stimulant of central chemoreceptors, it crosses the blood-brain barrier and results in increase H^+ concentration in brain interstitial fluid and thereby stimulating central chemoreceptors)
18. Apnea occurs after voluntary hyperventilation (Page no. 64, CO_2 washout)
19. Cyanosis is not seen in anemic hypoxia (Page no. 69 decrease in Hb concentration in anemia)
20. Cyanosis is a common occurrence in hypoxic hypoxia. (In hypoxic hypoxia there is increase in reduced Hb, so cyanosis results)
21. Histotoxic hypoxia cannot cause cyanosis (Because reduced Hb is either not produced or produced in very small amount)
22. Babies of diabetic mothers are prone to develop IRDS (Page no. 53)
23. Systemic circulation has a low PO_2 than pulmonary circulation (Page no. 56)
24. In venous blood, RBCs have higher hematocrit than in arterial (Page no. 59)
25. Lesions in I neurons does not abolish respiratory activity (Page no. 60)
26. Increase in H^+ ion concentration in blood cannot activate central chemoreceptors (Page no. 65)
27. O_2 and He mixture is used in SCUBA (to avoid N_2 narcosis, he being low density gas is less soluble in fat than N_2)
28. Relief of orthopnea on sitting up (lying down position increases pulmonary congestion and aggrevates dyspnea)
29. Headache is experienced while staying in an over-crowded room for long time (due to increased level of CO_2 accumulation in the room and thereby leading to O_2 depletion within the body)
30. Severe joint pain occurs in decompression sickness (N_2 bubbles in tissues and blood around the joint causes severe joint pain).

CARDIOVASCULAR SYSTEM

1. Bradycardia in raised intracranial tension (Page no. 107)
2. Tachycardia in old age (due to fall in vagal tone)
3. Physiological hypertrophy of the left ventricle (LV has to do more work than RV, so LV wall becomes thicker than RV)
4. Heart sounds are not produced during opening of valves (opening of valves is a slowly developing process and so produce no sound)
5. Myocardium is well perfused during diastole (Page no. 112)
6. Fainting during emotions (Page no. 120)
7. The thin walled and delicate capillaries are less prone to rupture (Page no. 78)
8. Dilated heart has to do more work than a non-dilated heart (Because when the radius of a cardiac chamber is increased, a greater tension must be developed in myocardium to produce any given pressure)
9. Veins are called capacitance vessels (Page no. 77)
10. Variation in arteriolar diameter has marked effect on the systolic blood pressure (Page no. 79; BP = CO × PR. Peripheral resistance inversely proportional to radius raised to the power of 4)
11. Cardiac muscle cannot be tetanized/Cardiac muscle shows no signs of fatigue (Page no. 85)
12. Atrial and ventricular muscles do not show autorhythmicity (potential in them is plateau potential, it is not spontaneous and is produced only by stimulus from pacemaker cells which is spontaneous)
13. During BP measurements, systolic BP should be first measured by palpatory method (Page no. 359; auscultatory gap)
14. Heart rate increases in inspiration (Page no. 107)
15. Increased stroke volume during exercise (due to skeletal muscle pump, there is increase in venous return leading to increased in stroke volume)
16. Pressing the carotid sinus increases the heart rate (baroreceptor reflex)
17. Extracellular concentration of calcium influences the force of conduction in cardiac muscle. (For cardiac muscle AP the source of calcium for muscle contraction is not only stores in sarcoplasmic reticulum, but also extracellular calcium which enters from ECF to ICF)
18. Cold clammy skin and rapid pulse occurs in hypovolemic shock (due to activation of baroreceptor reflex and continuous vasoconstriction due increased sympathetic activity)
19. Body of a patient in shock should not be covered with blanket (because if covered with blanket body temperature raises, leading to increased metabolic activity making the condition of shock worser).

GASTROINTESTINAL SYSTEM

1. Postprandial alkaline tide or alkaline urine after heavy meal (Page no. 131)
2. Bulky, clay colored stools in obstructive jaundice (Page no. 135; Stercobilinogen gives normal color to stool)
3. A patient suffering from aptyalism has high-risk of dental caries (Page no. 128)
4. Steatorrhea occurs in pancreatic insufficiency (Page no. 135)
5. Gastrin release though vagally mediated is not blocked by atropine (Because the transmitter secreted by the post-ganglionic vagal fibers that innervate the gastrin cells is 'GRP' and not ACh)
6. Gastric mucosa is resistant to autodigestion (Page no. 133; Mucosal barrier)
7. Alcohol intoxication can be avoided if it is consumed after ingestion of a drink rich in fat (Gastric emptying time is the slowest for a fat rich food)
8. Duodenal ulcer can be treated by vagotomy (Vagotomy results in decreased gastric juice secretion during all its phases)
9. Resection of large segment of ileum can result in steatorrhea (Page no. 149)
10. Achlorhydria is associated with iron deficiency anemia (Iron is readily absorbed in ferrous state, but most of the dietary iron is in ferric form and HCl is needed for its reduction)
11. Ranitidine or Omeprazole is given in peptic ulcer (Page no. 134)
12. Dizziness after a heavy meal in gastrectomized patient (Page no. 150, dumping syndrome)
13. Rapidly changing movement causes vomiting (Stimulation of vomiting center)
14. Loss of fluid from the colon in chronic diarrhea results in severe hypokalemia (Because net movement of K^+ is directly proportional to the potential difference between blood and intestinal lumen)
15. Appreciable amounts of feces continue to be passed during prolonged starvation (Large fraction of facal mass is of non-dietary origin)
16. Majority of bile reaches circulation (Page no. 138)
17. Misoprostol given to patients on treatment of arthritis with NSAIDs (Page no. 134)
18. Glucose is not formed by the action of salivary amylase on starch (Salivary amylase acts on alpha 1, 4 linkage, but spares alpha 1, 6 linkage, terminal alpha 1, 4 linkage and alpha 1, 4 linkage next to branching points. Hence, the end products of alpha amylase digestion are oligosaccharides, disaccharides and trisaccharides)

RENAL PHYSIOLOGY

1. PCT has a high rate of O_2 consumption. (PCT cells are rich in mitochondria)
2. High resistance is offered to blood flow in efferent arteriole (efferent arteriole diameter is smaller compared to afferent arteriole)
3. Chronic renal disease produces anemia (Erythropoietin production decreases)
4. Predicted renal threshold for glucose is more than the actual value (Page no. 165)
5. Hyperventilation is associated with alkaline urine (Hyperventilation causes decreased CO_2 in cells → decreased H^+ formation within tubular cells leading to decreased HCO_3^- reabsorption)
6. Angiotensin II plays an important role in the body response to hypovolemia. (Angiotensin II has generalized vasoconstrictor effect, stimulate aldosterone, and ADH secretion)
7. Increase in ANP secretion leads to natriuresis. (Increase in ANP leads to efferent arteriolar constriction resulting in increased glomerular capillary resistance and thereby increases GFR, resulting in natriuresis)
8. Hemoglobin is the main buffer system in the body (Hb is present in large amounts and it contains 38 histidine molecules)
9. There is increased frequency of micturition during nervousness (During emotional stress, the power of urinary bladder to elongate its fibers as its contents increase in suspension)
10. High protein diet increases the ability of kidney to concentrate the urine (Page no. 168)
11. Albuminuria in nephrotic syndrome (Page no. 176)
12. Splay in glucose titration curve (Page no. 165)
13. Hyperosmolarity in medullary interstitium (Page no. 167)
14. Plateau phase in cystometrogram (Page no. 173)
15. Renal medulla is exposed to hypoxic damage than cortex (Cortex has more blood supply than the medulla. O_2 extraction of the cortex is also less compared to the medulla)
16. PAH is used to determine the renal blood flow (Page no. 171).

ENDOCRINOLOGY

1. Iodine preparation is given before thyroidectomy (Iodides in high concentration decrease all phases of thyroid activity, they slightly decrease the size of the thyroid gland and decrease its blood supply. This decrease the necessary amount of surgery, the amount of bleeding)
2. Hypothyroid patients prefer hot environment (because of decreased heat production, hypothyroid are hypersensitive to cold and prefer hot environment).

3. Even though prolactin increases during pregnancy, there is no milk secretion (prolactin plays an important role in development of lobuloalveolar system, its role in milk production is minimal)
4. Epinephrine does not produce reflex bradycardia (Page no. 212)
5. High levels of aldosterone cause diuresis and natriuresis (Page no. 207)
6. Perimetry is indicated in acromegaly (due to pituitary tumor the optic chiasma is getting compressed)
7. Purple striae, truncal obesity, red cheeks and moon like face are seen in Cushing's syndrome (Page no. 210)
8. Centripetal distribution of fat in Cushings syndrome. (Page no. 210)
9. Polyuria, polydypsia and polyphagia in DM (Page no. 205)
10. Amenorrhea during postpartum lactation (Page no. 190)
11. Exophthalmos in hyperthyroidism (Page no. 196)
12. Myxodema and carotinemia in hypothyroidism (Page no. 196)
13. Hypothyroidism retards growth (Page no. 194)
14. Muscle weakness in both hypothyroidism and hyperthyroidism (Page no 194; hyperthyroidism cause weakness of muscle due to catabolism of proteins in physiological amounts, thyroid hormone is essential for skeletal maturation)
15. Use of T4 metabolites as cholesterol lowering agents (T4 metabolites increase breakdown of cholesterol in liver and increases excretion of cholesterol in bile)
16. Alteration of thyroid activity impairs fertility in women (Page no. 194; because of disordered cyclic ovarian activity)
17. Diabetes mellitus is usually seen in hyperthyroid patients (Thyroid hormones cause hyperglycemia)
18. A person suffering from hypothyroidism is advised to avoid cabbage in his diet (Cabbage is a goitrogen, which forms goitrin, an active antithyroid agent and it prevents incorporation of iodine with tyrosine)
19. Children with cretinism have short stature and mental defect (Page no. 194)
20. Milk ejection in a lactating mother in response to cry of the baby (Oxytocin secretion can be conditioned, the physical stimulation of nipples is no longer required)
21. Sexual precocity individuals are dwarf (Although androgen initially stimulate growth, yet ultimately terminates growth by causing epiphyseal closure, thereby decreasing linear growth)
22. Diabetic children fail to grow (Due to impaired glucose utilization)
23. Diabetic patient fails to gain weight inspite of polyphagia. (Due to impaired glucose utilization)
24. Bile increases calcium absorption from the GIT (Bile and bile salts increase the solubility of Ca salts)
25. Higher incidence of fractures after 40 years of age (After 40 years of age, there is normally a progressive loss of skeletal mass, leading to 'senile' osteoporosis)
26. Neuromuscular hyperexcitability is seen in tetany (Page no. 200)
27. Glucocorticoids are used in prevention of rejection of a tissue transplant. (Glucocorticoids in the late stages, decreases antibody formation by its destructive effect on fixed lymphoid tissues)
28. Osteoporosis is associated with glucocorticoid excess (Page no. 202)
29. Anemia in persons suffering from chronic adrenal insufficiency (Page no. 209)
30. Glucocorticoids have hyperglycemic effect (Page no. 208)
31. Hyperpigmentation in aldosteronism (High aldosterone levels leads to indirect stimulation of melanocyte stimulating hormone)
32. Dopamine is used in management of shock (Page no. 213)
33. Carpopedal spasm is seen in tetany (Decrease in Ca^{2+})
34. Injection of epinephrine produces a biphasic effect on BP (Page no. 212, Dales vasomotor reversal)
35. Non-pitting edema in hypothyroidism (Increased quantities of hyaluronic acid and chondritin sulfate bound with protein form excessive tissue gel in the interstitial spaces. Because of gel nature of excess fluid, the edema is non-pitting type)
36. Alloxan administration leads to DM and not DI (Pancreatic cell destruction)
37. In Conn's syndrome there is no peripheral edema (Due to aldosterone escape and here there is increased of ANP leading to increased Na^+ excretion, so no accumulation thereby no edema)
38. V_2 receptor mutation results in diabetes insipidus. (Vasopressin causes rapid insertion of aquaporin-2 on collecting duct through V_2 receptor).

REPRODUCTIVE SYSTEM

1. Oral contraceptives prevent pregnancy (Page no. 231)
2. Sterility in a man working in hot surroundings (Spermatogenesis requires a temperature considerably lower than that of the interior of the body, high temperature impairs spermatogenesis)
3. Androgen when given orally is ineffective. (It is inactivated in the liver by converting it into less potent androsterone and dehydroepiandrosterone)
4. Menstrual blood does not normally contain clots (Page no. 222; it is liquefied by fibrinolysin in the vagina)
5. There is usually swelling and tenderness of breasts prior to menstruation (These are cyclic changes occurring in the breasts under the influence of estrogen and progesterone)
6. LH surge is necessary for ovulation (Page no. 223)

7. Ovulation occurs around the 14th day of normal menstrual cycle (occurs due to a sudden rise in LH secretion secondary to rise in estrogen concentration)
8. Higher incidences of patent ductus arteriosus in children with history of fetal distress (decreased PO_2 of ductus blood in cases of fetal distress)
9. Removal of ovaries in the 6th week of pregnancy results in termination of pregnancy (because during the first 3 months corpus luteum in the ovaries secrete estrogen and progesterone, the hormone maintaining pregnancy and later only the placenta takes over).

CENTRAL NERVOUS SYSTEM

1. Acupuncture lessens pain (Page no. 271)
2. Gentle rubbing over the area reduces pain sensation (Page no. 271)
3. Discharge of postsynaptic neuron even after cessation of presynaptic impulse (Page no. 263; after discharge)
4. Over reaction to pain occurs in thalamic lesions (Thalamic syndrome)
5. Wounded soldiers in battlefield are unaware of pain (Page no. 271; stress analgesia)
6. Phantom limb (Page no. 259)
7. Clasp knife effect and clonus-physiological basis (Page no. 262)
8. Spinal man cannot stand unsupported (Page no. 287)
9. Rigidity occurs in lesion of basal ganglia (Page no. 301)
10. Pendular knee jerk in cerebellar lesion (Page no. 294)
11. Finger nose test is positive in cerebellar lesion (Page no. 294; damping function)
12. L-dopa in Parkinsonism (Page no. 302)
13. Resting tremors in basal ganglia dysfunctions (Page no. 302)
14. Cerebellar lesions affect the same side of the body (double crossing; each cerebellar hemisphere influences the opposite cortex; which in turn the motor cortex via the corticospinal tracts controls the movement of the opposite side of the body. Because of the double decussation, each cerebellar hemisphere controls the voluntary movements on its own side of the body)
15. Babinski's sign positive in UMN lesion (Page no. 276)
16. Stimulation of gamma efferent system causes reflex contraction of all muscles (Stimulation of gamma efferents shortens the contractile ends of intrafusal fibers which stretches nuclear bag portion of spindles, deforming the annulospiral endings and initiate impulses in the Ia fiber leading to reflex contraction of muscle)
17. Jendrassik's maneuver facilitates deep tendon reflex (Reinforcement acts by increasing the excitability of alpha motor neurons and by increasing the sensitivity of the muscle spindle primary sensory endings to stretch)
18. Ankle clonus in UMN lesion (in UMN lesion there is increased activity of facilitatory area leading to increased tone and also there is increased gamma efferent discharge leading to clonus)
19. Deep tendon reflex is exaggerated in spastic paralysis (decrease in supraspinal inhibition on gamma efferents)
20. REM sleep is called paradoxical sleep (Page no. 297).

SPECIAL SENSES

1. Vision is not possible over the optic disk (optic disk contains no light sensitive receptors)
2. Visual acuity is maximum over fovea (fovea is a rod free portion where the cones are densely packed and there are few cells and no blood vessels overlying the receptors)
3. High incidence of cataract in diabetes mellitus patients (due to the action of glucose on lens protein which makes them easily coagulable by light)
4. Retinal detachment damages photoreceptors. (Photoreceptors are mainly nourished by the capillary plexus in the choroid)
5. Blurring of vision when a person is inside water (when a person is inside water, no refraction occurs at the cornea as refractive index of water and cornea becomes the same)
6. Blurred vision following instillation of homatropine into the eye (local administration of homatropine causes mydriasis (dilatation of pupil) and cyclopegia (loss of accommodation)
7. Reading or close work becomes progressively difficult with advancing age (near point becomes progressively distant with advancing age)
8. Ultraviolet and infrared are not perceived by the human eye (eye responds to light of wavelength between 400 nm and 750 nm called visibility or sensitivity range of vision)
9. Cones are responsible for color vision (different color sensations are produced by stimulation of various combination of 3 types of receptors–cyanolabe, chlorolabe and erythrolabe)
10. Radiologists and aircraft pilots wear red goggles when in bright light. (They need maximum visual sensitivity in dim light. They can avoid having to wait 20 minutes in the dark to become dark adapted if they wear red goggles, light wavelength in the red end of the spectrum stimulate the rods to only a slight degree while permitting the cones to function reasonably well. Therefore, a person wearing red goggles can see in bright light, during the time it takes for the rods to become dark adapted)
11. Transient blue green color blindness occurs in patients taking sildenafil (viagra). (Drug inhibit retinal as well as penile form of phosphodiesterases) (Page no. 325).

CHAPTER

18

Calculations

Q1. Determine the absolute counts of neutrophils, eosinophils, and basophils from the data given below.

Data

a. Total leukocyte count = 7800/mm^3

b. Neutrophil count = 65%

c. Eosinophil count = 3.5%

d. Basophil count = 0.5%

Ans. Absolute neutrophil count = 7800/100 × 65 = 4875/mm^3

Absolute eosinophil count = 7800/100 × 3.5 = 273/mm^3

Absolute basophil count = 7800/100 × 0.5 = 39/mm^3

Q2. Determine the mean corpuscular hemoglobin (MCH) from the data given below.

Data

a. Hemoglobin concentration = 14.5 g/dl

b. RBC count = 4.8 million/mm^3

c. Packed cell volume = 42%

Ans. MCH = Hb (g/dl) × 10/RBC count (in millions/mm^3)

= 14.5 × 10/4.8 = 30 pg

Q3. Calculate the mean corpuscular volume (MCV) from the data given below.

Data

a. RBC count = 4.5 million/mm^3

b. Packed cell volume (PCV) = 40%

c. Hb concentration = 14 g/dl

Ans. MCV = PCV ×10/RBC count (in millions/mm^3)

= 40 × 10/4.5 = 88 μm^3

Q4. Calculate the mean corpuscular hemoglobin concentration from the data given below.

Data

a. Hemoglobin concentration = 9 g/dl

b. Packed cell volume (PCV) = 36%

c. RBC count = 3.4 million/mm^3

Ans. MCHC = Hb (g%)/PCV × 100 = 9/36 × 100 = 25%

Q5. Calculate the platelet count from the data given below.

Data

a. Number of platelets in 80 smallest squares = 34

b. Dilution of blood employed = 1 in 200 (1:200)

Ans. Number of platelets in 80 smallest squares = 34

Volume of these 80 squares = 1/50 mm^3

(volume of 1 smallest square = 1/4000 mm^3)

Thus, 1/50 mm^3 contains = 34 platelets

Therefore, 1 mm^3 contains 34 × 50 = 1700 platelets

Dilution employed is 1 in 200

Number of platelets in undiluted blood = 1700 × 200

= 340,000/mm^3

The platelet count is 3.4 lacs/mm^3.

Q6. Determine the reticulocyte count from the data given below.

Data

a. Number of RBCs in 50 oil immersion fields = 1500

b. Number of reticulocytes in 100 oil immersion fields = 45

Number of RBCs in 50 oil immersion fields = 1500

Therefore, number of cells in 100 oil immersion fields = 3000

Ans. Number of reticulocytes in 100 oil immersion field = 45 (data)

Thus, per 3000 RBCs, there are 45 reticulocytes

Therefore, per 100 RBCs, there are 45/3000 × 100 = 1.5 reticulocytes

The reticulocyte count is 1.5% of red cells.

Q7. Find out the physiological dead space from the data provided below.

Data

a. Tidal volume = 450 ml

b. Alveolar air PCO_2 = 40 mm Hg

c. Expired air PCO_2 = 26 mm Hg

Ans. Physiological dead space = [(Alveolar air PCO_2 – expired air PCO_2)/Alveolar air PCO_2] × Tidal volume

= [(40 – 26)/40] × 450 = 157 ml.

Q8. Find out the expiratory reserve volume (ERV); residual volume (RV); inspiratory reserve volume (IRV); and functional residual capacity (FRC) from the given data.

Data

a. Total lung capacity = 5200 ml

b. Tidal volume = 450 ml

c. Inspiratory capacity = 3000 ml

d. Vital capacity = 4000 ml

Ans. ERV = VC – IC = 4000 – 3000 = 1000 ml
RV = TLC – VC = 5200 – 4000 = 1200 ml
IRV = IC – TV = 3000 – 450 = 2550 ml
FRC = RV + ERV = 1200 + 1000 = 2200 ml

Q9. Determine the oxygen carrying capacity and oxygen content of arterial and venous blood samples from the data provided below.

Data

a. Percentage saturation of arterial blood with oxygen = 97%

b. Percentage saturation of venous blood with oxygen = 75%

c. Hemoglobin concentration = 14.5 g/dl

Ans. Oxygen carrying capacity of blood (ml/100 ml) = Hb (g%) × 1.34 = 14.5 × 1.34 = 19.43 ml/dl

Formula for O_2 content of blood = (Percentage saturation × Oxygen carrying capacity)/100

Oxygen content of arterial blood = (97 × 19.43)/100 = 18.84 ml/100 ml

Oxygen content of venous blood = (75 × 19.43)/100 = 14.57 ml/100 ml

Q10. Find out the breathing reserve and the dyspnea index from the data provided below.

Data

a. Respiratory rate = 12/min

b. Tidal volume = 500 ml

c. Maximum voluntary ventilation (MVV) = 130 liters (Syn: maximum voluntary volume)

Ans. Respiratory minute volume (RMV), i.e. volume of gas expired per minute = 500 × 12 = 6000 ml

Breathing reserve = MVV – RMV = 130 – 6 = 124 liters (It means that the ventilation can be increased from 6 l/min to 130 l/min with maximum effort).

Dyspnea index (breathing reserve percent) = [(MVV – RMV)/MVV] × 100 = [(130 – 6)/130] × 100 = 95%

(When the dyspnea index falls below 70% (dyspnea point), dyspnea is present. We are not conscious of breathing until ventilation is doubled. Breathing is not uncomfortable (i.e. dyspnea point is not reached) until ventilation increases 3 or 4 times the resting level).

Q11. Calculate the respiratory quotient from the data given below.

Data

a. Volume of expired air in 6 minutes = 30 liters

b. Percentage of CO_2 in expired air = 4.2%

c. Oxygen consumption in 6 minutes = 1470 ml

Ans. Volume of expired air in 6 minutes = 30 liters

Volume of expired air in 1 minute = 5 liters

Percentage of CO_2 in expired air = 4.2%

Therefore, 5000 ml of expired air in 1 minute contain = 5000 × 4.2 = 210 ml of CO_2

Oxygen consumed in 6 minutes = 1470 ml

Therefore, oxygen consumed in 1 minute = 1470/6 = 245 ml

Respiratory quotient (RQ) = (CO_2 output/min)/(O_2 consumed/min) = 210/245 = 0.85

Q12. Calculate the cardiac index of the individual from his data given below.

Data

a. Cardiac output = 5.20 liters/min

b. Body surface area (BSA) = 1.65 m^2

Ans. (Cardiac index is the cardiac output per m^2 BSA per minute)

Cardiac index = (Cardiac output/min)/BSA = 5.20/1.65 = 3.15

Cardiac index = 3.15 liters/min.

Q13. Calculate the heart rate from the ECG provided.

Ans. There are two methods to calculate the heart rate from an ECG.

1. Divide 1500 by the number of smallest squares between any two successive R waves:
   Assume there are 18 smallest squares between two R waves:
   Then the heart rate will be 1500/18 = 82/min.
2. Divide 300 by the number of large squares between any two successive R waves:
   Assume there are 4 large squares between two R waves:
   Then the heart rate will be 300/4 = 75/min.
   The constant 1500 and 300 are used because 1500 × 0.04 sec (each smallest square represents 0.04 sec) = 60 sec and 300 × 0.2 sec (each large square represents 0.2 sec) = 60 sec and the heart rate is been calculated in beats per 60 sec. These formula should be used only when the heart rate is regular.

Q14. Calculate the stroke volume and cardiac output from the data given below.

Data

a. Oxygen content of mixed venous blood = 14.8 ml/100 ml

b. Oxygen content of systemic arterial blood = 19.5 ml/100 ml

c. Heart rate = 70/min

d. Oxygen consumption per minute = 245 ml

Ans. (The cardiac output is calculated by applying Fick principle).

Cardiac output = (Oxygen consumption/Arteriovenous oxygen difference) × 100 = 245/(19.5 – 14.8) × 100 = (245/4.7) × 100 = 5200 ml

Stroke volume = Cardiac output/Heart rate = 5200/70 = 74 ml

Q15. Calculate the effective filtration pressure from the data given below.

Data

a. Glomerular capillary hydrostatic pressure = 55 mm Hg
b. Glomerular capillary blood osmotic pressure = 30 mm Hg
c. Bowman's capsular fluid pressure = 15 mm Hg
d. Bowman's capsular fluid osmotic pressure = 0 mm Hg.

Ans. ***Effective filtration pressure:*** Glomerular hydrostatic pressure **(55 mm Hg)** – Glomerular osmotic pressure **(30 mm Hg)** + Bowman capsule pressure **(15 mm Hg)**.

The effective filtration pressure is the function of two variables: the hydrostatic pressure gradient driving fluid out of the glomerular capillaries and into Bowman's capsule, and the colloid osmotic pressure gradient bringing fluid into the glomerular capillaries. The colloid osmotic pressure of capsular fluid is near zero because it normally contains little protein—only a few milligrams of albumin which is reabsorbed in the proximal tubules.

The glomerular hydrostatic pressure is about 55 mm Hg when the mean systemic arterial pressure is 100 mm Hg.
Thus, the effective filtration pressure = 55 – (30 + 15)
= 10 mm Hg

The glomerular capillary hydrostatic pressure is about 55 mm Hg when the mean systemic arterial pressure is 100 mm Hg.
Thus, the effective filtration pressure = 55 – (30 + 15)
= 10 mm Hg

Q16. Calculate the glomerular filtration rate (GFR) from the data provided below.

Data

a. Concentration of inulin in plasma (P) = 0.24 mg/ml
b. Concentration of inulin in urine (U) = 34 mg/ml
c. Rate of urine formation (V) = 0.9 ml/min

Ans. Plasma inulin clearance = (Concentration of inulin in urine × Volume of urine/min)/Concentration of inulin in plasma
$= (U_{IN} \times V)/P_{IN} = (34 \times 0.9)/0.24 = 127$ ml/min

The major determinant of GFR is the hydrostatic pressure within the glomerular capillaries. In addition, the renal blood flow (RBF) through the glomeruli has a great effect on GFR; when the rate of RBF increases, the GFR increases.

The term clearance refers to the volume of plasma from which a substance X is completely removed or 'cleared' per unit time, i.e. the ml of plasma that 'contained' the substance X that is present in one minute's urine. It is a theoretical volume rather than a volume that can be collected and directly measured. Its value can be calculated from measurable quantities. For example, inulin is only filtered and measures GFR, while p-aminohippuric acid (PAH; see below) is both filtered and secreted into the proximal tubules and measures renal blood flow (RBF).

Q17. Calculate the renal blood flow (RBF) from the data given below.

Data

a. Concentration of PAH in urine (UPAH) = 14 mg/ml
b. Concentration of PAH in plasma (PPAH) = 0.03 mg/ml
c. Rate of urine flow (V) = 1.5 ml/min
d. Hematocrit (Hct) = 43%

Ans. Plasma clearance of PAH
$= (U_{PAH} \times V)/P_{PAH} = (14 \times 1.5)/0.03 = 700$ ml/min
This plasma clearance of PAH is the effective renal plasma flow (ERPF).
The ERPF can be converted into actual renal plasma flow (RPF):
Actual RPF = ERPF/Extraction ratio =700/0.9
= 770 ml/min
(About 90% of PAH in the arterial blood is removed during a single passage through the kidneys, i.e. its extraction ratio is 0.9)
Hematocrit = 43% (given data)
Therefore, renal blood flow = [100/(100 – Hct)] × RPF
= [100/(100 – 43)] × 770
= (100/57) × 770 = 1350
The renal blood flow is 1350 ml per minute.

Q18. Calculate the urea clearance from the given data.

Data

a. Concentration of urea in urine (U) = 20 mg/ml
b. Concentration of urea in blood (B) = 38 mg/100 ml
c. Rate of urine flow (V) = 1.5 ml/min

Ans. Since the urine flow is less than 2.0 ml/min, the formula of 'standard' urea clearance is: $[(U \times \sqrt{V})/B] \times 100$
Urea clearance $= [(20 \times \sqrt{1.5})/38] \times 100$
$= [(20 \times 1.22)/38] \times 100$
= 64 ml/min

It has been shown empirically that with rapid flow of urine (2 ml per minute or more), the excretion of urea is maximum—hence called 'maximum' urea clearance. The formula for maximum clearance is UV/P. The value for maximum clearance is 65–100 ml per minute, while the normal value for standard clearance is 40–65 ml per minute.

CHAPTER

19 Question Bank

GENERAL PHYSIOLOGY

1. Transport across cell membrane (3)
2. Facilitated diffusion (4)
3. Compartment of body fluids (7)
4. Na^+– K^+ ATPase pump (5)
5. All or none response (11)
6. RMP: Ionic basis (9)
7. Action potential graph and ionic basis (9)
8. Latent period (10)
9. Refractory period (12)
10. Various channel blockers – Na, K, Ca (5)
11. Saltatory conduction (12)
12. Compound action potential (13)

CIRCULATING BODY FLUIDS

Short Notes

1. Functions of blood (20)
2. Plasma proteins-functions and values (20)
3. Factors affecting erythropoiesis (27)
4. Red cell indices (25)
5. ESR—clinical significance (335)
6. Hb—functions and variants (21)
7. Fate of Hb (22)
8. Heme-heme interaction (22)
9. Agranulocytosis (32)
10. Functions and properties of neutrophils (30)
11. Polycythemia (30)
12. Functions of platelets and their role in hemostasis (purpuras) (33)
13. Thalassemia (22)
14. Clotting factors (34)
15. Role of calcium in coagulation (35)
16. Platelet plug formation (33)
17. Hemophilia—types (36)
18. Arneth count (22)
19. Cellular immunity (41)
20. Humoral immunity (39)
21. Immunoglobulins (40)
22. Reticuloendothelial system (41)
23. Purpura (36)
24. Fibrinolytic system (35)
25. Blood group - ABO system (37)
26. Landsteiner's law (37)
27. Rh incompatibility (Hemolytic disease of newborn) (37)
28. Kernicterus (38)
29. Erythroblastosis fetalis (38)
30. Anticoagulants and their mechanism of action (37)
31. Cross matching (37)
32. Indications and complications of blood transfusion (38)

Essays

1. Erythropoiesis and factors affecting it (26)
2. Mechanism of blood coagulation: Intrinsic and extrinsic (33)
3. Anemia: Classification, causes and symptoms (28)
4. Formation and functions of lymph: Starling's law (42)

RESPIRATORY SYSTEM

Short Notes

1. Respiratory and non-respiratory functions of lungs (47)
2. Surfactants—functions, factors affecting synthesis, applications (52)
3. Artificial respiration (78)
4. Lung compliance (54)
5. Spirogram (50)
6. Lung volumes: TV, IRV, ERV, RV (50)
7. Lung capacities: VC, IC, FRC, TLC (50)
8. Timed vital capacity and its clinical significance (52)
9. FEV, difference between obstructive and restrictive lung diseases (52)
10. Physiological shunt and significance (56)
11. Dead space: Anatomical and physiological functions (55)
12. V/P ratio (Ventilation-perfusion ratio) (56)
13. Respiratory membrane and the factors affecting diffusion of gases (47)
14. Haldane effect (60)
15. Bohr effect (58)
16. Chloride shift (Hamburger phenomenon)—its significance (59)
17. Hering-Breuer reflex (63)
18. ODC—shift to right and left, factors affecting it (58)

19. CO_2 dissociation curve with graph (59)
20. Periodic breathing - Cheyne-Stokes respiration and Biot's breathing (70)
21. Cyanosis, definition and types (69)
22. Decompression sickness (Caisson's disease, Dysbarism) (72)
23. Acclimatization, mountain sickness (71)
24. Asphyxia (69)
25. Inspiratory RAMP signal (61)
26. Airway resistance, factors affecting it (47)

Essays

1. Regulation of respiration (Neural and chemical) (60)
2. Respiratory changes in exercise (73)
3. Hypoxia (65)
4. O_2 and CO_2 transport (57)
5. Adjustments in respiratory physiology at high altitude (71)

CARDIOVASCULAR SYSTEM

Short Notes

1. Action potential of cardiac muscle: Ionic basis and diagram (80)
2. Heart: Conducting system, AV nodal delay (81)
3. Pacemaker potential (81)
4. Regulation of heart rate (104)
5. Factors affecting BP (108)
6. Determinants of BP (109)
7. Arterial pulse (92)
8. Stokes-Adams syndrome (100)
9. WPW and LGL syndrome (100)
10. Wenckebach phenomenon (PR interval and its importance) (100)
11. Heart sounds and murmurs (93)
12. LV pressure changes with the graph (89)
13. Aortic pressure changes: Incisura (90)
14. Heart block (99)
15. JVP and its clinical significance (88)
16. Frank-Starling law (85)
17. Laplace's law: Application (78)
18. CSF formation and functions (114)
19. EDV- factors affecting it (86)
20. Fick principle: Measurement of CO (102)
21. Baroreceptor reflex (105)
22. Bainbridge reflex (106)
23. Bezold-Jarisch reflex (106)
24. Windkessel effect (77)
25. Marey's law (106)
26. Cushing reflex (107)
27. Vagal escape and vagal inhibition (104)
28. ECG: Waves and intervals (98)
29. Types of blood flow, Reynolds number and its significance (78)
30. Blood-brain barrier (115)
31. Triple response (117)
32. Axon reflex (118)
33. Special features of coronary circulation (112)
34. Cerebral circulation (113)
35. ECG leads (95)
36. Hypertension (111)

Essays

1. BP—definition, determinants, long-term and short-term regulation of BP (108)
2. Cardiac output and its regulation: Homeometric and heterometric auto regulation (102)
3. Cardiac cycle: LV pressure changes, volume tracing (86)
4. Shock: Definition and types (118)
5. CVS changes in exercise (124)

GASTROINTESTINAL SYSTEM

Short Notes

1. Nerve supply of GIT (127)
2. Saliva: Composition, functions, regulation of secretion (128)
3. Chorda tympani/Frey's syndrome (129)
4. Gastric juice: Composition and function (130)
5. Phases of gastric secretion-Vagovagal reflex (132)
6. Mechanism of HCl secretion and regulation (130)
7. Peptic ulcer (133)
8. Difference between duodenal and gastric ulcer (134)
9. Actions of gastrin and regulation of secretion (150)
10. Pancreatic juice: Composition, functions, control (134)
11. Secretin (151)
12. CCK: PZ (151)
13. GI hormones (150)
14. Functions of liver (136)
15. Functions of gallbladder (138)
16. Formation and composition of bile and its functions (137)
17. Enterohepatic circulation (138)
18. Phases of deglutition (important - 2nd phase) (140)
19. Gastric emptying time and the factors affecting it (142)
20. Hunger contractions (142)
21. MMC (142)
22. BER (141)
23. Vomiting mechanism (142)
24. Steatorrhea (135)
25. Achalasia cardia (141)
26. Mucosal barrier (133)
27. Functions of SI and LI (107)
28. Peristaltic movements of SI and LI (143)
29. Importance of dietary fibers (149)
30. Chylomicron (149)
31. Sham feeding (133)

Essays

1. Control and secretion of gastric juice (131)
2. Peptic ulcer: Causes, types, symptoms, complications (133)
3. Movements of small intestine (143)
4. Jaundice and its types (138)
5. GI hormones (130)
6. Digestion and absorption of carbohydrates: Full (145)
7. Fat digestion, absorption: Full (147)

RENAL PHYSIOLOGY

Short Notes

1. Functions of kidney (153)
2. JG apparatus (155)
3. Nephron (153)
4. Difference between cortical and juxtamedullary nephrons (155)
5. Peculiarities of renal circulation (157)
6. Autoregulation of renal blood flow (158)
7. GFR: Factors affecting, normal value, measurement (159)
8. Counter current mechanism (167)
9. Na^+ reabsorption (161)
10. Water reabsorption (164)
11. Glucose reabsorption (164)
12. Nephrotic syndrome (176)
13. Transport maximum(T_{max}) (164)
14. Tubuloglomerular feedback (158)
15. Glomerulotubular balance (163)
16. Cystometrogram (173)
17. Micturition reflex (173)
18. Abnormalities of micturition (174)
19. Bladder innervations (172)
20. Automatic and atonic bladder (174)
21. Tubular maximum for glucose (164)
22. Obligatory and facultative H_2O absorption (164)
23. Clearance tests (171)
24. Diuretics (175)
25. Acid-base balance (169)
26. Renin: Angiotensin Mechanism (156)
27. Splay (165)
28. Difference between osmotic and H_2O dieresis (175)
29. RFT, renal flow measurements (171)
30. Renal circulation (157)

Essays

1. GFR: Factors affecting (full essay) (159)
2. Mechanism of urine formation (159)
3. Urine concentrating mechanism (Counter current mechanism) (167)
4. Acidification of urine—factors influencing H^+ secretion (169)
5. Reabsorption of glucose, Na^+, H_2O (full essay) (161, 164)

TEMPERATURE REGULATION

Regulation of body temperature (178).

ENDOCRINOLOGY

Short Notes

1. Mechanism of hormone action, twenty messenger (182)
2. Somatomedin (185)
3. Hypothalamo-hypophyseal axis (184)
4. Acromegaly (187)
5. Gigantism (186)
6. Dwarfism (187)
7. Difference between pituitary and thyroid dwarf (187)
8. Synthesis of thyroid hormones (192)
9. Difference between T3 and T4 (193)
10. Action of growth hormone and regulation (185, 186)
11. Actions of thyroid hormone (193)
12. Hyperthyroidism (196)
13. Myxedema (196)
14. Antithyroid drugs (195)
15. Diabetes mellitus: Types, clinical features (204)
16. Cushing's syndrome (210)
17. Glucagon (206)
18. Adrenogenital syndrome (211)
19. Regulation of mineralocorticoid secretion (207)
20. Addison's disease (211)
21. Vitamin D actions (198)
22. Hormones of anterior pituitary (184)
23. PTH: Actions and regulations (198)
24. Hypocalcemic tetany (200)
25. Calcitonin: Actions (199)
26. Aldosterone escape (207)
27. Thyroid function tests (195)
28. Oxytocin: Action, regulation (190)
29. ADH: Action, regulation (190)
30. Dale's vasomotor reversal (212)
31. Regulation of glucocorticoid secretion (209)
32. Mechanism of action of aldosterone (207)
33. Addisonian crisis (211)
34. Diabetes insipidus: Types (205)
35. Prolactin (189)

Essays

1. TH: Synthesis, actions, regulation, disorders (192)
2. Insulin: Secretion, action, regulation (regulation of blood sugar level) (202)
3. Glucocorticoids: Action and regulation (208)
4. Calcium homeostasis (197)
5. ADH: Biosynthesis, action and regulation (191)
6. Mineralocorticoids: Function, regulation and abnormalities (207)

7. Hormonal regulation of glucose metabolism (186, 193, 203, 206, 208)
8. Hormonal physiology of growth (188)

REPRODUCTIVE SYSTEM

Short Notes

1. Spermatogenesis: Factors influencing it (216)
2. Blood-testis barrier (215)
3. Functions of sertoli cells (218)
4. Tests for male infertility (219)
5. Actions of testosterone and regulation (218)
6. Klinefelter Turners, Down syndrome (215)
7. Menstrual cycle graph with LH Surge (221)
8. Graffian follicle (221)
9. Actions of estrogen (224)
10. Actions of progesterone (224)
11. Fetoplacental unit (228)
12. Hormones of pregnancy, placental hormones (227, 229)
13. Milk ejection reflex/neuroendocrine reflex/sucking reflex (229)
14. Hormonal regulation of lactation (229)
15. Contraception (230)
16. Oral contraceptive pills and mini pills (232)
17. Cryptorchidism (219)
18. Pregnancy tests (226)
19. Ovulation (221)
20. Physiological changes during pregnancy (225)
21. Role of oxytocin in parturition (229)
22. IUCD (231)

Essays

Menstrual cycle: Its hormonal regulation (220)

NERVE MUSCLE PHYSIOLOGY

Short Notes

1. Structure of neuron: Diagram (233)
2. Classification of nerve fibers (234)
3. Neuromuscular junction and its inhibitors (238)
4. Wallerian degeneration (227)
5. Myasthenia gravis (240)
6. Motor unit (243)
7. Rigor mortis (244)
8. Role of calcium in muscle contraction (242)
9. Types of muscle fibers (244)
10. Isometric and isotonic contraction (244)
11. Sarcotubublar system (241)
12. Molecular basis of smooth muscle contraction (242)
13. Role in calmodulin in smooth muscle contraction (246)
14. Difference between action potential and end plate potential (258)
15. Diseases of neuromuscular junction (240)

Essays

Excitation contraction coupling (242)

CENTRAL NERVOUS SYSTEM

Short Notes

1. Synapse: Classification, functions, properties with synaptic delay (249)
2. Classification of receptors (257)
3. Properties of receptors, law of projection, Weber-Fechner law (257)
4. Summation and occlusion (255)
5. Phantom limb (259)
6. Generator potential (257)
7. Types of synaptic inhibition (pre, post and Renshaw cell) (253)
8. Reciprocal innervation (261)
9. Golgi bottle neuron (262)
10. Difference between EPSP, IPSP, Ionic basis (258)
11. Reflex arc with diagram (259)
12. Properties of reflex (263)
13. Adequate stimulus (263)
14. Monosynaptic reflex-stretch reflex (260)
15. Structure of muscle spindle and function (260)
16. Inverse stretch reflex (262)
17. Polysynaptic reflex-withdrawal reflex (262)
18. Crossed extensor reflex (262)
19. Pain-gait control theory, central analgesic system, modulation of pain (270)
20. Fast and slow pain (266)
21. Two-point discrimination and stereognosis (265)
22. Referred pain and theories (269)
23. Sensory homunculus (264)
24. Stages of complete transection of spinal cord (279)
25. Brown-Séquard syndrome (281)
26. Difference between UMN and LMN lesion (276)
27. Babinski's sign and its clinical importance (276)
28. Decerebrate and decorticate rigidity (288)
29. Functions of basal ganglia (301)
30. Functions of cerebellum (293)
31. Functions of hypothalamus (304)
32. ARAS (290)
33. Limbic system: Connections and functions (309)
34. Chorea, athetosis, ballism (302)
35. Tabes dorsalis (282)
36. Huntington's disease (302)
37. Parkinsonism: Cause and features (301)
38. Leadpipe rigidity and cogwheel rigidity (301)
39. Difference between spasticity and rigidity (274)
40. Difference between pyramidal and extrapyramidal tracts (274)

41. Extrapyramidal tract: Functions (273)
42. EEG: Waves, variation, uses (296)
43. Difference between REM and NREM sleep (299)
44. Motor homunculus (272)
45. Lesions of cerebellum (293)
46. Functional divisions of cerebellum (291)
47. Regulation of food intake (305)
48. Vestibular apparatus: Components, functions, mechanism of detection of linear and rotatory acceleration (282)
49. Mass reflex (264)
50. Speech: Areas involved, abnormalities (309)
51. Aphasia types (311)
52. Memory (312)
53. Conditioned reflexes: Types (312)
54. Epilepsy (296)

Essays

1. Properties of synapse and synaptic inhibition (255)
2. Touch pathway: Crude and fine (including pathway of face) (266, 267)
3. Pain, temperature pathway (theories of pain inhibition) (266)
4. Connections and functions of thalamus (Thalamic syndrome) (294)
5. Pyramidal tract: Components, functions, effect of lesions at various levels (especially at internal capsule) (272)
6. Basal ganglia: Connections, functions, disorders (Parkinsonism) (299)
7. Cerebellum: Connections, functions, disorders, symptoms of cerebellar dysfunction(reasons) (291)
8. Hypothalamus: Centers, connections and functions (303)

SPECIAL SENSES

Vision

Short Notes

1. Glaucoma (317)
2. Accomodation (323)
3. Near response (323)
4. Pupillary reflexes (322)
5. Errors of refraction (324)
6. Astigmatism (324)
7. Difference between rods and cones (318)
8. Electrical events in photoreceptors (318)
9. Color vision and theories—Young-Helmholtz theory (324)
10. Color blindness (325)
11. Dark adaptation (319)
12. Visual acuity and tests (320)
13. Night blindness (325)
14. Homonymous and heteronymous hemianopia (321)
15. Macular sparing (322)
16. Binocular vision and scotoma (322)
17. Strabismus (323)
18. Presbyopia (324)
19. Photopic and scotopic vision (320)
20. Near point and far point (324)
21. Argyll Robertson pupil (ARP) (323)
22. Reduced eye (320)

Essays

1. Visual pathway, effect of lesion at different levels (321)
2. Aqueous humor: Production, circulation and functions (317)

Hearing, Smell and Taste

Short Notes

1. Organ of Corti (326)
2. Auditory pathway (327)
3. Functions of middle ear (325)
4. Impedance matching (325)
5. Tympanic reflex (326)
6. Types of deafness: Conduction deafness and nerve deafness (328)
7. Rinne's, Weber's and Schwabach test (329)
8. Vestibulo-ocular reflex and nystagmus (329)
9. Theories of hearing (328)
10. Endocochlear potential (329)
11. Olfactory pathway (331)
12. Structure of taste bud (329)
13. Taste pathway (330)

LIST OF DIAGRAMS

General Physiology

Blood

Respiratory System

Cardiovascular System

3. JVP - phlebogram (88)
4. Pressure changes in LV correlated with phases of cardiac cycle (89)
5. Aortic pressure changes correlated with the phases of cardiac cycle (90)
6. ECG (98)
7. Sinoaortic reflex (105)

Gastrointestinal System

1. Layers of GIT (127)
2. Nerve supply of GIT (128)
3. Mechanism of HCl secretion (131)
4. Mucosal barrier (133)

Renal Physiology

1. Electron microscopic structure of nephron (154)
2. Juxtaglomerular apparatus (155)
3. Splay in glucose titration curve (165)
4. Innervation of urinary bladder (172)

Endocrinology

1. Negative feedback inhibition for growth hormone (186)
2. Synthesis of thyroid hormone (192)
3. Negative feedback inhibition for thyroid hormone (195)

Reproductive System

1. Phases of spermatogenesis (216)
2. Graph of menstrual cycle (221)

Nerve Muscle Physiology

1. Structure of neuron (233)
2. Neuromuscular junction (238)
3. Sarcomere (240)

Central Nervous System

1. Muscle spindle (260)
2. CS of spinal cord at thoracic level showing all ascending and descending tracts (264)
3. Presynaptic and postsynaptic inhibition (254)
4. Stretch and inverse stretch reflex (262)
5. Dorsal column pathway (266)
6. Lateral spinothalamic pathway (266)
7. Ventral (anterior) spinothalamic pathway (267)
8. Neuronal connections in basal ganglia (300)
9. Neuronal connections in cerebellum (292)
10. Pyramidal tract (272)

Special Senses

1. Structure of eye (316)
2. Visual pathway and field defects due to lesions at various levels (322)
3. Layers of retina (316)
4. Cross section of cochlea (326)
5. Structure of the organ of corti (327)
6. Structure of olfactory mucous membrane (331)
7. Structure of taste bud (329)
8. Taste pathway (330)

CHAPTER 20

Common Laboratory Values

CIRCULATING BODY FLUIDS

1. RBC count:
   Males: 5.4×10^6 /µL
   Females: 4.8×10^6 /µL
2. WBC count
   Total: 9,000 cells/µL (average)
   Range: 4000 – 11000 cells/µL

	Average	Range
3. Granulocyte		
• Neutrophils	5400 cells/µL	3000–6000 cells/µL
• Eosinophils	275 cells/µL	150–300 cells/µL
• Basophils	35 cells/µL	0–100 cells/µL
4. Lymphocytes	2750 cells/µL	1500–4000 cells/µL
5. Monocytes	540 cells/µL	300–600 cells/µL
6. Platelets	3,00,000 cells/µL	2,00,000–5,00,000 cells/µL

7. Hematocrit (Hct)
   Males : 47%
   Females : 42%
8. Hemoglobin (Hb)
   Males : 16 g/dL
   Females : 14 g/dL
9. Mean corpuscular volume (MCV)
   Males : 87 fL or μm^3
   Females : 87 fL or μm^3
10. Mean corpuscular hemoglobin (MCH)
   Males : 29 pg
   Females : 29 pg
11. Mean corpuscular hemoglobin concentration (MCHC)
   Males : 34 g/dL
   Females : 34 g/dL
12. Mean cell diameter (MCD)
   Males : 7.5 µm
   Females : 7.5 µm
13. Protein (Serum concentration)
   - Total : 6.0–8.0 g/dL
   - Albumin : 3.1–4.3 g/dL
   - Globulin : 2.6–4.1 g/dL
   - Fibrinogen : 1.5–4 g/dL
14. Bilirubin (Serum)
   Conjugated (direct) : up to 0.4 mg/dL
   Unconjugated (indirect) : 0.6 mg/dL
   Total (conjugated plus free) : up to 1.0 mg/dL
15. Normal bleeding time : 1–5 minutes
16. Normal clotting time : 3–6 minutes

   Note:
   a. Mean cell diameter is the mean diameter of 500 cells in smear.
   b. Cells with MCVs > 95 fL are called macrocytes; cells with MCVs < 80 fL are called microcytes; cells with MCHs < 25 g/dL are called hypochromic.
17. Glucose, fasting (plasma): 70–110 mg/dL
18. Normal serum concentrations
   - Sodium : 135–145 mEq/L
   - Potassium : 3.5–5.0 mEq/L
   - Phosphorous (inorganic): 2.6–4.5 mg/dL
19. Normal blood uric acid: 4 mg/dL (0.24 mmol//L)
20. Total blood cholesterol:150–200 mg/dL
21. HDL fraction
   Males: 30–60 mg/dL
   Females: 35–75 mg/dL
22. LDL fraction (30–39 years): 80–175 mg/dL
23. Normal prothrombin time: 11–16 second

RESPIRATORY SYSTEM

1. Arterial blood
   - pO_2: 95 mm Hg
   - pCO_2: 40 mm Hg
   - Hb saturation: 97%
   - O_2 content: 19.8 ml O_2/dL
2. Venous blood
   - pO_2: 40 mm Hg
   - pCO_2: 46 mm Hg
   - Hb saturation: 75%
   - O_2 content: 15.2 ml O_2/dL

	Males	*Females*
3. Tidal volume (TV)	0.5 L	0.5 L
4. Inspiratory reserve volume (IRV)	3.3 L	1.9 L
5. Expiratory reserve volume (ERV)	1.0 L	0.7 L
6. Residual volume (RV)	1.2 L	1.1 L
7. Vital capacity (VC)	4.8 L	3.1 L
8. Inspiratory capacity (IC)	3.8 L	2.4 L
9. Expiratory capacity (EC)	1.5 L	1.2 L
10. Functional residual capacity (FRC)	2.2 L	1.8 L
11. Total lung capacity (TLC)	6.0 L	4.2 L

12. Respiratory minute volume (rest): 6 L/min
13. Alveolar ventilation (rest): 4.2 L/min
14. Maximal voluntary ventilation: 125-170 L/min
15. Timed vital capacity: 83% of total in 1sec, 97 % in 3 sec
16. Work of quiet breathing: 0.5 kg-m/min
17. Maximal work of breathing: 10 kg-m/breath
18. Compliance of lungs alone: 0.22 L/cm of H_2O
19. Compliance of lungs and thoracic wall: 0.11 L/cm of H_2O
20. Normal respiratory rate: 14–16/min
21. Normal intrapleural pressure: 754–757 mm Hg
22. Normal intra-alveolar pressure: 759–761 mm Hg

CARDIOVASCULAR SYSTEM

1. Normal cardiac output: 5 L/min (4.5–6 L/min)
2. Cardiac index: 2.5–3.6 L/min/m^2 BSA
3. Stroke volume: 70–90 ml
4. Normal heart rate: 60–100/min
5. End-diastolic ventricular volume: 130 mL
6. ECG waves duration

ECG waves duration	Average	Range
• PR interval	0.18 s	0.12–0.20 s
• QRS duration	0.08 s	0.08–0.10 s
• QT interval	0.40 s	0.40–0.43 s
• ST interval	0.32 s	-

7. Conduction speeds in cardiac tissue
   - SA node : 0.05 m/s
   - Atrial pathways : 1 m/s
   - AV node : 0.05 m/s
   - Bundle of His : 1 m/s
   - Purkinje's system : 4 m/s
   - Ventricular muscle : 1 m/s
8. Average rate of impulse production
   - SA node : 72/min
   - AV node : 50/min
   - Ventricle : 30/min
9. Cardiac cycle
   - Atrial systole (0.1 sec)
   - Ventricular systole (0:3 sec)
   - Ventricular diastole (0.5 sec)
   - Atrial diastole (0.7 sec)
10. Ventricular systole (0.3 sec)—3 phases:
    - Isovolumetric (Isometric) ventricular contraction (0.05 sec)
    - Maximum (rapid) ejection phase (0.1 sec)
    - Reduced ejection phase (0.15 sec)
11. Ventricular diastole (0.5 sec)—4 phases
    - Protodiastole (0.04 sec)
    - Isovolumetric relaxation phase (0.06 sec)
    - Ventricular diastole proper (0.3 sec)
    - Last rapid filling phase (0.10 sec).
12. Resting blood flow and % of CO flow through various organs

Organ	*Blood flow (mL/min)*	*% of CO*
• Liver	1500	27.8
• Kidneys	1260	23.3
• Brain	750	13.9
• Skin	462	8.6
• Skeletal muscle	840	15.6
• Heart muscle	250	4.7
• Rest of body	336	6.2
• Whole of body	5400	100

13. Normal blood pressure
    - Systolic pressure: 100–140 mm Hg (average—120 mm Hg)
    - Diastolic pressure: 60–90 mm Hg (average—70 mm Hg)
    - Pulse pressure: 50 mm Hg
    - Mean arterial blood pressure: 90 mm Hg

GASTROINTESTINAL SYSTEM

1. Gastric emptying time: 3–4 hours
2. Normal pH of saliva: 7–8
3. Normal pH of gastric juice: 1–2
4. Normal pH of pancreatic juice: 6–7
5. Normal pH of hepatic duct bile: 7.8–8.6
6. Normal pH of gallbladder bile: 7.0–7.4

RENAL PHYSIOLOGY

1. Glomerular filtration rate (GFR): 125 mL/min or 180 L/day.
2. Filtration fraction: 0.16–0.2
3. Transport maximum (T_MG) for glucose
   Male: 375 mg/min Female: 300 mg/min
4. Renal threshold value for glucose: 300 mg/dL
   Actual renal threshold of:
   - Arterial blood: 200 mg/dL
   - Venous blood: 180 mg/dL
5. Renal blood flow:1273 mL/min
6. Actual renal plasma flow: 700 mL/min
7. Effective renal plasma flow: 625 mL/min(average)
8. Inulin clearance value: 125 mL
9. Normal plasma creatinine: 0.6–1.5 mg/dL

ENDOCRINOLOGY

1. Growth hormone (GH): 3 ng/mL (plasma)
2. Thyroid binding globulin (TBG): 7–17 mg/L (plasma)
3. Thyroxine (T4): 70–140 nmol/L (plasma)
4. Thyroxine (free) plasma: 9–22 pmol/L
5. Triiodothyronine (T3): 1.2–3.0 nmol/L (plasma)
6. Parathyroid hormone (PTH): 10–55 pg/mL
7. Plasma testosterone (free and bound)
   Adult male: 300–1000 ng/dL (10.4–34.7 nmol/L)
   Adult female: 30–70 ng/dL (1.04–2.43 nmol/L

8. Plasma progesterone
   Male: 0.3 ng/mL (1 nmol/L)
   Female: 0.9 ng/mL (3 nmol/L)—During the follicular phase of menstrual cycle
9. Plasma prolactin concentration
   Male: 5 ng/mL
   Female: 8 ng/mL
11. Insulin (plasma): 0.3–2 ng/mL
12. Hormonal levels in human maternal blood during normal pregnancy

Hormone	*Approx peak value*
• HCG	5 mg/mL
• Relaxin	1 ng/mL
• HCS	15 mg/mL
• Estradiol	16 ng/mL
• Estriol	14 ng/mL
• Progesterone	190 ng/mL
• Prolactin	200 ng/mL

REPRODUCTIVE SYSTEM

1. Normal sperm count: 80–120 million/mL (average—100 million/mL)
2. Average volume of semen per ejaculate: 2.5–3.5 mL
3. Testosterone secretion rate: 4–9 mg/day—(normal adult males)
4. Normal duration of menstrual flow: 3–5 days
5. Normal blood loss during menstruation: 30–80 mL

NERVE AND MUSCLE PHYSIOLOGY

1. RMP of neurons: –70 mV
2. RMP of skeletal muscle: –80 mV to –90 mV
3. RMP of cardiac muscle: –90 mV
4. RMP of smooth muscle: –55 mV
5. Normal synaptic delay: 0.5 ms

CENTRAL NERVOUS SYSTEM

1. EPSP: 60 mV to –6 mV
2. IPSP: –80 mV to –90 mV
3. Reaction time to monosynaptic system: 19–24 msec
4. Central delay: 0.6–0.9 msec
5. Important cortical areas
   - Primary motor area: 4
   - Premotor area: 6
   - Frontal eye field: 8
   - Prefrontal eye field: 9, 10, 11, 12
   - Broca's speech area: 44
   - Primary sensory area: 3, 1, 2
   - Primary auditory area: 41, 42
   - Primary visual area: 17
   - Visual association area: 18, 19
   - Wernicke's area: 22

SPECIAL SENSES

1. Aqueous humor
   - Refractive index: 1.336
   - pH: 7.1–7.3
2. Intraocular pressure: 10–20 mm Hg
3. Venous plexus pressure: 10–15 mm Hg
4. Number of rod cells: 120 million
5. Number of cone cells: 6 million
6. Dark adaptation
   - Fast response: 4–5 min
   - Slow response: 20–25 min
7. Normal frequency of human hearing: 20–20000 Hz

GENERAL

1. Normal body temperature: 37°C (98.6°F)
   - Hypothermia: < 35°C
   - Hyperthermia: >38°C
2. Normal temperature of the scrotum: 32°
3. Respiratory quotient

• Carbohydrate	1.00
• Fats	0.70
• Protein	0.82

4. CSF

• Glucose	70% of serum mg/dL
• Immunoglobulin G	< 40 mg/L
• Lactate	1.1–2.8 mmol/L
• Protein	<400 mg/L (< 40 mg/dL)

5. Normal lumbar CSF pressure: 70–180 mm CSF

Appendix

ANSWERS FOR CLINICAL QUESTIONS

Note: The weightage of clinical questions are often 10 marks or more. In this section, hints for the questions are given. Answers should be elaborated wherever necessary. Please go through the theory section for detailed explanation.

CIRCULATING BODY FLUIDS

1. a. In solution with a lower osmotic pressure (hypotonic) RBC swell, become spherical and eventually lose their hemoglobin (hemolysis). The hemoglobin of hemolyzed red cells dissolves in the plasma.
b. Osmosis, page no 25
c. Diffusion, vesicular transport

2. a. Mismatched blood transfusion
b. Hemolytic jaundice
c. Cross matching of blood before transfusion

3. a. Thrombocytopenic purpura
b. Easy or excessive bruising (purpura), superficial bleeding into the skin that appears as a rash of pinpoint-sized reddish-purple spots (petechiae), usually on the lower legs, bleeding from the gums or nose, blood in urine or stools, unusually heavy menstrual flow

4. a. Secondary polycythemia
b. Hypoxia
c. Treatment of secondary polycythemia depends on its cause. Supplemental oxygen can be provided for individuals with chronic hypoxia. Other therapies can be directed toward treating the cause of polycythemia. Polycythemia can cause increase in viscosity of blood and increased susceptibility to thrombosis.

5. a. Iron deficiency anemia
b. Spoon-shaped nails, pallor, breathlessness, weakness, palpitation
c. Iron supplementation, deworming

6. a. Rh incompatibility
b. No antibodies against the fetal RBCs during the first birth
c. Anti-Rh immunoglobulin during pregnancy

7. a. Iron defiency anemia. Picca; persistent eating of non edible substances like earth, paint, charcoal can lead to worm infestation and thus iron deficiency anemia
b. Deficiency of Vit B_{12}, congenital causes like hereditary spherocytosis

8. a. Hemophilia
b. Clotting factors should be supplemented
c. Vasoconstriction, platelet plug formation, coagulation of blood

9. a. ABO incompatibility should be there
b. 3 months no previous blood transfusion
c. Cross matching of blood should be done, screening for infectious diseases like HIV, hepatitis B, hepatitis C

10. a. AIDS (acquired immunodeficiency syndrome).
b. Caused by a virus called HIV (human immunodeficiency virus). The disease alters the attacks immune cells called CD-4 cells, which are a subset of T cells, making people much more vulnerable to infections and diseases.
c. Most of the symptoms of HIV infection are the result of infections caused by bacteria, viruses, fungi, and/or parasites. These conditions do not normally develop in individuals with healthy immune systems, which protect the body against infection.

11. a. Hemolytic jaundice due to mismatched transfusion
b. ABO or Rh incompatibity
c. Cross matching before transfusion

12. a. Aplastic anemia

RESPIRATORY SYSTEM

1. a. Decompression sickness
b. Nitrogen is decompressed and escapes from tissues at a faster rate. Being gas it forms bubbles while escaping

rapidly from tissues. The gas blocks the blood vessels producing tissue ischemia and sometimes

c. Slow ascent to top of sea

2. a. High altitude sickness
 b. Acute hypoxia
 c. Oxygen therapy, slow and stepwise ascent of mountain

3. a. Breathing reserve – 90 ml (see page 68, 416)
 b. Page no 68

4. a. 250 ml
 b. 1.4
 c. Page no 56

5. a. High altitude sickness
 b. Breathlessness, irritability, muscle cramps
 c. Slow ascent of mountain

CARDIOVASCULAR SYSTEM

1. a. Myocardial infarction/Ischemic heart disease
 b. Imbalance between oxygen supply and demand
 c. Referred pain (from dermatomes)

2. a. Congestive cardiac failure
 b. Jugular venous pressure is elevated so the neck veins are prominent
 c. P waves are tall because of right ventricular hypertrophy (p pulmonale)

3. a. Physiological bradycardia, see page no 103
 b. Sympathetic stimulation of nervous system
 c. Page no 126

4. a. Vasovagal syncope
 b. To increase the venous return to heart, page no 122

5. a. Blood transfusion
 b. Blood and crystalloids
 c. Inotropes

6. a. Anaphylactic shock
 b. Type 1 hypersensitivity reaction
 c. Adrenaline injection to cause vasoconstriction and counter effects of histamine release which causes hypotension

7. a. Hypovolemic shock
 b. Page no 124
 c. Page no 122

8. a. Hydrocephalus
 b. Obstruction to the CSF flow
 c. Decrease the CSF production by acetazolamide; carbonic anhydrase inhibitor

GASTROINTESTINAL SYSTEM

1. a. Duodenal ulcer
 b. Acidity causes erosion of duodenal mucosa
 c. Page no 134

2. a. Hepatitis
 b. Liver functions test, imaging studies

3. a. Cholestatic jaundice
 b. Posthepatic obstruction
 c. Page no 139

4. a. Gastric ulcer
 b. Page no 134

RENAL PHYSIOLOGY

1. a. Nephrotic syndrome
 b. No

2. a. Atonic bladder.
 b. Page no 174
 c. Page no 172

3. a. Effective filtration pressure - 10 mm Hg (see page 417)

TEMPERATURE REGULATION

1. a. Heat stress
 b. Page no 180
 c. Rest, drink water, keep patient in cool environment

ENDOCRINOLOGY

1. a. Diabetus insipidus
 b. The main symptom of diabetes insipidus is polyuria, excessive thirst
 c. Page no 192

2. a. Acromegaly
 b. Excessive production of growth hormone
 c. Page no 187

3. a. Cushing's syndrome
 b. Excessive production of glucocorticoids
 c. Page no 211

4. a. Hypocalcemic tetany
 b. Laryngeal stridor, facial muscle irritability and carpopedal spasms, Chvostek's sign
 c. Page no 200

5. a. Hyperthyroidism
 b. Serum thyroid hormones, TSH (thyroid profile), thyroid imaging, radioactive iodine
 c. Antithyroid drugs

6. a. Hyperthyroidism
   b. Increased production of thyroid hormones (T3, T4)
   c. Serum thyroid hormones, TSH, thyroid imaging

7. a. Hypothyroidism
   b. Decreased production of thyroid hormones
   c. Serum thyroid hormone levels, TSH

8. a. Diabetes mellitus
   b. Page no 206

9. a. Diabetic mellitus
   b. Page no 206

NERVE MUSCLE PHYSIOLOGY

1. a. Rigor mortis
   b. The muscle contracts when the myosin shifts, but the lack of ATP prevents it from detaching, and the muscle remains contracted.
   c. Rigor mortis helps in determining the time of death. Starting between two and six hours following death, rigor mortis begins with the eyelids, neck and jaw.

2. a. Myasthenia gravis
   b. Myasthenia gravis (MG) is a relatively rare autoimmune disorder in which antibodies form against nicotinic acetylcholine (ACh) postsynaptic receptors at the neuromuscular junction (NMJ) of the skeletal muscles
   c. Neostigmine is a cholinesterase inhibitor

3. a. Refractory period
   b. Absolute and Relative refractory period
   c. Page no 12

4. a. d-tubocurarine
   b. The main toxin of curare, d-tubocurarine occupies the same position on the receptor as ACh with an equal or greater affinity, and elicits no response, making it a competitive antagonist. The antidote for curare poisoning is an acetylcholinesterase inhibitor (anti-cholinesterase), such as physostigmine or neostigmine.

5. a. Neurotoxin venom in snake
   b. The neurotoxins in snake venom disrupt synaptic transmission. They can either inhibit the release of neurotransmitter from exocytosis of synaptic vesicle at the presynaptic site or bind to the neurotransmitter receptor at postsynaptic site.

CENTRAL NERVOUS SYSTEM

1. a. Cerebellar lesion
   b. Cerebellar degeneration, infarction, trauma, hemorrhage

2. Dorsal column lesion

3. a. UMN lesion
   b. The hyperexcitability of the stretch reflex produces spasticity, clonus, and the increase of deep tendon reflexes.

4. a. Stroke, page no 276
   b. Aphasia is caused by damage to one or more of the language areas of the brain. A stroke that affects the left side of the brain may lead to aphasia

5. a. Paraplegia, UMN lesion
   b. Spinal cord injury

6. a. Parkinsonism
   b. Page no 301
   c. Page no 301, 302

7. a. Motion sickness
   b. Page no 285

8. a. Parkinsonism
   b. Page no 301
   c. Page no 302

9. a. Cerebellar lesion
   b. Page no 293, 294

SPECIAL SENSES

1. a. Conductive deafness
   b. Rinne's test, Weber's test
   c. Causes of conductive hearing loss includes cerumen (ear wax obstruction), foreign body in ear canal, atresia of ear canal, middle ear fluid or infection, tympanic membrane perforation, etc.

2. a. Hypermetropia
   b. This vision problem occurs when light rays entering the eye focus behind the retina, rather than directly on it
   c. Convex lens

3. a. Myopia
   b. Concave lens

4. a. Color blindness
   b. Ishihara color vision test

5. a. Glaucoma
   b. Page no 317
   c. Beta adrenergic blockers

6. a. Cataract
   b. The lens epithelium is believed to undergo age-related changes, particularly a decrease in lens epithelial cell density and an aberrant differentiation of lens fiber cells. Consequently, progressive oxidative damage to the lens with aging takes place, leading to opacity and cataract development
   c. Surgical extraction along with intraocular lens implantation

7. a. Myopia
   b. If the patient can read the top most letter from a distance of 6 meters, his vision is 6/60. If he can read second line his vision is 6/36. If he can read third line his vision is 6/24. Numerator is constant. It denotes the distance at which the patient is normally examined, which is 6 meters. Denominator: Letters designed for 24 meters distance can be read at 6 meters only. What normal person can read at 24 meters can be read at 6 meters only.
   c. Concave lens

BIBLIOGRAPHY

1. A Textbook of Practical Physiology: CL Ghai
2. Comprehensive Textbook of Medical Physiology: GK Pal
3. Concise Medical Physiology: Chaudhuri
4. Essentials of Medical Physiology: Indu Khurana
5. Essentials of Medical Physiology:Sembulingam
6. Fundamentals of Physiology: L Prakasam Reddy
7. Review of Medical Physiology: William F Ganong
8. Textbook of Medical Physiology: Guyton and Hall
9. Textbook of Physiology: AK Jain
10. Textbook of Physiology: Berne and Levy
11. Textbook of Physiology: Mahapatra
12. Understanding Medical Physiology: RL Bijlani

Index

Page numbers followed by *f* refer to figure, *fc* refer to flowchart and *t* refer to table

M

N

O

P

T

U

V

W

X

Y

Z